Clinical Diabetes

Clinical Diabetes

Edited by **Rex Slavin**

hayle
medical

New York

Published by Hayle Medical,
30 West, 37th Street, Suite 612,
New York, NY 10018, USA
www.haylemedical.com

Clinical Diabetes
Edited by Rex Slavin

International Standard Book Number: 978-1-63241-404-5 (Hardback)

Printed in the United States of America.

Contents

Preface

Every book is initially just a concept; it takes months of research and hard work to give it the final shape in which the readers receive it. In its early stages, this book also went through rigorous reviewing. The notable contributions made by experts from across the globe were first molded into patterned chapters and then arranged in a sensibly sequential manner to bring out the best results.

This book unravels the recent studies in the area of clinical diabetes. It provides interesting topics for research which readers can take up. Diabetes is a chronic disease which is caused either due to improper functioning of pancreas or if body cannot utilize the produced insulin effectively. It is one of the most prevalent diseases at present. This book is a compilation of chapters that discuss the most vital concepts and emerging trends in the area of diabetes. It includes contributions of experts and scientists which will provide innovative insights into this field. Researchers and students studying this discipline will be assisted by this book.

It has been my immense pleasure to be a part of this project and to contribute my years of learning in such a meaningful form. I would like to take this opportunity to thank all the people who have been associated with the completion of this book at any step.

Editor

Blood Glucose Fluctuations in Type 2 Diabetes Patients Treated with Multiple Daily Injections

Feng-fei Li,[1] Li-yuan Fu,[2] Wen-li Zhang,[1] Xiao-fei Su,[1] Jin-dan Wu,[1] Jin Sun,[1] Lei Ye,[3] and Jian-hua Ma[1]

[1]Department of Endocrinology, Nanjing First Hospital, Nanjing Medical University, Nanjing 210012, China
[2]Nanjing University of Chinese Medicine, Nanjing 210023, China
[3]National Heart Research Institute Singapore, National Heart Centre Singapore, Singapore 169606

Correspondence should be addressed to Jian-hua Ma; majianhua@china.com

Academic Editor: Harald Sourij

To compare blood glucose fluctuations in type 2 diabetes mellitus (T2DM) patients were treated using three procedures: insulin intensive therapy which is continuous subcutaneous insulin infusion (CSII), MDI3 (three injections daily), and MDI4 (four injections daily). T2DM patients were hospitalized and were randomly assigned to CSII, aspart 30-based MDI3, and glargine based MDI4. Treatments were maintained for 2-3 weeks after the glycaemic target was reached. After completing the baseline assessment, 6-day continuous glucose monitoring (CGM) was performed before and after completion of insulin treatment. Treatment with CSII provided a greater improvement of blood glucose fluctuations than MDI (MDI3 or MDI4) therapy either in newly diagnosed or in long-standing T2DM patients. In long-standing diabetes patients, the MDI4 treatment group had significantly greater improvement of mean amplitude glycemic excursion (MAGE) than the MDI3 treatment group. However, in patients with newly diagnosed diabetes, there were no significant differences in the improvement of MAGE between MDI3 and MDI4 groups. Glargine based MDI4 therapy provided better glucose fluctuations than aspart 30-based MDI3 therapy, especially in long-standing T2DM patients, if CSII therapy was not available.

1. Introduction

Intensive insulin therapy may be necessary if conventional therapies were no longer sufficient to maintain glycemic control in patients with type 2 diabetes mellitus (T2DM) [1]. Intensive insulin therapy consists of continuous subcutaneous insulin infusion (CSII) using an insulin pump and multiple daily injections (MDIs). Several studies have demonstrated that early implementation of a short course of intensive insulin therapy may dramatically improve beta-cell function in most patients with newly diagnosed T2DM. This improvement of β-cell function might be responsible for the remission described in newly diagnosed T2DM patients [2–5]. However, the clinical response to short-term CSII may be variable, and this is probably a reflection of the heterogeneity of T2DM. Some have suggested that patients with higher late-phase insulin secretion may be able to benefit most in improvement of beta-cell function with CSII intervention [6]. Very recently, the OpT2mise group confirmed that even patients with long-standing T2DM for many years, despite previous use of MDI, are still able to achieve further significant improvement of the mean glycated haemoglobin (HbA1c) with CSII and with decreased blood glucose fluctuations [7].

CSII has become common practice in the world. Although MDI is inferior in control patient blood sugar levels compared with CSII, many people with T2DM are still struggling to keep their blood glucose values in target range by MDI. MDIs are three or more injections daily with long-acting or short-acting insulin. However, the knowledge of CSII or MDI therapy (three or more injections daily) for T2DM patients favouring better glucose fluctuation control is still limited.

We, therefore, performed a randomised, parallel-group trial using continuous glucose monitoring (CGM) to assess the blood glucose fluctuations in T2DM patients, who achieved euglycemic control treated with two procedures of intensive insulin therapy, that is, MDI, aspart 30-based MDI3 (three injections daily), and glargine based MDI4 (four injections daily).

2. Methods

This was a randomised, parallel-group study consisting of a run-in period and a 2- to 3-week randomised phase. Patients with newly diagnosed and long-standing T2DM were enrolled from eight centres in China between February, 2010, and December, 2014. The patients with the age of 18–80 years were required to have HbA1c values ranging from 9.0% to 12.0%. Patients were excluded if they were positive for antiglutamic acid decarboxylase antibodies, pregnant, or planning to become pregnant. Patients with maturity onset diabetes in youth and mitochondria diabetes mellitus, with cognitive disorder, or with abuse of alcohol or drugs were also excluded [8]. There was a 4- to 6-day run-in period of diet alone. The protocol and informed consent document were approved by institutional Ethics Committee approval at each of the study centres. All patients gave written informed consent.

All patients were admitted to hospitals. Fasting blood samples were collected for measuring FPG and insulin in all patients before and after treatment (2 days after insulin cessation). Fasting blood samples were obtained for insulin and C-peptide determination. Continuous glucose monitoring (CGM) data were obtained with Medtronic Minimed CGM Gold (Medtronic Incorporated, Northridge, USA) for at least 6 days before randomization and after treatments, as described in a previous study [9].

After completing the baseline assessment and 3 days of CGM, patients (with newly diagnosed T2DM) were randomly assigned into CSII group (CSII N, hereafter), aspart 30-based, three injections daily, group (MDI3 N, hereafter), and glargine based, four injections daily, group (MDI4 N, hereafter). Long-standing T2DM patients were also randomly assigned into the previously mentioned three groups (CSII L, MDI3 L, and MDI4 L, hereafter). Patients in CSII group were provided with aspart (Novo Nordisk, Bagsvaerd, Denmark) using Medtronic insulin pump (Northridge, CA). Initial insulin doses were calculated as 0.4–0.5 IU/kg and were equally administered as basal and bolus injection. Insulin doses were subsequently adapted by the treating physician according to blood glucose values obtained by self-monitoring. Patients in MDI3 group were injected aspart 30 (Novo Nordisk, Bagsvaerd, Denmark) before each meal. Patients in MDI4 group were injected aspart before each meal and glargine (Sanofi-Aventis Pharmaceuticals, Paris, France) at bedtime. Premeal doses were also calculated as 0.4–0.5 IU/kg and distributed evenly throughout every premeal. Euglycemic control was achieved if the fasting capillary blood glucose was less than 6.1 mmol/L and capillary blood glucose at 2 h after each of three meals was less than 8.0 mmol/L [8]. Investigators titrated insulin doses on an individual-patient basis at the titration algorithm (if the fasting blood glucose level was less than 4.4 mmol/L, the insulin dose was reduced 2 units; if the fasting blood glucose level was within 4.4 to 6.1 mmol/L, the insulin dose was unchanged; if the fasting blood glucose level was within 6.2 to 7.8 within 7.9 to 10.0, and >10.0 mmol/L, the insulin dose was increased subsequently by 2, 4, and 6 units, resp.). When euglycemic control was achieved, treatments were remained unchanged and maintained for 2-3 weeks.

The 24 h mean amplitude of glycemic excursions (MAGE) and other plasma glucose fluctuation parameters such as the 24 h mean blood glucose (MBG), the standard deviation (SD) of the MBG, the percentage time duration (%), and the incremental area under curve (AUC) of plasma glucose >10.0 mmol/L and <3.9 mmol/L was calculated, and hypoglycemia episodes were also recorded. MAGE was calculated for each patient by measuring the arithmetic mean of the ascending and descending excursions between consecutive peaks and nadirs for the same 24 h period; only absolute excursion values >1 SD were considered [10]. HbA1c was measured centrally at the Department of Endocrinology, Nanjing First Hospital, Nanjing Medical University. Radioimmunoassay was used for measurement of insulin (Beijing Technology Company, Beijing, China). 8-iso prostaglandin $F_{2\alpha}$ (8-iso $PGF_{2\alpha}$) was measured using an enzyme immunoassay method (Cayman Chemical Co., Ann Arbor, MI). Tumor necrosis factor-α (TNF-α) was measured using the human-specific Milliplex map kit according to the manufacturer's instructions (Millipore, St. Charles, MO, USA). Interleukin-6 (IL-6) was determined using commercially available Enzyme-Linked Immunosorbent Assay kits according to manufacturer's instructions (R&D Systems, Minneapolis, MN, USA). Routine clinical laboratory tests were done in the central laboratory units of the eight participating centres. Basal β-cell function and insulin resistance were estimated by homoeostasis model assessment-B (HOMA-B) and (HOMA-IR), which were calculated as previously described [8, 11].

The primary endpoint was the between-group differences of 24 h MAGE. Secondary endpoints were the effect of different interventions on oxidative stress, inflammatory levels, and β-cell function in these patients. The MAGE, 24 h MBG, AUC for hypoglycemia (defined as sensor glucose values <3.9 mmol/L) and hyperglycemia (sensor glucose values >10 mmol/L), and time spent in hypoglycemia and hyperglycemia were also analyzed.

2.1. *Statistical Analysis.* Data were analyzed with the SPSS PASW Statistics 18 Package. Normally distributed and continuous variables are presented as mean (standard deviation, SD). Nonnormally distributed variables were presented as median (IQR) and logarithmically transformed before analysis. The independent samples t-test was used to compare each group difference. Significance was defined as $P < 0.05$.

This study was registered with Chinese Clinical Trial Registry, number ChiCTR-TRC-11001218.

3. Results

Table 1 gives the baseline characteristics of the 116 newly diagnosed patients and the 127 patients with long-standing

TABLE 1: Baseline characteristics of newly diagnosed and long-standing T2DM patients.

	CSII group	MDI3 group	MDI4 group
N	$n = 39$	$n = 38$	$n = 39$
L	$n = 43$	$n = 41$	$n = 43$
Age (years)			
N	55.10 ± 10.02	52.95 ± 9.63	52.56 ± 9.97
L	59.68 ± 8.22	57.67 ± 10.82	58.89 ± 11.85
Men			
N	19 (49%)	18 (47%)	19 (49%)
L	25 (58%)	21 (51%)	23 (53%)
Duration of diabetes (years)			
N	No	No	No
L	12.34 ± 2.07	11.33 ± 1.14	13.28 ± 2.54
Body mass index (kg/m^2)			
N	24.55 ± 2.90	25.72 ± 3.62	25.03 ± 2.84
L	24.73 ± 3.43	25.17 ± 3.29	24.66 ± 2.84
HbA1c (%)			
N	9.65 ± 1.81	9.99 ± 1.75	10.13 ± 1.93
L	8.38 ± 1.68	8.18 ± 1.58	8.66 ± 1.73
Systolic blood pressure (mm Hg)			
N	126.77 ± 12.55	127.05 ± 16.44	131.03 ± 15.56
L	129.12 ± 12.76	127.41 ± 15.28	132.33 ± 11.17
Diastolic blood pressure (mm Hg)			
N	81.10 ± 9.84	81.64 ± 10.15	81.25 ± 6.78
L	82.72 ± 10.46	83.67 ± 11.41	83.06 ± 11.10
Fasting plasma glucose (mmol/L)			
N	10.47 ± 2.62	11.07 ± 3.01	11.24 ± 2.94
L	9.32 ± 2.22	8.66 ± 2.75	9.56 ± 2.35
Fasting plasma insulin (mU/L)			
N	5.58 ± 2.95	7.40 ± 8.84	6.79 ± 2.91
L	5.97 ± 2.86	6.01 ± 4.19	6.11 ± 3.15
Fasting plasma C-peptide (pmol/L)			
N	2.23 ± 0.77	1.98 ± 1.07	2.36 ± 1.12
L	1.94 ± 0.60	2.41 ± 1.11	2.02 ± 0.62

Data are mean (SD) or n (%). N: newly diagnosed T2DM patients group; L: long-standing T2DM patients group.

T2DM patients. The 116 newly diagnosed patients were allocated randomly to the CSII N (39), the MDI3 N (38), and the MDI4 N groups (39); and the 127 long-standing T2DM patients were randomly allocated to the CSII L (43), the MDI3 L (41), and the MDI4 L groups (43). There were no significant demographic differences between the different groups at baseline (Table 1).

3.1. The Effects of Transient Intensive Insulin Therapy on Metabolic Control

3.1.1. Glycemic Control. Significant improvement in blood glucose control was achieved in both CSII and MDI groups (fasting capillary blood glucose was <6.1 mmol/L and capillary blood glucose at 2 h after each of three meals was <8.0 mmol/L). Patients in the CSII group reached glycemic goals significantly earlier than in the MDI groups, in the newly diagnosed T2DM patients (4.26 ± 1.88 days in CSII N group, 6.17 ± 2.36 days in MDI3 N group, and 5.81 ± 2.46 days in MDI4 N group; $P < 0.05$ for CSII N group versus MDI3 N group or MDI4 N group; $P > 0.05$ for MDI3 N group versus MDI4 N group) and also in the long-standing T2DM patients (CSII L group 5.45 ± 2.76 days, MDI3 L group 6.39 ± 3.81 days, and MDI4 N group 6.28 ± 2.19 days; $P < 0.05$ for CSII L group versus MDI3 L group or MDI4 L group; $P > 0.05$ for MDI3 L group versus MDI4 L group). In addition, there were no differences in the mean daily insulin doses in all groups (36.91 ± 10.87 IU/day in the CSII N group, 38.45 ± 13.62 IU/day in the MDI3 N group, 37.86 ± 15.90 IU/day in the MDI4 N group, 38.20 ± 17.47 IU/day in the CSII L group, 40.14 ± 18.54 IU/day in the MDI3 L group, and 41.01 ± 20.77 IU/day in the MDI4 L group).

3.1.2. Oxidative Stress and Inflammatory Profile. To determine the effect of transient insulin intensive therapy on oxidative stress, we measured 8-PGF$_{2\alpha}$, a well-recognized

TABLE 2: Oxidative stress and inflammatory profile of newly diagnosed and long-standing T2DM patients.

	CSII N group	MDI3 N group	MDI4 N group
8-PGF$_{2\alpha}$ (pg/mL)			
N			
Before therapy	8.11 ± 2.77	9.46 ± 0.89	10.15 ± 2.34
After therapy	6.12 ± 2.66**	7.00 ± 1.93**	6.70 ± 2.53**
L			
Before therapy	8.07 ± 2.89	8.58 ± 3.14	8.46 ± 1.75
After therapy	4.10 ± 2.93**	5.17 ± 3.88**	4.16 ± 2.10**
TNF-α (pg/mL)			
N			
Before therapy	19.59 ± 4.56	18.01 ± 7.41	17.11 ± 6.32
After therapy	9.08 ± 5.14**	10.26 ± 3.33*	8.13 ± 5.00**
L			
Before therapy	13.46 ± 2.99	14.53 ± 3.23	11.55 ± 4.58
After therapy	6.08 ± 1.14*†	8.70 ± 2.34*	6.25 ± 2.37**†
IL-6 (pg/mL)			
N			
Before therapy	4.51 ± 1.87	5.08 ± 1.12	6.03 ± 4.52
After therapy	2.17 ± 1.43*	2.60 ± 0.78*	2.90 ± 1.84*
L			
Before therapy	3.66 ± 2.19	4.12 ± 1.88	3.73 ± 2.00
After therapy	2.62 ± 2.16**†	4.32 ± 1.45*	3.01 ± 2.55**†

Data are mean ± (SD). $^*P < 0.05$, $^{**}P < 0.01$ versus the same item before therapy; $^†P < 0.05$ versus MDI3 N group after therapy. N: newly diagnosed T2DM patients group; L: long-standing T2DM patients group.

biomarker of oxidative stress. Compared to baseline, serum 8-PGF$_{2\alpha}$ levels were significantly decreased in all groups after transient intensive therapy (Table 2). There was no significant difference between any of the treatment groups.

In order to determine the effect transient intensive insulin therapy on inflammation, we measured serum levels of TNF-α and IL-6 reflecting the inflammatory profile in patients with T2DM [12]. Patients in all groups had higher inflammatory cytokine levels at baseline. After transient intensive insulin treatment, we found an improvement of inflammatory cytokines in all groups ($P < 0.01$) (Table 2). CSII and MDI4 therapies had greater decrease of serum levels of IL-6 and TNF-α compared to MDI3 therapy in long-standing T2DM patients ($P < 0.05$) (Table 2).

3.2. The Effects of Transient Intensive Insulin Therapy on Blood Glucose Fluctuation Control. We collected CGM data at baseline and on 5 days after euglycemic control achieved. The 24 h mean glucose concentrations were significantly decreased after therapy either in newly diagnosed T2DM (Table 3) or in long-standing T2DM patients (Table 4). Of patients who achieved the target glycaemic goals, the 24 h mean glucose concentration was similar in all groups ($P < 0.01$). However, in newly diagnosed T2DM patients, the MAGE in the CSII group was significantly decreased compared to both MDI groups (CSII N group 4.51 ± 1.92 mmol/L, MDI3 N group 5.05 ± 1.97 mmol/L, MDI4 N group 4.94 ± 2.21 mmol/L, $P < 0.05$ versus MDI3 N group and MDI4 N group). There was no statistically significant difference between MDI3 N

group and MDI4 N group ($P > 0.05$). The incremental AUC (>10 mmol/L) detected by CGM was not significantly decreased (0.29 ± 0.57 mmol/L per day) in CSII N group compared with the MDI3 N group (0.27 ± 0.37 mmol/L per day) and MDI4 N group (0.27 ± 0.35 mmol/L per day) ($P > 0.05$ versus MDI3 N group and MDI4 N group). The time spent in normal glycaemia (%) (between 3.9 and 10.0 mmol/L) in CSII N group was not significantly increased compared to MDI3 N group and MDI4 N group (85% ± 16 in CSII N group, 83% ± 13 mmol/L per day in MDI3 N group, and 84% ± 15 mmol/L per day in MDI4 N; $P > 0.05$ versus MDI3 N group and MDI4 N group).

Long-standing T2DM patients also achieved significantly better improvement of MAGE in CSII therapy compared with the MDI3 or MDI4 treatment group (CSII L group 4.62 ± 2.97 mmol/L, MDI3 L group 6.27 ± 1.83 mmol/L, and MDI4 L group 5.16 ± 1.98 mmol/L; $P < 0.01$ versus MDI3 L group; $P < 0.05$ versus MDI4 L group). In addition, our results showed that patients in MDI4 L group had significantly improved MAGE compared to patients in MDI3 L treatment group ($P < 0.05$). The incremental AUC (>10 mmol/L) in patients treated with CSII therapy was not significantly different (16% ± 17) compared with MDI3 L group (19% ± 10) and MDI4 L group (18% ± 15) ($P > 0.05$ versus MDI3 L group and MDI4 L group). Again, the time duration in normoglycemia (%) (>3.9 and <10.0 mmol/L) in the CSII L treatment group and that in MDI4 L group were significantly increased compared to the MDI3 L group (83% ± 17 in CSII L group and 79% ± 11 in MDI4 L group,

TABLE 3: Blood glucose fluctuations of newly diagnosed T2DM patients.

	CSII N group	MDI3 N group	MDI4 N group
24 h MBG (mmol/L)			
Before therapy	11.55 ± 2.63	12.51 ± 2.73	12.20 ± 2.74
After therapy	$7.70 \pm 1.79^{**}$	$7.55 \pm 1.13^{**}$	$7.44 \pm 1.40^{**}$
MAGE			
Before therapy	7.11 ± 2.87	6.87 ± 2.01	6.31 ± 3.62
After therapy	$4.51 \pm 1.92^{*}$	$5.05 \pm 1.97^{*}$	$4.94 \pm 2.21^{*}$
The time spent (>10 mmol/L) (%)			
Before therapy	62 ± 31	67 ± 29	66 ± 31
After therapy	$14 \pm 17^{**}$	$14 \pm 13^{**}$	$12 \pm 14^{**}$
The time spent in <3.9 mmol/L (%)			
Before therapy	2 ± 4	1.8 ± 5	2.6 ± 6
After therapy	$0.32 \pm 0.8^{**}$	$0.4 \pm 0.8^{**}$	$0.7 \pm 0.3^{**}$
The time spent in normal glycaemia (%)			
Before therapy	38 ± 31	33 ± 29	38 ± 36
After therapy	$85 \pm 16^{**}$	$83 \pm 13^{**}$	$84 \pm 15^{**}$
The AUC (>10 mmol/L) (mmol/L per day)			
Before therapy	2.55 ± 1.99	2.84 ± 2.29	2.81 ± 2.02
After therapy	$0.29 \pm 0.57^{**}$	$0.27 \pm 0.37^{**}$	$0.27 \pm 0.35^{**}$
The AUC for <3.9 mmol/L (mmol/L per day)			
Before therapy	0.02 ± 0.08	0.01 ± 0.05	0.02 ± 0.09
After therapy	$0.00 \pm 0.00^{**}$	$0.00 \pm 0.02^{**}$	$0.00 \pm 0.03^{**}$

Data are mean $\pm$ (SD). $^{*}P < 0.05$, $^{**}P < 0.01$ versus the same item before therapy.

TABLE 4: Blood glucose fluctuations of long-standing T2DM patients.

	CSII N Group	MDI3 N Group	MDI4 N Group
24 h MBG (mmol/L)			
Before therapy	10.80 ± 2.82	10.00 ± 2.60	11.43 ± 3.19
After therapy	$7.69 \pm 2.24^{**}$	$7.65 \pm 1.15^{**}$	$8.07 \pm 1.40^{**}$
MAGE			
Before therapy	6.56 ± 2.77	6.95 ± 2.74	6.48 ± 3.15
After therapy	$4.62 \pm 2.97^{*\dagger}$	$6.27 \pm 1.83^{*}$	$5.16 \pm 1.98^{*\dagger}$
The time spent (>10 mmol/L) (%)			
Before therapy	60 ± 32	65 ± 27	62 ± 36
After therapy	$16 \pm 17^{**}$	$19 \pm 10^{**}$	$18 \pm 15^{**}$
The time spent in <3.9 mmol/L (%)			
Before therapy	3 ± 9	4 ± 5	1 ± 2
After therapy	$0.2 \pm 0.2^{**\dagger}$	$0.4 \pm 0.1^{**}$	$0.2 \pm 0.3^{**\dagger}$
The time spent in normal glycaemia (%)			
Before therapy	39 ± 31	33 ± 29	38 ± 36
After therapy	$83 \pm 17^{**\dagger}$	$73 \pm 10^{**}$	$79 \pm 11^{**\dagger}$
The AUC (>10 mmol/L) (mmol/L per day)			
Before therapy	2.34 ± 2.12	2.77 ± 1.73	2.93 ± 2.50
After therapy	$0.25 \pm 0.60^{**}$	$0.37 \pm 0.27^{**}$	$0.28 \pm 0.09^{**}$
The AUC for <3.9 mmol/L (mmol/L per day)			
Before therapy	0.02 ± 0.08	0.02 ± 0.04	0.06 ± 0.02
After therapy	$0.00 \pm 0.00^{**}$	$0.00 \pm 0.00^{**}$	$0.00 \pm 0.00^{**}$

Data are mean $\pm$ (SD). $^{*}P < 0.05$, $^{**}P < 0.01$ versus the same item before therapy; $^{\dagger}P < 0.05$ versus MDI3 N group after therapy.

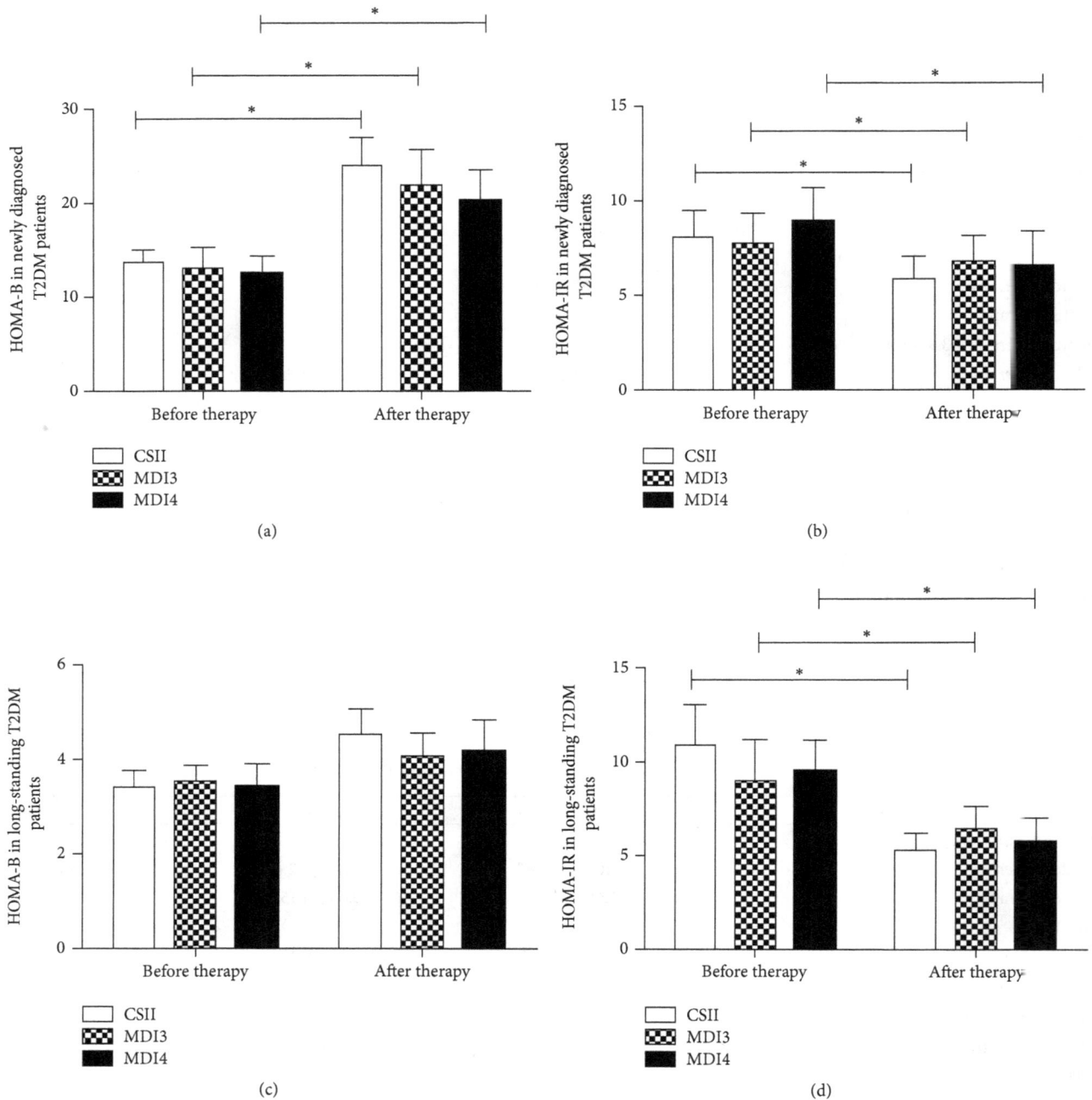

(a)

(b)

(c)

(d)

FIGURE 1: The effect of transient insulin intensive therapy on β-cell function and insulin resistance.

$P < 0.05$ CSII L group and MDI4 L group versus MDI3 L group).

There were no serious hypoglycemic episodes, defined as an event requiring the assistance of another person or other resuscitative treatments, in any treatment group. However, the time spent in hypoglycemia (<3.9 mmol/L) (%) detected by CGM was significantly decreased by the use of transient insulin intensive treatment either in newly diagnosed (Table 3) or in advanced T2DM patients compared with the baseline before treatment (Table 4).

3.3. The Effect of Transient Insulin Intensive Therapy on β-Cell Function and Insulin Resistance. In newly diagnosed T2DM patients, the HOMA-B and HOMA-IR were similar among the three treatment groups before treatment. After 2-3 weeks of intensive treatment, the HOMA-B was significantly increased in the newly diagnosed T2DM patients in both CSII and MDI treatments ($P < 0.05$) (Figure 1(a)), accompanied by the improvement in insulin resistance ($P < 0.05$) (Figure 1(b)). Similarly, in long-standing T2DM patients, the HOMA-IR significantly improved after CSII and MDI therapy ($P < 0.05$) (Figure 1(c)). However, the HOMA-B was not dramatically increased ($P > 0.05$), even in patients treated with CSII therapy group (Figure 1(d)).

4. Discussion

We have conducted a prospective study on a relatively large number of patients and demonstrated using CGMS that glargine based MDI4 provided better control with less blood glucose fluctuations compared to aspart 30-based MDI3 in long-standing T2DM patients. We also confirmed that treatment with CSII provided a greater improvement of blood glucose fluctuations than either glargine based MDI4 or glargine based MDI3 in newly diagnosed T2DM or long-standing T2DM patients.

CSII and MDI are commonly used forms of intensive insulin therapies. CSII provide precise insulin delivery throughout the day and simulates the function of the islet cells more closely. Use of CSII therapy is now regarded as a safe and valuable alternative in patients with newly diagnosed T2DM. Two to three weeks of early CSII therapy in patients with newly diagnosed T2DM in Chinese population achieved prolonged glycaemic remission, as well as recovery and maintenance of β-cell function compared with treatment with oral hypoglycemic agents [8]. Insulin replacement could achieve optimum glycaemic control for 1 year, which might attribute to the increase in acute insulin response, the improvement of qualitative insulin secretion, the reduction in glucotoxicity, and the amelioration of the lipid profile [2, 3, 5, 8]. Furthermore, the early restoration of β-cell function and amelioration of insulin resistance might alter the natural history of T2DM [8, 13]. OpT2mise study revealed that, for patients with poorly controlled T2DM, despite using multiple daily injections of insulin, pump treatment can be considered as a safe and valuable treatment option [7]. OpT2mise study enrolled patients from Canada, Europe, Israel, South Africa, and USA. They found that the mean HbA1c of patients in CSII group decreased by −0.7% compared with that in MDI group at 6 months, accompanied by improved blood glucose fluctuations measured by CGM [7].

The goals of intensive therapy can also be achieved by MDI. MDIs are three or more injections daily with intermediate and long-acting insulin. The remission rates after 1 year were significantly higher in the MDI groups than in the oral hypoglycemic agents group [8]. In contrast, study indicated that CSII was superior to MDI with four injections daily in improving HbA1c and postmeal glucose AUC [14].

However, near-normal glucose control is more difficult to achieve, partly because of the limitations of the glycemic profile obtained from intermittent fingerpricks [15]. The intermittent finger pricks were included in a total of three fasting capillary blood glucose monitoring and capillary blood glucose monitoring tests 2 h after each of three meals [8]. Thus, 24 h blood glycemic excursions are undoubtedly missed by these point-to-point glimpses of blood glucose. CGM provides a unique opportunity to examine the 24 h glucose excursions in T2DM when patients achieved euglycemic control.

In the present pilot study, we expected to see a better improvement of blood glucose fluctuations in CSII group compared with MDI group. It is now believed that 2 h glucose concentration may be a better predictor for cardiovascular disease in patients with onset T2DM [16]. Large glucose fluctuations may cause the overproduction of superoxide by the mitochondrial electron-transport chain, which induces a subsequent nitrosative stress [18]. Our data showed a remarkable improved MAGE with CSII therapy compared to MDIs therapy in newly diagnosed T2DM patients. In addition, there was no difference between MDI3 and MDI4 therapy in improvement of MAGE. In contrast, in long-standing T2DM patients, there was better improvement of MAGE in CSII and MDI4 therapy compared to MDI3 therapy. Consistent with this finding, CSII and MDI4 therapy also decreased oxidation stress and inflammation markers in long-standing T2DM patients. It has been demonstrated that repeated fluctuations of glucose increased circulating levels of inflammatory cytokines compared with sustained hyperglycemia [19]. Daniele et al. demonstrated that the inflammatory score, an integrated quantification of TNF-α, IL-6, monocyte chemoattractant protein-1, fractalkine, osteopontin, and APN, is increased in patients with T2DM and correlated with hyperglycemia [12].

In addition, our data showed that MDI3 therapy achieved similar improvement of glucose fluctuations either in newly diagnosed T2DM patients or in long-standing T2DM patients. We also did not observe the differences in the incremental AUC (glucose > 10 mmol/L) or the incremental AUC (glucose < 3.9 mmol/L) either in newly diagnosed T2DM patients or in long-standing T2DM patients treated with MDI4 therapy. However, newly diagnosed T2DM patients treated with MDI4 therapy achieved increased improvement of MAGE compared with those in long-standing T2DM patients (4.64 ± 2.21 versus 5.16 ± 1.98 mmol/L, $P < 0.05$), as well as the increasing tendency of the time spent in normal glycaemia (glucose < 10 mmol/L and >3.9 mmol/L) ($85 \pm 15\%$ versus $73 \pm 21\%$, $P > 0.05$). We could infer that the reason for the differences might partially account the declined β-cell function in long-standing T2DM patients compared with new diagnosed T2DM patients (Figures 1(a) and 1(c)). Very recently, Jia et al. indicated that intensive premixed insulin therapy (thrice daily) could further decrease HbA1c level in Asian patients with T2DM who were treated with premixed insulin (twice daily) previously [20]. Our data showed that intensive premixed insulin therapy (thrice daily) could achieve improvement of MAGE in long-standing T2DM patients, which might contribute to the decline of HbA1c level in patients with T2DM treated with intensive premixed insulin therapy [20]. In addition, we also found that long-standing T2DM patients treated with MDI4 therapy achieved greater improvement of MAGE compared with those of MDI3 therapy. A possible explanation might be that MDI4 could more closely mimic physiological insulin secretion compared with MDI3 therapy. However, we have no data for glargine based MDI4 to know if it had favourable outcomes on blood glucose fluctuations control in patients with long-standing T2DM.

Our study has several limitations. First, the study period was 4 years long, from February, 2010, to 24 December, 2014, so the group was heterogeneous. Second, we did not measure the late-phase insulin secretion of β-cell. Preserved late-phase insulin secretion might be the key factor in the identification of the patients with established T2DM who can benefit from CSII therapy [6]. Furthermore, the decline in HOMA-IR might partially account the elimination of the deleterious effects of hyperglycemia and the better improvement of blood glucose fluctuations. However, our data could not answer the mechanisms which underline the phenomena. We have now addressed this as another limitation.

In conclusion, CSII results in favourable outcomes on blood glucose fluctuations control either in newly diagnosed patients with T2DM or in patients with long-standing T2DM compared with MDI therapy. In addition, our data suggested that glargine based MDI4 could be considered as a practicable treatment option, if CSII therapy was not available.

Conflict of Interests

No competing financial interests exist.

Acknowledgments

This research was funded by Nanjing Public Health Bureau project (no. YKK11110), Nanjing Committee of Science and Technology project (no. 201201108), and Jiangsu Provincial Department of Science and Technology project (no. BL2014010).

References

[1] M. Riddle, G. Umpierrez, A. DiGenio et al., "Contributions of basal and postprandial hyperglycemia over a wide range of A1C levels before and after treatment intensification in type 2 diabetes," *Diabetes Care*, vol. 34, pp. 2508–2514, 2011.

[2] H. Ilkova, B. Glaser, A. Tunçkale, N. Bagriaçik, and E. Cerasi, "Induction of long-term glycemic control in newly diagnosed type 2 diabetic patients by transient intensive insulin treatment," *Diabetes Care*, vol. 20, no. 9, pp. 1353–1356, 1997.

[3] Y. Li, W. Xu, Z. Liao et al., "Induction of long-term glycemic control in newly diagnosed type 2 diabetic patients is associated with improvement of β-cell function," *Diabetes Care*, vol. 27, no. 11, pp. 2597–2602, 2004.

[4] R. Retnakaran and D. J. Drucker, "Intensive insulin therapy in newly diagnosed type 2 diabetes," *The Lancet*, vol. 371, no. 9626, pp. 1725–1726, 2008.

[5] E. A. Ryan, S. Imes, and C. Wallace, "Short-term intensive insulin therapy in newly diagnosed type 2 diabetes," *Diabetes Care*, vol. 27, no. 5, pp. 1028–1032, 2004.

[6] R. Retnakaran, N. Yakubovich, Y. Qi, C. Opsteen, and B. Zinman, "The response to short-term intensive insulin therapy in type 2 diabetes," *Diabetes, Obesity & Metabolism*, vol. 12, no. 1, pp. 65–71, 2010.

[7] Y. Reznik, O. Cohen, R. Aronson et al., "Insulin pump treatment compared with multiple daily injections for treatment of type 2 diabetes (OpT2mise): a randomised open-label controlled trial," *The Lancet*, vol. 384, no. 9950, pp. 1265–1272, 2014.

[8] J. Weng, Y. Li, W. Xu et al., "Effect of intensive insulin therapy on beta-cell function and glycaemic control in patients with newly diagnosed type 2 diabetes: a multicentre randomised parallel-group trial," *The Lancet*, vol. 371, no. 9626, pp. 1753–1760, 2008.

[9] J. Zhou, H. Li, X. Ran et al., "Reference values for continuous glucose monitoring in Chinese subjects," *Diabetes Care*, vol. 32, no. 7, pp. 1188–1193, 2009.

[10] F. J. Service, G. D. Molnar, J. W. Rosevear, E. Ackerman, L. C. Gatewood, and W. F. Taylor, "Mean amplitude of glycemic excursions, a measure of diabetic instability," *Diabetes*, vol. 19, no. 9, pp. 644–655, 1970.

[11] D. R. Matthews, J. P. Hosker, A. S. Rudenski, B. A. Naylor, D. F. Treacher, and R. C. Turner, "Homeostasis model assessment: insulin resistance and beta-cell function from fasting plasma glucose and insulin concentrations in man," *Diabetologia*, vol. 28, no. 7, pp. 412–419, 1985.

[12] G. Daniele, R. Guardado Mendoza, D. Winnier et al., "The inflammatory status score including IL-6, TNF-α, osteopontin, fractalkine, MCP-1 and adiponectin underlies whole-body insulin resistance and hyperglycemia in type 2 diabetes mellitus," *Acta Diabetologica*, vol. 51, no. 1, pp. 123–131, 2014.

[13] D. LeRoith, V. Fonseca, and A. Vinik, "Metabolic memory in diabetes—focus on insulin," *Diabetes/Metabolism Research and Reviews*, vol. 21, no. 2, pp. 85–90, 2005.

[14] J. Wainstein, M. Metzger, M. Boaz et al., "Insulin pump therapy vs. multiple daily injections in obese Type 2 diabetic patients," *Diabetic Medicine*, vol. 22, no. 8, pp. 1037–1046, 2005.

[15] E. Boland, T. Monsod, M. Delucia, C. A. Brandt, S. Fernando, and W. V. Tamborlane, "Limitations of conventional methods of self-monitoring of blood glucose: lessons learned from 3 days of continuous glucose sensing in pediatric patients with type 1 diabetes," *Diabetes Care*, vol. 24, no. 11, pp. 1858–1862, 2001.

[16] DECODE Study Group, "Glucose tolerance and cardiovascular mortality: comparison of fasting and 2-hour diagnostic criteria," *Archives of Internal Medicine*, vol. 161, no. 3, pp. 397–405, 2001.

[17] M. Coutinho, H. C. Gerstein, Y. Wang, and S. Yusuf, "The relationship between glucose and incident cardiovascular events. A metaregression analysis of published data from 20 studies of 95,783 individuals followed for 12.4 years," *Diabetes Care*, vol. 22, no. 2, pp. 233–240, 1999.

[18] M. Brownlee, "The pathobiology of diabetic complications: a unifying mechanism," *Diabetes*, vol. 54, no. 6, pp. 1615–1625, 2005.

[19] K. Esposito, F. Nappo, R. Marfella et al., "Inflammatory cytokine concentrations are acutely increased by hyperglycemia in humans: role of oxidative stress," *Circulation*, vol. 106, no. 16, pp. 2067–2072, 2002.

[20] W. Jia, X. Xiao, Q. Ji et al., "Comparison of thrice-daily premixed insulin (insulin lispro premix) with basal-bolus (insulin glargine once-daily plus thrice-daily prandial insulin lispro) therapy in east Asian patients with type 2 diabetes insufficiently controlled with twice-daily premixed insulin: an open-label, randomised, controlled trial," *The Lancet Diabetes & Endocrinology*, vol. 3, pp. 254–262, 2015.

2

JNK1 Deficient Insulin-Producing Cells Are Protected against Interleukin-1β-Induced Apoptosis Associated with Abrogated Myc Expression

Michala Prause,[1,2] **Christopher Michael Mayer,**[3]
Caroline Brorsson,[4] **Klaus Stensgaard Frederiksen,**[5] **Nils Billestrup,**[2]
Joachim Størling,[4] **and Thomas Mandrup-Poulsen**[1,6]

[1]*Immuno-Endocrinology Lab, Endocrinology Research Section, Department of Biomedical Sciences, University of Copenhagen, 2200 Copenhagen N, Denmark*
[2]*Section of Cellular and Metabolic Research, Department of Biomedical Sciences, University of Copenhagen, 2200 Copenhagen N, Denmark*
[3]*Hagedorn Research Institute, Novo Nordisk, 2760 Måløv, Denmark*
[4]*Copenhagen Diabetes Research Center, Herlev University Hospital, 2730 Herlev, Denmark*
[5]*Biopharmaceuticals Research Unit, Novo Nordisk, 2760 Måløv, Denmark*
[6]*Department of Molecular Medicine and Surgery, Karolinska Institutet, 17177 Stockholm, Sweden*

Correspondence should be addressed to Michala Prause; michalapr@sund.ku.dk

Academic Editor: Hiroshi Okamoto

The relative contributions of the JNK subtypes in inflammatory β-cell failure and apoptosis are unclear. The JNK protein family consists of JNK1, JNK2, and JNK3 subtypes, encompassing many different isoforms. INS-1 cells express JNK1α1, JNK1α2, JNK1β1, JNK1β2, JNK2α1, JNK2α2, JNK3α1, and JNK3α2 mRNA isoform transcripts translating into 46 and 54 kDa isoform JNK proteins. Utilizing Lentiviral mediated expression of shRNAs against JNK1, JNK2, or JNK3 in insulin-producing INS-1 cells, we investigated the role of individual JNK subtypes in IL-1β-induced β-cell apoptosis. JNK1 knockdown prevented IL-1β-induced INS-1 cell apoptosis associated with decreased 46 kDa isoform JNK protein phosphorylation and attenuated Myc expression. Transient knockdown of Myc also prevented IL-1β-induced apoptosis as well as caspase 3 cleavage. JNK2 shRNA potentiated IL-1β-induced apoptosis and caspase 3 cleavage, whereas JNK3 shRNA did not affect IL-1β-induced β-cell death compared to nonsense shRNA expressing INS-1 cells. In conclusion, JNK1 mediates INS-1 cell death associated with increased Myc expression. These findings underline the importance of differentiated targeting of JNK subtypes in the development of inflammatory β-cell failure and destruction.

1. Introduction

Inflammatory β-cell inhibition and apoptosis are increasingly accepted as key contributors to failing insulin secretion leading to type 1 and type 2 diabetes [1, 2]. Interleukin-1, a 17 kDa proinflammatory cytokine and mediator of inflammation, fever, and acute-phase responses [1, 3], inhibits β-cell function *in vitro* and *in vivo* by signaling via NFκB and mitogen activated protein kinases (MAPK) to activate endoplasmic reticulum and mitochondrial death pathways [4–7]. The

MAPK family encompasses the extracellular signal-regulated kinase (ERK), c-Jun N-terminal kinase (JNK), and p38 cascades. The precise contribution of the JNK pathway to stress-induced β-cell failure is not fully understood, especially with regard to the differential roles of the JNK subtypes, JNK1, JNK2, and JNK3.

The JNK proteins control the expression of immediate early genes such as AP-1 transcription factor family members and are important regulators of both apoptosis and survival, depending on the biological context [8, 9]. Three mammalian genes encoding for JNK have been identified: *jnk1, jnk2,* and *jnk3,* located on different chromosomes [10, 11]. JNK1 and JNK2 are expressed in a large variety of tissues regulating cell proliferation, differentiation, inflammation, autoimmunity, obesity, and tumorigenesis [12]. JNK3 expression was thought to be restricted to the brain, heart, and testes [13, 14]; however, more recently, JNK3 was found to be expressed also in human and mouse pancreatic β-cells [15]. All three JNK subtypes control cellular apoptosis. Mice deficient in a single JNK allele survive, as do $jnk1^{-/-}jnk3^{-/-}$ and $jnk2^{-/-}jnk3^{-/-}$ mice, whereas combined genetic disruption of *jnk1* and *jnk2* alleles causes early embryonic death due to severe dysregulation of apoptosis in the brain [14]. Additionally, $jnk1^{-/-}/jnk2^{-/-}$ mouse embryonic fibroblasts (MEFs) are protected against UV-induced apoptosis, indicating that JNK1 and JNK2 are required for a normal apoptotic response to UV exposure [16]. Furthermore, $jnk3^{-/-}$ mice are protected from stroke, neuronal death, and oxidative stress [17]. Supporting these direct observations of the importance of JNK in proapoptotic signalling, cell-permeable JNK inhibitory protein-1 (JIP-1) derived JNK inhibitory peptides or the JNK inhibitory small molecule SP600125 decrease intracellular JNK signalling and improve cell survival *in vitro* and *in vivo* [18–22].

Splicing of the *jnk* genes gives rise to more than twelve different transcript variants [13, 23] translating into proteins with and without a COOH-terminal extension to generate both 46 kDa and 54 kDa isoform proteins with a high level of homology [24]. Initially, the different JNK subtypes were thought to have largely redundant functions, but different tissue distribution, substrate preferences, and expression patterns support that the JNK subtypes also have nonredundant functions and are involved in distinct cellular processes [10, 12, 13, 23, 25]. However, little is known about how the individual JNK isoforms and subtypes mediate apoptosis. Apart from phosphorylating and activating members of the activating protein-1 (AP-1) transcription factor family, JNK proteins regulate other proteins involved in cell proliferation and apoptosis, including p53, Myc, and members of the Bcl-2 family of proteins [6, 26, 27].

The precise contribution of the individual JNK subtypes in mediating IL-1β-induced β-cell apoptosis is largely unknown, although a protective role of JNK3 in IL-1β, TNF-α, and IFN-γ-induced β-cell apoptosis via Akt2 signaling has been suggested [15, 28]. In these studies, no differentiation was made between the roles of the JNK subtypes in the signaling pathways of the three individual proinflammatory cytokines. Since JNK subtype activation is stimulus dependent and as IL-1β is indispensable in the proapoptotic combination of inflammatory cytokines, the action of TNF-α and INF-γ being mainly to synergize with IL-1β, it is important to investigate the differential role of the JNK subtypes in stimulus-specific pancreatic β-cell signalling.

Here, we investigated the individual roles of JNK1, JNK2, and JNK3 in IL-1β-induced apoptosis in insulin-producing INS-1 cells and provide evidence for a critical role of JNK1 in mediating IL-1β-induced β-cell apoptosis, whereas JNK2 but not JNK3 conferred protection.

2. Materials and Methods

2.1. Cell Culture and Reagents. The clonal rat β-cell line INS-1 [29] (gift from Wollheim, Geneva, Switzerland) and INS-1 cell lines stably expressing shRNA [30] were grown in RPMI-1640 medium with 11 mmol/L glucose (Invitrogen, Nærum, Denmark) supplemented with 50 μmol/L β-mercaptoethanol, 100 U/mL penicillin, 100 μg/mL streptomycin, and 10% heat-inactivated fetal bovine serum (FBS) (Invitrogen). Cells were incubated in a humidified atmosphere of 5% CO_2 at 37°C. Recombinant mouse IL-1β was from BD Bioscience Pharmingen (San Diego, CA, USA).

JNK1(F-3) mouse monoclonal antibody raised against amino acid 1-384 of full length JNK1 p46 human origin was purchased from Santa Cruz Technologies (Santa Cruz, CA, USA, catalog number: sc-1648, used at 1:1000 dilution). JNK2 rabbit polyclonal antibody raised against a synthetic peptide for human JNK2 (catalog number: #4672, used at 1:1000 dilution), JNK3 rabbit monoclonal antibody raised against a synthetic peptide for human JNK3 (catalog number: #55A8, used at 1:1000 dilution), P-JNK (Thr183/Tyr185) polyclonal rabbit antibody raised against a synthetic phosphopeptide corresponding to residues surrounding Thr183/Tyr185 of human SAPK/JNK (catalog number: #9251, used at 1:1000 dilution), T-JNK polyclonal rabbit antibody raised against a recombinant human JNK2 fusion protein (catalog number: #9252, used at 1:1000 dilution), cleaved caspase 3 (Asp175) rabbit polyclonal antibody raised against amino terminal residues adjacent to Asp175 in human caspase 3 (catalog number: #9661, used at 1:500 dilution), Myc (D84C12) rabbit monoclonal antibody raised against synthetic peptide corresponding to amino-terminal residues of c-Myc (catalog number: #5605, used at 1:1000 dilution), and β-tubulin (9F3) rabbit monoclonal antibody raised against human β-tubulin (catalog number: #2128, used at 1:1000 dilution) were all from Cell Signalling (Beverly, MA, USA). The mouse monoclonal β-actin antibody raised against β-cytoplasmic actin N-terminal peptide, Ac-Asp-Asp-Asp-Ile-Ala-Ala-Leu-Val-Ile-Asp-Asn-Gly-Ser-Gly-Lys, conjugated to Keyhole Limpet Haemocyanin (KLH) was obtained from Abcam (Cambridge, UK, catalog number: ab6276, used at 1:10000 dilution). The specificity of the JNK antibodies was previously verified against recombinant JNK1, JNK2, and JNK3 protein using Western blot analysis [30].

HEK293FT cells, used to produce Lentivirus, were cultured in D-MEM medium (Invitrogen) supplemented with 100 U/mL penicillin, 10 nM MEM nonessential amino acids, 1 mM sodium pyruvate, and 10% FBS (Invitrogen) (complete D-MEM).

HT1080 cells, used for virus titration, were cultured in D-MEM medium (Invitrogen) supplemented with 100 U/mL penicillin, 100 μg/mL streptomycin, and 10% FBS (Invitrogen).

2.1.1. Lentivirus Expressing shRNA and INS-1 Stable Cell Line Production. INS-1 cell lines, stably expressing JNK1, JNK2, or JNK3 shRNAs, nonsense shRNA, or empty vector, were created as described in [31]. In brief, INS-1 cells were transduced with an MOI of 5 with virus generated by transfection of HEK293FT cells with the Lentiviral vectors pLKO.1 JNK1 (TRCN0000055115), pLKO.1 JNK2 (TRCN0000012590), pLKO.1 JNK3 (TRCN0000012634), or empty vector (all from Open Biosystems, Thermo Scientific, St. Leon-Rot, Germany) or pLKO.1 nonsense (SHC002) (Sigma, Brondby, Denmark). All constructs contained a puromycin-resistance gene as mammalian selection marker, and stably transduced INS-1 cells were selected using 1 μg/mL puromycin (Sigma). INS-1 cell lines were passaged a minimum of three times and tested for knockdown efficiency and specificity compared to empty vector and nonsense shRNA expressing INS-1 cell lines.

2.2. Microarray Analysis. Total RNA was isolated using Trizol (Sigma) followed by RNeasy Mini Elute Kit (Qiagen, Hilden, Germany) purification. 1 μg of total RNA was used to prepare targets by One-Cycle Target labeling kit (Affymetrix, Santa Clara, CA, USA) following the instructions of the manufacturer. Hybridization cocktails were hybridized onto Rat Genome 230 2.0 GeneChips, containing 31,099 rat gene probes, at 45°C for 17 h (60 Rpm) in a Hybridization Oven 640 (Affymetrix). GeneChips were rinsed and stained in a GeneChip fluidics station 450 using the fluidics protocol "EukGE-WS2v5_450" (Affymetrix). Chips were scanned in a GeneChip scanner 3000 (Affymetrix). For all conditions, three separate experiments were analyzed on separate arrays; that is, a total of 36 arrays were used. Array data is available at Arrayexpress [31] (https://www.ebi.ac.uk/arrayexpress), accession number E-MTAB-3146.

2.2.1. Microarray Data Preprocessing and Visualization. To adjust for nonspecific hybridization, optical effects, and comparability, probe intensities were combined and normalized using the RMA method. All intensities were $\log_2$-transformed. Significant differential expression was assessed using the moderated t-statistics for pairwise comparison between conditions implemented in the LIMMA package. The comparisons performed were 45 min IL-1β exposed JNK1 knockdown (KD) INS-1 cells adjusted for nonexposed JNK1 KD versus 45 min IL-1β exposed NS control INS-1 cells adjusted for nonexposed NS control INS-1 cells; 45 min IL-1β exposed JNK2 KD INS-1 cells adjusted for nonexposed JNK2 KD versus 45 min IL-1β exposed NS control INS-1 cells adjusted for nonexposed NS control INS-1 cells; and 45 min IL-1β exposed JNK3 KD INS-1 cells adjusted for nonexposed JNK3 KD versus 45 min IL-1β exposed NS control INS-1 cells adjusted for nonexposed NS control INS-1 cells. Genes were considered to be significantly regulated if the $\log_2$ fold change was >1 or < −1 and the P value was <0.05. Only probes that could be mapped to gene identifiers using the "rat2302.db" probe annotation package were considered for further analysis.

For clustering analysis, we used hierarchical clustering as implemented in the heatmap.2 function in the gplots r package. Briefly, the mean $\log_2$ expression value for three replicates of the 12 conditions was calculated for each probe. Overrepresented biological processes among groups of regulated genes were identified by hypergeometric testing of gene ontology (GO) terms using DAVID [32, 33]. Only GO terms reaching a Benjamini corrected P value <0.05 were considered significantly overrepresented.

2.3. cDNA and qRT-PCR. INS-1 cells were exposed to 150 pg/mL IL-1β or vehicle over either a 12 h (stable shRNA cell line experiments) or 24 h (INS-1 cell line experiments) time course and total RNA was isolated using the RNeasy kit (Qiagen) and quantified on a NanoDrop 1000 microvolume spectrophotometer. The RNA was treated with recombinant shrimp DNase (Affymetrix), and first strand cDNA was synthesized from 2 μg of RNA using the High Capacity cDNA Reverse Transcription Kit (Applied Biosystems, Carlsbad, CA, USA) following the manufacturer's protocol. Quantitative RT-PCR was performed in a 10 μL volume using 0.5 μL of premixed Taqman primer/probes (Applied Biosystems), 5 μL 2x Taqman Universal Master Mix (Applied Biosystems), and 4.5 μL template (20 ng) and run on a 384-well plate in triplicate on the Applied Biosystems Prism 7900HT real-time PCR machine for 40 cycles. The results were analyzed using SDS 2.4 software (Applied Biosystems). The following primer/probes were purchased from Applied Biosystems: Hprt1 (Rn01527840_m1), RN18S1 (Hs03928990_g1), JNK1 (Rn01453358_m1), JNK2 (Rn00569058_m1), JNK3 (Rn00563035_m1), Jun (Rn00572991_s1), Trp53 (Rn00755717_m1), Junb (Rn00572994_s1), Jund (Rn00824678_s1), and Myc (Rn00561507_m1). The primer/probe sequences for the JNK isoforms are listed in Table 1 and synthesized by Integrated DNA Technologies (IDT, Berchem, Belgium). We utilized the human isoform-specific primer and probe sequences determined by Dreskin et al. [34] and modifying them based upon a cross species homology comparison between human and mouse, as the rat JNK isoform sequences were not published. Relative transcript quantities were calculated by the standard curve method and normalized to the average of the housekeeping genes 18S and Hprt1. The appropriate housekeeping genes were selected by analyzing the mRNA expression of four common housekeeping genes, GAPDH, PPIA, 18S, and Hprt1, in INS-1 cells after 12 and 24 h exposures to IL-1β. The two genes used were the least variable following IL-1β treatment.

2.4. Transfection Studies. INS-1 cells (0.8×10^6 cells/well for Western blotting and 0.075×10^6 cells/well for Cell Death Detection Assay) were transfected with siRNA directed against rat Myc (Sigma), negative control siRNA (mission siRNA universal negative control, Sigma), or vehicle. The cells were transfected using DharmaFECT4 (Thermo Scientific, Denmark) according to the manufacturer's protocol, with a final concentration of siRNA of 50 nmol/L. The cells were incubated for 22 h with siRNA or vehicle and then exposed to IL-1β (150 pg/mL) or left nonexposed for 24 h. Protein was isolated and analyzed by Western blotting and apoptotic cell death was measured by the Cell Death Detection ELISA^{PLUS} (Roche, Hvidovre, Denmark).

2.5. Western Blot Analysis. INS-1 cells or INS-1 cell lines stably expressing shRNA were grown to 80–90% confluence,

TABLE 1: Rat JNK isoform-specific primers.

Isoform	Sense primer (5′-3′)	Antisense primer (5′-3′)	Probe
JNK1α1	GAGAAATGGTTTGCCACA	ACTGCTGCACCTGTGCTA	(VIC)-TTGAACAGCTCGGAACACCTTGTCCTG-(TAMRA)
JNK1α2	GAGAAATGGTTTGCCACA	ACTGCTGCACCTAAAGGA	(VIC)-TTGAACAGCTCGGAACACCTTGTCCTG-(TAMRA)
JNK1β1	GGAGAAATGATCAAAGGTG	ACTGCTGCACCTGTGCTA	(VIC)-TTGAACAGCTCGGAACACCTTGTCCTG-(TAMRA)
JNK1β2	GGAGAAATGATCAAAGGTG	ACTGCTGCACCTAAAGGA	(VIC)-TTGAACAGCTCGGAACACCTTGTCCTG-(TAMRA)
JNK2α1	GAGAGCTGGTGAAAGGTT	TTACTGCTGCATCTGTGC	(VIC)-AAAGTTATTGAACAGCTAGGAACACCATCC-(TAMRA)
JNK2α2	GAGAGCTGGTGAAAGGTT	ACTGCTGCATCTGAAGGC	(VIC)-AAAGTTATTGAACAGCTAGGAACACCATCC-(TAMRA)
JNK2β1	GAAATGGTCCTCCATAAAG	TTACTGCTGCATCTGTGC	(VIC)-AAAGTTATTGAACAGCTAGGAACACCATCC-(TAMRA)
JNK2β2	GAAATGGTCCTCCATAAAG	ACTGCTGCATCTGAAGGC	(VIC)-AAAGTTATTGAACAGCTAGGAACACCATCC-(TAMRA)
JNK3α1	GCCCTCACCTTCAGCACAG	AGGCAGGCGGCTAGTCAC	(VIC)-AGCAGTGAGAGTCTCCCTCCATCCTCGT-(TAMRA)
JNK3α2	GCCCTCACCTTCAGGTG	AGGCAGGCGGCTAGTCAC	(VIC)-AGCAGTGAGAGTCTCCCTCCATCCTCGT-(TAMRA)

exposed to IL-1β (150 pg/mL) or vehicle for up to 24 h, washed in ice-cold PBS, and lysed for 15 min on ice using 1x lysis buffer (Cell Signaling). The protein concentration was measured by the Bradford method (Bio-Rad, Copenhagen, Denmark). 30–40 micrograms of total protein were mixed with 4x LDS sample buffer (Invitrogen), heated for 5 min at 70°C, and loaded on 10% NuPAGEBis-Tris gel (Invitrogen). Proteins were blotted onto nitrocellulose filter membranes (Invitrogen). Ponceau staining measuring total protein was used as loading control. The blots were blocked for 1 h in 1x tris-buffered saline (pH 7.6) containing 0.1% Tween 20 and 5% BSA and afterwards incubated overnight at 4°C with primary antibody. Blots were rinsed and incubated with a rabbit secondary horseradish peroxidase-conjugated antibody for 1 h. Immune complexes were detected by chemiluminescence using Super Signal West Dura Extended Duration Substrate (Thermo Scientific), and images were captured digitally by use of the Fuji LAS3000 platform (Fujifilm, Tokyo, Japan) or the Alpha Innotech FlourChem Q imaging platform (Kem-En-Tec, Taastrup, Denmark).

2.6. Cell Death Detection Assay. Apoptotic cell death was measured by the detection of DNA-histone complexes released from the nucleus to the cytosol of cells by using Cell Death Detection ELISA^{PLUS} (Roche) as described by the manufacturer. In brief, 0.075×10^6 INS-1 cells stably expressing JNK1, JNK2, JNK3, nonsense shRNA, or empty vector were cultured 24 h prior to exposure to IL-1β (150 pg/mL) or vehicle. After an additional 24 h, the culture medium was removed and cells lysed in 200 μL 1x lysis buffer for 30 min at room temperature. The lysate was then centrifuged for 10 min at 200 ×g, incubated with anti-DNA peroxidase and anti-histone-biotin, and added to streptavidin-coated

wells for 2 h at room temperature. Absorbance was measured after addition of peroxidase substrate ABTS (2.2-azino-bis-3-ethylbenzthiazoline-6-sulfonate) at 405 and 490 nm.

2.7. Statistical Analysis. All statistical analyses were performed at raw data using GraphPad Prism (GraphPad Software Inc., San Diego, CA, USA). Where the figures show normalized data, the mean of the controls of the individual experiment was set to 1 and the error bars show the standard error calculated from the raw data. Statistical significance was determined using one- or two-way ANOVA with *post hoc* tests, or Student's *t*-test as appropriate. P values less than or equal to 0.05 were considered statistically significant.

3. Results

3.1. JNK Isoform Expression and Activity in INS-1 Cell. The JNK family of proteins consists of more than 10 isoforms. In order to determine which isoforms are expressed in the INS-1 cell model, we created rat-specific primers and probes (Table 1), utilizing the human isoform-specific primer and probe sequences determined by Dreskin et al. [34] and modifying them based upon a cross species homology comparison between human and mouse, as the rat JNK isoform sequences have not been published. Utilizing quantitative RT-PCR, we found that the INS-1 cells expressed JNK1α1, JNK1β1, JNK2α1, JNK2α2, JNK3α1, and JNK3α2. JNK1α2 and JNK1β2 were expressed at very low levels and JNK2β1 and JNK2β2 were not expressed in INS-1 cells (data not shown). We chose to examine IL-1β-induced regulation of the six isoforms with the higher level of expression in the INS-1 cell line. We exposed INS-1 cells to 150 pg/mL of IL-1β or vehicle for 2 to 24 h. We used 150 pg/mL IL-1β to induce apoptosis in the

INS-1 cells as titration experiments showed that this was the lowest concentration sufficient to induce maximal apoptosis (data not shown). Utilizing RT-PCR, we found that JNK1α1, JNK1β1, JNK2α1, and JNK2α2 were not regulated by IL-1β, whereas JNK3α1 was significantly upregulated at 8 h and JNK3α2 was upregulated from 8 to 24 h (Figures 1(a)–1(f)). Comparison of the data obtained with JNK isoform-specific primers with data obtained with nonisoform-specific Taqman primers confirmed that JNK1 and JNK2 were not regulated by IL-1β, whereas JNK3 was upregulated from 6 to 12 h (Supplementary Figures 1A–1C, in Supplementary Material available online at http://dx.doi.org/10.1155/2016/1312705).

We next asked if IL-1β altered JNK protein expression in INS-1 cells. As there are no available commercial JNK isoform-specific antibodies, we used JNK1, JNK2, or JNK3 subtype specific antibodies. We exposed INS-1 cells to 150 pg/mL IL-1β for 4 to 24 h to measure the expression and regulation of the JNK subtype proteins by Western blot analysis. The JNK1 subtype encompasses JNK1α1 and JNK1β1 isoforms translating into 46 kDa and JNK1α2 and JNK1β2 isoforms translating into 54 kDa isoform proteins, respectively. We found that only JNK1 46 and 54 kDa isoform proteins expressions were significantly regulated in that they were decreased by IL-1β in a time-dependent manner (Figure 2(a)). The JNK2 subtype includes JNK2α1 and JNK2α2 translating into 46 kDa and 54 kDa isoform proteins, respectively. The JNK2 antibody reacts only with the 54 kDa isoform protein, compatible with JNK2α2 being the predominating JNK2 isoform expressed in INS-1 cells (unpublished data). The JNK3 subtype specific antibody reacts only with the 54 kDa protein isoform corresponding to JNK3α2; however, JNK3α1 that translates into a 46 kDa protein isoform and JNK3α2 are expressed at equally high levels in INS-1 cells (unpublished data). However, the observed IL-1β-induced JNK3 mRNA expression did not translate into increased JNK3 54 kDa isoform protein expression (Figure 2(a)). Of note, detection of IL-1β-regulated JNK3α1 isoform protein expression was not possible with this JNK3 subtype antibody.

Finally, we exposed INS-1 cells to 150 pg/mL IL-1β or vehicle for 0.5 to 24 h to measure JNK phosphorylation as a measure of JNK activity. JNK 46 and 54 kDa isoforms were both significantly phosphorylated after 0.5 to 6 h of IL-1β exposure, with maximum peak phosphorylation of the isoforms after 0.5 to 1 h of IL-1β exposure (Figure 2(b)).

In summary, IL-1β increased JNK3α1 and JNK3α2 mRNA expression and decreased JNK1 subtype protein expression in INS-1 cells. Furthermore, IL-1β-induced JNK phosphorylation peaks after 0.5 to 6 h of stimulation.

3.2. JNK Knockdown INS-1 Cell Lines. To investigate the differential roles of the JNK subtypes in IL-1β-induced cell death, we produced stable INS-1 knockdown cell lines expressing shRNAs directed against JNK1, JNK2, or JNK3, as well as nontarget (nonsense, NS) shRNA and empty vector (EV) controls. The JNK knockdown cell lines were tested for knockdown specificity and efficiency by Western blot analysis using JNK subtype specific antibodies (Figure 3(a)). We achieved specific knockdown of the intended JNK subtypes

by approximately ~80% JNK1, ~75% JNK2, and ~45% JNK3 knockdown compared to control NS (NS shRNA) INS-1 cells (Figure 3(a)).

We next wished to measure early response JNK activity in the stable JNK knockdown INS-1 cell lines to investigate how knockdown of the individual JNK subtype affected total phosphorylation status of the different JNK isoforms (46 or 54 kDa). We exposed the stable JNK knockdown INS-1 cells to 150 pg/mL IL-1β or vehicle for 0.5 h (Figure 3(b)) as we detected peak JNK phosphorylation at this time point in nontransduced INS-1 cells (Figure 2(b)). Though the JNK knockdown INS-1 cell lines showed specific JNK1, JNK2, or JNK3 knockdown (Figure 3(b)), this did not affect the total level of JNK (all JNK subtypes) (Figure 3(b)). Interestingly, JNK1 knockdown (JNK1 shRNA) INS-1 cells showed significantly reduced IL-1β-induced phosphorylation of the 46 kDa isoforms compared to control NS expressing INS-1 cells. Phosphorylations of the 46 kDa isoforms in JNK2 knockdown (JNK2 shRNA) and JNK3 knockdown (JNK3 shRNA) INS-1 cells were not different compared to the control NS INS-1 cells (Figure 3(b)). There were no differences in phosphorylation of the 54 kda JNK isoforms between 0.5 h IL-1β exposed NS and JNK1, JNK2, or JNK3 knockdown INS-1 cell lines (Figure 3(b)). To summarize, only JNK1 knockdown reduced early IL-1β-mediated activity of the 46 kDa JNK isoforms as determined by phosphorylation in INS-1 cells.

3.3. JNK1 Knockdown Attenuates IL-1β-Induced Caspase 3 Activation and Apoptosis in INS-1 Cells. Next, to investigate the functional impact of knockdown of the individual JNK subtypes, we exposed the stable JNK knockdown and control cell lines to 150 pg/mL of IL-1β or vehicle for 24 h, after which apoptosis markers were measured by Elisa and Western blotting. IL-1β-induced apoptosis was observed in the control NS and EV expressing INS-1 cells. In contrast, knockdown of JNK1 prevented IL-1β-induced apoptosis, measured as decreased levels of cytoplasmic nucleosomes (Figure 4(a)). JNK1 knockdown also attenuated IL-1β-induced caspase 3 cleavage (Figure 4(b)). Interestingly, knockdown of JNK2 significantly potentiated IL-1β-induced apoptosis and caspase 3 activation, while JNK3 knockdown did not significantly affect IL-1β-induced apoptosis or cleavage of caspase 3 compared to NS cells.

Since the JNK members had differential effects on IL-1β-induced apoptosis, we next determined if there were unique early response gene clusters regulated by each JNK member. INS-1 cells stably expressing shRNAs directed against JNK1, JNK2, JNK3, or NS were exposed to 150 pg/mL of IL-1β or vehicle for 45 min. mRNA expression was analyzed by microarray analysis. When we compared the normalized gene expression profile of the 45 min IL-1β exposed JNK1, JNK2, or JNK3 knockdown INS-1 cells with the gene expression profile of 45 min IL-1β exposed NS INS-1 cells, adjusted for their IL-1β nonexposed control conditions, 74, 144, and 134 genes, respectively, were found to be differentially regulated (Supplementary Tables 1–3). The JNK1 knockdown INS-1 cell line gene expression pattern was significantly different from that of JNK2 or JNK3 knockdown and NS INS-1 cells

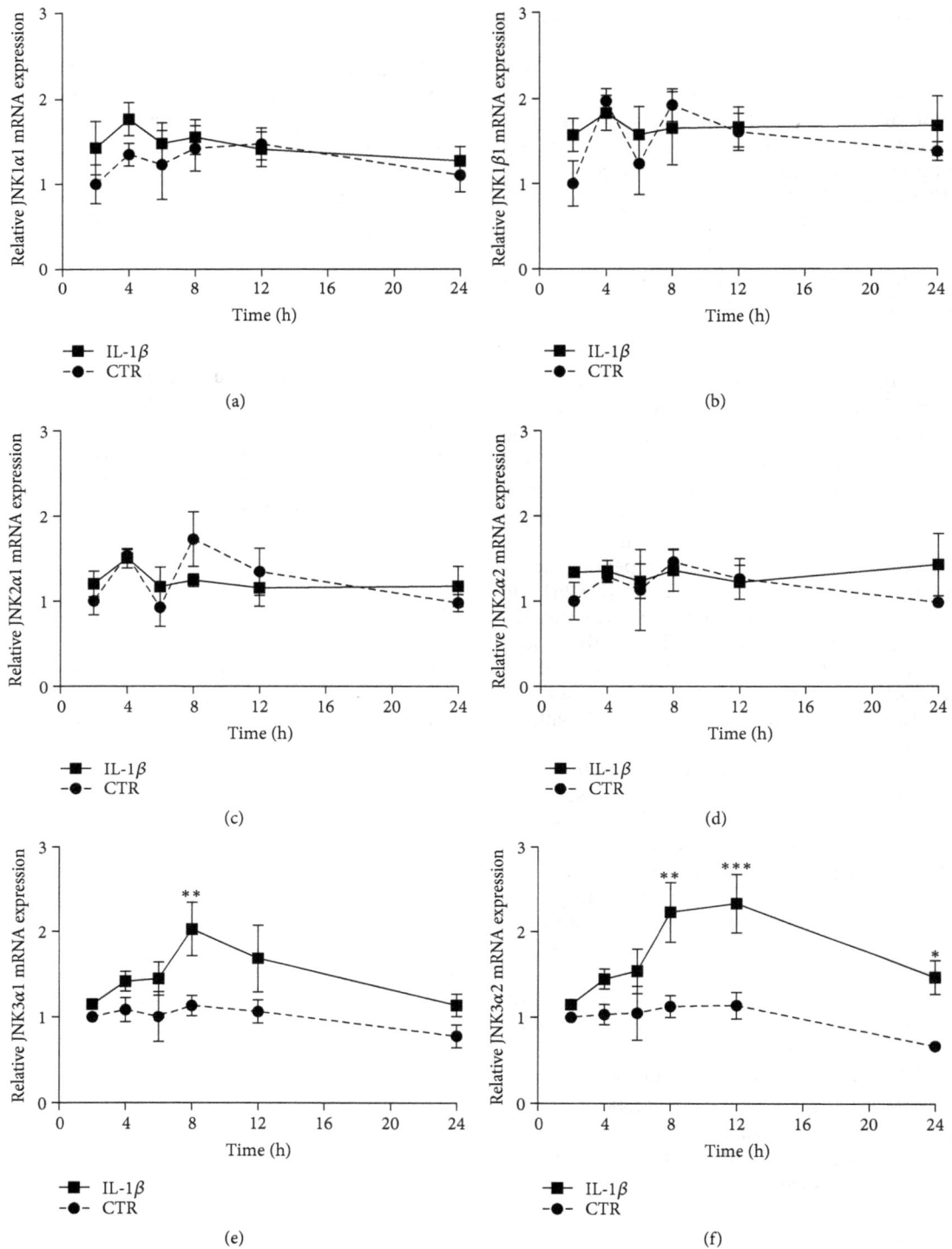

FIGURE 1: JNK isoform expression in INS-1 cell. INS-1 cells were exposed to 150 pg/mL IL-1β (square) or vehicle (circle) for 2 to 24 h. Relative mRNA of the JNK isoforms was measured using quantitative RT-PCR and normalized to the average of 18S and hprt1. (a) Relative JNK1α1 mRNA expression, (b) relative JNK1β1 mRNA expression, (c) relative JNK2α1 mRNA expression, (d) relative JNK2β2 mRNA expression, (e) relative JNK3α1 mRNA expression, and (f) relative JNK3α2 mRNA expression. Data are means ± SEM of n = 4 independent experiments. $^*P < 0.05$, $^{**}P < 0.01$, and $^{***}P < 0.001$.

(a)

(b)

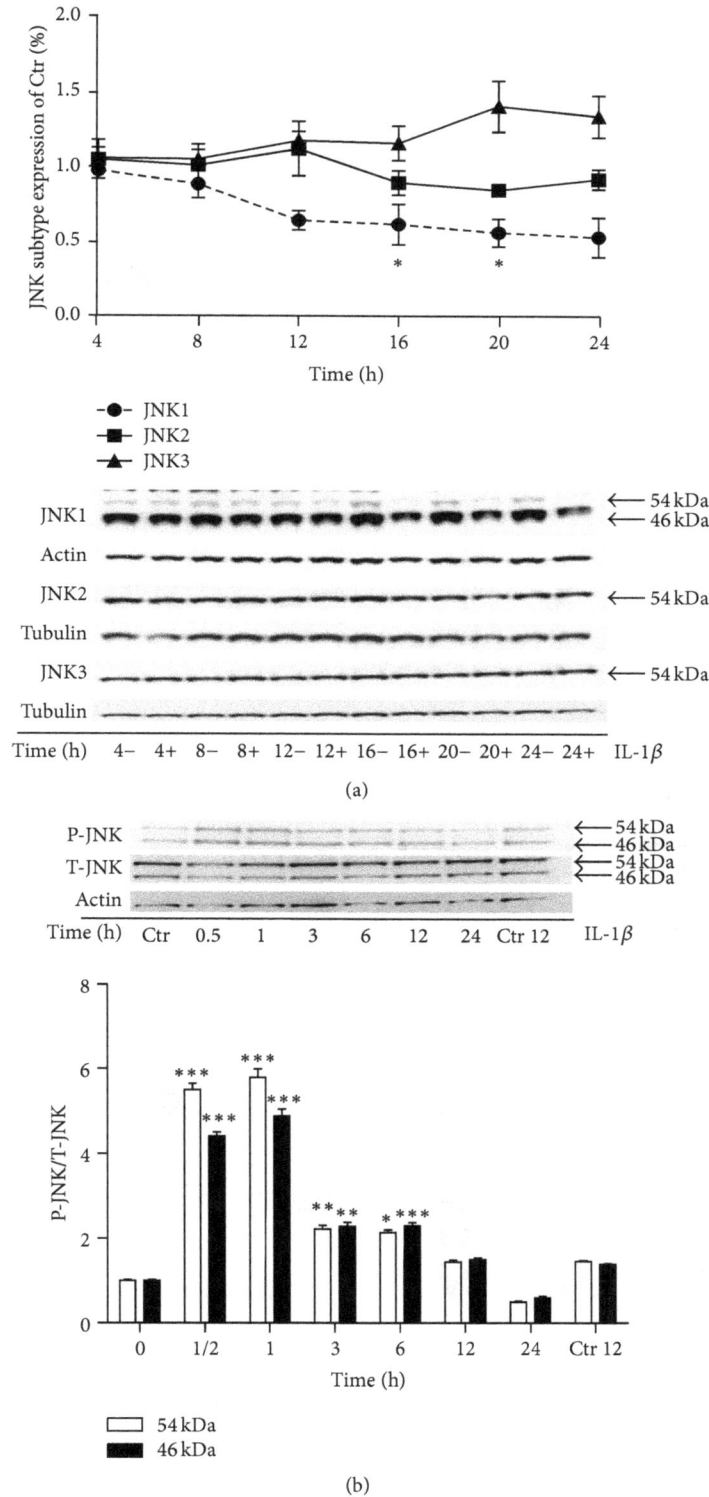

FIGURE 2: IL-1β reduces JNK1 but not JNK2 or JNK3 protein expression and increases P-JNK after 0.5 h of exposure in INS-1 cells. (a) INS-1 cells were exposed to 150 pg/mL IL-1β or vehicle for 4 to 24 h. JNK subtypes protein expression, JNK1 (circle), JNK2 (square), and JNK3 (triangle), were measured by immunoblotting and normalized to actin or tubulin. Data are shown as % IL-1β-regulated JNK subtype expression of their respective nonexposed controls. Data are shown as means of $n = 3$–5 independent experiments $\pm$ SEM; $^*P < 0.05$ versus 4 h time point. (b) INS-1 cells were exposed to 150 pg/mL IL-1β or vehicle for 0.5 to 24 h. INS-1 cells exposed for IL-1β for 12 h were lysed at an earlier time point paralleled with the 12 h vehicle ctrl. P-JNK was measured by immunoblotting and normalized to T-JNK. Data are shown as means of $n = 4$ independent experiments $\pm$ SEM; $^*P < 0.05$, $^{**}P < 0.01$, and $^{***}P < 0.001$ versus vehicle (0 h). Representative gels are shown.

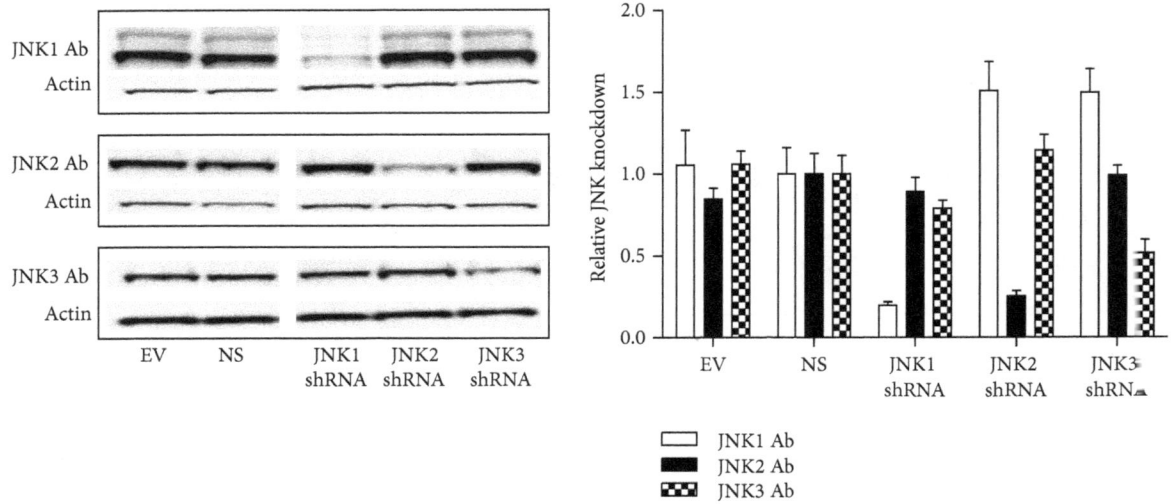

(a)

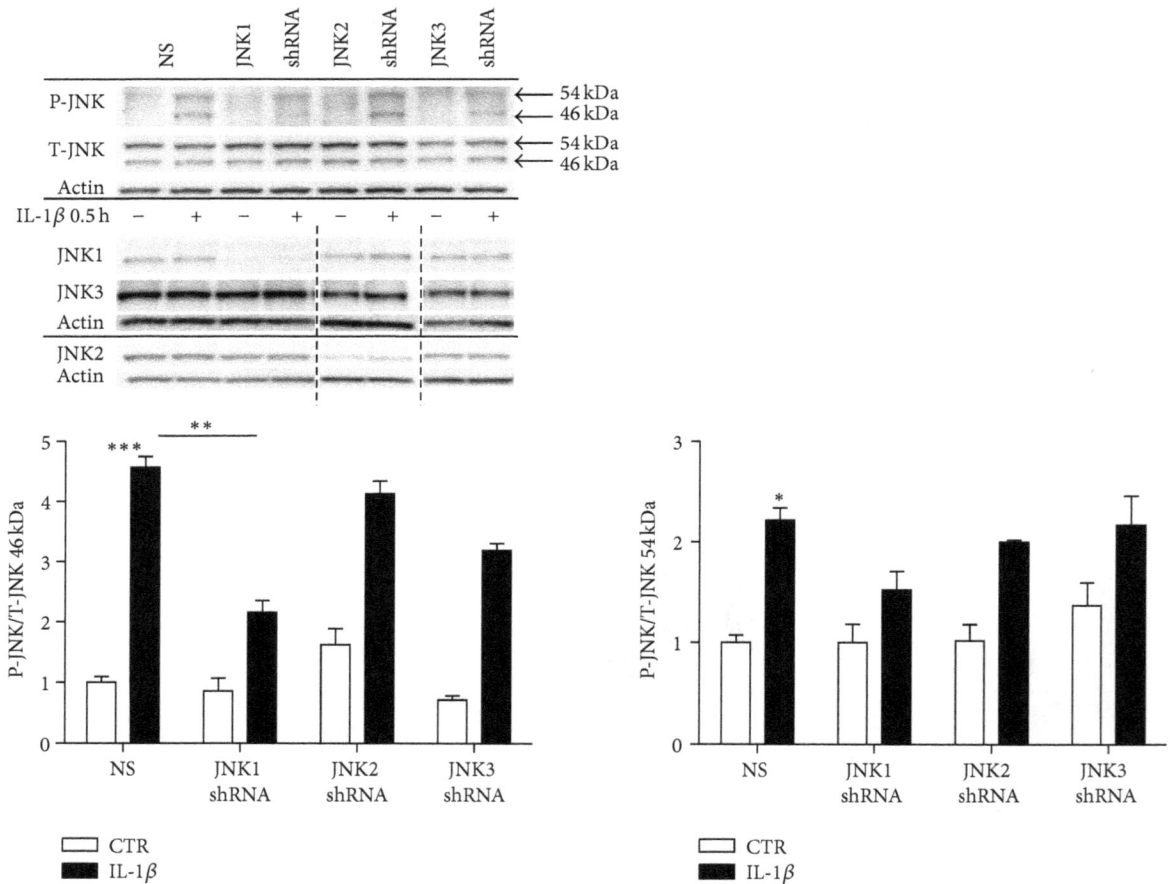

(b)

FIGURE 3: Phosphorylated JNK in individual JNK subtype knockdown INS-1 cell lines exposed to IL-1β for 0.5 h. INS-1 cells were transduced with Lentivirus containing shRNA directed against JNK1, JNK2, or JNK3 and nonsense (NS) or empty vector (EV) controls. Cells stably expressing the shRNA plasmids were selected with puromycin. (a) Stable INS-1 cell lines expressing shRNA for JNK1, JNK2, JNK3, nonsense shRNA, or empty vector controls were cultured for 4 days, protein was isolated, and JNK1, JNK2, and JNK3 protein knockdown expression was analyzed by immunoblotting. Data are shown as means ± SEM of $n = 3$ independent experiments. Representative blots are shown. (b) Stable INS-1 cell lines expressing shRNA for JNK1, JNK2, JNK3, nonsense shRNA, or empty vector were exposed to 150 pg/mL IL-1β (closed bars) or vehicle (open bars) for 0.5 h. P-JNK was assessed with immunoblotting and normalized to T-JNK. Data were quantified in respect to 46 kDa and 54 kDa P-JNK/T-JNK. Data are shown as means ± SEM of $n = 3$ independent experiments. Specific knockdowns of the individual JNK subtypes, JNK1, JNK2, or JNK3, are shown with their respective actin. Blots were cut as indicated by the dotted black line. $^{*}P < 0.05$, $^{**}P < 0.01$, and $^{***}P < 0.001$ versus IL-1β exposed NS. Representative gels are shown.

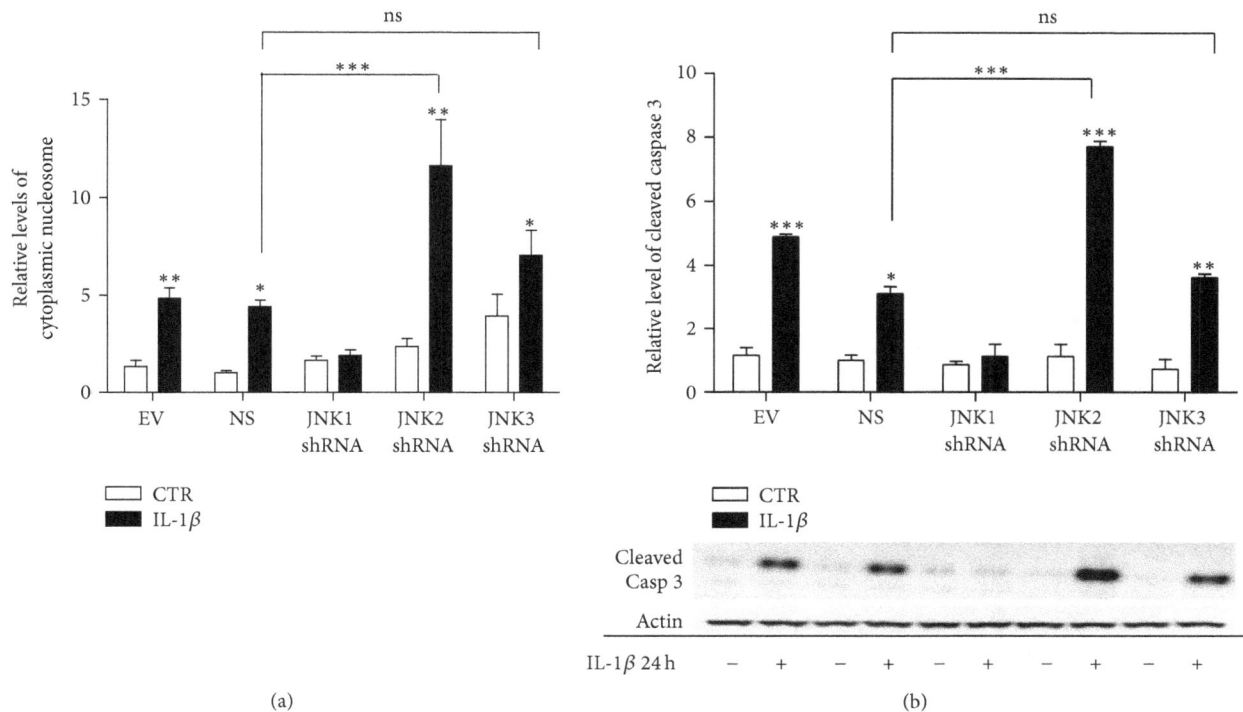

FIGURE 4: JNK1 knockdown attenuates IL-1β-induced caspase 3 activation and apoptosis in INS-1 cells. Stable INS-1 cell lines expressing shRNA for JNK1, JNK2, JNK3, nonsense shRNA, or empty vector controls were exposed to 150 pg/mL IL-1β (closed bars) or vehicle (open bars) for 24 h. (a) Apoptosis was measured as the relative levels of cytoplasmic nucleosomes in INS-1 stable cell lines lysates using the Roche Cell Death detection Elisa kit. Data are shown as means ± SEM of $n = 5$ independent experiments. (b) Cleaved caspase 3 was assessed with immunoblotting and normalized to actin. Data are shown as means ± SEM of $n = 4$ independent experiments; $^{*}P < 0.05$, $^{**}P < 0.01$, and $^{***}P < 0.001$, comparing caspase 3 activity in the presence with the activity in the absence of IL-1β, unless otherwise indicated. Representative gels are shown.

(Supplementary Figure 2). However, overall, there were no significant clusters or pathway associations to cast light on the potential pathways or early IL-1β-induced mechanisms underlying the unique actions of the JNK subtypes, and we therefore decided to proceed with a candidate gene approach to understand the mechanisms of action of the JNK subtypes.

3.4. JNK1 Knockdown Attenuates the Increase of Myc mRNA Expression by IL-1β. We therefore next analyzed in the JNK knockdown cells specific JNK-related signalling molecules known to be regulated by the JNK proteins to determine if the regulation of these genes by IL-1β is mediated specifically by JNK1. INS-1 cells stably expressing shRNA directed against JNK1, JNK2, or JNK3, or the NS or EV controls, were exposed to 150 pg/mL of IL-1β for 2, 6, and 12 h. IL-1β upregulated Jun mRNA from 2 to 12 h, Trp53 mRNA at 6 and 12 h, Junb mRNA from 2 to 12 h, Jund mRNA at 2 h, and Myc mRNA at 12 h (Figures 5(a)–5(e)). These findings indicate that many of the common JNK-related signalling proteins are regulated by IL-1β. Interestingly, there was a temporal difference in the regulation of the mRNA transcripts, as Jun and Junb were upregulated at all time points, whereas Myc was upregulated only at 12 h and Jund was upregulated significantly only at 2 h.

Knockdown of JNK1, JNK2, or JNK3 did not affect the regulation of Trp53 or Junb mRNA expression by IL-1β. This

indicates that these mRNA transcripts are not regulated by JNK1, JNK2, or JNK3 specifically, either due to redundancy in the actions of the JNK members or due to the fact that they are not regulated by the JNK proteins in INS-1 cells. JNK1 knockdown increased basal Jun mRNA expression at 2 h (Figure 5(a)) and attenuated the upregulation of Myc by IL-1β at 12 h (Figure 5(e)), indicating that JNK1 may be involved in the basal regulation of Jun and that it specifically mediates the regulation of Myc mRNA expression by IL-1β.

3.5. JNK1 Knockdown Attenuated the IL-1β-Induced Increase of Myc Protein Levels. Next, we wished to determine if IL-1β regulates the levels of Myc protein and if JNK1 mediates this regulation in response to IL-1β. INS-1 cells were exposed to 150 pg/mL of IL-1β or vehicle for 4 to 24 h, and protein was analyzed by Western blot analysis. IL-1β increased the total amount of Myc protein from 12 to 24 h (Figure 6(a)). The increase in total Myc protein by IL-1β corresponded to the timing of the upregulation of Myc mRNA by IL-1β, which we noted at 12 h (Figure 5(e)). Next, we exposed the INS-1 cells stably expressing shRNA directed against JNK1, JNK2, or JNK3, or the NS or EV controls to 150 pg/mL of IL-1β or vehicle for 16 h. Knockdown of JNK1 prevented IL-1β induction of total Myc protein expression (Figure 6(b)). This indicates that JNK1 mediates IL-1β regulation of total

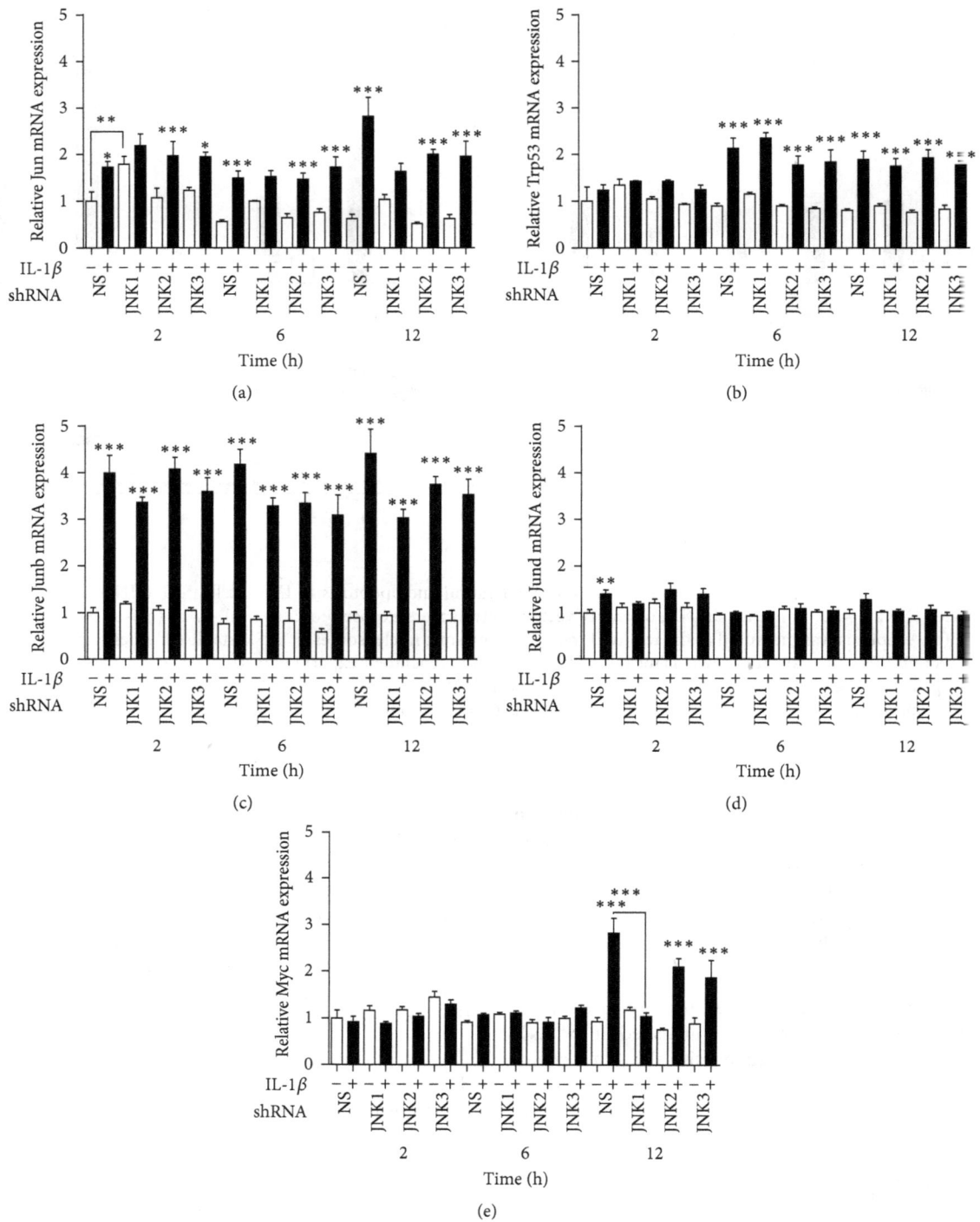

FIGURE 5: JNK1 knockdown attenuates the regulation of Myc mRNA expression by IL-1β. Stable INS-1 cell lines expressing shRNA for JNK1, JNK2, JNK3, nonsense shRNA, or empty vector controls were exposed to 150 pg/mL IL-1β (closed bars) or vehicle (open bars) for 2, 6, and 12 h. Relative mRNA expression were measured using quantitative RT-PCR and normalized to the average of 18S and Hprt1. (a) Relative Jun mRNA expression, (b) relative Trp53 mRNA expression, (c) relative Junb mRNA expression, (d) relative Jund mRNA expression, and (e) relative Myc mRNA expression. Data are shown as means ± SEM of 3–5 independent experiments. $^{*}P < 0.05$, $^{**}P < 0.01$, and $^{***}P < 0.001$, comparing expression in the presence with expression in the absence of IL-1β, unless otherwise indicated.

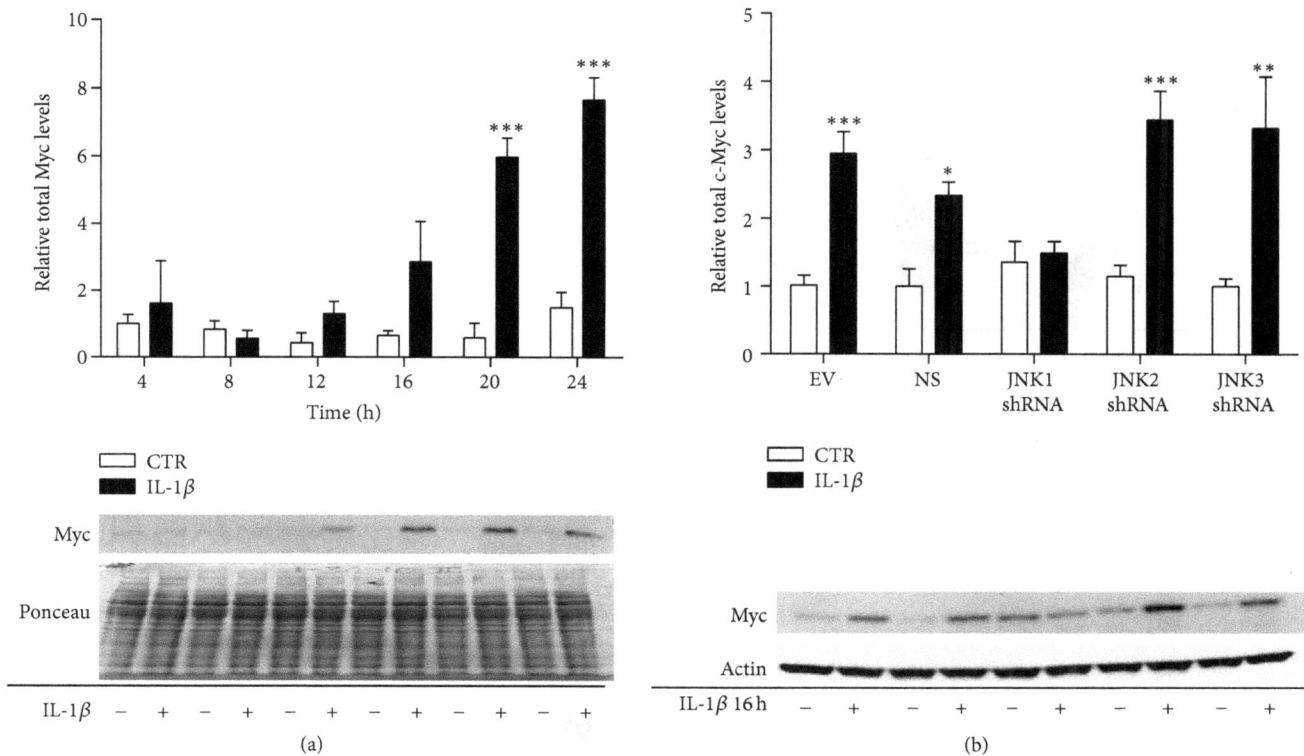

FIGURE 6: JNK1 knockdown prevents the regulation of total Myc protein by IL-1β. INS-1 cells were exposed to 150 pg/mL IL-1β (closed bars) or vehicle (open bars) for 4 to 24 h. Protein was isolated and (a) total Myc protein levels were analyzed by immunoblotting. Total protein was used as the loading control. Data are shown ± SEM of n = 3-4 independent experiments. INS-1 cells stably expressing shRNA directed against JNK1, JNK2, JNK3, or the nonsense or empty vector controls were exposed to 150 pg/mL IL-1β (black bars) or left unexposed (white bars) for 16 h. Protein was isolated, and (b) total Myc protein levels were analyzed by immunoblotting. Actin was used as the loading control. Data are shown ± SEM of n = 5 independent experiments. $^{**}P$ < 0.01 and $^{***}P$ < 0.001 comparing Myc levels in the presence with Myc levels in the absence of IL-1β, unless otherwise indicated.

Myc protein levels. These results, taken together with the data in Figure 5(e), indicate that JNK1 mediates inflammatory regulation of Myc transcription and translation in INS-1 cells.

3.6. Myc Knockdown Attenuates IL-1β-Induced Apoptosis in INS-1 Cells. The Myc protein has been shown previously to be involved in JNK-mediated apoptosis triggered by UV irradiation or antineoplastic drugs [26, 35]. We therefore wished to determine if Myc mediates IL-1β-induced apoptosis in the INS-1 β-cell model. INS-1 cells were transiently transfected with either siRNA directed against Myc or a control NS oligonucleotide sequence and then exposed to 150 pg/mL of IL-1β or vehicle for 24 h (Figure 7). Transfection with siRNA directed against Myc decreased the total level of Myc by ~2.8-fold detected by Western blot analysis (Figure 7(a)) and, interestingly, attenuated the IL-1β-induced caspase 3 activation by ~3.2-fold (Figure 7(b)). In addition, transfection of INS-1 cells with Myc siRNA attenuated IL-1β-induced apoptosis by ~1.6-fold (Figure 7(c)). This indicates that Myc may mediate IL-1β-induced apoptosis in the INS-1β-cell line and, taken together with the previous results, that the JNK1-Myc pathway is an important mediator of IL-1β-induced apoptosis.

4. Discussion

Few studies have investigated the differential roles of the JNK subtypes in cellular apoptosis, or if there are specific downstream signaling proteins utilized by a specific JNK subtype to mediate its actions. It is known that IL-1β does not induce apoptosis in most cells but the pancreatic β-cells belong to the exceptions. Many studies have shown that JNK plays an important role in cellular apoptosis and specifically in cytokine and IL-1β-induced β-cell apoptosis [19] most using the nonspecific JNK inhibitor SP600125 [36]. We show here that JNK1α1, JNK1β1, JNK2α1, JNK2α2, JNK3α1, and JNK3α2 isoforms are expressed in INS-1 cells whereas only the JNK3 isoforms mRNA is regulated by IL-1β. When we analyzed JNK1, JNK2, and JNK3 subtype protein expression, only JNK1 subtype was significantly downregulated by IL-1β after 24 h of exposure. We believe that this downregulation of JNK1 subtype is not mediated by proteases after cell lysis since we use a broad protease inhibitor cocktail in our lysis buffer. The reduced JNK1 subtype expression may though be a side effect of apoptosis due to caspase 3-mediated cleavage; however, in other stress-induced apoptotic cell lines, JNK protein expression is shown to be caspase-independent [37, 38]. Gene expression profiling

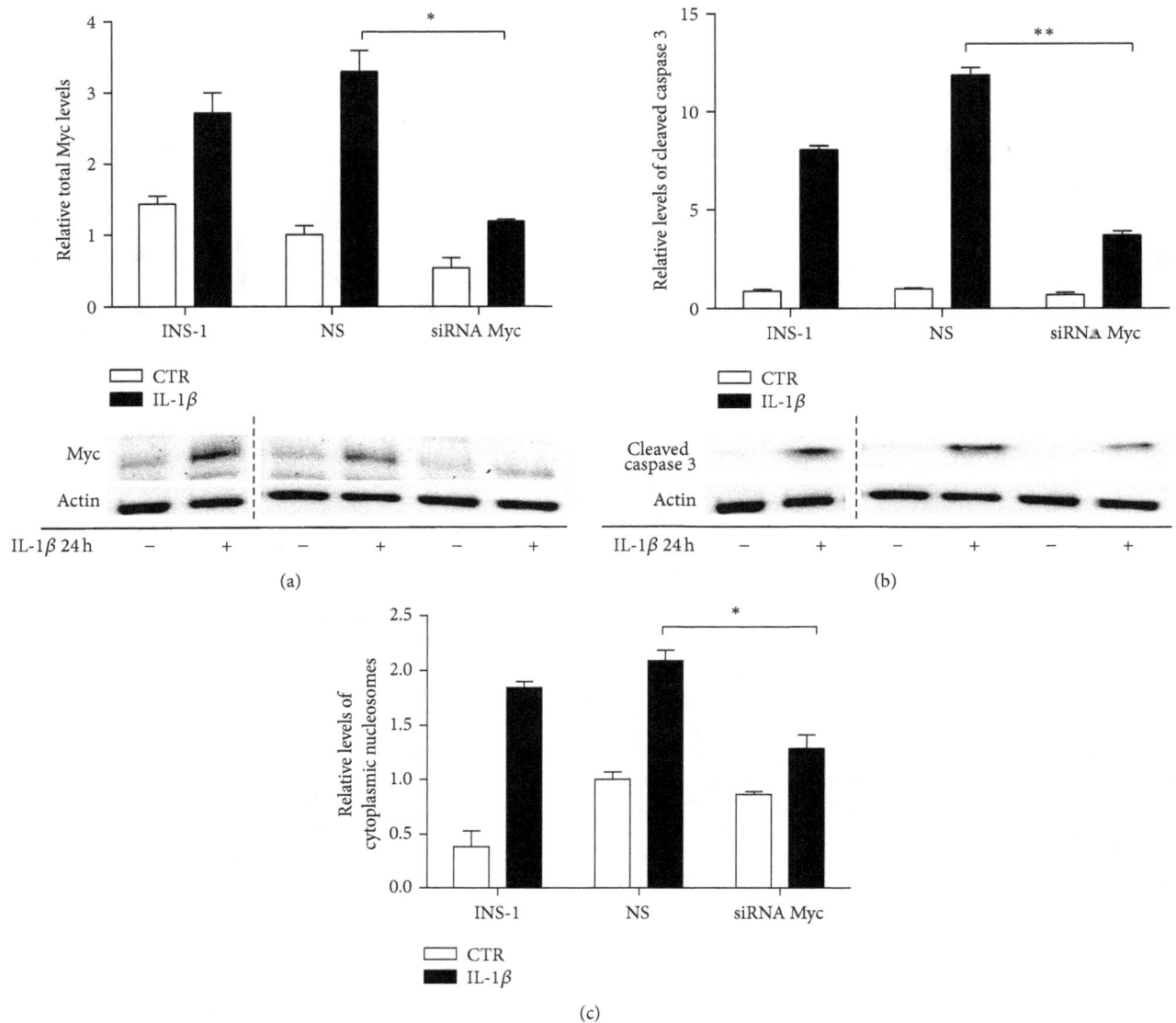

FIGURE 7: Myc knockdown attenuates IL-1β-induced apoptosis in INS-1 cells. INS-1 cells were transfected with siRNA directed against Myc, a scrambled siRNA control (NS) or vehicle (INS-1) for 16 h. Thereafter, cells were exposed to 150 pg/mL IL-1β (closed bars) or vehicle (open bars) for 24 h. (a) Total Myc protein levels and (b) cleaved caspase 3 were analyzed by immunoblotting. Actin was used as the loading control. Data are shown as means ± SEM of 3-4 independent experiments. Blots shown are representative. (c) Apoptosis was measured as relative levels of cytoplasmic nucleosomes in lysates measured by the Roche Cell Death Elisa kit. Data are shown as means ± SEM of 3-4 independent experiments. $^*P < 0.05$ and $^{**}P < 0.01$ versus IL-1β exposed NS.

studies followed by functional characterization of candidate genes have demonstrated that the exposure of insulin-producing cell lines, fluorescence-activated cell-sorted primary rodent β-cells, intact rodent islets, and human islets to proinflammatory cytokines induces not only upregulation of proapoptotic/downregulation of antiapoptotic genes, but also a protective response including downregulation of proapoptotic/upregulation of antiapoptotic genes, with a high degree of concordance between the different model systems [39, 40]. These findings suggest that inflammatory attack on the pancreatic β-cell induces a race between deleterious and protective responses, of which the deleterious pathways

eventually prevail [41]. We believe that the observed decrease in JNK1 content following 16 h of exposure to IL-1β is a late compensatory negative feedback mechanism serving to suppress signaling via JNK1; however, this late suppression in JNK1 content is insufficient to prevent apoptosis.

We selectively knocked down the three JNK subtypes to understand their individual contributions. Knockdown of JNK1 completely prevented IL-1β-induced INS-1 cell apoptosis, while JNK2 knockdown potentiated cytokine-induced INS-1 cell apoptosis. This is an interesting observation as JNK2 has been shown to inhibit JNK1 signaling [42], and thus knockdown of JNK2 may act to increase JNK1 activity.

Knockdown of JNK3 did not significantly affect IL-1β-induced apoptosis compared to NS cells but an increase could be observed, but not in levels of cleaved caspase 3. JNK3 has been suggested as being protective against cytokine-induced INS-1E cell death [15]. Both JNK1 and JNK2 knockdown protected INS-1E cells against apoptosis by 40 and 60%, respectively, in that study. We found complete protection of apoptosis by JNK1 knockdown and found that JNK2 knockdown potentiated the effect of IL-1β. Our study and [15] differed in the following respects: we utilized INS-1 cells stably expressing shRNA, whereas Abdelli et al. used transiently siRNA transfected INS-1E cells. However, the key difference between these studies is the inflammatory stimulus used. Abdelli et al. used a cytokine combination, containing 10 ng/mL IL-1β, 25 ng/mL TNF-α, and 150 ng/mL IFN-γ, while we exposed INS-1 cells to only IL-1β at 150 pg/mL. TNF-α receptor is a death-domain containing receptor and activates caspase 8 directly. The TNFR also signals through JNK and NFκB, as does the IL-1 receptor. IFN-γ signals through the JAK-STAT pathway. Thus, using a cytokine combination, confounding pathways and downstream signaling molecules are activated compared to testing IL-1β alone. However, as we only achieved ~50% knockdown of JNK3 in this study, new studies with more efficient JNK3 knockdown might acknowledge JNK3 as a protective protein.

We also investigated early IL-1β-induced JNK phosphorylation as a surrogate for JNK activity in the JNK knockdown INS-1 cells. Here, we only observed significant reduction of phosphorylation of the 46 kDa isoform in 0.5 h IL-1β exposed JNK1 knockdown INS-1 cells when compared to NS INS-1 cells. This was not surprising to us as the major JNK1 isoforms expressed in INS-1 cells translate into 46 kDa proteins and as we achieved a high JNK1 knockdown efficiency in the JNK1 knockdown INS-1 cell line. Despite high specific knockdown of the individual JNK subtypes in the shRNA expressing INS-1 cell lines, we did not see any changes in total levels of JNK. The total JNK antibody recognizes all three JNK subtypes and therefore a reduction in only one subtype is unlikely to affect the total amount of JNK. The reduced 46 kDa phosphorylation might explain the decreased IL-1β-induced apoptosis in JNK1 knockdown INS-1 cells as inhibition of total JNK activity decreases intracellular JNK signalling and improves rodent β-cell survival in vitro in response to cytokines [5, 18, 19, 43]. We did not observe altered 54 kDa isoform phosphorylation between 0.5 h IL-1β exposed NS and JNK1, JNK2, or JNK3 perhaps indicating that IL-1β-induced phosphorylation in the individual JNK knockdown subtype INS-1 cells is covered by the remaining JNK isoforms.

There are many potential downstream targets of JNK1 that activate apoptosis, such as the mitochondrial stress pathway and caspase activation, but there are few studies analyzing if there are specific signaling proteins or transcription factors that are uniquely regulated by each JNK subtype. We performed microarray mRNA expression profiling to investigate the genes regulated by the JNK subtypes. There were no differences in basal gene expression levels in JNK1, JNK2, or JNK3 shRNA expressing INS-1 cells when compared to NS shRNA expressing INS-1 cells, indicating that individual JNK subtype knockdown does not initiate differential basal gene regulation. Exposure of the cells to IL-1β for 45 min initiated differential gene regulation; however, no significant clusters were identified. This indicates that the JNK subtypes might mediate their major differential effect by modulating activity of proteins rather than affecting early IL-1β-induced gene transcription in β-cells. Using a transcription factor candidate gene expression analysis, we found that Myc was specifically regulated by JNK1 after 12 h of IL-1β exposure. We found that Myc mRNA and total protein levels were specifically downregulated in JNK1 knockdown INS-1 cells and that knockdown of Myc decreased IL-1β-induced apoptosis and cleaved caspase 3. In addition to activating Myc expression, JNK proteins are known to increase the stability of the Myc protein [44] that normally has a short half-life of approximately 30 minutes. Our data also suggests that JNK1 increases the stability of total Myc, as Myc protein levels were increased in wild-type INS-1 cells by IL-1β from 16 h to 24 h; additionally, we found that Myc mRNA expression was increased at 12 h. This increase could be due to an increased stability of the mRNA transcript, as opposed to transcriptional activation, given that there is a delayed increase in Myc mRNA expression relative to other JNK-regulated genes, such as Jun, Junb, and Jund, which were all increased at 2 h.

Myc is involved in mediating numerous cellular functions, including cell proliferation, growth, differentiation, and apoptosis [45]. There is much debate as to how Myc regulates these opposing cellular processes, but it seems to be through a complex and intricate balance between Myc and its protein interaction partner MAX, as well as other signaling pathways [45]. There are also numerous pathways through which Myc can promote cellular death. Myc induces the expression of the tumor suppressor protein cyclin-dependent kinase inhibitor 2A, which stabilizes p53, an important regulator of apoptosis, by sequestering the E3 ubiquitin-protein ligase, mouse double minute 2 homolog, in turn degrading p53 [46]. Myc also induces the proapoptotic BH3-only protein, Bim, and blocks the expression of the antiapoptotic proteins Bcl-2 and Bcl-xl. Myc has been shown to promote intrinsic cell death by destabilizing via the Bax protein [47]. Thus, Myc knockdown in cisplatin-induced apoptosis in A549 human lung carcinoma cells blocked cytochrome C release and prevented Bax oligomerization [48]. Another potential death promoting mechanism is through the p53-p21 pathway. Myc binds to the cell cycle gene p21CIP1 promoter, thereby preventing p53-induced transcription [49]. p53 induction of p21CIP1 drives the cell into senescence, and blocking p21 upregulation redirects the actions of p53 to activate apoptotic pathways [49]. p53 was significantly upregulated in INS-1 cells following IL-1β treatment; however, when we analyzed p21CIP1 mRNA expression in the INS-1 cells stably expressing JNK1 shRNA, we did not observe a decrease in expression, and thus we do not favor this mechanism of action.

In nonstressed islets, Myc expression is low [50] and β-cell specific Myc overexpression markedly increases β-cell apoptosis [51]. Here, we suggest that Myc is a key mediator of IL-1β-induced apoptosis in the INS-1 cell model. We additionally propose that JNK1 specifically regulates Myc, implicating Myc as a potential downstream relay of the apoptotic effect of JNK1. Further experiments are likewise required to verify the direct involvement of Myc in mediating the apoptotic actions of JNK1, such as overexpression of JNK1 combined with Myc knockdown.

5. Conclusion

In summary, this study suggests that JNK1 is a key mediator of IL-1β-induced INS-1 cell apoptosis, that the transcription factor Myc is regulated specifically by JNK1, and that Myc may mediate the apoptotic actions of JNK1. Future studies are required to investigate if the JNK1-Myc pathway is involved in cytokine-induced apoptosis in other cell types to determine if this is a pancreatic β-cell specific effect or a more general cellular effect. We propose that the JNK1-Myc pathway may be a target for protecting pancreatic β-cells from inflammatory stress, and thus a potential treatment target in diabetes.

Conflict of Interests

The authors declare that there is no conflict of interests regarding the publication of this paper.

Acknowledgments

This study is supported by Novo Nordisk and the Novo Nordisk Foundation and the PhD Program for Molecular Metabolism. The authors are thankful to Fie Hillesø for expert technical assistance.

References

[1] T. Mandrup-Poulsen, L. Pickersgill, and M. Y. Donath, "Blockade of interleukin 1 in type 1 diabetes mellitus," *Nature Reviews Endocrinology*, vol. 6, no. 3, pp. 158–166, 2010.

[2] C. A. Dinarello, M. Y. Donath, and T. Mandrup-Poulsen, "Role of IL-1beta in type 2 diabetes," *Current Opinion in Endocrinology, Diabetes and Obesity*, vol. 17, no. 4, pp. 314–321, 2010.

[3] C. A. Dinarello, "Interleukin-1 in the pathogenesis and treatment of inflammatory diseases," *Blood*, vol. 117, no. 14, pp. 3720–3732, 2011.

[4] L. G. Grunnet, R. Aikin, M. F. Tonnesen et al., "Proinflammatory cytokines activate the intrinsic apoptotic pathway in β-cells," *Diabetes*, vol. 58, no. 8, pp. 1807–1815, 2009.

[5] A. Ammendrup, A. Maillard, K. Nielsen et al., "The c-Jun amino-terminal kinase pathway is preferentially activated by interleukin-1 and controls apoptosis in differentiating pancreatic beta-cells," *Diabetes*, vol. 49, no. 9, pp. 1468–1476, 2000.

[6] E. N. Gurzov, F. Ortis, D. A. Cunha et al., "Signaling by IL-1β+IFN-γ and ER stress converge on DP5/Hrk activation: a novel mechanism for pancreatic β-cell apoptosis," *Cell Death & Differentiation*, vol. 16, no. 11, pp. 1539–1550, 2009.

[7] M. Y. Donath, J. Størling, L. A. Berchtold, N. Billestrup, and T. Mandrup-Poulsen, "Cytokines and β-cell biology: from concept to clinical translation," *Endocrine Reviews*, vol. 29, no. 3, pp. 334–350, 2008.

[8] M. Hibi, A. Lin, T. Smeal, A. Minden, and M. Karin, "Identification of an oncoprotein- and UV-responsive protein kinase that binds and potentiates the c-Jun activation domain," *Genes and Development*, vol. 7, no. 11, pp. 2135–2148, 1993.

[9] R. J. Davis, "Signal transduction by the JNK group of MAP kinases," *Cell*, vol. 103, no. 2, pp. 239–252, 2000.

[10] T. Kallunki, B. Su, I. Tsigelny et al., "JNK2 contains a specificity-determining region responsible for efficient c-Jun binding and phosphorylation," *Genes and Development*, vol. 8, no. 24, pp. 2996–3007, 1994.

[11] B. Dérijard, M. Hibi, I.-H. Wu et al., "JNK1: a protein kinase stimulated by UV light and Ha-Ras that binds and phosphorylates the c-Jun activation domain," *Cell*, vol. 76, no. 6, pp. 1025–1037, 1994.

[12] A. M. Bode and Z. Dong, "The functional contrariety of JNK," *Molecular Carcinogenesis*, vol. 46, no. 8, pp. 591–598, 2007.

[13] S. Gupta, T. Barrett, A. J. Whitmarsh et al., "Selective interaction of JNK protein kinase isoforms with transcription factors," *The EMBO Journal*, vol. 15, no. 11, pp. 2760–2770, 1996.

[14] C.-Y. Kuan, D. D. Yang, D. R. Samanta Roy, R. J. Davis, P. Rakic, and R. A. Flavell, "The Jnk1 and Jnk2 protein kinases are required for regional specific apoptosis during early brain development," *Neuron*, vol. 22, no. 4, pp. 667–676, 1999.

[15] S. Abdelli, J. Puyal, C. Bielmann et al., "JNK3 is abundant in insulin-secreting cells and protects against cytokine-induced apoptosis," *Diabetologia*, vol. 52, no. 9, pp. 1871–1880, 2009.

[16] C. Tournier, P. Hess, D. D. Yang et al., "Requirement of JNK for stress-induced activation of the cytochrome c-mediated death pathway," *Science*, vol. 288, no. 5467, pp. 870–874, 2000.

[17] D. D. Yang, C.-Y. Kuan, A. J. Whitmarsh et al., "Absence of excitotoxicity-induced apoptosis in the hippocampus of mice lacking the Jnk3 gene," *Nature*, vol. 389, no. 6653, pp. 865–870, 1997.

[18] C. Bonny, A. Oberson, S. Negri, C. Sauser, and D. F. Schorderet, "Cell-permeable peptide inhibitors of JNK: novel blockers of β-cell death," *Diabetes*, vol. 50, no. 1, pp. 77–82, 2001.

[19] S. Abdelli, A. Abderrahmani, B. J. Hering, J. S. Beckmann, and C. Bonny, "The c-Jun N-terminal kinase JNK participates in cytokine- and isolation stress-induced rat pancreatic islet apoptosis," *Diabetologia*, vol. 50, no. 8, pp. 1660–1669, 2007.

[20] G. Spigolon, C. Veronesi, C. Bonny, and A. Vercelli, "c-Jun N-terminal kinase signaling pathway in excitotoxic cell death following kainic acid-induced status epilepticus," *European Journal of Neuroscience*, vol. 31, no. 7, pp. 1261–1272, 2010.

[21] Y. Zhao, G. Spigolon, C. Bonny, J. Culman, A. Vercelli, and T. Herdegen, "The JNK inhibitor D-JNKI-1 blocks apoptotic JNK signaling in brain mitochondria," *Molecular and Cellular Neuroscience*, vol. 49, no. 3, pp. 300–310, 2012.

[22] D. A. Cunha, P. Hekerman, L. Ladrière et al., "Initiation and execution of lipotoxic ER stress in pancreatic β-cells," *Journal of Cell Science*, vol. 121, no. 14, pp. 2308–2318, 2008.

[23] P. Wang, Y. Xiong, C. Ma, T. Shi, and D. Ma, "Molecular cloning and characterization of novel human JNK2 (MAPK9) transcript variants that show different stimulation activities on AP-1," *BMB Reports*, vol. 43, no. 11, pp. 738–743, 2010.

[24] R. K. Barr and M. A. Bogoyevitch, "The c-Jun N-terminal protein kinase family of mitogen-activated protein kinases (JNK MAPKs)," *International Journal of Biochemistry and Cell Biology*, vol. 33, no. 11, pp. 1047–1063, 2001.

[25] M. A. Bogoyevitch, "The isoform-specific functions of the c-Jun N-terminal kinases (JNKs): differences revealed by gene targeting," *BioEssays*, vol. 28, no. 9, pp. 923–934, 2005.

[26] K. Noguchi, C. Kitanaka, H. Yamana, A. Kokubu, T. Mochizuki, and Y. Kuchino, "Regulation of c-Myc through phosphorylation at Ser-62 and Ser-71 by c-Jun N-terminal kinase," *The Journal of Biological Chemistry*, vol. 274, no. 46, pp. 32580–32587, 1999.

[27] X. Deng, L. Xiao, W. Lang, F. Gao, P. Ruvolo, and W. S. May Jr., "Novel role for JNK as a stress-activated Bcl2 kinase," *The Journal of Biological Chemistry*, vol. 276, no. 26, pp. 23681–23688, 2001.

[28] S. Abdelli and C. Bonny, "JNK3 maintains expression of the insulin receptor substrate 2 (IRS2) in insulin-secreting cells: functional consequences for insulin signaling," *PLoS ONE*, vol. 7, no. 5, Article ID e35997, 2012.

[29] M. Asfari, D. Janjic, P. Meda, G. Li, P. A. Halban, and C. B. Wollheim, "Establishment of 2-mercaptoethanol-dependent differentiated insulin-secreting cell lines," *Endocrinology*, vol. 130, no. 1, pp. 167–178, 1992.

[30] M. Prause, D. P. Christensen, N. Billestrup, and T. Mandrup-Poulsen, "JNK1 protects against glucolipotoxicity-mediated beta-cell apoptosis," *PLoS ONE*, vol. 9, no. 1, Article ID e87067, 2014.

[31] G. Rustici, N. Kolesnikov, M. Brandizi et al., "ArrayExpress update—trends in database growth and links to data analysis tools," *Nucleic Acids Research*, vol. 41, no. 1, pp. D987–D990, 2013.

[32] D. W. Huang, B. T. Sherman, and R. A. Lempicki, "Systematic and integrative analysis of large gene lists using DAVID bioinformatics resources," *Nature Protocols*, vol. 4, no. 1, pp. 44–57, 2008.

[33] D. W. Huang, B. T. Sherman, and R. A. Lempicki, "Bioinformatics enrichment tools: paths toward the comprehensive functional analysis of large gene lists," *Nucleic Acids Research*, vol. 37, no. 1, pp. 1–13, 2009.

[34] S. C. Dreskin, G. W. Thomas, S. N. Dale, and L. E. Heasley, "Isoforms of jun kinase are differentially expressed and activated in human monocyte/macrophage (THP-1) cells1," *Journal of Immunology*, vol. 166, no. 9, pp. 5646–5653, 2001.

[35] K. Noguchi, H. Yamana, C. Kitanaka, T. Mochizuki, A. Kokubu, and Y. Kuchino, "Differential role of the JNK and p38 MAPK pathway in c-myc- and s-myc-mediated apoptosis," *Biochemical and Biophysical Research Communications*, vol. 267, no. 1, pp. 221–227, 2000.

[36] J. Bain, L. Plater, M. Elliott et al., "The selectivity of protein kinase inhibitors: a further update," *Biochemical Journal*, vol. 408, no. 3, pp. 297–315, 2007.

[37] C. Widmann, S. Gibson, and G. L. Johnson, "Caspase-dependent cleavage of signaling proteins during apoptosis. A turn-off mechanism for anti-apoptotic signals," *Journal of Biological Chemistry*, vol. 273, no. 12, pp. 7141–7147, 1998.

[38] A. Poehlmann, K. Reissig, P. Schönfeld et al., "Repeated H_2O_2 exposure drives cell cycle progression in an in vitro model of ulcerative colitis," *Journal of Cellular and Molecular Medicine*, vol. 17, no. 12, pp. 1619–1631, 2013.

[39] A. K. Cardozo, M. Kruhøffer, R. Leeman, T. Ørntoft, and D. L. Eizirik, "Identification of novel cytokine-induced genes in pancreatic β-cells by high-density oligonucleotide arrays," *Diabetes*, vol. 50, no. 5, pp. 909–920, 2001.

[40] B. Kutlu, A. K. Cardozo, M. I. Darville et al., "Discovery of gene networks regulating cytokine-induced dysfunction and apoptosis in insulin-producing INS-1 cells," *Diabetes*, vol. 52, no. 11, pp. 2701–2719, 2003.

[41] D. L. Eizirik and T. Mandrup-Poulsen, "A choice of death—the signal-transduction of immune-mediated beta-cell apoptosis," *Diabetologia*, vol. 44, no. 12, pp. 2115–2133, 2001.

[42] J. Liu, Y. Minemoto, and A. Lin, "c-Jun N-terminal protein kinase 1 (JNK1), but not JNK2, is essential for tumor necrosis factor alpha-induced c-Jun kinase activation and apoptosis," *Molecular and Cellular Biology*, vol. 24, no. 24, pp. 10844–10856, 2004.

[43] C. Bonny, A. Oberson, M. Steinmann, D. F. Schorderet, P. Nicod, and G. Waeber, "IB1 reduces cytokine-induced apoptosis of insulin-secreting cells," *Journal of Biological Chemistry*, vol. 275, no. 22, pp. 16466–16472, 2000.

[44] K. Noguchi, A. Kokubu, C. Kitanaka, H. Ichijo, and Y. Kuchino, "ASK1-signaling promotes c-Myc protein stability during apoptosis," *Biochemical and Biophysical Research Communications*, vol. 281, no. 5, pp. 1313–1320, 2001.

[45] S. Pelengaris, M. Khan, and G. Evan, "c-MYC: more than just a matter of life and death," *Nature Reviews Cancer*, vol. 2, no. 10, pp. 764–776, 2002.

[46] C. J. Sherr, "Divorcing ARF and p53: an unsettled case," *Nature Reviews Cancer*, vol. 6, no. 9, pp. 663–673, 2006.

[47] P. Juin, A. Hunt, T. Littlewood et al., "c-Myc functionally cooperates with Bax to induce apoptosis," *Molecular and Cellular Biology*, vol. 22, no. 17, pp. 6158–6169, 2002.

[48] X. Cao, R. L. Bennett, and W. S. May, "c-Myc and caspase-2 are involved in activating bax during cytotoxic drug-induced apoptosis," *Journal of Biological Chemistry*, vol. 283, no. 21, pp. 14490–14496, 2008.

[49] J. Seoane, H.-V. Le, and J. Massagué, "Myc suppression of the $p21^{Cip1}$ Cdk inhibitor influences the outcome of the p53 response to DNA damage," *Nature*, vol. 419, no. 6908, pp. 729–734, 2002.

[50] J.-C. Jonas, D. R. Laybutt, G. M. Steil et al., "High glucose stimulates early response gene c-Myc expression in rat pancreatic beta cells," *The Journal of Biological Chemistry*, vol. 276, no. 38, pp. 35375–35381, 2001.

[51] D. R. Laybutt, G. C. Weir, H. Kaneto et al., "Overexpression of c-Myc in β-cells of transgenic mice causes proliferation and apoptosis, downregulation of insulin gene expression, and diabetes," *Diabetes*, vol. 51, no. 6, pp. 1793–1804, 2002.

3

Vascular Endothelial Growth Factor Gene Polymorphism (rs2010963) and Its Receptor, Kinase Insert Domain-Containing Receptor Gene Polymorphism (rs2071559), and Markers of Carotid Atherosclerosis in Patients with Type 2 Diabetes Mellitus

Sebastjan Merlo,[1] Jovana Nikolajević Starčević,[2] Sara Mankoč,[2] Marija Šantl Letonja,[3] Andreja Cokan Vujkovac,[4] Marjeta Zorc,[2] and Daniel Petrovič[2]

[1]Institute of Oncology Ljubljana, Zaloška 2, Sl-1000 Ljubljana, Slovenia
[2]Institute of Histology and Embryology, Faculty of Medicine, University in Ljubljana, Vrazov trg 2, Sl-1000 Ljubljana, Slovenia
[3]General Hospital Rakičan, Ulica dr. Vrbnjaka 6, Sl-9000 Murska Sobota, Slovenia
[4]General Hospital Slovenj Gradec, Gosposvetska Cesta 1, Sl-2380 Slovenj Gradec, Slovenia

Correspondence should be addressed to Daniel Petrovič; dp.petrovic@gmail.com

Academic Editor: Ronald G. Tilton

Background. The current study was designed to reveal possible associations between the polymorphisms of the vascular endothelial growth factor (VEGF) gene (rs2010963) and its receptor, kinase insert domain-containing receptor (KDR) gene polymorphism (rs2071559), and markers of carotid atherosclerosis in patients with type 2 diabetes mellitus (T2DM). *Patients and Methods.* 595 T2DM subjects and 200 control subjects were enrolled. The carotid intima-media thickness (CIMT) and plaque characteristics (presence and structure) were assessed ultrasonographically. Biochemical analyses were performed using standard biochemical methods. Genotyping of VEGF/KDR polymorphisms (rs2010963, rs2071559) was performed using KASPar assays. *Results.* Genotype distributions and allele frequencies of the VEGF/KDR polymorphisms (rs2010963, rs2071559) were not statistically significantly different between diabetic patients and controls. In our study, we demonstrated an association between the rs2071559 of KDR and either CIMT or the sum of plaque thickness in subjects with T2DM. We did not, however, demonstrate any association between the tested polymorphism of VEGF (rs2010963) and either CIMT, the sum of plaque thickness, the number of involved segments, hsCRP, the presence of carotid plaques, or the presence of unstable carotid plaques. *Conclusions.* In the present study, we demonstrated minor effect of the rs2071559 of KDR on markers of carotid atherosclerosis in subjects with T2DM.

1. Introduction

Type 2 diabetes mellitus (T2DM) is considered a major epidemic of this century. It is estimated that its prevalence will increase worldwide from 371 million people in 2013 to 552 million people in 2030 [1]. T2DM is associated with accelerated progression of atherosclerosis, the major cause of vascular complications leading to increased morbidity and mortality [2].

Chronic, low-grade inflammation has been demonstrated to be involved in the pathogenesis of atherosclerosis in subjects at high risk to develop cardiovascular disease [3–7]. Among immune cells infiltrating atherosclerotic lesions, polymorphonuclear neutrophil leukocytes with their products were reported to have an important role in the development and progression of atherosclerosis [8–11]. Marino and coworkers have recently reported that both circulating and intraplaque polymorphonuclear neutrophil leukocytes from subjects with carotid atherosclerosis are active producers of different inflammatory mediators including the vascular endothelial growth factor (VEGF) [11].

Several environmental and genetic factors (i.e., hypoxia, hyperglycemia, oxidative stress, ischemia, and gene polymorphisms of VEGF) influence plasma VEGF levels [12–16]. Among several polymorphisms of the VEGF gene, the rs2010963 (−634C/G polymorphism of the VEGF gene) and few others were reported to affect serum VEGF levels [13–15]. Moreover, rs2010963 was demonstrated to be associated with several disorders, such as diabetic retinopathy, diabetic nephropathy, myocardial infarction, and impaired prognosis in patients with chronic heart failure [13–15, 17]. Despite these findings, however, data about VEGF polymorphisms and their possible association with carotid atherosclerosis in patients with diabetes mellitus are limited [18–20]. Additionally, CIMT is highly heritable and associated with stroke and myocardial infarction, making it a promising quantitative intermediate phenotype for genetic studies of vascular disease [21].

The present study was thus designed to investigate the association between polymorphisms of the VEGF gene (rs2010963) and the KDR gene (rs2071559) and markers of carotid atherosclerosis (such as carotid intima-media thickness (CIMT), the number of affected segments of carotid arteries, and the sum of plaques thickness) in patients with T2DM.

2. Material and Methods

The study protocol was approved by the Slovene Medical Ethics Committee in September 2010 (Protocol number 128/09/2010). After an informed consent for the participation in the study was obtained, a detailed interview was made.

This cross-sectional study included 595 subjects with T2DM and 200 subjects without T2DM (control group). They were selected among patients admitted to the diabetes outpatient clinics of the General Hospitals Murska Sobota and Slovenj Gradec, Slovenia. Subjects in the control group were not allowed to have T2DM, and they were the staff of the General Hospital Murska Sobota. Subjects with T2DM and control subjects were excluded if they had homozygous familial hypercholesterolaemia or a previous cardiovascular event such as myocardial infarction or a cerebral stroke.

All ultrasound examinations were performed by two experienced doctors blinded to the participants' diabetes status. The CIMT, defined as the distance from the leading edge of the lumen-intima interface to the leading edge of the media-adventitia interface, was measured, as described previously [22]. Plaques were defined as a focal intima-media thickening and divided into 5 types according to their echogenic/echolucent characteristics, as previously described [22]. The interobserver reliability for carotid plaque characterization was found to be substantial ($\kappa = 0.64$, $p < 0.001$).

The genomic DNA was extracted from 100 μL of whole blood using a FlexiGene DNA isolation kit, in accordance with the recommended protocol (Qiagene GmbH, Hilden, Germany).

For VEGF rs2010963 polymorphism competitive allele specific PCR (KASP) was conducted on an ABI Step-One System (Applied Biosystems, Foster City, CA). The reaction mixture (5 μL) contained 2.5 μL 2x KASPar reaction Mix (v3), 0.07 μL Assay Mix, 1.43 μL of distilled water Dnase/RNase-free (Gibco, Invitrogen Life Technologies), and 10 ng of extracted genomic DNA (1 μL). Thermal cycling employed the following conditions: hot-start enzyme activation (15 min at 94°C), denaturation (20 sec at 94°C) followed by 10 cycles of touchdown over 65–57°C for 60 sec (dropping 0.8°C per cycle), and final 26 cycles (20 sec at 94°C and 60 sec at annealing temperature 57°C). For rs2071559 (KDR) everything was the same with the exception of thermal conditions. Hot-start enzyme activation (15 min at 94°C) and denaturation (20 sec at 94°C) were followed by 15 cycles of touchdown over 55–65°C for 60 sec (dropping 0.8°C per cycle) and final 26 cycles (20 sec at 93°C and 60 sec at annealing temperature 58°C).

In addition, the fasting serum VEGF levels were analyzed in 70 subjects with T2DM and in 33 subjects with T2DM. For the determination of the fasting serum VEGF concentration (isoform VEGF 165), a solid phase sandwich ELISA using two kinds of high specific antibodies (hVEGF Assay Kit, IBL Co., Ltd. Aramachi, Takasaki-shi, Gunma, Japan) was used. The respective CV (%) were between 3 and 5.5 for interassay measurements and between 2.6 and 5.3 for intra-assay measurements.

Continuous variables are expressed as means ± standard deviations. Continuous clinical data were compared using unpaired Student's t-test or analysis of variance (ANOVA). The Pearson χ^2 test was used to compare discrete variables. A two-tailed p value of less than 0.05 was considered statistically significant. A statistical analysis was performed using the SPSS program for Windows version 21 (SPSS Inc., Chicago, Ilinois, USA).

3. Results

Patients with T2DM were older, had a greater waist circumference, and had higher fasting glucose and HbA1c levels compared to controls, whereas there were no differences in BMI and systolic and diastolic blood pressure between patients with T2DM and control subjects (Table 1). Patients with T2DM had lower total, HDL, and LDL cholesterol levels and a higher triglyceride level compared to controls (Table 1). Plasma levels of inflammatory markers (i.e., hs-CRP and fibrinogen) were higher in patients with T2DM compared to controls (Table 1). Additionally, there was higher percentage of men, statin therapy, and antihypertensive therapy and lower percentage of smokers in T2DM group compared to control group (Table 1).

The genotype distributions in both patients with T2DM and controls were in Hardy-Weinberg equilibrium for both VEGF gene polymorphisms [rs2010963: T2DM (genotype frequencies: CC genotype 8.7%, CG genotype 47.1%, and GG genotype 44.2%; $\chi^2 = 3.48$; $p = 0.06$) and controls (genotype frequencies: CC genotype 9%, CG genotype 48%, and GG genotype 43%; $\chi^2 = 1.46$; $p = 0.22$)]. The genotype distributions in both patients with T2DM and controls

TABLE 1: Baseline characteristics of subjects with T2DM and subjects without T2DM (control group).

	Subjects with T2DM $n = 595$	Control group $n = 200$	p
Age (years)	62.39 ± 9.61	60.07 ± 9.18	0.008
Male sex (%)	338 (56.8)	92 (46.0)	0.008
Diabetes duration (years)	11.25 ± 7.88	—	—
Cigarette smoking (%)	53 (8.91)	34 (17.0)	0.002
Waist circumference (cm)	108.65 ± 12.88	93.31 ± 13.18	<0.001
BMI (kg/m^2)	31.00 ± 4.74	27.90 ± 4.42	0.16
SBP (mm Hg)	147.1 ± 19.80	143.3 ± 16.6	0.86
DBP (mm Hg)	85.78 ± 11.60	84.7 ± 11.6	0.19
Fasting glucose (mmol/L)	8.04 ± 2.57	5.27 ± 0.87	<0.001
HbA1c (%)	7.89 ± 3.56	4.79 ± 0.29	<0.001
Total cholesterol (mmol/L)	4.70 ± 1.18	5.36 ± 1.08	<0.001
HDL cholesterol (mmol/L)	1.20 ± 0.35	1.43 ± 0.37	<0.001
LDL cholesterol (mmol/L)	2.63 ± 0.94	3.24 ± 0.98	<0.001
Triglycerides (mmol/L)	1.9 (1.2–2.7)	1.3 (0.9–1.9)	<0.001
hs-CRP (mg/L)	3.5 ± 1.18	2.2 ± 1.18	<0.001
CIMT (μm)	958 ± 194	890 ± 212	0.007
Statin therapy (%)	375 (63.0)	62 (31.0)	<0.001
Antihypertensive agents (%)	499 (83.9)	58 (29%)	<0.001

Continuous variables were expressed as means ± standard deviations when normally distributed and as median (interquartile range) when asymmetrically distributed. Categorical variables were expressed as frequency (percentage). BMI: body mass index; SBP: systolic blood pressure; DBP: diastolic blood pressure; HbA1c: glycated haemoglobin; hs-CRP: high sensitivity C-reactive protein.

were in Hardy-Weinberg equilibrium for the KDR gene polymorphism [rs2071559: T2DM (genotype frequencies: CC genotype 22.0%, CT genotype 51.9%, and TT genotype 26.1%; $\chi^2 = 0.97$; $p = 0.33$) and controls (genotype frequencies: CC genotype 30.0%, CT genotype 48.0%, and TT genotype 22.0%; $\chi^2 = 0.63$; $p = 0.23$)]. No statistically significant differences in the VEGF rs2010963 and KDR rs2071559 genotype distribution frequencies were observed between T2DM patients and controls.

The observed minor allele frequency (MAF) distributions were mostly in agreement with the 1000 Genomes Project data in the European population. The C allele frequency of the VEGF rs2010963 showed no significant difference ($p = 0.79$) between patients with T2DM and controls (32.3% versus 33%). However, the C allele frequency of the KDR rs2071559 polymorphism was significantly lower ($p = 0.04$) in T2DM subjects as compared to the controls (49% versus 54%).

Higher VEGF serum levels were demonstrated in subjects with T2DM with the CC genotype (rs2010963) compared to those with other (CG + GG) genotypes (Table 2). Moreover, higher VEGF serum levels were found in subjects with the CC genotype (rs2071559) compared to those with other (CT + TT) genotypes (Table 2).

The comparison of atherosclerosis parameters was performed with regard to different genotypes of the VEGF polymorphism (rs2010963) upon enrolment. In our study, we did not demonstrate any association between the rs2010963 and either CIMT, the sum of plaque thickness, the number of involved segments, hsCRP or the presence of carotid plaques, or the presence of unstable carotid plaques (Tables 3 and 4). We did, however, demonstrate an association between the rs2071559 and either CIMT or the sum of plaque thickness in subjects with T2DM (Table 3).

4. Discussion

In our study, we demonstrated an association between the rs2071559 of KDR and CIMT in subjects with T2DM, whereas we did not demonstrate an association between tested polymorphism of VEGF (rs2010963) and CIMT. Variations in the VEGF gene were reported to be weakly associated with CIMT [19]. None of the single genotyped polymorphisms (−2578A>C rs699947, −634C>G rs2010963, and +936C>T rs3025039) were significantly associated with overall IMT in the study reported by Kangas-Kontio and coworkers [19]. The haplotype CCC, however, was associated with higher overall CIMT in women and the haplotype CCT with higher CIMT in the internal carotid artery in men [19].

Additionally, we also demonstrated an association between the rs2071559 of KDR and the sum of plaque thickness in subjects with T2DM, whereas no association between tested polymorphism of VEGF (rs2010963) and markers of carotid atherosclerosis was demonstrated. The rs2010963 polymorphism of the VEGF gene was not demonstrated to exert a significant influence on the risk of subclinical atherosclerosis manifested by the presence of endothelial dysfunction by brachial artery reactivity and increased CIMT in a series of patients with rheumatoid arthritis [23]. Contrary, the importance of VEGF and its receptor (VEGFR1) was reported by Russell and coworkers [24]. They analyzed 34 intact carotid endarterectomy specimens and compared histologically stable and unstable plaques. In unstable plaques (cap rupture/thinning) increased VEGF and receptor (VEGFR1) staining as well as increased microvessel density was demonstrated in comparison with stable carotid plaques [24]. Additionally, Marino and coworkers have recently reported that both circulating and intraplaque polymorphonuclear neutrophils (PMN) from subjects with carotid atherosclerosis are active producers of VEGF, IL-8, and elastase [11]. Moreover, an evidence is provided that these PMN have an increased ability to produce VEGF (at mRNA levels) in comparison to cells from healthy subjects. Additionally, increased VEGF mRNA occurs in both intraplaque and circulating PMN, at rest as well as after stimulation, suggesting that such functional

TABLE 2: VEGF serum levels in subjects with and without T2DM with regard to the rs2010963 and rs2071559 genotypes.

rs2010963	Mean (95% CI)		p	Linear trend analysis	
	CC (52)	CG + GG (543)		F	p
VEGF (ng/L)	63.5 ± 29.2	46.1 ± 22.3	<0.01	3.22	0.03
rs2071559	Mean (95% CI)		p	Linear trend analysis	
	CC (131)	CT + TT (464)		F	p
VEGF (ng/L)	69.4 ± 25.1	40.9 ± 28.3	<0.01	3.70	0.02

TABLE 3: Comparison of markers of carotid atherosclerosis (CIMT, sum of plaque thickness, and number of involved segments) in subjects with T2DM at the beginning of the study with regard to the rs2010963 and rs2071559 genotypes.

rs2010963	Mean (95% CI)			p	Linear trend analysis	
	CC (52)	CG (280)	GG (263)		F	p
CIMT (μm)	1045 ± 192 (969–1121)	996 ± 210 (964–1026)	1026 ± 210 (995–1058)	0.27	2.29	0.13
Sum of plaque thickness (mm)	7.58 ± 4.52 (5.67–9.49)	7.79 ± 4.28 (7.09–8.48)	8.11 ± 4.73 (7.35–8.88)	0.76	0.009	0.93
Number of involved segments	2.67 ± 1.51 (2.07–3.26)	2.48 ± 1.70 (2.24–2.73)	2.54 ± 1.60 (2.31–2.77)	0.84	0.34	0.56
rs2071559	Mean (95% CI)			p	Linear trend analysis	
	CC (131)	TC (309)	TT (155)		F	p
CIMT (μm)	1053 ± 186 (1012–1092)	1029 ± 200 (987–1070)	988 ± 219 (958–1019)	0.04	5.64	0.04
Sum of plaque thickness (mm)	8.81 ± 4.30 (7.83–9.78)	8.27 ± 4.50 (7.26–9.29)	7.31 ± 4.48 (6.61–8.00)	0.03	5.91	0.02
Number of involved segments	2.87 ± 1.41 (0.94–1.65)	2.38 ± 1.60 (0.95–1.73)	2.24 ± 1.70 (0.98–1.46)	0.64	0.22	0.83

TABLE 4: Comparison of markers of carotid atherosclerosis (presence of carotid plaques, presence of unstable plaques) in subjects with T2DM at the beginning of the study with regard to the rs2010963 and rs2071559 genotypes.

	rs2010963				rs2071559			
	CC (52)	CG (280)	GG (263)	p	CC (131)	TC (309)	TT (155)	p
Presence of carotid plaques n (%)	46 (88.5)	229 (81.8)	223 (84.7)		117 (89.3)	250 (80.9)	133 (85.8)	
OR (95% CI)	*	0.68 (0.46–2.57)	0.72 (0.41–1.26)	0.45	*	0.57 (0.53–2.06)	0.68 (0.34–1.34)	0.15
$p^{\dagger}$	—	0.70	0.24		—	0.59	0.26	
Presence of unstable carotid plaques n (%)	27 (51.9)	143 (51.1)	121 (46.0)		69 (52.7)	142 (46.0)	77 (49.7)	
OR (95% CI)	*	1.09 (0.22–3.66)	0.97 (0.38–2.50)	0.45	*	0.55 (0.14–2.18)	0.67 (0.20–2.26)	0.42
$p^{\dagger}$	—	0.56	0.59		—	0.39	0.51	

*Reference genotype is CC.

$^{\dagger}p$ value for logistic regression analysis.

changes are systemic and not limited to cells infiltrating the vascular wall [11]. In contrast to these findings, we did not demonstrate an effect of VEGF/KDR polymorphisms on the presence of either plaques or unstable plaques, since no difference in genotype distribution was present.

In our study, the effect of either rs2071559 of KDR or rs2010963 on VEGF serum levels was demonstrated. These findings are in accordance with our previous studies in which

subjects with recent MI history (up to 9 months after MI) were enrolled [13, 16, 25]. Moreover, increased plasma VEGF levels demonstrated in the stable phase after MI correlated with inflammation cytokines (IL-8 and IL-6), but not with atherosclerotic burden [25].

In contrast to the minor effect of the rs2071559 of KDR and the absence of the rs2010963 of the VEGF, an association of either rs2071559 or rs2010963 with MI has recently been reported in Caucasians with T2DM [13, 16, 24]. Our present findings and previous reports are additional evidence that markers of carotid atherosclerosis and atherothrombotic events (i.e., MI) are most probably not regulated via similar genetical/biological mechanisms.

To conclude, in our study we demonstrated a minor effect of the rs2071559 of KDR on markers of carotid atherosclerosis (CIMT, sum of plaque thickness) in subjects with T2DM, whereas we failed to demonstrate an effect of tested polymorphism of the VEGF gene (rs2010963) on markers of carotid atherosclerosis.

Conflict of Interests

The authors declare that there is no conflict of interests regarding the publication of this paper.

Acknowledgment

The authors thank Mrs. Brina Beškovnik, BA, for revising the English.

References

[1] M. Laakso and J. Kuusisto, "Insulin resistance and hyperglycaemia in cardiovascular disease development," *Nature Reviews Endocrinology*, vol. 10, no. 5, pp. 293–302, 2014.

[2] P. R. Moreno and V. Fuster, "New aspects in the pathogenesis of diabetic atherothrombosis," *Journal of the American College of Cardiology*, vol. 44, no. 12, pp. 2293–2300, 2004.

[3] L. Guasti, F. Marino, M. Cosentino et al., "Simvastatin treatment modifies polymorphonuclear leukocyte function in high-risk individuals: a longitudinal study," *Journal of Hypertension*, vol. 24, no. 12, pp. 2423–2430, 2006.

[4] F. Marino, L. Guasti, M. Cosentino et al., "Angiotensin II type 1 receptor expression in polymorphonuclear leukocytes from high-risk subjects: changes after treatment with simvastatin," *Journal of Cardiovascular Pharmacology*, vol. 49, no. 5, pp. 299–305, 2007.

[5] L. Guasti, F. Marino, M. Cosentino et al., "Prolonged statin-associated reduction in neutrophil reactive oxygen species and angiotensin II type 1 receptor expression: 1-year follow-up," *European Heart Journal*, vol. 29, no. 9, pp. 1118–1126, 2008.

[6] N. Khuseyinova and W. Koenig, "Biomarkers of outcome from cardiovascular disease," *Current Opinion in Critical Care*, vol. 12, no. 5, pp. 412–419, 2006.

[7] P. N. Hopkins, "Molecular biology of atherosclerosis," *Physiological Reviews*, vol. 93, no. 3, pp. 1317–1542, 2013.

[8] A. Mócsai, "Diverse novel functions of neutrophils in immunity, inflammation, and beyond," *The Journal of Experimental Medicine*, vol. 210, no. 7, pp. 1283–1299, 2013.

[9] R. Baetta and A. Corsini, "Role of polymorphonuclear neutrophils in atherosclerosis: current state and future perspectives," *Atherosclerosis*, vol. 210, no. 1, pp. 1–13, 2010.

[10] M. Van Leeuwen, M. J. J. Gijbels, A. Duijvestijn et al., "Accumulation of myeloperoxidase-positive neutrophils in atherosclerotic lesions in LDLR$^{-/-}$ mice," *Arteriosclerosis, Thrombosis, and Vascular Biology*, vol. 28, no. 1, pp. 84–89, 2008.

[11] F. Marino, M. Tozzi, L. Schembri et al., "Production of IL-8, VEGF and elastase by circulating and intraplaque neutrophils in patients with carotid atherosclerosis," *PLoS ONE*, vol. 10, no. 4, Article ID e0124565, 2015.

[12] T. Awata, K. Inoue, S. Kurihara et al., "A common polymorphism in the 5′-untranslated region of the VEGF gene is associated with diabetic retinopathy in type 2 diabetes," *Diabetes*, vol. 51, no. 5, pp. 1635–1639, 2002.

[13] D. Petrovič, R. Verhovec, M. Globočnik Petrovič, J. Osredkar, and B. Peterlin, "Association of vascular endothelial growth factor gene polymorphism with myocardial infarction in patients with type 2 diabetes," *Cardiology*, vol. 107, no. 4, pp. 291–295, 2007.

[14] M. G. Petrovič, P. Korošec, M. Košnik et al., "Local and genetic determinants of vascular endothelial growth factor expression in advanced proliferative diabetic retinopathy," *Molecular Vision*, vol. 14, pp. 1382–1387, 2008.

[15] P. van der Meer, R. A. de Boer, H. L. White et al., "The VEGF +405 CC promoter polymorphism is associated with an impaired prognosis in patients with chronic heart failure: a MERIT-HF substudy," *Journal of Cardiac Failure*, vol. 11, no. 4, pp. 279–284, 2005.

[16] S. Kariž and D. Petrovič, "Minor association of kinase insert domain-containing receptor gene polymorphism (rs2071559) with myocardial infarction in Caucasians with type 2 diabetes mellitus: case-control cross-sectional study," *Clinical Biochemistry*, vol. 47, no. 16-17, pp. 192–196, 2014.

[17] P. Douvaras, D. G. Antonatos, K. Kekou et al., "Association of VEGF gene polymorphisms with the development of heart failure in patients after myocardial infarction," *Cardiology*, vol. 114, no. 1, pp. 11–18, 2009.

[18] E. Alioglu, U. Turk, S. Cam, A. Abbasaliyev, I. Tengiz, and E. Ercan, "Polymorphisms of the methylenetetrahydrofolate reductase, vascular endothelial growth factor, endothelial nitric oxide synthase, monocyte chemoattractant protein-1 and apolipoprotein E genes are not associated with carotid intima-media thickness," *Canadian Journal of Cardiology*, vol. 25, no. 1, pp. e1–e5, 2009.

[19] T. Kangas-Kontio, J. M. Tapanainen, H. Huikuri et al., "Variation in the vascular endothelial growth factor gene, carotid intima-media thickness and the risk of acute myocardial infarction," *Scandinavian Journal of Clinical and Laboratory Investigation*, vol. 69, no. 3, pp. 335–343, 2009.

[20] C. Giannarelli, M. Alique, D. T. Rodriguez et al., "Alternatively spliced tissue factor promotes plaque angiogenesis through the activation of HIF-1α and VEGF signaling," *Circulation*, vol. 130, pp. 1274–1286, 2014.

[21] L. Paternoster, N. A. Martinez-Gonzalez, R. Charleton, M. Chung, S. Lewis, and C. L. M. Sudlow, "Genetic effects on carotid intima-media thickness: systematic assessment and meta-analyses of candidate gene polymorphisms studied in more than 5000 subjects," *Circulation: Cardiovascular Genetics*, vol. 3, no. 1, pp. 15–21, 2010.

[22] J. Nikolajevic Starcevic, M. Santl Letonja, Z. J. Praznikar, J. Makuc, A. C. Vujkovac, and D. Petrovic, "Polymorphisms XbaI (rs693) and EcoRI (rs1042031) of the ApoB gene are associated with carotid plaques but not with carotid intima-media thickness in patients with diabetes mellitus type 2," *Vasa*, vol. 43, no. 3, pp. 171–180, 2014.

[23] L. Rodríguez-Rodríguez, M. García-Bermúdez, C. González-Juanatey et al., "Vascular endothelial growth factor A and cardiovascular disease in rheumatoid arthritis patients," *Tissue Antigens*, vol. 77, no. 4, pp. 291–297, 2011.

[24] D. A. Russell, C. R. Abbott, and M. J. Gough, "Vascular endothelial growth factor is associated with histological instability of carotid plaques," *British Journal of Surgery*, vol. 95, no. 5, pp. 576–581, 2008.

[25] B. Eržen, M. Šilar, and M. Šabovič, "Stable phase post-MI patients have elevated VEGF levels correlated with inflammation markers, but not with atherosclerotic burden," *BMC Cardiovascular Disorders*, vol. 14, no. 1, pp. 166–170, 2014.

4

An Innovative Australian Outreach Model of Diabetic Retinopathy Screening in Remote Communities

Nicola M. Glasson,[1] Lisa J. Crossland,[2] and Sarah L. Larkins[1]

[1]College of Medicine and Dentistry, James Cook University, 1 James Cook Drive, Townsville City, QLD 4811, Australia
[2]Discipline of General Practice, University of Queensland, Level 8 Health Sciences Building, Royal Brisbane Hospital, Herston, QLD 4029, Australia

Correspondence should be addressed to Nicola M. Glasson; nicola.glasson@my.jcu.edu.au

Academic Editor: Ahmed Ibrahim

Background. Up to 98% of visual loss secondary to diabetic retinopathy (DR) can be prevented with early detection and treatment. Despite this, less than 50% of Australian and American diabetics receive appropriate screening. Diabetic patients living in rural and remote communities are further disadvantaged by limited access to ophthalmology services. *Research Design and Methods.* DR screening using a nonmydriatic fundal camera was performed as part of a multidisciplinary diabetes service already visiting remote communities. Images were onforwarded to a distant general practitioner who identified and graded retinopathy, with screen-positive patients referred to ophthalmology. This retrospective, descriptive study aims to compare the proportion of remote diabetic patients receiving appropriate DR screening prior to and following implementation of the service. *Results.* Of the 41 patients in 11 communities who underwent DR screening, 16.3% had received appropriate DR screening prior to the implementation of the service. In addition, 36.2% of patients had never been screened. Following the introduction of the service, 66.3% of patients underwent appropriate DR screening ($p = 0.00025$). *Conclusion.* This innovative model has greatly improved accessibility to DR screening in remote communities, thereby reducing preventable blindness. It provides a holistic, locally appropriate diabetes service and utilises existing infrastructure and health workforce more efficiently.

1. Introduction

In 2013, there were 382 million people with diabetes worldwide and it is predicted that this will increase to 592 million people by 2035 [1]. Diabetic retinopathy (DR) is the most serious ocular complication of diabetes and is the leading cause of preventable blindness in working age populations [2]. DR accounted for 5% of global blindness in 2002, approximately five million people worldwide [3]. It is estimated that up to 50% of people with proliferative DR who do not receive timely treatment will become legally blind within five years [4]. Although up to 98% of visual loss secondary to DR can be prevented with early detection and treatment, once it has progressed, vision loss is often permanent [5]. Despite this, comprehensive DR screening rates are poorly achieved globally, with less than 50% of Australian and American diabetic patients receiving appropriate screening [6, 7]. The number of people with diabetes living in rural areas is increasing worldwide and is expected to reach 145 million people by 2035 [1]. Patients living in rural and remote areas have poorer access to specialist ophthalmology services [8, 9]. Indigenous people worldwide are particularly vulnerable to eye disease, with blindness six times higher in Indigenous Australians than for non-Indigenous Australians [1, 10]. Impaired vision affects national economies through loss of productivity and earning capacity as well as having significant negative social impacts on communities worldwide, with vision impaired individuals relying heavily on social support [1].

A review of international rural remote DR screening models by the authors found that the vast majority of published models use ophthalmologists as the primary image graders. Given the growing number of diabetic patients worldwide, poor achievement of screening recommendations, and limited access to ophthalmology services in rural

TABLE 1: The documented diabetic population in remote communities visited by the screening program.

Remote community	2012		2013		2014	
	Documented diabetic population (n)	Patients screened (n)	Documented diabetic population (n)	Patients screened (n)	Documented diabetic population (n)	Patients screened (n)
1	37	11	46	12	No screening*	
2	10(2013)	4	No screening		No screening*	
3	3(2013)	3	3	4	No screening*	
4	8	5	8(2012)	7	8(2012)	4
5	10	2	10(2012)	1	10	6
6	15	5	16	8	14	7
7	39	13	49	18	35	17
8	32	9	22	17	27	10
9	7(2013)	1	7	1	13	8
10	26	10	26	10	18	9
11	15	5	14	5	15	6
Total	**202**	**68**	**201**	**83**	**140**	**67**
Diabetic population screened (%)		**33.7%**		**41.3%**		**47.9%**

Note: where no data was available on the diabetic population in a particular community from a specific year, the diabetic population is used from a previous year and indicated with the year in subscript.

Note: the diabetic population was documented from community health records. Lists were obtained from a chronic disease database and updated by PHCs and the regional diabetes educator. Patients were excluded if they were deceased or had moved from the district.

*These communities were screened early in 2015 due to changeover of the eye screening coordinator.

and remote communities, there is a recognised need for innovative approaches to the delivery of DR screening. This has led to trials utilising nonophthalmologist graders, with numerous studies demonstrating the efficacy of nonophthalmologist graders in detecting DR [4, 11–15]. This paper presents the results of the evaluation of an innovative remote outreach DR screening (RODRS) service delivered in remote communities in a state of Australia. The service aims to improve rates of DR screening for patients in remote settings with previously limited access to screening.

2. The Remote Outreach DR Screening (RODRS) Service

2.1. Existing Service. In 2012, the RODRS service was implemented in a Hospital District and Health Service in a state of Australia. Prior to 2012, visiting ophthalmologists and optometrists performed the majority of DR screening in the district. The implementation of the service was prompted by concerns that diabetic patients living in the region were not undergoing DR screening, and to utilise visiting ophthalmology services more efficiently. Optometrists and ophthalmologists service four rural and three remote communities in the region, with ophthalmologists visiting the district triannually (Figure 1). The RODRS program visits 11 remote communities in the district annually. These remote communities have nurse-led clinic facilities with visiting general practice services and three communities have visiting optometry and ophthalmology services. The documented diabetic population in each community ranges from 3 to 49 people and is listed in Table 1.

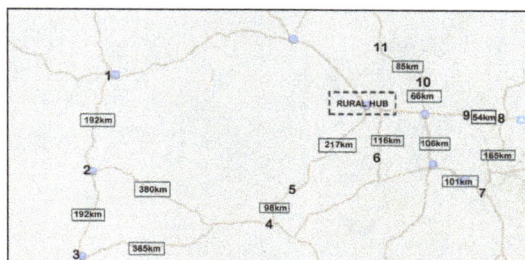

○ Locations of visiting optometry and ophthalmology services

FIGURE 1: Remote communities visited by the RODRS program (listed 1 to 11).

2.2. Service Promotion and Patient Identification. Figure 2 presents a graphical representation of the outreach screening process. Diabetic patients are identified from a State Health chronic disease database. Patient lists are then sent to each primary health care centre (PHC) and the regional diabetes educator, who adjusts lists adding patients and removing those no longer living in the district. Diabetic patients are contacted by community health from the rural hub or by their local PHC to invite them for annual screening. Posters are displayed in community public areas and local health workers raise awareness of the screening visit. On the day of screening, local health workers visit residents in their homes to remind them of the visiting service and provide transport to clinics if required.

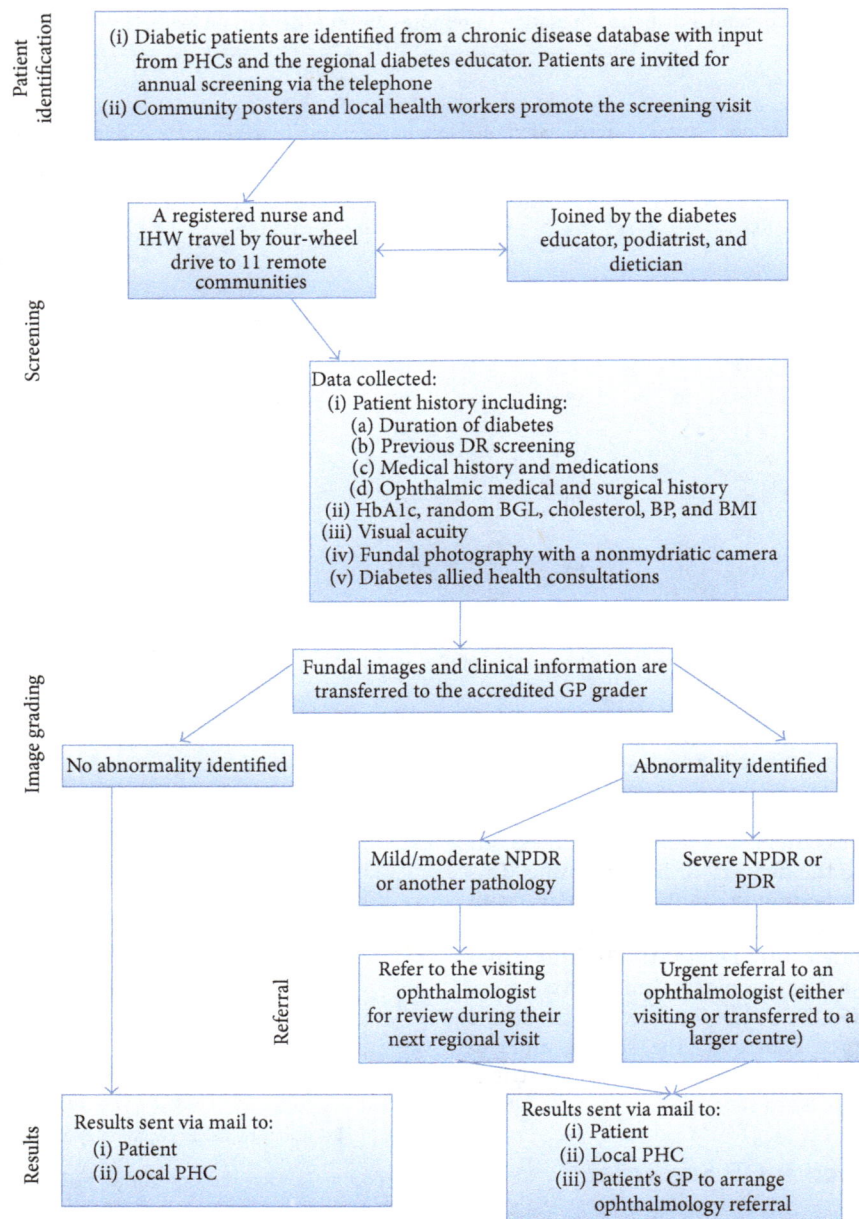

FIGURE 2: The remote outreach DR screening pathway.

2.3. Screening Visit. A registered nurse and Indigenous health worker (Indigenous refers to Aboriginal peoples and/or Torres Strait Islanders) (IHW) based in the rural hub travel via four-wheel drive to 11 remote communities with a fundal camera. This forms part of an existing chronic disease network in the district. Remote communities are located between 117 km and 693 km (approximately 1.5 to 7 hours' drive) from the rural hub, which itself is located 687 km from the closest major regional hospital and 1176 km from the state capital [16]. DR screening is performed in PHCs (except for one community where it is hospital-based). A brief patient history, random blood glucose level (BGL),

HbA1c, cholesterol level, blood pressure (BP), and body mass index (BMI) are collected. A visual acuity using a Snellen chart is then performed, with pinhole if required. Patients then undergo fundal photography by a registered nurse using an automated nonmydriatic camera (centervue DRS). One 45° fundal photograph centred on the macula and with view of the optic nerve is captured of each eye. If an adequate image cannot be acquired, patients undergo dilation with tropicamide (Mydriacyl) 0.5% unless contraindicated. A visiting diabetes educator, podiatrist, and dietician also attend most remote clinics to provide a comprehensive diabetes service.

2.4. Image Grading and Feedback of Results. Clinical information and fundal images are transferred to an urban, regional, or locally based rural general practitioner (GP) accredited to perform DR image grading (four GPs involved). Participating GPs completed a four-hour online DR upskilling program through The University of Queensland Masters of Medicine (General Practice) program followed by an accreditation assessment through The Royal Australian and New Zealand College of Ophthalmologists (RANZCO) Queensland Faculty [17, 18]. GPs complete a 50-patient (100 eyes) exam and must achieve at least 75% concordance with an ophthalmologist reviewer for accreditation [17, 18]. Accreditation was provided through Flinders University for one participating GP. For 2012-13 GP image grading was provided by a distant accredited GP; however, in 2014 it was performed by a locally based rural accredited GP, in collaboration with the visiting ophthalmologist.

The GP grader assesses the adequacy of the image, evaluates the image for the presence of DR or other pathology, grades DR (if present) according to the Wisconsin system, and nominates an appropriate management plan (Figure 2) [19]. An urban-based "buddy" ophthalmologist provides support to the GP grader and visits the region triannually. If no pathology is detected by the GP grader, screening results are sent to the PHC for filing, with a copy sent to the patient. If pathology is identified, results are sent to the PHC, the patient, and the patient's nominated GP to arrange ophthalmology referral. Those patients with mild or moderate nonproliferative DR (NPDR) are referred to the visiting ophthalmologist, to be seen during their triannual visit in the community closest to them (Figure 2). The "buddy" ophthalmologist is notified of any patients with severe NPDR or proliferative DR (PDR), and depending on the timing of their next visit to the region, the patient will either be reviewed by the regional ophthalmology team or urgently transferred to a larger centre with permanent ophthalmology services. Patients for whom an adequate image cannot be obtained are generally referred to the visiting ophthalmologist, as this may indicate another pathology such as cataract.

3. Method

3.1. Study Design. This retrospective, descriptive screening record audit had three aims:

(i) to identify the proportion of patients with documented diabetes mellitus (type 1/type 2) residing in 11 remote communities who underwent DR screening with the RODRS service,

(ii) to compare the proportion of those patients screened by the program who underwent appropriate DR screening prior to and following the implementation of the RODRS service,

(iii) to identify the proportion of screened patients with mild, moderate, or severe NPDR and PDR.

A further paper explores the acceptability of the program to patients, health professionals, and other key stakeholders.

3.2. Setting and Participants. Data was collected at PHCs during DR screening visits to 11 remote communities in a state of Australia. Eligible participants were patients with type 1 or type 2 diabetes mellitus aged 18 years or older, attending DR screening in remote communities between April 2012 and December 2014. Patients were excluded from participation if they had no perception of light in either eye, were terminally ill or deemed too unwell to participate, or had a physical or mental disability that prevented either screening or treatment. All eligible patients attending DR screening clinics were invited to take part in the study and all patients consented to participate ($n = 142$). However, one patient was screened with gestational diabetes mellitus and therefore was excluded from analysis. The Australian National Health and Medical Research Council (NHMRC) developed national guidelines for the recommended frequency of DR screening [19]. The guidelines recommend that all patients with diabetes (type 1 and type 2) undergo at least biennial screening. However, patients at high risk of DR, including Indigenous Australians and patients living in rural and remote communities, should be considered for annual examinations. In this paper "appropriate" refers to screening frequency in line with the NHMRC guidelines.

3.3. Intervention. The RODRS service was implemented in a Hospital District and Health Service in 2012.

3.4. Outcomes. A retrospective analysis of State Health screening data was conducted. The main outcome measures included (i) the proportion of the documented diabetic population living in remote communities who underwent DR screening with the program, (ii) the proportion of those patients screened by the program who underwent appropriate screening (in line with the NHMRC guidelines [19]) prior to and following the intervention, (iii) the quality of images captured by the screening team, (iv) the proportion of screening episodes with DR detected and the type of DR identified, and (v) the proportion of screening episodes which required ophthalmology referral. Clinical data on DR screening prior to the intervention was based on self-report. All other information was collected and accessed from State Health records.

3.5. Analysis. All screening data were entered initially into an Excel database, cleaned, and then imported into and analysed using SPSS (version 22). Histograms were viewed to assess the normality of continuous variables. Summary statistics are presented as frequency (percentage) for categorical variables and mean (standard deviation) for continuous variables that were normally distributed; otherwise median and interquartile ranges were reported. Where appropriate Chi-square tests (gender, ethnicity, and DR detection in high risk patients), Mann-Whitney U (age, HbA1c), and an independent sample t-test (systolic and diastolic BP) were used to assess bivariate associations. A McNemar's test was performed to determine a p value for proportions screened prior to and following implementation of the model. A p value of ≤ 0.05 was considered to be statistically significant.

3.6. Ethics Approval and Consent. In accordance with advice from the Human Research Ethics Committee (HREC), the

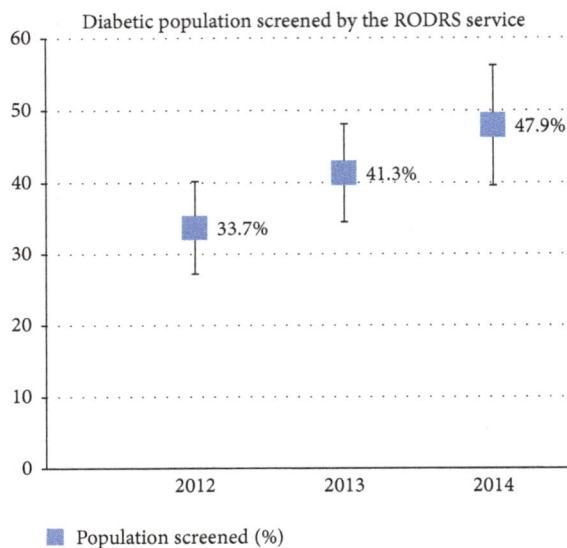

FIGURE 3: The proportion of the total documented diabetic population (residing in 11 remote communities) screened each year with 95% confidence intervals shown.

above project was compliant with the NHMRC guidance "ethical considerations in quality assurance and evaluation activities" and therefore was not recommended for HREC review (HREC/15/QRBW/122). Informed consent was obtained from all participants.

4. Results

4.1. Diabetic Population Screened. A total of 218 screening episodes were recorded across 11 remote communities between April 2012 and December 2014. The program screened 141 patients with 47 patients (33.3%) screened twice and 15 patients (10.6%) screened three times. Of the 11 remote communities visited by the screening team, eight communities were visited three times, two communities were visited twice, and one community was visited once. The proportion of the total documented diabetic population (residing in 11 remote communities) screened by the program significantly increased throughout the operation of the service from 33.7% in 2012 to 47.9% in 2014 (Table 1; Figure 3). The odds ratio for being screened in 2014 compared with 2012 was 2 (95% CI 1.49–2.68; $p = 0.00003$).

4.2. Participant Demographics. A total of 141 patients were identified as eligible for participation in this study. Of these 58.2% of diabetic patients were male (Table 2). Indigenous patients comprised 23.5% of patients screened, with most Indigenous patients identifying as Australian Aboriginal. Patients ranged from 18 to 90 years of age, with a median age of 63 years. The median duration of diabetes was 6 years with 32.1% of patients considered at high risk of DR (duration of diabetes more than 10 years) [2, 20]. This is similar to the national diabetes profile with diabetes slightly more common in males than females (5.1% of males and 4.2% of females), although the rate of diabetes is highest amongst those aged

TABLE 2: Participant demographics.

	$n = 141$
Gender	
Male	82 patients (58.2%)
Female	59 patients (41.8%)
Indigenous status	
Non-Indigenous	101 patients (76.5%)
Indigenous	
Australian Aboriginal	26 patients (19.7%)
Aboriginal & Torres Strait Islander	4 patients (3.0%)
South Sea Islander	1 patient (0.8%)
Total	**31 patients (23.5%)**
Age	
Median	63 years
Interquartile range	19
Duration of diabetes	
Median	6 years
Interquartile range	9
Duration >10 years	45 patients (32.1%)

Note: one missing record for duration of diabetes, nine missing records for Indigenous status.

TABLE 3: Clinical characteristics based on total screening episodes.

	$n = 218$
HbA1c	
Median	7.1%
Interquartile range	2
HbA1c ≥7%	71 patients (51.8%)
HbA1c ≥8% (high risk of DR)	39 patients (28.5%)
Hypertension	
Systolic BP	
Mean ± SD	140.5 mmHg (±20.3)
≥130 mmHg	97 patients (69.8%)
≥150 mmHg (high risk of DR)	36 patients (25.9%)
Diastolic BP	
Mean ± SD	82.9 mmHg (±12.0)
≥85 mmHg	64 patients (46.0%)
≥90 mmHg (high risk of DR)	45 patients (32.4%)

Note: four patients were missing one to two data variables.

75 to 84 years, slightly older than the population screened in this study [21].

4.3. Clinical Characteristics. The median HbA1c of diabetic patients screened by the program was 7.1%. Overall, 51.8% of patients had an HbA1c ≥ 7% indicating poor glycaemic control and 28.5% of patients had an HbA1c ≥ 8% (associated with increased risk of DR) (Table 3) [2, 20, 22]. Systolic BP ranged from 100 mmHg to 212 mmHg with a mean systolic BP of 140.5 mmHg. Diastolic BP ranged from 54 mmHg to 120 mmHg, with an average diastolic BP of 82.9 mmHg. Most patients had suboptimal BP control with 69.8% of patients with a systolic BP reading ≥ 130 mmHg and 46% of patients

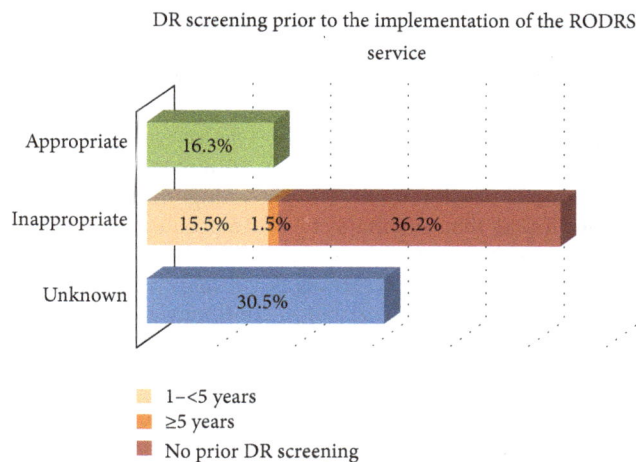

FIGURE 4: Patient reported DR screening prior to the implementation of the model ($n = 141$). Note: unknown included those patients who were not aware if they had undergone screening previously and those who had undergone screening but were unsure of the date.

with a diastolic BP $\geq$ 85 mmHg [22]. In addition, many patients were considered at high risk of DR with a systolic BP $\geq$ 150 mmHg (25.9%) or a diastolic BP $\geq$ 90 mmHg (32.4%) [2, 20].

4.4. DR Screening Rates. Of the 141 patients screened by the program, 16.3% had received appropriate DR screening prior to the implementation of the service (screening in line with recommendations made in the NHMRC guidelines), but 36.2% of patients had never been screened (Figure 4) [19]. Following the introduction of the program, 66.3% of eligible patients received appropriate screening (odds ratio 1.93; 95% CI of 1.42–2.64; $p = 0.00025$). (Note: A total of 92 patients were included in the analysis of appropriate screening following the implementation of the model (49 patients excluded). A total of 36 patients were excluded as rescreening could not be evaluated for the following reasons: (i) screened in a community only visited once by the program (one community), (ii) screened for the first time in 2014, or (iii) screened for the first time in 2013 in those communities not visited in 2014 (two communities). A further 13 patients who were deceased or had moved from the community were excluded.) Commonly recorded reasons for not attending community screening included previous screening by an ophthalmologist or optometrist, working or travelling out of town, illness/hospitalisation, or unable to be contacted. There was no significant difference between those patients who underwent appropriate screening with the model based on gender (1.216; 1 df; $p = 0.27$), Indigenous status (0.007; 1 df; $p = 0.93$), age ($z = -1.84$; $p = 0.07$), HbA1c ($z = -0.37$; $p = 0.71$), systolic BP ($t = -0.29$; $p = 0.77$), or diastolic BP ($t = -0.74$; $p = 0.46$).

4.5. Image Quality. A total of 13.9% of screening episodes required rescreening due to inadequate images (Table 5). Further analysis demonstrated that the vast majority of

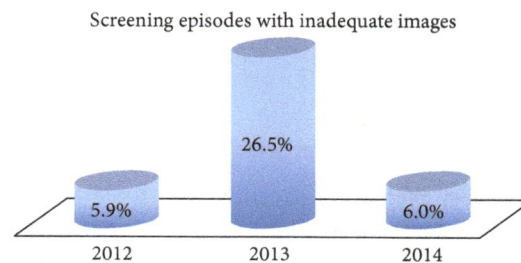

FIGURE 5: The proportion of screening episodes requiring rescreening due to inadequate images (according to GP management plan) by year.

TABLE 4: Appearance of fundi (GP grader).

| | Left eye ($n = 218$) | Right eye ($n = 218$) | Screening episodes ($n = 218$) |
	n (%)	n (%)	n (%)
No DR detected	142 (66.7%)	143 (66.2%)	126 (58.9%)
DR detected			
Mild NPDR	22 (10.3%)	24 (11.1%)	27 (12.6%)
Moderate NPDR	11 (5.2%)	14 (6.5%)	18 (8.4%)
Severe NPDR	2 (0.9%)	1 (0.5%)	2 (0.9%)
Proliferative DR	5 (2.3%)	1 (0.5%)	5 (2.3%)
Total detected	40 (18.7%)	40 (18.5%)	52 (24.3%)
Inadequate image	31 (14.6%)	33 (15.3%)	36 (16.8%)

Note: data was missing from two to five records.
Note: where the diagnosis differed between images of the right eye and left eye, the screening episode was categorised according to the most serious diagnosis. Where a patient had one inadequate image and the other image identified DR, the screening episode was categorised as DR.

inadequate images occurred in 2013, with a rate as high as 26.5% of screening episodes (Figure 5) and traced to a faulty camera. Following camera servicing, this decreased to 6% of screening episodes.

4.6. Diabetic Retinopathy Detection and Referral. Table 4 describes the proportion of screening episodes where images were normal, abnormal, or inadequate and required reimaging. A total of 58.9% of screening episodes were normal, 24.3% had DR detected, and 16.8% produced inadequate images. The majority of patients with DR had mild to moderate NPDR detected (21%); however, in 3.2% of screening episodes sight-threatening DR was detected (defined by severe NPDR or PDR). GP graders identified diabetic maculopathy in 5.6% of screening episodes, with all cases detected in 2014.

There was no statistically significant association between detection of DR and the absence or presence of appropriate DR screening prior to the implementation of the service (0.525; 1 df; $p = 0.47$). DR was detected more often in patients with a duration of diabetes more than 10 years and an HbA1c $\geq$ 8%, cut-offs previously shown to increase the risk of DR [2, 20]. A total of 51.6% of patients with diabetes longer than 10 years had DR detected, compared with 25.2% of patients with no DR detected (7.798; 1 df; $p = 0.005$). In

TABLE 5: GP management plan.

	Screening episodes (n = 218) n (%)
No action	**125 (57.9%)**
Ophthalmology referral	
Refer to "buddy" ophthalmologist	55 (25.5%)
Urgent referral	6 (2.8%)
Total	**61 (28.2%)**
Inadequate image	**30 (13.9%)**

Note: data was missing from two records.

Note: where the management plan differed between the right and the left eyes, the screening episode was categorised according to the most urgent management plan. Where a patient had one inadequate image and the other image identified pathology requiring ophthalmology referral, the screening episode was categorised as an ophthalmology referral.

Note: differences in the number of patients with inadequate images between Tables 4 and 5 is due to some patients being identified for ophthalmology referral due to detection of another pathology.

screening episodes where the patient's HbA1c was ≥8%, DR was detected more often (47.1%, compared to 23.4% with no DR) (10.602; 1 df; 0.001). There was no statistically significant association between a diastolic BP ≥ 90 mmHg (0.363; 1 df; $p = 0.547$) or a systolic BP ≥ 150 mmHg (3.447; 1 df; $p = 0.063$) and detection of DR.

A total of 28.2% of screening episodes were referred to the "buddy" ophthalmologist for review of DR or secondary to identification of another pathology. This included 2.8% of screening episodes for urgent referral (Table 5).

4.7. Other Pathology. Pathology other than DR was detected in 15.1% of screening episodes. Cataract was the most commonly identified pathology and clouded fundal photographs. Macular degeneration and hypertensive retinopathy were also detected.

5. Discussion

The implementation of the RODRS service has significantly improved patient access to DR screening. Appropriate screening has quadrupled from 16.3% to 66.3% of patients. This is above the national population average for appropriate DR screening and is a significant achievement in remote populations with minimal to no access to optometry and ophthalmology services [6]. Since the introduction of the program, screening of the eligible diabetic population living in remote communities has become more comprehensive, increasing from 33.7% to 47.9% across its three years of operation. International rural and remote DR screening programs reported population coverage ranging from 39% to 85% [23–31]. Indeed, achieving high rates of screening is particularly challenging in these study communities given the transient and highly mobile nature of the population, the fact that patients are often employed away from townships, the delivery of screening only once annually, and the lack of a fully coordinated approach to screening with visiting optometry and ophthalmology services. Low health literacy

and limited patient contact with local health services are also recognised barriers to achieving comprehensive population coverage. It is hoped that with continued service promotion and improved community awareness, patient uptake will continue to improve.

Despite limited ophthalmology resources, a review of international rural remote DR screening models by the authors found that the majority of programs use ophthalmologists as the primary image graders. Most countries are not adequately meeting screening recommendations and the number of people with diabetes continues to rise [6, 7, 32, 33]. Further to this, evidence suggests that on average 70% of fundal images captured show no retinopathy [17]. There is thus a need to explore innovative approaches to DR screening within a range of settings. Previous studies have demonstrated the efficacy of GP graders, with an Australian pilot of DR grading by general practitioners demonstrating good sensitivity (87%) and specificity (95%) [1]. During the operation of the RODRS service, just 28.2% of patients required ophthalmology referral for DR. This model may thus provide a more efficient solution to managing limited specialist ophthalmology resources in rural and remote areas.

Many international rural remote DR screening models have identified the successful integration of screen-positive patients with ophthalmology follow-up to be particularly challenging [34, 35]. A benefit of the RODRS program is the integration of screen-positive patients with specialist follow-up through the use of a "buddy" ophthalmologist, who supports the GP grader and provides visiting services to the region. The RODRS program also integrated DR screening with other diabetes care, providing a holistic multidisciplinary diabetes service that enables patients to easily complete their annual cycle of care. The significance of this is demonstrated by data released by the National Diabetes Strategic Advisory Group indicating that just 18% of Australian diabetics had a claim made by their GP for an annual cycle of care [36, 37]. It is hoped that provision of a coordinated approach to diabetes care will increase the proportion of diabetic patients undergoing annual DR screening and completing their annual cycle of care.

The RODRS service is inherently unique in its delivery, using local health professionals to screen diabetic patients and a local GP to grade images. This community-based approach enables the service to tailor itself to the needs of the local population and workforce. Also notable are the high screening rates amongst the Indigenous population comprising 23.5% of patients screened. Providing a service that meets the needs of the local Indigenous community is vitally important given that just 20% of Indigenous Australians undergo appropriate DR screening and rates of blindness are six times higher than for non-Indigenous Australians [10].

DR was detected in 24.3% of screening episodes. This is consistent with other rural remote Australian studies with reported detection rates ranging from 11% to 45%, but with the majority of programs reporting rates of 16 to 18% [23, 24, 38, 39]. This is significant and exemplifies the benefits of the program in detecting abnormality and avoiding preventable blindness. Diabetic maculopathy was identified in 5.6% of screening episodes. All cases were detected in 2014, following a changeover of GP graders. This could be explained by differing terminology amongst GP graders, with some graders believing they should only report diabetic macula oedema. Other Australian rural remote models have reported rates of diabetic macula oedema ranging from 0.2% to 2.8%, whilst international studies reported rates of clinically significant macula oedema ranging from 4.4% to 6.1% [23, 28, 38, 40–42].

The recent release of the consultation paper for the development of the Australian National Diabetes Strategy has highlighted improved eye screening as a key challenge for the future [36]. Models such as this one provide a successful approach both to screening and comprehensive ongoing management of patients with DR. Further research is needed to identify the generalisability of this model in terms of infrastructure, payment models, and incentives for quality. The Australian Medical Services Advisory Committee (MSAC), the group that advises government on additional medical services nationally, has recently recommended a Medicare Benefits Schedule (MBS) item number for nonmydriatic retinal photography in primary care settings, significantly improving the feasibility of this model of care in Australian communities [43].

6. Limitations

Some patient records were missing clinical information. No data was available on the proportion of screen-positive patients who actually underwent follow-up by an ophthalmologist.

7. Conclusion

Given the increasing number of remote Australians with diabetes, the development and trial of efficient workforce solutions for DR screening are of growing importance. This innovative model has significantly improved patient access to DR screening. It utilises existing infrastructure and the local health workforce to develop a community-driven and delivered service that meets the needs of the local population. It integrates DR screening into an already existing multidisciplinary diabetes service, providing comprehensive and holistic diabetes care.

Abbreviations

DR: Diabetic retinopathy
RODRS: Remote outreach diabetic retinopathy screening
GP: General practitioner
PHC: Primary health care centre
IHW: Indigenous health worker
BGL: Blood glucose level
BP: Blood pressure
BMI: Body mass index
NPDR: Nonproliferative DR
PDR: Proliferative DR
NHMRC: National Health and Medical Research Council.

Conflict of Interests

The authors declare that they have no financial conflict of interests. However, the primary author has a personal relationship with an ophthalmologist who participated in this study.

Authors' Contribution

Lisa J. Crossland was primarily involved in the design of this study, including the design of data collection tools, with input from Nicola M. Glasson and Sarah L. Larkins. Nicola M. Glasson participated in data collection. Lisa J. Crossland and Nicola M. Glasson entered data. Data analysis was performed by Nicola M. Glasson and Sarah L. Larkins. Nicola M. Glasson drafted the paper which was critically reviewed by Lisa J. Crossland and Sarah L. Larkins. All authors approved the final paper.

Acknowledgments

This model of care was adapted from a DR screening model developed by the University of Queensland Discipline of General Practice. We would like to acknowledge the dedication of the RODRS team and thank them for their assistance in completing this paper. We would also like to acknowledge the GP graders and "buddy" ophthalmologist, many of whom worked without remuneration.

References

[1] IDF, *International Diabetes Federation: IDF Diabetes Atlas*, 6th edition, 2013, http://www.idf.org/diabetesatlas.

[2] Q. Mohamed, M. C. Gillies, and T. Y. Wong, "Management of diabetic retinopathy: a systematic review," *Journal of the American Medical Association*, vol. 298, no. 8, pp. 902–916, 2007.

[3] World Health Organization, "Priority eye diseases diabetic retinopathy," 2015, http://www.who.int/blindness/causes/priority/en/index5.html.

[4] L. Verma, G. Prakash, H. K. Tewari, S. K. Gupta, G. V. S. Murthy, and N. Sharma, "Screening for diabetic retinopathy by nonophthalmologists: an effective public health tool," *Acta Ophthalmologica Scandinavica*, vol. 81, no. 4, pp. 373–377, 2003.

[5] C. A. McCarty, C. W. Lloyd-Smith, S. E. Lee, P. M. Livingston, Y. L. Stanislavsky, and H. R. Taylor, "Use of eye care services by people with diabetes: the Melbourne Visual Impairment Project," *British Journal of Ophthalmology*, vol. 82, no. 4, pp. 410–414, 1998.

[6] D. J. McCarty, C. L. Fu, C. A. Harper, H. R. Taylor, and C. A. McCarty, "Five-year incidence of diabetic retinopathy in the Melbourne Visual Impairment Project," *Clinical and Experimental Ophthalmology*, vol. 31, no. 5, pp. 397–402, 2003.

[7] S. Garg and R. M. Davis, "Diabetic retinopathy screening update," *Clinical Diabetes*, vol. 27, no. 4, pp. 140–145, 2009.

[8] A. C. Madden, D. Simmons, C. A. McCarty, M. A. Khan, and H. R. Taylor, "Eye health in rural Australia," *Clinical and Experimental Ophthalmology*, vol. 30, no. 5, pp. 316–321, 2002.

[9] C. B. Estopinal, S. Ausayakhun, S. Ausayakhun et al., "Access to ophthalmologic care in Thailand: a regional analysis," *Ophthalmic Epidemiology*, vol. 20, no. 5, pp. 267–273, 2013.

[10] H. R. Taylor, *National Indigenous Eye Health Survey*, Indigenous Eye Health Unit, Centre for Eye Research Australia and Vision CRC, 2009, http://www.vision2020australia.org.au/uploads/resource/29/NationalIndigenousEyeHealthSurvey.pdf.

[11] D. Askew, P. J. Schluter, G. Spurling et al., "Diabetic retinopathy screening in general practice: a pilot study," *Australian Family Physician*, vol. 38, no. 8, pp. 650–656, 2009.

[12] M. Bhargava, C. Y.-L. Cheung, C. Sabanayagam et al., "Accuracy of diabetic retinopathy screening by trained non-physician graders using non-mydriatic fundus camera," *Singapore Medical Journal*, vol. 53, no. 11, pp. 715–719, 2012.

[13] Z. Georgievski, K. Koklanis, A. Fenton, and I. Koukouras, "Victorian orthoptists' performance in the photo evaluation of diabetic retinopathy," *Clinical and Experimental Ophthalmology*, vol. 35, no. 8, pp. 733–738, 2007.

[14] N. Germain, B. Galusca, N. Deb-Joardar et al., "No loss of chance of diabetic retinopathy screening by endocrinologists with a digital fundus camera," *Diabetes Care*, vol. 34, no. 3, pp. 580–585, 2011.

[15] V. Sundling, P. Gulbrandsen, and J. Straand, "Sensitivity and specificity of Norwegian optometrists' evaluation of diabetic retinopathy in single-field retinal images—a cross-sectional experimental study," *BMC Health Services Research*, vol. 13, no. 1, article 17, 2013.

[16] RACQ, "Travel distance calculator," 2015, http://www.racq.com.au/travel/trip-planner.

[17] G. K. P. Spurling, D. A. Askew, N. E. Hayman, N. Hansar, A. M. Cooney, and C. L. Jackson, "Retinal photography for diabetic retinopathy screening in Indigenous primary health care: the Inala experience," *Australian and New Zealand Journal of Public Health*, vol. 34, supplement 1, pp. S30–S33, 2010.

[18] D. A. Askew, L. Crossland, R. S. Ware et al., "Diabetic retinopathy screening and monitoring of early stage disease in general practice: design and methods," *Contemporary Clinical Trials*, vol. 33, no. 5, pp. 969–975, 2012.

[19] The National Health and Medical Research Council (NHMRC), *Guidelines for the Management of Diabetic Retinopathy*, Australian Diabetes Society for the Department of Health and Aging, 2008, https://www.nhmrc.gov.au/_files_nhmrc/publications/attachments/di15.pdf.

[20] R. M. Schiffelers, M. H. A. M. Fens, J. M. van Blijswijk, D. I. Bink, and G. Storm, "Targeting the retinal microcirculation to treat diabetic sight problems," *Expert Opinion on Therapeutic Targets*, vol. 11, no. 11, pp. 1493–1502, 2007.

[21] ABS, "Australian Health Survey: Updated Results, 2011-2012. 4364.0.55.003," 2013, http://www.abs.gov.au/ausstats/abs@.nsf/Lookup/4364.0.55.003main+features12011-2012.

[22] Royal Australian College of General Practitioners and Diabetes Australia, "General practice management of type 2 diabetes—2014-15," March 2015, http://www.racgp.org.au/your-practice/guidelines/diabetes/.

[23] C. J. Barry, I. J. Constable, I. L. McAllister, and Y. Kanagasingam, "Diabetic screening in Western Australia: a photographer's perspective," *Journal of Visual Communication in Medicine*, vol. 29, no. 2, pp. 66–75, 2006.

[24] C. A. Harper, P. M. Livingston, C. Wood et al., "Screening for diabetic retinopathy using a non-mydriatic retinal camera in rural Victoria," *Australian and New Zealand Journal of Ophthalmology*, vol. 26, no. 2, pp. 117–121, 1998.

[25] S. J. Lee, C. A. McCarty, C. Sicari et al., "Recruitment methods for community-based screening for diabetic retinopathy," *Ophthalmic Epidemiology*, vol. 7, no. 3, pp. 209–218, 2000.

[26] A. McKenzie and J. Grylls, "Diabetic retinal photographic screening: a model for introducing audit and improving general practitioner care of diabetic patients in a rural setting," *Australian Journal of Rural Health*, vol. 7, no. 4, pp. 237–239, 1999.

[27] E. Reda, P. Dunn, C. Straker et al., "Screening for diabetic retinopathy using the mobile retinal camera: the Waikato experience," *New Zealand Medical Journal*, vol. 116, no. 1180, p. U562, 2003.

[28] P. Romero, R. Sagarra, J. Ferrer, J. Fernández-Ballart, and M. Baget, "The incorporation of family physicians in the assessment of diabetic retinopathy by non-mydriatic fundus camera," *Diabetes Research and Clinical Practice*, vol. 88, no. 2, pp. 184–188, 2010.

[29] N. Hautala, R. Aikkila, J. Korpelainen et al., "Marked reductions in visual impairment due to diabetic retinopathy achieved by efficient screening and timely treatment," *Acta Ophthalmologica*, vol. 92, no. 6, pp. 582–587, 2014.

[30] R. Lemmetty and K. Mäkelä, "Mobile digital fundus screening of type 2 diabetes patients in the Finnish county of South-Ostrobothnia," *Journal of Telemedicine and Telecare*, vol. 15, no. 2, pp. 68–72, 2009.

[31] T. Peto and C. Tadros, "Screening for diabetic retinopathy and diabetic macular edema in the United Kingdom," *Current Diabetes Reports*, vol. 12, no. 4, pp. 338–345, 2012.

[32] R. McKay, C. A. McCarty, and H. R. Taylor, "Diabetic retinopathy in Victoria, Australia: the visual impairment project," *British Journal of Ophthalmology*, vol. 84, no. 8, pp. 865–870, 2000.

[33] P. P. Goh, M. A. Omar, and A. F. Yusoff, "Diabetic eye screening in Malaysia: findings from the National Health and Morbidity Survey 2006," *Singapore Medical Journal*, vol. 51, no. 8, pp. 631–634, 2010.

[34] S. J. Lee, P. M. Livingston, C. A. Harper, C. A. McCarty, H. R. Taylor, and J. E. Keeffe, "Compliance with recommendations from a screening programme for diabetic retinopathy," *Australian and New Zealand Journal of Ophthalmology*, vol. 27, no. 3-4, pp. 187–189, 1999.

[35] D. B. Mak, A. J. Plant, and I. McAllister, "Screening for diabetic retinopathy in remote Australia: a program description and evaluation of a devolved model," *Australian Journal of Rural Health*, vol. 11, no. 5, pp. 224–230, 2003.

[36] The National Diabetes Strategy Advisory Group, "A strategic framework for action: consultation paper for the development of the Australian National Diabetes Strategy," 2015, http://www.diabetesaustralia.com.au/Documents/DA/Media%20Releases/National%20Diabetes%20Strategy%20Consultation%20Paper.pdf.

[37] Australian Institute of Health and Welfare (AIHW), "Annual Cycle of Care," May 2015, http://www.aihw.gov.au/diabetes-indicators/annual-cycle-of-care/.

[38] R. B. Murray, S. M. Metcalf, P. M. Lewis, J. K. Mein, and I. L. McAllister, "Sustaining remote-area programs: retinal camera use by Aboriginal health workers and nurses in a Kimberley partnership," *Medical Journal of Australia*, vol. 182, no. 10, pp. 520–523, 2005.

[39] S. J. Lee, C. Sicari, C. A. Harper et al., "Examination compliance and screening for diabetic retinopathy: a 2-year follow-up study," *Clinical and Experimental Ophthalmology*, vol. 28, no. 3, pp. 149–152, 2000.

[40] R. Ling, V. Ramsewak, D. Taylor, and J. Jacob, "Longitudinal study of a cohort of people with diabetes screened by the Exeter Diabetic Retinopathy Screening Programme," *Eye*, vol. 16, no. 2, pp. 140–145, 2002.

[41] S. McHugh, C. Buckley, K. Murphy et al., "Quality-assured screening for diabetic retinopathy delivered in primary care in Ireland: an observational study," *British Journal of General Practice*, vol. 63, no. 607, pp. e134–e140, 2013.

[42] P. Massin, A. Chabouis, A. Erginay et al., "OPHDIAT: a telemedical network screening system for diabetic retinopathy in the Île-de-France," *Diabetes and Metabolism*, vol. 34, no. 3, pp. 227–234, 2008.

[43] Medical Services Advisory Committee, "Public summary document: application 1181—non-mydriatic retinal photography in people with diagnosed diabetes," 2014, http://www.msac.gov .au/internet/msac/publishing.nsf/Content/1181-public.

5

Protective Effects of Celastrol on Diabetic Liver Injury via TLR4/MyD88/NF-κB Signaling Pathway in Type 2 Diabetic Rats

Li-ping Han, Chun-jun Li, Bei Sun, Yun Xie, Yue Guan, Ze-jun Ma, and Li-ming Chen

2011 Collaborative Innovation Center of Tianjin for Medical Epigenetics, Key Laboratory of Hormone and Development, Ministry of Health, Metabolic Disease Hospital and Tianjin Institute of Endocrinology, Tianjin Medical University, Tianjin 300070, China

Correspondence should be addressed to Li-ming Chen; xfx22081@vip.163.com

Academic Editor: Giovanni Annuzzi

Immune and inflammatory pathways play a central role in the pathogenesis of diabetic liver injury. Celastrol is a potent immunosuppressive and anti-inflammatory agent. So far, there is no evidence regarding the mechanism of innate immune alterations of celastrol on diabetic liver injury in type 2 diabetic animal models. The present study was aimed at investigating protective effects of celastrol on the liver injury in diabetic rats and at elucidating the possible involved mechanisms. We analyzed the liver histopathological and biochemical changes and the expressions of TLR4 mediated signaling pathway. Compared to the normal control group, diabetic rats were found to have obvious steatohepatitis and proinflammatory cytokine activities were significantly upregulated. Celastrol-treated diabetic rats show reduced hepatic inflammation and macrophages infiltration. The expressions of TLR4, MyD88, NF-κB, and downstream inflammatory factors IL-1β and TNFα in the hepatic tissue of treated rats were downregulated in a dose-dependent manner. We firstly found that celastrol treatment could delay the progression of diabetic liver disease in type 2 diabetic rats via inhibition of TLR4/MyD88/NF-κB signaling cascade pathways and its downstream inflammatory effectors.

1. Introduction

Diabetic liver damage was mainly caused by fatty infiltration of the liver leading to nonalcoholic fatty liver disease (NAFLD). NAFLD is the hepatic manifestation of the metabolic syndrome and covers a disease spectrum ranging from simple steatosis with no inflammation to steatosis with varying degrees of inflammation (steatohepatitis, NASH) to fibrosis, cirrhosis, and hepatocellular carcinoma [1, 2]. Among them, NASH is an important turning point and the complex cellular components of the innate immune system play an essential role in perpetuating and modulating the inflammatory response in the liver [3].

The Toll-like receptors (TLRs) family is one of the best-characterized pattern recognition receptor families and is responsible for sensing invading pathogens outside of the cell [4, 5]. Once a molecular pattern has been recognized by the TLRs, downstream signaling is initiated, resulting in the innate immune and inflammatory responses. TLR4 is one of the receptors which is related to whole-body, low-grade chronic inflammatory diseases [6] and contributes to macrophage infiltration in experimental models of diabetes-related liver injury [7]. NF-κB is a ubiquitous and well-known transcription factor responsible for the rapid induction of many cytokines implicated in the immune and inflammation [8]. There is evidence showing that NF-κB is activated in NASH and liver fibrosis models in vivo and in vitro [9, 10]. Moreover, the TLR4 signaling pathway can activate NF-κB and induce the expression of proinflammatory genes [11]. Therefore, downregulation of the expression of TLR4/NF-κB signaling pathways and its downstream inflammatory effectors might represent a novel treatment strategy for reducing diabetic liver injury.

Celastrol ($C_{29}H_{38}O_4$) is a pharmacologically active pentacyclic-triterpene extract from the roots of traditional Chinese herbal plant *Tripterygium wilfordii* Hook.f. (TwHF, thunder god vine). Recent research reported that celastrol had potent anti-inflammatory and immunosuppressive properties. To date, celastrol has been widely used for the treatment of various diseases, such as cancer, neurodegenerative disease, and autoimmune diseases [12–15]. The latest research reported that celastrol was able to effectively alleviate high-fat mediated cardiovascular disease and diabetic nephropathy [16, 17]. But there is still a lack of data describing the anti-inflammatory and immunosuppressive activities of celastrol on diabetic liver injury. The present study was conducted using rat model of T_2DM induced by high-fat diet combined with low-dose STZ to investigate the effects of celastrol on hepatic tissues and explore its possible mechanisms.

2. Materials and Methods

2.1. Animals. This study was carried out in strict accordance with the recommendations in the Guide for the Care and Use of Laboratory Animals of the National Institutes of Health. The protocol was approved by the Animal Care and Use Committee on the Ethics of Animal Experiments of Tianjin Medical University (Tianjin, China). All steps were taken to avoid animal suffering at each stage of the experiment. Seventy-five healthy male Sprague-Dawley rats, 4~5 weeks of age, weighing 161 ± 9 g, were purchased from Beijing HFK Technology Co., Ltd. (Beijing, China). All of the rats were housed under pathogen-free conditions and were provided with rat chow and water ad libitum. The animals were maintained at a controlled temperature (22°C ± 2°C), humidity (55% ± 10%), and photoperiod (12 h light/dark cycles). The animals were acclimatized to the laboratory for 1 week before the experiments. 15 rats were randomly selected as normal control group (NC group) and fed with a conventional diet. The remaining 60 rats were given high-fat diet (formula is sucrose 10%, lard 10%, cholesterol 1%, and sodium cholate 0.3%, and the rest is composed of the basic diet, irradiated by cobalt-50, provided by HFK Technology Co., Ltd., Beijing, China). After 8 weeks of feeding, fasting plasma glucose (FPG) and insulin (FINS, Radioimmunoassay), and triglycerides, total cholesterol levels were measured, and HOMA-IR and HOMA-β were assessed by homeostasis model (HOMA-IR = FPG × FINS/22.5, HOMA-β = 20 × FINS/(FPG − 3.5)). When insulin resistance occurred, STZ 30 mg/kg (pH 4.32) intravenously was injected to induce rat model of T_2DM. 15 normal rats were intravenously injected with sodium citrate buffer. The tail blood glucose was measured, which is greater than 16.7 mmol/L to be thought successful. The diabetic rats were randomly assigned to four groups: rats receiving vehicle only (DM group) and three groups of rats receiving different doses of celastrol.

2.2. Celastrol Solution. Purified celastrol was purchased from Sigma Chemical Co. (Sigma, St. Louis, MO, USA) and stored at −20°C. Celastrol was freshly dissolved in 10% dimethyl sulfoxide (DMSO) before use in the experiments, and vehicle (distilled water containing 10% DMSO) was used as a control. Treatment rats were administered by oral gavage with low-dose celastrol (100 μg/kg, CL group), medium-dose celastrol (200 μg/kg, CM group), and high-dose celastrol (500 μg/kg, CH group) once daily for 8 weeks.

2.3. Biochemical Analysis. Rats were sacrificed under anesthesia by i.p. injection of sodium pentobarbital. We measured liver weight and calculated liver index (liver weight/body weight). After centrifugation of the blood samples, the serum concentrations of glucose, alanine aminotransferase, aspartate aminotransferase, blood urea nitrogen, creatinine, total cholesterol, triglyceride, and high density lipoprotein cholesterol were measured using an automatic clinical analyzer (7600A-020, HITACHI Ltd., Tokyo, Japan). Serum IL-1β and TNFα levels were measured using an enzyme-linked immunosorbent assay (ELISA) kit (Cusabio Biotech, USA). Liver tissue was analyzed for total cholesterol and triglyceride contents (Jiancheng Bioengineering Institute, Nanjing, China), according to the manufacturer's instructions.

2.4. Histopathological Evaluations. Sections from the livers were removed and fixed in 10% neutral-buffered formalin and embedded in paraffin and stained with hematoxylin-eosin and Masson's trichrome (MT) for histological analysis.

2.5. Immunohistochemistry Staining. The sectioned slides were stained according to standard protocols described previously. Paraffin-embedded sections of hepatic tissue were deparaffinized, dehydrated, and stained immunohistochemically for detection of mouse monoclonal anti-CD68 antibody (diluted 1 : 200 in PBS; Abcam, UK), mouse monoclonal anti-TLR4 antibody (diluted 1 : 100 in PBS; Abcam, UK), rabbit polyclonal anti-MyD88 antibody (diluted 1 : 100 in PBS; Bioworld technology, Co. Ltd., Nanjing, China), rabbit polyclonal anti-NF-κBp65 antibody (diluted 1 : 1000 in PBS; Abcam, UK), rabbit polyclonal anti-IL-1β antibody (diluted 1 : 100 in PBS; Abcam, UK), and rabbit polyclonal anti-TNFα antibody (diluted 1 : 100 in PBS; Abcam, UK) by sequential incubation. A peroxidase-linked secondary antibody and diaminobenzidine (Sungene Biotech Co., Ltd., Tianjin, China) were used to detect specific immunostaining. The slides were rinsed twice and counterstained with hematoxylin. As negative controls for nonspecific binding of the secondary antibody, sections from the same samples were processed without the primary antibody.

2.6. Real-Time Reverse Transcription Polymerase Chain Reaction (RT-PCR). All primers were synthesized by AuGCT Biotechnology (Beijing, China). The primer for rat glyceraldehyde-3-phosphate dehydrogenase gene was used as housekeeping gene. The real-time PCR primer sequences used for PCR were shown in Table 1. Total RNA was isolated from the liver sections with TRIzol reagent (Invitrogen Life Technologies, Carlsbad, CA, USA). cDNA synthesis was performed using the High-Capacity cDNA Reverse Transcription kit (Applied Biosystems, Foster City, CA, USA) according to the manufacturer's instructions. Real-time PCR was performed in 10 μL that contained 5 μL of 2×SYBR Green Premix Ex TaqTM (Takara Biotechnology, Japan), 1 μL of cDNA, 3 μL of distilled water, and 0.5 μL of each primer. PCR was carried out in a thermal cycler (Bio-Rad, Hercules, CA, USA). Initial denaturation was carried out at 95°C for 3 min, followed by 45 cycles of denaturation for 10 s at 95°C, annealing for 30 s at

TABLE 1: Sequences of real-time PCR primers.

Primer name	Sequence	Annealing temperature	Size
TLR4	Forward 5′-ATGAGGACTGGGTGAGAAAC-3′ Reverse 5′-CACCACCACAATAACTTTCC-3′	52°C	161 bp
MyD88	Forward 5′-TGGTGGTTGTTTCTGACGAT-3′ Reverse 5′-CGCAGATAGTGATGAACCGT-3′	58.4°C	165 bp
NF-κB	Forward 5′-AAAAACGCATCCCAAGGTGC-3′ Reverse 5′-AAGCTCAAGCCACCATACCC-3′	52°C	185 bp
IL-1β	Forward 5′-GGACAGAACATAAGCCAACA-3′ Reverse 5′-CTTTCATCACACAGGACAGG-3′	61.4°C	127 bp
TNFα	Forward 5′-TCCCAGGTTCTCTTCAAGG-3′ Reverse 5′-GTACATGGGCTCATACCAG-3′	61.4°C	177 bp
GAPDH	Forward 5′-GCAAGTTCAACGGCACAG-3′ Reverse 5′-GCCAGTAGACTCCACGACAT-3′	52°C	218 bp

PCR: polymerase chain reaction; TLR4: Toll-like receptor 4; MyD88: myeloid differentiation factor 88; NF-κB: nuclear factor-kappa B; IL-1β: interleukin-1 beta; TNFα: tumor necrosis factor alpha; GAPDH: glyceraldehyde-3-phosphate dehydrogenase.

the appropriate temperature, and extension for 20 s at 72°C. The mRNA levels were normalized against the mRNA levels of the housekeeping gene GAPDH. Gene expression and data analysis were monitored using the CFX Manager Software (version 1.6, Bio-Rad, CA, USA). Relative quantification was performed using the $2^{-\Delta\Delta Ct}$ method which results in ratios between target genes and a housekeeping reference gene.

2.7. Western Blotting Analysis. Proteins were extracted using RIPA buffer (Thermo, USA), according to the manufacturer's instructions, and the protein concentrations were measured using a BCA protein assay kit (Thermo, USA). An equal amount of protein from each sample was subjected to sodium dodecyl sulfate- (SDS-) polyacrylamide gel electrophoresis and then transferred to polyvinylidene difluoride (PVDF) membranes (Millipore, USA). Membranes were blocked with 5% milk for 2 h at room temperature and incubated overnight at 4°C with primary antibodies, including TLR4 (1 : 1000), MyD88 (1 : 1000), NF-κBp65 (1 : 1000), phospho-IκBα (p-IκBα, 1 : 500), IL-1β (1 : 1000), TNFα (1 : 1000), and internal control β-actin (1 : 10000, Sungene Biotech Co., Ltd., Tianjin, China). Membranes were washed twice for 10 min in 1×TBST and then incubated with HRP-conjugated secondary antibodies (goat anti-rabbit IgG: 1 : 12500; goat anti-mouse IgG: 1 : 12500, Sungene Biotech Co., Ltd., Tianjin, China) for 2 h. Membranes were then washed twice for 10 min in 1×TBST. Proteins were visualized by ECL (Millipore, USA), and blots were scanned in dark room. Densitometry analysis of bands was performed with the Image J software.

2.8. Statistical Analysis. Statistical analysis was performed by using SPSS 17.0 version (IBM SPSS Statistics, IBM Corporation, Armonk, NY, USA) and GraphPad Prism 5.0 software (GraphPad Software, Inc., La Jolla, Calif, USA). Quantitative data were expressed as mean ± standard error of the mean (SEM). The significance of the data obtained was evaluated using the one-way analysis of variance (*one-way ANOVA*),

followed by *LSD*-test. A value of $P < 0.05$ was considered statistically significant.

3. Results

3.1. Parameters after 8-Week High-Fat Feeding. Compared with the NC group, total cholesterol and triglycerides levels and the indexes of HOMA-IR and HOMA-β of high-fat rats were significantly higher, but there were no changes for blood glucose. These results showed that insulin resistance occurred after 8-week high-fat feeding (Table 2).

3.2. Effects of Celastrol on Physical and Biochemical Parameters in Rats. Physical and biochemical parameters for the different groups of rats are shown in Table 3. Compared with the NC group, the body weights of diabetic rats were significantly lower, and blood glucose, serum and liver TC, TG levels, and liver index were significantly higher. Rats given celastrol had no changes in blood glucose, serum lipid, and body weights but showed lower liver TC, TG contents, and liver index in the CH group. No significant differences were observed for ALT, AST, BUN, and SCr levels in all groups of rats.

3.3. Effects of Celastrol on Histological Changes of Hepatic Tissues in Rats. As shown in H&E staining sections in Figure 1(a), there was clear structure of hepatic lobule, and hepatocytes radially arranged around the central vein, no obvious inflammatory cell infiltration and Kupffer cells proliferation in the NC group. Hepatic lobular structure generally disappeared, and diffuse large bubble-like hepatocyte steatosis and ballooning with obvious inflammatory cell infiltration around portal area were observed in the DM group. Lesions in treatment group were less than that in the DM group, particularly in the CH group. Masson's trichrome staining (Figure 1(b)) showed weak coloration which appeared along the vascular wall of the portal vein and portal area in the NC group. However, diabetic rats showed more

TABLE 2: Glucose and islet function parameters after 8-week high fat feeding.

Group	FPG (mmol/L)	TG (mmol/L)	TC (mmol/L)	FINS (mIU/L)	HOMA-IR	HOMA-β
NC	5.7 ± 0.5	1.3 ± 0.4	2.0 ± 0.2	25.1 ± 4.1	6.5 ± 1.7	230.7 ± 28.7
High-fat	6.1 ± 0.7	3.0 ± 0.7[a]	3.2 ± 0.5[a]	31.6 ± 6.1[a]	8.6 ± 2.3[a]	259.8 ± 42.1[a]

FPG: fasting plasma glucose; TG: triglycerides; TC: total cholesterol; FINS: fasting insulin; IR: insulin resistance. Data are expressed as mean ± SEM, [a]$P < 0.05$ versus NC group.

TABLE 3: Physical and biochemical parameters for rats evaluated in this study.

	NC	DM	DM + CL	DM + CM	DM + CH
Glucose (mmol/L)	6.0 ± 0.2	28.2 ± 3.0[a]	25.3 ± 7.1[a]	26.8 ± 6.1[a]	25.0 ± 4.2[a]
Body weight (g)	442.7 ± 43.8	298.6 ± 37.1[a]	309.4 ± 24.2[a]	303.4 ± 29.5[a]	311.3 ± 30.8[a]
Liver index (g/100 g)	2.67 ± 0.23	4.51 ± 0.35[a]	4.42 ± 0.55[a]	4.27 ± 0.44[a]	3.9 ± 0.27[a,b]
Serum TG (mmol/L)	1.5 ± 1.2	4.4 ± 1.8[a]	4.1 ± 2.1[a]	3.7 ± 2.2[a]	3.5 ± 1.4[a]
Serum TC (mmol/L)	2.2 ± 1.2	6.9 ± 0.9[a]	6.5 ± 2.0[a]	6.4 ± 1.7[a]	6.0 ± 2.1[a]
HDL-C (mmol/L)	0.6 ± 0.1	0.5 ± 0.1	0.5 ± 0.1	0.6 ± 0.1	0.6 ± 0.2
ALT (U/L)	49.7 ± 9.5	55.1 ± 5.1	52.0 ± 9.4	52.7 ± 8.9	50.8 ± 9.1
AST (U/L)	105.1 ± 18.4	109.4 ± 8.4	112.6 ± 9.7	104.3 ± 13.6	104.8 ± 10.5
BUN (mmol/L)	10.9 ± 2.0	10.7 ± 1.6	10.5 ± 1.6	10.9 ± 1.2	9.8 ± 1.8
SCr (μmol/L)	32.8 ± 4.4	31.3 ± 3.3	30.6 ± 3.7	31.4 ± 3.2	30.7 ± 4.1
Liver TG (mg/gprot)	95.8 ± 18.6	412.4 ± 57.8[a]	388.3 ± 38.1[a]	342.4 ± 45.8[a]	228.3 ± 27.5[a,b]
Liver TC (mg/gprot)	40.3 ± 10.1	134.4 ± 25.1[a]	112.5 ± 20.4[a]	103.2 ± 17.5[a]	88.3 ± 12.4[a,b]

TG: triglycerides; TC: total cholesterol; HDL-C: high density lipoprotein cholesterol; ALT: alanine aminotransferase; AST: aspartate aminotransferase; BUN: blood urea nitrogen; SCr: serum creatinine; NC: normal control; DM: diabetes mellitus; DM + CL: diabetes with low-dose celastrol; DM + CM: diabetes with medium-dose celastrol; DM + CH: diabetes with high-dose celastrol. Data are expressed as mean ± SEM, [a]$P < 0.05$ versus NC group; [b]$P < 0.05$ versus DM group.

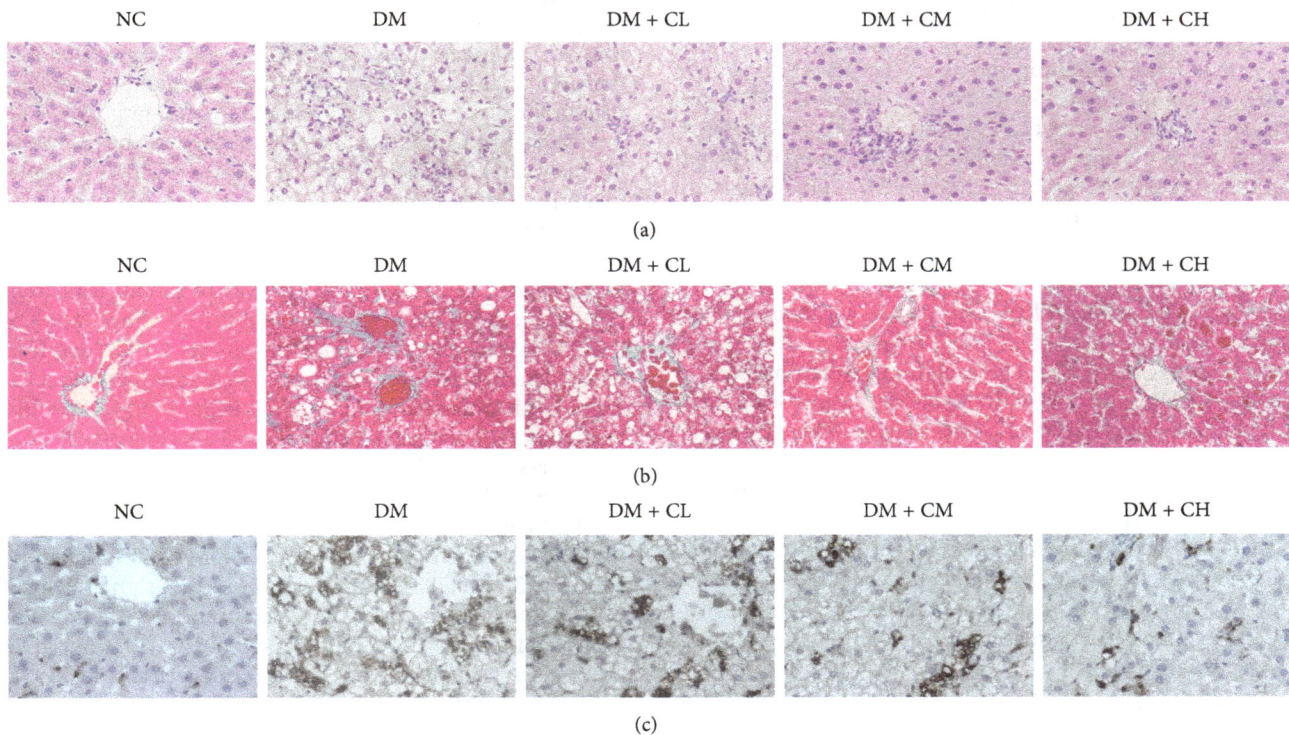

FIGURE 1: Celastrol exhibited protective effects on livers in diabetic rats. (a) H&E staining (×400) showed hepatic steatosis with lobular inflammation and ballooning of hepatocytes in diabetic rats. Alleviation of the infiltration of inflammatory cells and hepatic steatosis were observed in diabetic rats treated with celastrol. (b) Masson's staining (×400) showed mild fibrosis changes around perisinusoidal spaces and the portal area in diabetic rats. The degree of fibrosis decreased in celastrol-treated rats. (c) Immunohistochemistry staining of CD68. More Kupffer cells infiltration was detected in diabetic rats and was downregulated by celastrol administration.

fibrosis changes around perisinusoidal spaces and the portal area. The degree of fibrosis observed in hepatic tissues was much lower in celastrol-treated rats than diabetic rats. As a macrophage-specific marker, CD68 staining showed that there was more Kupffer cells infiltration in diabetic rats than in the NC rats. Celastrol administration decreased CD68 expression, particularly in the CH group (Figure 1(c)).

3.4. Effects of Celastrol on Expressions of TLR4 and Downstream Signaling Ligand MyD88 of Hepatic Tissues in Rats. TLR4 expression was observed only in a few hepatocytes in the NC group with immunohistochemical staining. In contrast, higher expression of TLR4 was observed in the cytoplasm and membranes of hepatocytes and Kupffer cells in the DM group and lower expression in celastrol treatment group, especially in the CH group. Similar patterns of expression were observed for MyD88 in the cytoplasm (Figures 2(a) and 2(b)). RT-PCR and Western Blotting analysis showed that TLR4, MyD88 mRNA, and protein levels in the hepatic tissues of the DM group were significantly increased compared with those of the NC group. Additionally, levels of all transcripts and expressions were decreased in rats in celastrol treatment groups. Moreover, celastrol administration decreased expressions in a dose-dependent manner (Figures 2(c)–2(f)).

3.5. Effects of Celastrol on Expressions of NF-κB and p-IκBα of Hepatic Tissues in Rats. NF-κB staining was observed with immunohistochemical staining only in a few hepatocytes in the NC group. In contrast, higher expression was observed in the nucleus in the DM group and lower expression in celastrol treatment group, especially in the CH group. RT-PCR and Western Blotting showed that NF-κBp65 and p-IκBα expressions in the DM group were significantly increased compared with those in the NC group. Additionally, expressions were decreased in celastrol treatment groups in a dose-dependent manner (Figures 3(a)–3(d)).

3.6. Effects of Celastrol on Expressions of Downstream Inflammatory Cytokines IL-1β and TNFα of Hepatic Tissues and Serum in Rats. IL-1β and TNFα staining were observed in the cytoplasm. Compared with the NC rats, there were more positive expressions in diabetic rats, all with reduced staining observed in rats treated with different doses of celastrol, especially in the CH group (Figures 4(a) and 4(b)). Similar to immunohistochemical staining, IL-1β, TNFα mRNA, and protein levels in the hepatic tissues and serum contents in the DM group were significantly increased compared with those in the NC group and were decreased in celastrol administration rats in a dose-dependent manner (Figures 4(c)–4(h)).

4. Discussion

Diabetes mellitus often coexists with different metabolic-related syndromes, such as dyslipidemia, hypertension, and NAFLD [7]. In our present study, experimental type 2 diabetes' rat model was induced by 8-week high-fat feeding combined with low-dose STZ injection [18]. Therefore, our experimental diabetic model is very similar to the pathogenesis of type 2 diabetes. Our observation documented that diabetic rats showed increased glucose combined with insulin resistance and abnormal lipid profiles, liver pathological changes including obvious inflammation and fibrosis, and more macrophage infiltration compared with normal rats, in line with steatohepatitis changes. But serum ALT and AST levels were not obviously increased, because of relative early stage of NAFLD. The earlier stage of NASH may only show mild pathological changes and may not result in the elevated liver enzymes. The latest research demonstrated that celastrol (100 μg–1 mg/kg) was able to effectively suppress weight and improve lipid accumulation in organs including the kidney, liver, and adipose tissue in db/db mice [17, 19]. In our study, we applied relative low three dosages of celastrol (100 μg/kg, 200 μg/kg, and 500 μg/kg) according to previous literature [17, 19]. After 8 weeks of administration, although there were no significant differences in serum glucose, triglycerides, and total cholesterol levels compared with the nontreatment group, the levels of triglycerides and total cholesterol of hepatic tissue were significantly decreased and the liver pathological changes were differently lessened in the treatment groups in a dose-dependent manner. The results showed that early use of celastrol could improve lipid metabolism disorders in liver and delay the progression of diabetic fatty liver disease.

TLR4 signaling pathway is more common pathway factor and has an important regulatory role in stimulating the immune and inflammatory response-related genes expression in the liver, which is activated by accumulation of fatty acids of the liver, particularly saturated fatty acids [3, 20]. Csak et al. found that inactivation of TLR4 in methionine-/choline-deficient mice resulted in a marked attenuation of steatohepatitis induced by a diet [21]. Consequently, targeting TLR4 provides a promising intervention strategy for the prevention or treatment of diabetic fatty liver disease [3]. T_2DM displays insulin resistance, abnormal glucose and lipid, oxidative stress, and so forth, leading to an increase of endogenous and exogenous ligands of TLR4 such as FFAs, LPS, and endotoxin, and activates TLR4 signaling pathway to induce liver injury [22], in line with our results. As mentioned above, we found that TLR4 were expressed generally on hepatocytes and Kupffer cells in diabetic liver and the consistent upregulation with immunohistochemical staining, RT-PCR, and Western Blotting, and the treatment with celastrol significantly reduced the expressions of TLR4. Similar results were also shown in Kim's research [17].

TLR4 is initiated through two different pathways, the MyD88-dependent pathway and the MyD88-independent pathway [3]. MyD88 is a critical downstream signaling ligand of TLR4 receptor complex and also is an important adapter protein of NF-κB signaling pathway, contributing to the expression of inflammatory genes. Spruss et al. showed that a significant increase of MyD88 mRNA in high-fat- and fructose-induced hepatic steatosis but inactivation of TLR4 led to a significant decrease in MyD88 mRNA level [23]. Miura et al. proved that the absence of MyD88 prevented hepatic steatosis [24]. Therefore, MyD88 served as the key TLR4 adaptor protein, linking the receptors to downstream kinases in fatty liver disease. Our study showed that TLR4 and MyD88 gene and

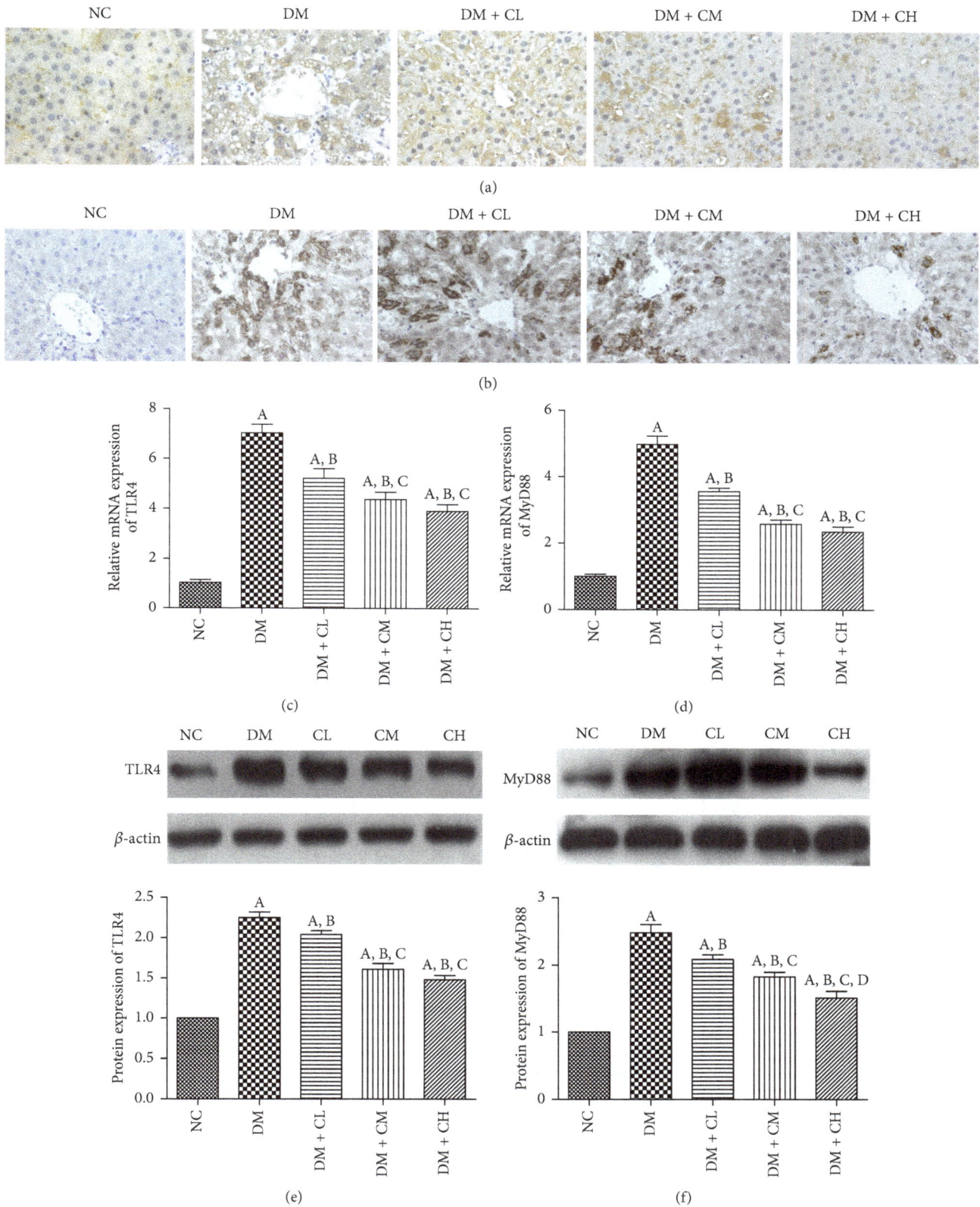

FIGURE 2: Celastrol administration downregulated the expressions of the TLR4 and MyD88 in diabetic rats liver. (a-b) Immunohistochemical staining of TLR4 and MyD88 (×400). (c-d) Relative mRNA expression levels of TLR4 and MyD88. (e-f) Relative protein expression levels of TLR4 and MyD88 were analyzed by Western Blotting, and the ratio of TLR4/actin and MyD88/actin was shown. The results are expressed as mean ± SEM, [A] $P < 0.05$ versus NC group; [B] $P < 0.05$ versus DM group; [C] $P < 0.05$ versus CL group; [D] $P < 0.05$ versus CM group.

(a)

(b)

(c)

(d)

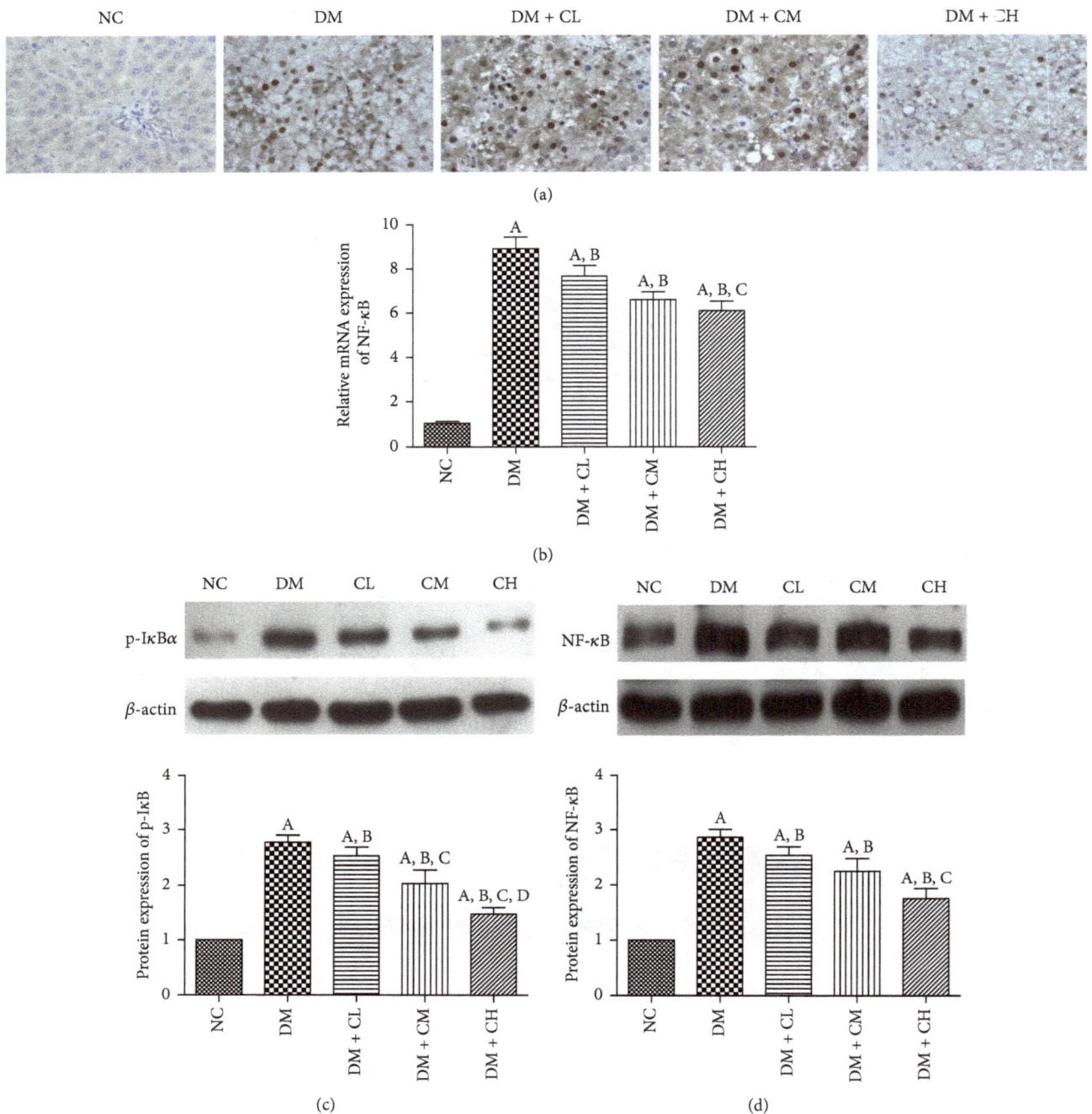

FIGURE 3: Celastrol administration downregulated NF-κB and p-IκBα expressions in diabetic rats liver. (a) Immunohistochemical staining of NF-κB ($\times$400). (b) Relative mRNA expression levels of NF-κB. (c-d) Relative protein expression levels of p-IκBα and NF-κBp65 were analyzed by Western Blotting, and the ratio of NF-κB/actin and p-IκBα/actin was shown. The results are expressed as mean $\pm$ SEM, [A]$P < 0.05$ versus NC group; [B]$P < 0.05$ versus DM group; [C]$P < 0.05$ versus CL group; [D]$P < 0.05$ versus CM group.

protein expressions were consistently increased in diabetic rat liver and suppressed with celastrol administration, indicating that anti-inflammatory effect of celastrol might be through TLR4/MyD88-dependent signal transduction pathway.

NF-κB activation is essential for hepatic inflammatory recruitment in steatohepatitis, uniformly found in human NASH and animal models [25–27]. NF-κBp65 subunit binds

to its inhibitory counterpart IκBα and other IκB proteins to form P65-IκB trimer which is located in the cytoplasm as an inactive complex. Following IκBα phosphorylation and degradation, the activated NF-κBp65 is disassociated from IκBα and shifts to nuclei where it binds to specific DNA motifs to regulate transcriptional activity of its target genes [28]. Therefore, IκBα phosphorylation is an indispensable process,

(a)

(b)

(c)

(d)

(e)

(f)

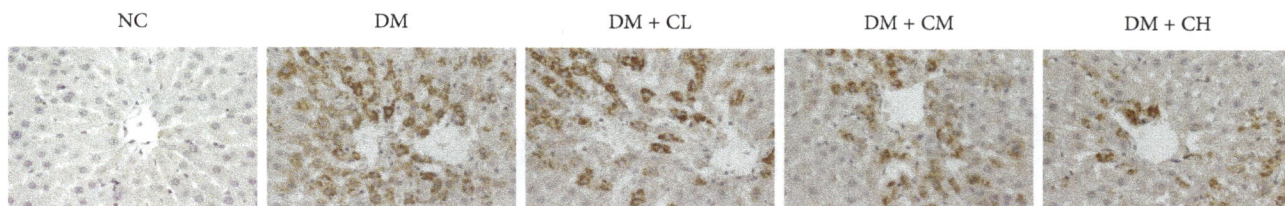

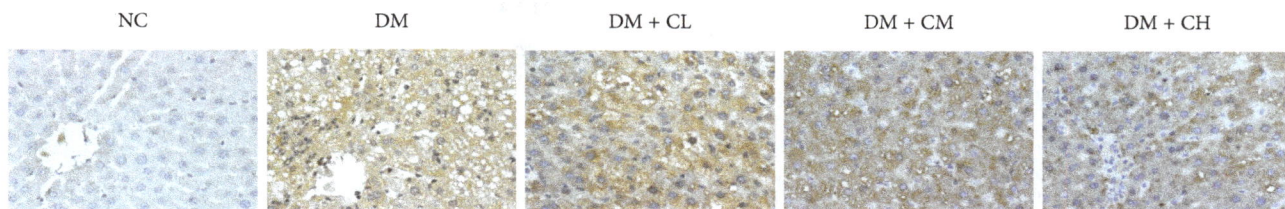

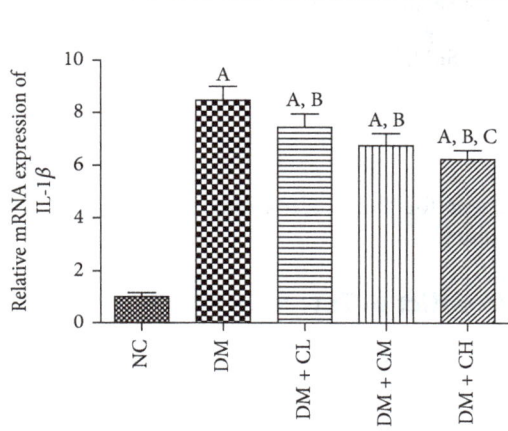

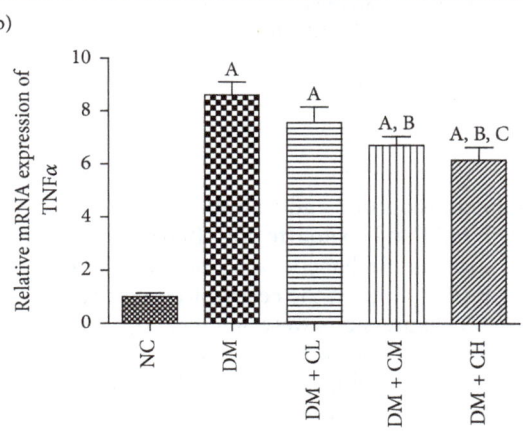

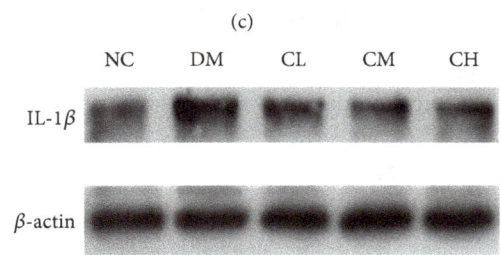

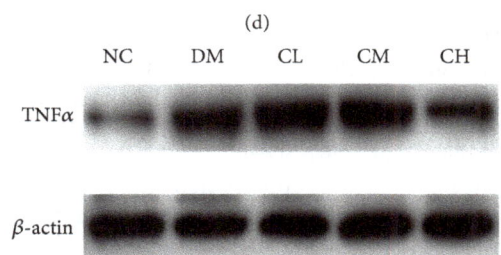

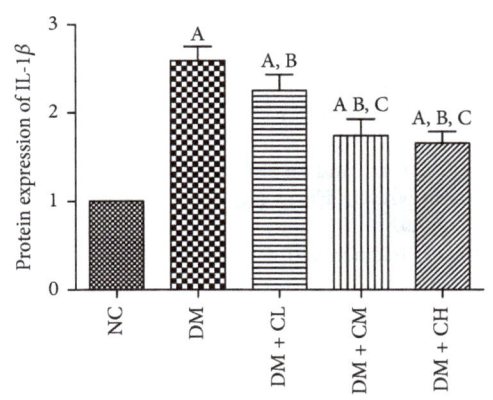

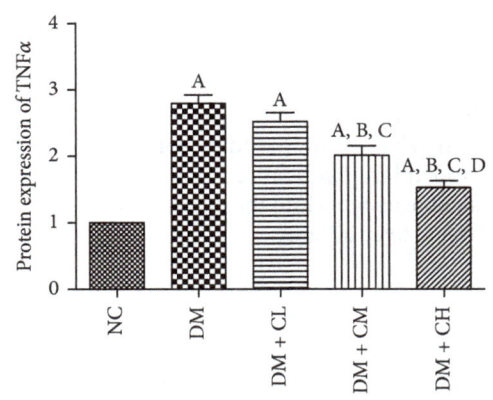

FIGURE 4: Continued.

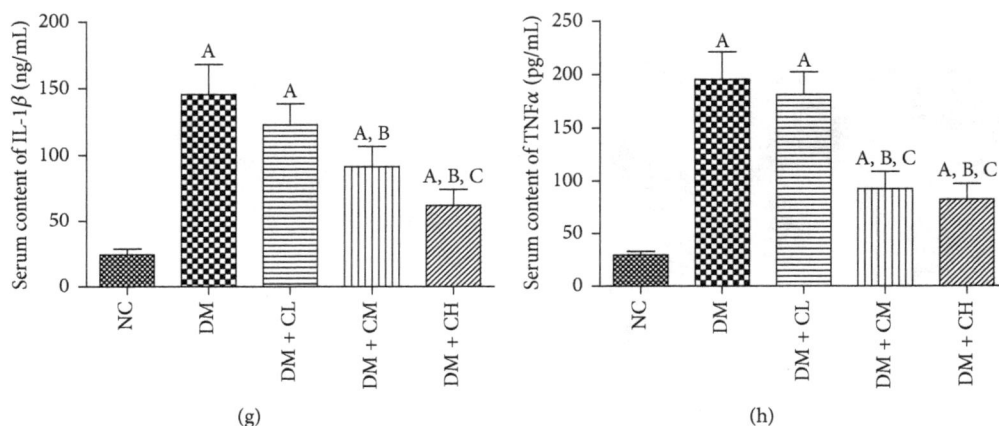

(g)   (h)

FIGURE 4: Celastrol administration downregulated downstream inflammatory cytokine IL-1β and TNFα expressions in diabetic rats liver. (a-b) Immunohistochemical staining of IL-1β and TNFα ($\times$400). (c-d) Relative mRNA expression levels of IL-1β and TNFα. (e-f) Relative protein expression levels of IL-1β and TNFα were analyzed by Western Blotting, and the ratio of IL-1β/actin and TNFα/actin was shown. (g-h) Serum contents of IL-1β and TNFα. The results are expressed as mean $\pm$ SEM, [A]$P < 0.05$ versus NC group; [B]$P < 0.05$ versus DM group; [C]$P < 0.05$ versus CL group; [D]$P < 0.05$ versus CM group.

which leads to the translocation and activation of NF-κBp65. In our study we found that hepatocyte NF-κBp65 was higher expressed in the nuclei in the diabetic rats, along with upregulated p-IκBα expressions. But in the celastrol-treated rats, p-IκBα and NF-κBp65 expressions were significantly reduced and NF-κBp65 was rarely seen in the nuclei. NF-κB was downstream activator of TLR4, involved in TLR4/MyD88-dependent signaling pathway and induced transcriptional expression of multiple proinflammatory chemokines (e.g., TNFα and IL-1β) associated with liver inflammation [6]. Moreover, proinflammatory chemokines could also upregulate the activity of NF-κB to form a positive feedback regulation mechanism and enhance inflammatory response further [29]. Our study showed that celastrol could inhibit the activation of NF-κB and subsequently suppress signaling cascades that avoid the release of inflammatory response factors TNFα and IL-1β.

In the present study, TLR4/MyD88/NF-κB-mediated inflammatory pathways were activated during the progression of diabetic liver disease, resulting in macrophages and other killer cell chemotaxes and aggregation and celastrol could significantly attenuate liver inflammation immune response. But, as a limitation of this study, our approach is only an initial experiment in vivo; further studies will be required in vitro in order to explore its definite mechanisms, which should provide valuable insights into the development of new treatments for diabetic liver injury.

5. Conclusion

In summary, our study firstly confirmed that celastrol provided a protective effect against target organ damage in type 2 diabetes rats through inhibition of proinflammatory development in hepatic tissue. These findings suggest that the TLR4/MyD88/NF-κB signaling cascade pathways may be a useful new therapeutic target and celastrol is a promising

agent for the pharmacological treatment of diabetic liver injury.

Conflict of Interests

The authors have no conflict of interests to report regarding the publication of this paper.

Acknowledgment

This work was supported by grants from the National Natural Science Foundation of China (no. 81273915).

References

[1] D. G. Tiniakos, M. B. Vos, and E. M. Brunt, "Nonalcoholic fatty liver disease: pathology and pathogenesis," *Annual Review of Pathology: Mechanisms of Disease*, vol. 5, pp. 145–171, 2010.

[2] H. Tilg and A. R. Moschen, "Evolution of inflammation in non-alcoholic fatty liver disease: the multiple parallel hits hypothesis," *Hepatology*, vol. 52, no. 5, pp. 1836–1846, 2010.

[3] V. Bieghs and C. Trautwein, "Innate immune signaling and gut-liver interactions in non-alcoholic fatty liver disease," *Hepatobiliary Surgery and Nutrition*, vol. 3, no. 6, pp. 377–385, 2014.

[4] M. Ganz and G. Szabo, "Immune and inflammatory pathways in NASH," *Hepatology International*, vol. 7, no. 2, pp. 771–781, 2013.

[5] O. Takeuchi and S. Akira, "Pattern recognition receptors and inflammation," *Cell*, vol. 140, no. 6, pp. 805–820, 2010.

[6] N. Wang, H. Wang, H. Yao et al., "Expression and activity of the TLR4/NF-κB signaling pathway in mouse intestine following administration of a short-term high-fat diet," *Experimental and Therapeutic Medicine*, vol. 6, no. 3, pp. 635–640, 2013.

[7] H. Wang, Q. Zhang, Y. Chai et al., "1,25(OH)$_2$D$_3$ downregulates the Toll-like receptor 4-mediated inflammatory pathway and ameliorates liver injury in diabetic rats," *Journal of Endocrinological Investigation*, vol. 38, no. 10, pp. 1083–1091, 2015.

[8] R. G. Baker, M. S. Hayden, and S. Ghosh, "NF-κB, inflammation, and metabolic disease," *Cell Metabolism*, vol. 13, no. 1, pp. 11–22, 2011.

[9] G. C. Farrell, D. van Rooyen, L. Gan, and S. Chitturi, "NASH is an inflammatory disorder: pathogenic, prognostic and therapeutic implications," *Gut and Liver*, vol. 6, no. 2, pp. 149–171, 2012.

[10] L.-W. Chong, Y.-C. Hsu, Y.-T. Chiu, K.-C. Yang, and Y.-T. Huang, "Antifibrotic effects of triptolide on hepatic stellate cells and dimethylnitrosamine-intoxicated rats," *Phytotherapy Research*, vol. 25, no. 7, pp. 990–999, 2011.

[11] Y. Wang, Q. Tu, W. Yan et al., "CXCl95 suppresses proliferation and inflammatory response in LPS-induced human hepatocellular carcinoma cells via regulating TLR4-MyD88-TAK1-mediated NF-κB and MAPK pathway," *Biochemical and Biophysical Research Communications*, vol. 456, no. 1, pp. 373–379, 2015.

[12] P. P. Li, W. He, P. F. Yuan, S. S. Song, J. Lu, and W. Wei, "Celastrol induces mitochondria-mediated apoptosis in hepatocellular carcinoma Bel-7402 cells," *The American Journal of Chinese Medicine*, vol. 43, no. 1, pp. 137–148, 2015.

[13] S. Shrivastava, M. K. Jeengar, V. S. Reddy, G. B. Reddy, and V. Naidu, "Anticancer effect of celastrol on human triple negative breast cancer: possible involvement of oxidative stress, mitochondrial dysfunction, apoptosis and PI3K/Akt pathways," *Experimental and Molecular Pathology*, vol. 98, no. 3, pp. 313–327, 2015.

[14] Y. Wang, L. Cao, L. Xu et al., "Celastrol ameliorates EAE induction by suppressing pathogenic T cell responses in the peripheral and central nervous systems," *Journal of Neuroimmune Pharmacology*, vol. 10, no. 3, pp. 506–516, 2015.

[15] S. H. Venkatesha, B. Astry, S. M. Nanjundaiah, H. Yu, and K. D. Moudgil, "Suppression of autoimmune arthritis by Celastrus-derived Celastrol through modulation of pro-inflammatory chemokines," *Bioorganic & Medicinal Chemistry*, vol. 20, no. 17, pp. 5229–5234, 2012.

[16] C. Wang, C. Shi, X. Yang, M. Yang, H. Sun, and C. Wang, "Celastrol suppresses obesity process via increasing antioxidant capacity and improving lipid metabolism," *European Journal of Pharmacology*, vol. 744, pp. 52–58, 2015.

[17] J. E. Kim, M. H. Lee, D. H. Nam et al., "Celastrol, an NF-κB inhibitor, improves insulin resistance and attenuates renal injury in db/db mice," *PLoS ONE*, vol. 8, no. 4, Article ID e62068, 2013.

[18] D. A. Nugent, D. M. Smith, and H. B. Jones, "A review of islet of Langerhans degeneration in rodent models of type 2 diabetes," *Toxicologic Pathology*, vol. 36, no. 4, pp. 529–551, 2008.

[19] J. Liu, J. Lee, M. Salazar Hernandez, R. Mazitschek, and U. Ozcan, "Treatment of obesity with celastrol," *Cell*, vol. 161, no. 5, pp. 999–1011, 2015.

[20] S. Huang, J. M. Rutkowsky, R. G. Snodgrass et al., "Saturated fatty acids activate TLR-mediated proinflammatory signaling pathways," *Journal of Lipid Research*, vol. 53, no. 9, pp. 2002–2013, 2012.

[21] T. Csak, A. Velayudham, I. Hritz et al., "Deficiency in myeloid differentiation factor-2 and toll-like receptor 4 expression attenuates nonalcoholic steatohepatitis and fibrosis in mice," *American Journal of Physiology—Gastrointestinal and Liver Physiology*, vol. 300, no. 3, pp. G433–G441, 2011.

[22] A. Takaki, D. Kawai, and K. Yamamoto, "Molecular mechanisms and new treatment strategies for non-alcoholic steatohepatitis (NASH)," *International Journal of Molecular Sciences*, vol. 15, no. 5, pp. 7352–7379, 2014.

[23] A. Spruss, G. Kanuri, S. Wagnerberger, S. Haub, S. C. Bischoff, and I. Bergheim, "Toll-like receptor 4 is involved in the development of fructose-induced hepatic steatosis in mice," *Hepatology*, vol. 50, no. 4, pp. 1094–1104, 2009.

[24] K. Miura, Y. Kodama, S. Inokuchi et al., "Toll-like receptor 9 promotes steatohepatitis by induction of interleukin-1β in mice," *Gastroenterology*, vol. 139, no. 1, pp. 323.e7–334.e7, 2010.

[25] X. Sun, F. Han, J. Yi, L. Han, and B. Wang, "Effect of aspirin on the expression of hepatocyte NF-κB and serum TNF-α in streptozotocin-induced type 2 diabetic rats," *Journal of Korean Medical Science*, vol. 26, no. 6, pp. 765–770, 2011.

[26] V. Gangarapu, K. Yıldız, A. T. Ince, and B. Baysal, "Role of gut microbiota: obesity and NAFLD," *Turkish Journal of Gastroenterology*, vol. 25, no. 2, pp. 133–140, 2014.

[27] A. Dela Peña, I. Leclercq, J. Field, J. George, B. Jones, and G. Farrell, "NF-κB activation, rather than TNF, mediates hepatic inflammation in a murine dietary model of steatohepatitis," *Gastroenterology*, vol. 129, no. 5, pp. 1663–1674, 2005.

[28] S.-S. Dang, B.-F. Wang, Y.-A. Cheng, P. Song, Z.-G. Liu, and Z.-F. Li, "Inhibitory effects of saikosaponin-d on CCl4-induced hepatic fibrogenesis in rats," *World Journal of Gastroenterology*, vol. 13, no. 4, pp. 557–563, 2007.

[29] W. Z. Mehal, "The inflammasome in liver injury and non-alcoholic fatty liver disease," *Digestive Diseases*, vol. 32, no. 5, pp. 507–515, 2014.

6

Coupling of the Functional Stability of Rat Myocardium and Activity of Lipid Peroxidation in Combined Development of Postinfarction Remodeling and Diabetes Mellitus

S. A. Afanasiev, D. S. Kondratieva, T. Yu. Rebrova, R. E. Batalov, and S. V. Popov

Federal State Budgetary Scientific Institution "Research Institute for Cardiology", 111a Kievskaya Street, Tomsk 634012, Russia

Correspondence should be addressed to D. S. Kondratieva; dina@cardio-tomsk.ru

Academic Editor: Gregory Giamouzis

Coupling of the functional stability of rat myocardium and activity of lipid peroxidation processes in combined development of postinfarction remodeling and diabetes mellitus has been studied. The functional stability of myocardium was studied by means of the analysis of inotropic reaction on extrasystolic stimulus, the degree of left ventricular hypertrophy, and the size of scar zone. It was shown that in combined development of postinfarction cardiac remodeling of heart (PICR) with diabetes mellitus (DM) animal body weight decreased in less degree than in diabetic rats. Animals with combined pathology had no heart hypertrophy. The amplitude of extrasystolic contractions in rats with PICR combined with DM had no differences compared to the control group. In myocardium of rats with PICR combined with DM postextrasystolic potentiation was observed in contrast with the rats with PICR alone. The rats with combined pathology had the decreased value of TBA-active products. Thus, the results of study showed that induction of DM on the stage of the development of postinfarction remodeling increases adaptive ability of myocardium. It is manifested in inhibition of increase of LPO processes activity and maintaining of force-interval reactions of myocardium connected with calcium transport systems of sarcoplasmic reticulum of cardiomyocytes.

1. Introduction

Diabetes mellitus (DM) is one of the threatening factors which increases the risk of cardiovascular accidents during cardiovascular diseases [1]. Metabolic changes developing during diabetes mellitus aggravate disorders of functional state of cardiomyocytes in heart failure (HF) [2–4]. It is caused to a great extent by change of energy metabolism, which is an additional trigger of functional and structural disorders of heart muscle. In turn, remodeling of the cardiomyocyte membranes with advanced glycation end products and free radical oxidation is essential factor in development of diabetes mellitus [5, 6]. All these factors contribute to the disorder of electrical stability of membranes and the ionic balance of heart cells. These changes may define mainly cardiomyocyte contractility. The key structure, responding to intracellular transport of Ca^{2+} and, accordingly, to inotropic response of cardiomyocytes, is sarcoplasmic reticulum (SR) [7]. It has been shown that disorder of SR functions is accompanied by the inversion of force-frequency and force-interval dependences of myocardium [8, 9]. The interrelation between change of Ca^{2+} homeostasis in cardiomyocytes and progression of HF is revealed: disorder of intracellular Ca^{2+} transport precedes the depression of mechanical performance of heart [10–12].

An important role in disorder of ion transport systems of cardiomyocytes is played by lipid peroxidation (LPO) processes [13]. Intensification of LPO is nonspecific cell reaction to pathological actions. Development of HF and DM is accompanied with considerable increase of LPO activity [14, 15]. So, it is shown that LPO products act on lipid phase of membranes making it penetrable for hydrogen and calcium ions. It results in uncoupling of oxidative phosphorylation in mitochondria which leaves cell in the state of energy deficiency. At that state the excess amount of Ca^{2+} entering the cytoplasm is not able to be withdrawn from myoplasm and, subsequently, damages cellular structures.

In contrast to clinical data, which unambiguously points to the decrease of stability of diabetic heart to ischemia, results of experimental studies are sufficiently contradictory.

So, in number of researches one notes paradoxically high myocardial resistance to ischemia (in vivo and in vitro) in adult animals with short-term streptozotocin-induced diabetes [16–18]. Our preliminary study also revealed facts of the maintenance of the myocardial contractility in combined development of HF and DM. Mechanisms of this phenomenon remain subject for scientific research. States of Ca^{2+} transport systems of cardiomyocyte SR and activity of LPO processes in combined development of HF and DM have been studied insufficiently.

2. Materials and Methods

The study was performed on adult male Wistar rats 200–220 g. Four groups of animals were formed: first group consisted of intact rats ($n = 12$), second group of the rats with postinfarction cardiac remodeling (PICR) ($n = 11$), third group of the rats with induced DM ($n = 8$), and the IV group of the rats with DM induced 2 weeks after coronary occlusion ($n = 8$). By the time of the experiment all animals were of the same age. Myocardial infarction was induced by means of occlusion of the left anterior descending artery [19]; then the animals were housed under standard vivarium conditions. Diabetes mellitus was induced by single injection of 60 mg/kg dose of streptozotocin ("Sigma," USA) abdominally, diluted ex tempore with 0.01 M/L citrate buffer (pH 4.5). Rats of the IV group were taken in the experiment 6 weeks after induction of diabetes. Concentration of glucose in blood serum was defined by enzymatic-colorimetric test ("Biocon Diagnostic," Germany).

The development of heart and left ventricle hypertrophy was estimated by corresponding mass ratio [20]. For that reason the ratios of heart mass to animal body mass and left ventricle mass to heart mass were defined. Size of postinfarction scars of animal heart was estimated by the method of planimetry and calculated in percentages from area of free wall of left ventricle [21].

In the day of experiment animal blood has been sampled in a tube with heparin (10 : 1). Blood samples were centrifuged at 3000 rpm for 10 min. Obtained serum was dispensed for aliquots and stored in liquid nitrogen until the investigation moment.

Contractile activity was studied on papillary muscles. For that animals under Rausch-narcosis were immobilized with displacement of cervical region of the vertebral column and then their chests were opened. Isolated heart was washed in the specialized flow chamber through aorta with Krebs-Henseleit solution of the following composition (in mM): NaCl: 120; KCl: 4.8; $CaCl_2$: 2.0; $MgSO_4$: 1.2; KH_2PO_4: 1.2; $NaHCO_3$: 20.0; glucose: 10.0 ("Sigma," USA). Then, papillary muscles were isolated and placed in the temperature-stabilized (36°C) flow chamber. Perfusion of muscles has been performed with Krebs-Henseleit solution. Oxygenation of solution has been performed with carbogen (O_2: 95%, CO_2: 5%). Contractile activity of muscles was estimated in isometric mode, using "Force transducer KG-Series" transducer (Scientific Instruments GmbH, Germany). Tension developed by muscle calculated on diameter of isolated muscle (mN/mm^2) was estimated. Stimulation of muscles was performed with rectangular electrical pulses with duration of 5 ms and frequency of 0.5 Hz. Before the beginning of the research muscles had been adapted to the perfusion conditions and isometric mode in 60 minutes.

It is known that functional state of isolated myocardial strips can be estimated by changing the mode of their electrical stimulation. At extrasystolic impact, we registered extrasystolic contraction which characterizes excitability of sarcolemma [22] and postextrasystolic contraction which reflects the ability of cardiomyocyte sarcoplasmic reticulum (SR) to accumulate Ca^{2+} ions which additionally enter the myoplasm at extraordinary excitation and define amplitude of postextrasystolic contractions [22]. In our work, extrasystolic impact was made by additional single electrical pulse on 0.2, 0.225, 0.25, 0.5, 0.75, 1.0, and 1.5 s (extrasystolic interval) from the beginning of the regular cycle. Amplitudes of extrasystolic (ES) and postextrasystolic (PES) contraction were expressed as percentages of the amplitude of regular (basic) cycle. We analyzed the dependence of changes of ES and PES contraction amplitude on the duration of extrasystolic interval.

LPO activity in blood serum was estimated by measuring the concentration of TBA-active products (TBAAP) acquired in reaction with 2-thiobarbituric acid (TBA) [23]. The concentration of primary products of LPO-dien conjugates (DC) was measured in the hexane extracts of serum samples with spectrophotometer at 232 nm [24].

Data is presented in the form of median and interquartile range (Me (Q1; Q3)). Student's criterion has been used for normal distribution of values. Study data is presented as M ± SD, where M is mean value and SD is standard deviation. Reliability of differences of obtained data was estimated using Mann-Whitney U test for independent samples in the case of distribution which differs from normal one. Differences at value $p < 0.05$ have been considered statistically significant.

3. Results and Discussion

Results reflecting values of mass indices obtained in considered groups are presented in Table 1. It can be seen that the animals with PICR (the II group) had decreased (on 18.8%) body weight and hypertrophied (on 90%) heart compared to those of intact animals. Induction of diabetes (the III group) led to decreased animal body weight by 56%, $p < 0.05$, but in this case without heart hypertrophy. In combined development of PICR with DM (the IV group), animal body weight was 26% less than the one of the animals from the I group. These animals as well as the animals in the III groups did not have heart hypertrophy. It appeared that size of scar zone in II and IV groups did not differ. Blood glucose level of the animals of III and IV groups exceeded that of intact rats by 4.5 and 3 times, accordingly.

In our study, the remodeling of myocardium both after coronary artery occlusion (the II group) and after development of hyperglycemia (the III group) led to a change in inotropic reaction of papillary muscles on extrasystolic actions compared to the control group (Figure 1). So, amplitude of ES contractions of papillary muscles of the PICR

TABLE 1: Body and heart weights of rats after coronary artery occlusion and diabetes induction.

Number	Group	n	Body weight, g	Glucose, mol/L	Heart weight/body weight, mg/g	Left ventricle weight/heart weight, mg/mg	Scar area, %
I	Control	12	298 ± 23.7	6 ± 0.37	3.29 ± 0.21	0.645 ± 0.013	—
II	PICR	11	$242 \pm 11.17^{***\#}$	$7 \pm 0.13^{\#}$	$6.27 \pm 0.33^{***\#}$	$0.687 \pm 0.016^{**}$	51.3 ± 8.9
III	DM	8	$160 \pm 14.8^{*}$	$27 \pm 2.75^{*}$	3.77 ± 0.31	0.676 ± 0.014	—
IV	PICR + DM	8	$221 \pm 4.51^{*}$	$18 \pm 1.79^{*}$	3.37 ± 0.11	0.673 ± 0.019	46.1 ± 2.7

Note. PICR: rats with postinfarction cardiac remodeling. $^{*}p < 0.01$, $^{**}p < 0.05$ compared with control, $^{\#}p < 0.05$ compared with PICR. Scar area was calculated as a percentage from area of free wall of left ventricle.

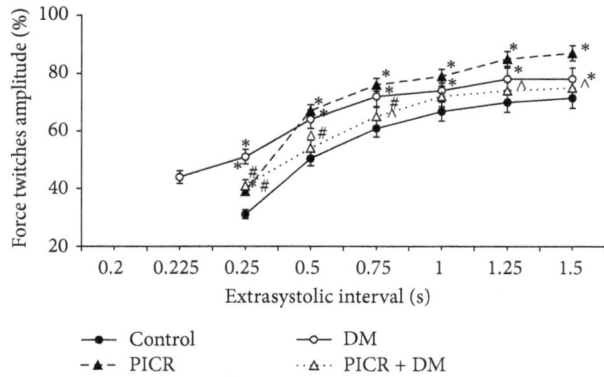

FIGURE 1: Extrasystolic contractions of papillary muscles of rats with postinfarction heart failure and diabetes mellitus. Note: the force twitches amplitude expressed in percentage of base contraction. $^{*}p < 0.001$ compared with control, $^{\#}p < 0.05$ compared with DM, and $^{\wedge}p < 0.05$ compared with PICR.

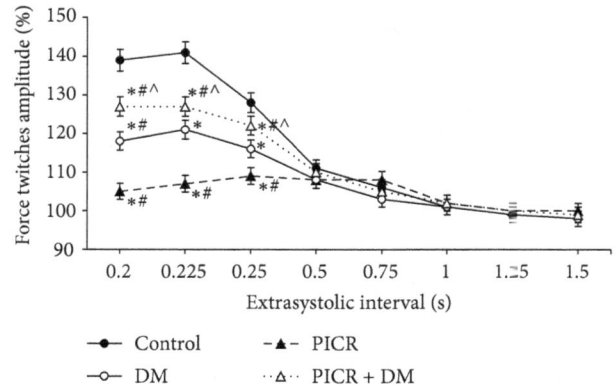

FIGURE 2: Postextrasystolic contractions of papillary muscles of rats with postinfarction heart failure and diabetes mellitus Note: $^{*}p < 0.001$ compared with control, $^{\#}p < 0.05$ compared with DM, and $^{\wedge}p < 0.05$ compared with PICR.

rats (the II group) on short extrasystolic intervals was 8% higher than that of intact animals ($p < 0.05$). After the longest ES interval, this difference increased and reached 16% ($p < 0.05$). Amplitude increase of ES contractions of papillary muscles of PICR testifies the increased intracellular amount of Ca^{2+} taking part in ES contraction. It is known that ischemic damage of heart is characterized by the suppression of ATP-sensitive processes including the work of intracellular ion transport systems. It leads to the increase in intracellular concentrations of Na^{+} and Ca^{2+} [25–27]. ES contractions of papillary muscles of the rats from the III group have their own peculiarities. So, independent ES contraction appeared already at ES interval of 0.225 s. In the rest of the groups ES contraction appeared only at ES interval of 0.25 s. It is known that ES action causes inotropic response only if it happens in the phase of relative refractivity [22]. From these positions result obtained in the III group shows that development of diabetes leads to a shortened phase of absolute refractivity and hence to an increased excitability of cardiomyocytes. The fact that the amplitude of ES contractions in the III group on short extrasystolic intervals was 20% higher than that in the I group (intact animals) testifies in favor of that. At long intervals these differences decreased to 7% (Figure 1).

Result obtained by studying the IV group differs from the case of II or III group. In case of combined development of ischemic and diabetic damage of myocardium we obtained

essentially less manifested change of ES contraction dynamics.

It is known that stimulating pulse which falls on the 3rd phase of action potential is not able to induce contractile response. However, it initiates additional income of external calcium ions in the myoplasm. This Ca^{2+} is accumulated in SR and takes part in the first PES cycle of contraction-relaxation [22]. For this reason amplitude of PES contraction exceeds amplitude of regular cycle. In our research extraordinary impetus at ES interval of 0.2 s did not cause ES contraction of the myocardium of intact rats (the I group). But we registered 39% increase of PES contraction amplitude compared to the amplitude of regular contraction (Figure 2). With appearance of ES contraction and increase of its amplitude we observed decrease of ES contraction amplitude. For intact animals PES potentiation of contraction was absent on the longest ES intervals (Figure 2).

As we can see from Figure 2 in the II group of rats PES potentiation of contraction of papillary muscles was not observed no matter what the duration of ES interval was. This fact can testify essential decrease of Ca^{2+} storing function of SR. Probably, in conditions of postinfarction remodeling of rat myocardium the function of Ca^{2+} transport systems of SR is damaged [11, 28, 29]. While studying the papillary muscles of the rats of the III group, PES potentiation of contraction was essentially lower than in the I group (intact animals) and was 21–16% (Figure 2). In combined postinfarction and

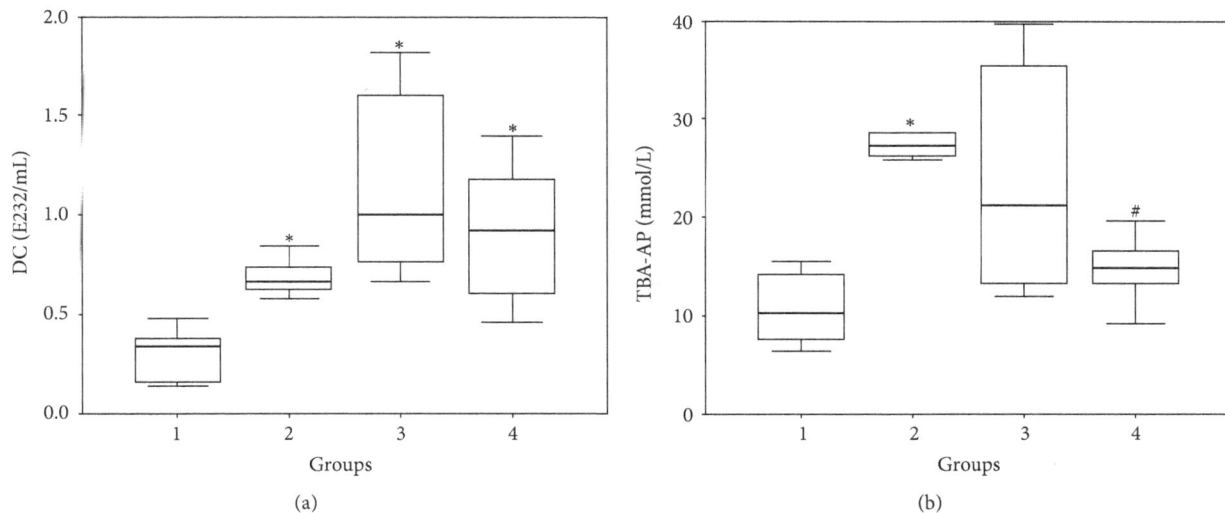

FIGURE 3: Concentration of DC (a) and TBA-AP (b) in blood plasma of the experimental animals (Me (Q1; Q3)). Note: (1) group: control, (2) group: PICR, (3) group: DM, and (4) groups: PICR + DM. $^*p < 0.01$ compared with group 1 (control) and $^\#p < 0.01$ compared with group 2 (PICR).

diabetic remodeling of myocardium (IV group) on the short ES intervals, the increase in PES contraction was 27–19% (Figure 2). This result testifies maintenance of Ca^{2+} storing ability of SR.

It is known that higher activity of peroxidation process is important component of damage of cardiomyocytes due to myocardium infarction [30]. Alteration of the lipid bilayer of membranes with oxygen radicals is considered to be one of the mechanisms of distortion of intracellular Ca^{2+} homeostasis and contractile activity of cardiomyocytes. Previously we have shown that higher activity of LPO is also maintained during postinfarction remodeling of heart. Moreover, in simulation of PICR, the dynamics of changes in LPO, the products (TBAAP and DC) in myocardial tissue, and blood serum of rats coincided [31]. On this basis it is possible to define TBAAP and DC concentration in blood serum and to extrapolate it on myocardium.

It is known that activation of free radical oxidation of lipids is also noted at DM [15]. Data obtained at determination of TBAAP and DC concentration in blood serum of animals included in the present research is presented in Figure 3. It can be seen that the PICR animals blood (the II group) contained reliably more LPO products than the intact animal group. Simulation of DM (the III group) also promoted reliable increase of TBAAP and DC concentration. Intensified generation of active oxygen forms and activation of LPO processes at the following pathologies is known fact and is noted in the works of many authors [13–15]. Active oxygen forms in pathologically high concentrations go into reaction and damage both lipids and proteins of cellular membranes and components of blood serum. Literature contains data about decreased activity of proteins and enzymes including Ca^{2+}-ATPase of cardiomyocytes [13] in pathologies accompanying activation of free radical processes. These results are quite matched with data obtained at estimation of inotropic reaction of papillary muscles of the animals of

II and III groups on extrasystolic action. This reaction can be a consequence of decrease in activity of Ca^{2+}-ATPase and contractile proteins as the result of structural damage caused by active forms of oxygen, violation of lipid bilayer of membrane, and leakage of Ca^{2+} from sarcoplasmic reticulum.

Combining development of PICR and DM in theory should cause more manifested LPO activation. However, for animals with combined pathology (the IV group) we obtained paradoxical result. Thus, the value of TBAAP appeared reliably lower than in the II group. Also, the downward trend in DC concentration takes place. Obtained data is well-matched with the results characterizing contractile ability of papillary muscles of the animals of the IV group. Decreased TBAAP concentration testifies the decreased intensity of passing of concluding stages of lipid peroxidation reaction. The fact of negligible decrease in DC testifies that intensity of the first LPO stages remains on sufficiently high level. Metabolites of fat acids forming on these stages can take part in formation of other LPO products [32].

Our data testify that induction of diabetes on the background of postinfarction remodeling paradoxically promotes maintaining functional activity of Ca^{2+} transport systems of SR. It may be connected with the fact that glycosylation products increase rigidity of cardiomyocytes membranes on the background of developing hyperglycemia. Enhancement of adaptive reactions at combined development of postinfarction and diabetic damage of myocardium can be connected with peculiarities of intracellular energy metabolism at given pathological states. So, increase of glucose level during the first stages of development of postinfarction cardiosclerosis allows activating glycolysis processes in cardiomyocytes. It is known that positive effect of glucose on the heart functioning in the experimental myocardial ischemia is connected with increase of glycolytic production of ATP [33, 34]. In combination with inhibition of LPO activity, shift of energy metabolism to glycolytic production of ATP can help to obtain higher functional activity of Ca^{2+} transport system of SR at combined pathology. Data obtained by us corresponds to the results of other researchers. So, it was shown that ATP which is formed in glycolysis process is the irreplaceable source of energy for Ca^{2+} transport system of SR [35]. Increase of ischemic resistivity of myocardium was described for animals with short term of streptozotocin stimulated diabetes in vivo and in vitro [16, 36].

Thus, results of present study showed that in the experimental conditions induction of DM on the stage of formation of postinfarction remodeling increases adaptive ability of myocardium. It is manifested in inhibition of increase in LPO processes activity and maintaining of force-interval reactions of myocardium connected with calcium transport systems of cardiomyocyte SR.

Conflict of Interests

The authors declare that there is no conflict of interests regarding the publication of this paper.

References

[1] M. J. Garcia, P. M. McNamara, T. Gordon, and W. B. Kannell, "Morbidity and mortality in diabetics in the Framingham population. Sixteen year follow up study," *Diabetes*, vol. 23, no. 2, pp. 105–111, 1974.

[2] S. Boudina, S. Sena, H. Theobald et al., "Mitochondrial energetics in the heart in obesity-related diabetes: direct evidence for increased uncoupled respiration and activation of uncoupling proteins," *Diabetes*, vol. 56, no. 10, pp. 2457–2466, 2007.

[3] J. Buchanan, P. K. Mazumder, P. Hu et al., "Reduced cardiac efficiency and altered substrate metabolism precedes the onset of hyperglycemia and contractile dysfunction in two mouse models of insulin resistance and obesity," *Endocrinology*, vol. 146, no. 12, pp. 5341–5349, 2005.

[4] S.-Y. Li, X. Yang, A. F. Ceylan-Isik, M. Du, N. Sreejayan, and J. Ren, "Cardiac contractile dysfunction in Lep/Lep obesity is accompanied by NADPH oxidase activation, oxidative modification of sarco(endo)plasmic reticulum Ca^{2+}-ATPase and myosin heavy chain isozyme switch," *Diabetologia*, vol. 49, no. 6, pp. 1434–1446, 2006.

[5] A. Ziegelhöffer, I. Waczulíková, M. Ferko, L. Šikurová, J. Mujkošová, and T. Ravingerová, "Involvement of membrane fluidity in endogenous protective processes running on subcellular membrane systems of the rat heart," *Physiological Research*, vol. 61, supplement 2, pp. S11–S21, 2012.

[6] B. Ziegelhöffer-Mihalovičová, I. Waczulíková, L. Šikurová, J. Styk, J. Čársky, and A. Ziegelhöffer, "Remodelling of the sarcolemma in diabetic rat hearts: the role of membrane fluidity," *Molecular and Cellular Biochemistry*, vol. 249, no. 1-2, pp. 175–182, 2003.

[7] A. T. Roe, M. Frisk, and W. E. Louch, "Targeting cardiomyocyte Ca^{2+} homeostasis in heart failure," *Current Pharmaceutical Design*, vol. 21, no. 4, pp. 431–448, 2014.

[8] R. R. Lamberts, N. Hamdani, T. W. Soekhoe et al., "Frequency-dependent myofilament Ca^{2+} desensitization in failing rat myocardium," *The Journal of Physiology*, vol. 582, no. 2, pp. 695–709, 2007.

[9] S. V. Popov, D. S. Kondratieva, S. A. Afanasiev, and B. N. Kozlov, "Changes in mechanical restitution of isolated myocardium in patients with ischemic heart disease and diabetes mellitus," *Frontiers in Pathology and Genetics*, vol. 1, no. 3, pp. 25–29, 2013.

[10] I. A. Hobai and B. O'Rourke, "Decreased sarcoplasmic reticulum calcium content is responsible for defective excitation-contraction coupling in canine heart failure," *Circulation*, vol. 103, no. 11, pp. 1577–1584, 2001.

[11] S. E. Lehnart, L. S. Maier, and G. Hasenfuss, "Abnormalities of calcium metabolism and myocardial contractility depression in the failing heart," *Heart Failure Reviews*, vol. 14, no. 4, pp. 213–224, 2009.

[12] Q. Lou, V. V. Fedorov, A. V. Glukhov, N. Moazami, V. G. Fast, and I. R. Efimov, "Transmural heterogeneity and remodeling of human ventricular excitation-contraction coupling in human heart failure," *Circulation*, vol. 123, no. 17, pp. 1881–1890, 2011.

[13] A. C. Köhler, C. M. Sag, and L. S. Maier, "Reactive oxygen species and excitation-contraction coupling in the context of cardiac pathology," *Journal of Molecular and Cellular Cardiology*, vol. 73, pp. 92–102, 2014.

[14] H. Tsutsui, S. Kinugawa, and S. Matsushima, "Oxidative stress and heart failure," *The American Journal of Physiology—Heart and Circulatory Physiology*, vol. 301, no. 6, pp. H2181–H2190, 2011.

[15] D. Wu, C.-X. Gong, X. Meng, and Q.-L. Yang, "Correlation between blood glucose fluctuations and activation of oxidative stress in type 1 diabetic children during the acute metabolic disturbance period," *Chinese Medical Journal*, vol. 126, no. 21, pp. 4019–4022, 2013.

[16] H. Chen, W.-L. Shen, X.-H. Wang et al., "Paradoxically enhanced heart tolerance to ischaemia in type 1 diabetes and role of increased osmolarity," *Clinical and Experimental Pharmacology and Physiology*, vol. 33, no. 10, pp. 910–916, 2006.

[17] T. Ravingerová, A. Adameová, J. Matejíková et al., "Subcellular mechanisms of adaptation in the diabetic myocardium: relevance to ischemic preconditioning in the nondiseased heart," *Experimental & Clinical Cardiology*, vol. 15, no. 4, pp. 68–76, 2010.

[18] I. Waczulíková, A. Ziegelhöffer, Z. Országhová, and J. Čársky, "Fluidising effect of resorcylidene aminoguanidine on sarcolemmal membranes in streptozotocin-diabetic rats: blunted adaptation of diabetic myocardium to Ca^{2+} overload," *Journal of Physiology and Pharmacology*, vol. 53, no. 4, part 2, pp. 727–739, 2002.

[19] D. S. Kondrat'eva, S. A. Afanas'ev, and S. V. Popov, "Expression of Ca^{2+}-ATPase in sarcoplasmic reticulum in rat cardiomyocytes during experimental postinfarction cardiosclerosis and diabetes mellitus," *Bulletin of Experimental Biology and Medicine*, vol. 156, no. 6, pp. 750–752, 2014.

[20] N. Satoh, T. Sato, M. Shimada, K. Yamada, and Y. Kitada, "Lusitropic effect of MCC-135 is associated with improvement of sarcoplasmic reticulum function in ventricular muscles of rats with diabetic cardiomyopathy," *Journal of Pharmacology and Experimental Therapeutics*, vol. 298, no. 3, pp. 1161–1166, 2001.

[21] M. A. Usacheva, E. V. Popkova, E. A. Smirnova, V. A. Saltykova, and L. M. Belkina, "Adaptation of the cardiovascular system to postinfarction cardiosclerosis in rats with congenital adrenoreactivity of the myocardium," *Bulletin of Experimental Biology and Medicine*, vol. 144, no. 6, pp. 775–779, 2007.

[22] D. V. Vassallo, E. Q. Lima, P. Campagnaro, A. N. Faria, and J. G. Mill, "Mechanisms underlying the genesis of post-extrasystolic

potentiation in rat cardiac muscle," *Brazilian Journal of Medical and Biological Research*, vol. 28, no. 3, pp. 377–383, 1995.

[23] E. N. Korobeinikova, "Modification of the definition of lipid peroxidation products in the reaction with thiobarbituric acid," *Laboratory Work*, no. 7, pp. 8–10, 1989.

[24] J. L. Bolland and H. P. Koch, "The course of antioxidant reaction in polyisoprenes and allied compounds. Part IX. The primary thermal oxidation product of ethyl linoleate," *Journal of the Chemical Society*, no. 7, pp. 445–447, 1945.

[25] J. Inserte, D. Garcia-Dorado, V. Hernando, I. Barba, and J. Soler-Soler, "Ischemic preconditioning prevents calpain-mediated impairment of Na^+/K^+-ATPase activity during early reperfusion," *Cardiovascular Research*, vol. 70, no. 2, pp. 364–373, 2006.

[26] R. Sniecinski and H. Liu, "Reduced efficacy of volatile anesthetic preconditioning with advanced age in isolated rat myocardium," *Anesthesiology*, vol. 100, no. 3, pp. 589–597, 2004.

[27] K. Tanonaka, K. Motegi, T. Arino, T. Marunouchi, N. Takagi, and S. Takeo, "Possible pathway of Na^+ flux into mitochondria in ischemic heart," *Biological and Pharmaceutical Bulletin*, vol. 35, no. 10, pp. 1661–1668, 2012.

[28] S. E. Lehnart, X. H. T. Wehrens, A. Kushnir, and A. R. Marks, "Cardiac ryanodine receptor function and regulation in heart disease," *Annals of the New York Academy of Sciences*, vol. 1015, pp. 144–159, 2004.

[29] J. Palomeque, M. V. Petroff, L. Sapia, O. A. Gende, C. Mundiña-Weilenmann, and A. Mattiazzi, "Multiple alterations in Ca^{2+} handling determine the negative staircase in a cellular heart failure model," *Journal of Cardiac Failure*, vol. 13, no. 2, pp. 143–154, 2007.

[30] M. K. Misra, M. Sarwat, P. Bhakuni, R. Tuteja, and N. Tuteja, "Oxidative stress and ischemic myocardial syndromes," *Medical Science Monitor*, vol. 15, no. 10, pp. RA209–RA219, 2009.

[31] T. I. Rebrova, D. S. Kondrat'eva, S. A. Afanas'ev, and E. I. Barzakh, "Activity of lipid peroxidation and functional state of the myocardium in remodeling of rat heart after experimental myocardial infarction," *Kardiologiia*, vol. 47, no. 6, pp. 41–45, 2007.

[32] C. Schneider, "An update on products and mechanisms of lipid peroxidation," *Molecular Nutrition & Food Research*, vol. 53, no. 3, pp. 315–321, 2009.

[33] H. Ardehali, H. N. Sabbah, M. A. Burke et al., "Targeting myocardial substrate metabolism in heart failure: potential for new therapies," *European Journal of Heart Failure*, vol. 14, no. 2, pp. 120–129, 2012.

[34] T. Doenst, T. D. Nguyen, and E. D. Abel, "Cardiac metabolism in heart failure: implications beyond ATP production," *Circulation Research*, vol. 113, no. 6, pp. 709–724, 2013.

[35] A. V. Zima, J. Kockskämper, and L. A. Blatter, "Cytosolic energy reserves determine the effect of glycolytic sugar phosphates on sarcoplasmic reticulum Ca^{2+} release in cat ventricular myocytes," *Journal of Physiology*, vol. 577, no. 1, pp. 281–293, 2006.

[36] T. Nawata, N. Takahashi, T. Ooie, K. Kaneda, T. Saikawa, and T. Sakata, "Cardioprotection by streptozotocin-induced diabetes and insulin against ischemia/reperfusion injury in rats," *Journal of Cardiovascular Pharmacology*, vol. 40, no. 4, pp. 491–500, 2002.

7

Association between Self-Reported Habitual Snoring and Diabetes Mellitus: A Systemic Review and Meta-Analysis

Xiaolu Xiong,[1] Anyuan Zhong,[2] Huajun Xu,[3] and Chun Wang[4]

[1]Department of Endocrinology, Drum Tower Clinical Medical College of Nanjing Medical University,
53 North Zhongshan Road, Nanjing 210008, China
[2]Department of Respiratory Diseases, The Second Affiliated Hospital of Soochow University, 1055 Sanxiang Road,
Suzhou 215004, China
[3]Department of Otolaryngology, Shanghai Jiao Tong University Affiliated Sixth People's Hospital,
Otolaryngology Institute of Shanghai Jiao Tong University, 600 Yishan Road, Shanghai 200233, China
[4]Department of Geriatrics, Drum Tower Clinical Medical College of Nanjing Medical University, 53 North Zhongshan Road,
Nanjing 210008, China

Correspondence should be addressed to Huajun Xu; sunnydayxu2010@sjtu.edu.cn and Chun Wang; wcglyy@163.com

Academic Editor: Geoff Werstuck

Aim. Several studies have reported an association between self-reported habitual snoring and diabetes mellitus (DM); however, the results are inconsistent. *Methods*. Electronic databases including PubMed and EMBASE were searched. Odds ratios (ORs) and 95% confidence intervals (CIs) were used to assess the strength of the association between snoring and DM using a random-effects model. Heterogeneity, subgroup, and sensitivity analyses were also evaluated. Begg's, Egger's tests and funnel plots were used to evaluate publication bias. *Results*. A total of eight studies (six cross sectional and two prospective cohort studies) pooling 101,246 participants were included. Of the six cross sectional studies, the summary OR and 95% CI of DM in individuals that snore compared with nonsnorers were 1.37 (95% CI: 1.20–1.57, $p < 0.001$). There was no heterogeneity across the included studies ($I^2 = 2.9\%$, $p = 0.408$). When stratified by gender, the pooled OR (95% CI) was 1.59 (1.20–2.11) in females ($n = 12298$), and 0.89 (0.65–1.22) in males ($n = 4276$). Of the two prospective studies, the pooled RR was 1.65 (95% CI, 1.30–2.08). *Conclusions*. Self-reported habitual snoring is statistically associated with DM in females, but not in males. This meta-analysis indicates a need to paying attention to the effect of snoring on the occurrence of DM in females.

1. Introduction

Diabetes mellitus (DM) is becoming a major global public health problem. Compared with 1980s, the proportion of diabetes of both men (9.8% versus 8.3%) and women (9.2% versus 7.5%) increased in 2008 [1]. It is worthwhile to note that over 438 million individuals are expected to be at risk of developing DM by 2030 [2]. Besides its high prevalence, growing research also suggests that DM could induce adverse health implication [3, 4]. Similarly, habitual snoring is a common and early symptom of obstructive sleep apnea (OSA) and affects ~33% of the general population [5]. Snoring has long been considered a nuisance especially for bed partners and brought social burden (i.e., traffic accident and poor school performance) [6–8]. An increasing amount of evidence has also suggested that habitual snoring might be associated with health-related complications, including endothelial dysfunction, vascular injury, stroke, and cardiovascular diseases [6, 9–12].

Many studies have assessed the association between self-reported habitual snoring and DM. However, conflicting results have been reported. Importantly, habitual snoring might help doctors identify individuals at a higher risk of developing DM. Therefore, the relationship between these two common diseases should be evaluated comprehensively.

To our knowledge, a quantitative analysis evaluating the association between self-reported habitual snoring and DM susceptibility is not available. Thus, it is essential to perform a meta-analysis to clarify this potential association. The purpose of the current study was to identify the association between self-reported snoring and DM by performing pooled risk estimates.

2. Materials and Methods

We performed this meta-analysis according to the recommendations of Meta-analysis Of Observational Studies in Epidemiology (MOOSE) statement [13].

2.1. Literature Search Strategy. To identify studies that assessed the relationship between self-reported snoring and susceptibility to DM, we searched electronic databases systemically, including PubMed and EMBASE in May 2015. No language and human study restriction were imposed. The following combinations of MeSH terms and text word terms were used (snoring or snorer or self-reported snoring) and (diabetes or diabetic or diabetes mellitus or hyperglycemia). We also checked the reference lists of relevant articles that might be appropriate for inclusion in the meta-analysis. The searches were conducted by Drs. Xiong and Zhong, respectively.

2.2. Inclusion and Exclusion Criteria. Studies that met the following criteria were included: (1) studies that evaluated self-reported snoring and the risk of DM; (2) prospective observational, retrospective, cohort, cross-sectional, or case-controlled studies; (3) subjects without a diagnosis of DM at baseline or who were excluded from the final statistical analysis; (4) odds ratios (ORs) or risk ratios (RRs) and 95% confidence intervals (CIs) which were provided for comparing snorers to nonsnorers; (5) snoring status which was defined using the question "To the best of your knowledge, do you snore now or have you snored previously?" and habitual snoring which was defined by each study; (6) the definition of diabetes which was mainly according to a history of diagnosis made by a physician, fasting serum glucose levels, oral glucose tolerance test (OGTT), or the use of medicine to treat DM. Studies were excluded if (1) it was not a full-text paper (i.e., no reviews, abstracts, letters, or comments); (2) snoring was not measured using a questionnaire; (3) it analyzed subjects with gestational diabetes mellitus; (4) no variables were adjusted.

2.3. Data Extraction. Two authors (Drs. Xiong and Zhong) extracted the data from the included studies to a standard sheet independently. The data extracted includes the first author and year of publication, country of origin, source of the study, study design, sample size, percentage of female participants, age range, OR or RR with 95% CI, adjusted variables, the measurement used to assess snoring, and the diagnosis of DM. If there were discrepancies in the basic information of the included studies, a third reviewer (Dr. Xu) examined the inconsistent extracted data. If there were additional queries or if further details were needed, the authors of the original studies were contacted via email.

2.4. Quality Assessment. The methodological quality of all included studies was assessed according to the Newcastle-Ottawa scale (NOS) guidelines (http://www.ohri.ca/programs/clinical_epidemiology/oxford.asp). A study was awarded a maximum of one star for each numbered item within the selection and outcome categories. Therefore, a maximum of four, three, and two stars were given for selection, outcome, and comparability, respectively. More stars indicated a higher quality study. We recognized one star as one score, and the score of each study was presented in Table 1.

2.5. Statistical Analysis. ORs, RRs, and 95% CIs were used to assess the relationship between self-reported snoring and DM across the included studies. The ORs were transformed into RRs using the formula $RR = OR/[(1 - P_o) + (P_o * OR)]$ (P_o is the incidence of the outcome of interest in the nonexposed group). If an included study reported various adjustments for covariates, the most fully adjusted OR/RR was used in pooled analysis. Heterogeneity was examined using Cochrane Q tests and the I^2 statistic [14]. If between-study heterogeneity existed ($p < 0.10$ or $I^2 > 50\%$), a random-effects model was used; otherwise a fixed-effect model was applied [15]. Subgroup analysis was performed to assess the effect of significant group differences according to gender. Sensitivity analysis was performed to test the robustness of the results by omitting one study each time. Potential publication bias was assessed using Begg's rank correlation and Egger linear regression tests [16]. Unless stated otherwise, $p < 0.05$ was considered to be statistically significant. All the above-mentioned statistical analyses were performed using the STATA software (version 12.0, Stata Corp., College Station, TX, USA).

3. Results

3.1. Literature Search Results. A total of 497 potentially relevant references were retrieved from the PubMed and EMBASE databases. 31 duplicates were removed. After first reviewing the titles and abstracts, 449 studies were further excluded for various reasons. The remaining 17 papers were reviewed fully, and a further nine reported papers were excluded for evaluating self-reported snoring and gestational DM ($n = 5$), self-reported snoring and metabolic syndrome ($n = 2$), and self-reported snoring and hemoglobin A1c levels, glucose, and insulin metabolism ($n = 2$). Finally, eight studies were enrolled in the qualitative synthesis, among which six were included in the meta-analysis. The detailed search process is presented in Figure 1.

3.2. Characteristics of the Included Studies. A total of eight studies (including six cross-sectional and two prospective cohort studies) pooling 101,246 participants were included. The mean age of the participants at baseline ranged from 20 to 85 years. The percentage of female subjects ranged from 48.8% to 100%, except for one study that enrolled only male subjects. Three of the included studies were performed in the United States [17, 22, 23], three were conducted in Sweden [1, 18, 21], and one was undertaken in each of Finland [19]

TABLE 1: Characteristics of included studies in this meta-analysis.

(a)

First author Year	Country	Source and study type	Sample size	Female (%)	Age range	OR or RR (95% CI)	Adjusted variables
Sabanayagam 2012 [17]	America	Population-based Cross-sectional	6522	48.8	20–85	1.44 (1.16–1.79)[a]	Age, sex, ethnicity, education, smoking, alcohol, physical activity, BMI, depression, SBP, CRP, and TC
Valham 2009 [18]	Sweden	Population-based Cross-sectional	7905	51.2	25–79	Female: 1.58 (1.02–2.44)[a] Male: 0.92 (0.64–1.33)[a]	Smoking, age, BMI, and waist circumference
Renko 2005 [19]	Finland	Population-based Cross-sectional	593	58.7	61–63	1.93 (1.04–3.57)[a]	Age, weight gain, smoking, alcohol dependence, and physical inactivity
Marchesini 2004 [20]	Italy	Population-based Cross-sectional	1890	78	20–65	1.31 (0.95–1.81)[a] Female: 1.62 (1.11–2.36)[a] Male: 0.81 (0.45–1.50)[a]	Age, sex, and BMI
Lindberg 2007 [21]	Sweden	Population-based Cross-sectional	6779	100%	20–99	No EDS: 1.36 (0.87–2.13)[a] EDS: 1.82 (0.97–3.43)[a]	Age, BMI, smoking, physical activity, and alcohol dependency
Enright 1996 [22]	America	Population-based Cross-sectional	5201	57%	≥65	Women: 1.34 (0.10–1.65)[a]	Age and being married
Al-Delaimy 2002 [23]	America	Population-based Prospective cohort	69852	100%	40–65	1.63 (1.29–2.07)[b]	Age, high TC, high BP, smoking, BMI, physical activity, alcohol use, postmenopausal hormone use, family history of diabetes, sleeping position, sleep time, years of shift-work, and WHR
Elmasry 2000 [1]	Sweden	Population-based Prospective cohort	2504	0%	30–69	Nonobese: 1.06 (0.36–3.1)[a] Obese: 7.0 (2.9–16.9)[a]	Age, weight gain, smoking, alcohol dependence, and physical inactivity

(b)

Definition of snoring	Assessment/definition of DM	Presence of comorbidities	NOS score
Questionnaire answer: never or rare, occasionally as nonhabitual snorers; frequently as habitual snorers	Serum glucose ≥ 126 mg/dL after fasting for a minimum of 8 hours, a plasma glucose ≥ 200 mg/dL for those who fasted <8 hours or HbA1c ≥ 6.5%, a self-reported DM or current use of oral hypoglycemic medication or insulin	(—)	7
Questionnaire answer: always or often as habitual snorers; sometimes, never, or almost never as nonhabitual snorers	Questionnaire answer: "Do you suffer from DM?"	(—)	8
Questionnaire answer: those who reported snoring every or almost every night were classified as habitual snorers	Previously diagnosed DM, OGTT according to WHO criteria in 1998	(—)	7
Questionnaire answer: occasional or habitual as habitual snorers	Previously diagnosed DM, OGTT according to WHO criteria in 1998	Hypertension, hyperlipidemia	7
Questionnaire answer: how often they snored using a five-point scale; snoring was defined as a score of 3–5	Questionnaire answer: "Do you have diabetes?" and/or attended regular medical examinations for diabetes	Hypertension	7
Questionnaire answer: yes or no or don't know; yes as habitual snorers	History of DM, current use of insulin or oral hypoglycemic medication, fasting glucose ≥ 140 mg/dL, or 2-hour postload glucose ≥ 200 mg/dL.	Hypertension, carotid disease, and arthritis	7
Questionnaire answer: regularly as habitual snorers; occasionally or never	Classic symptoms associated with an elevated plasma glucose level or no symptoms, but at least two elevated plasma glucose values on different occasions; or treatment with hypoglycemic medication	(—)	8
Questionnaire answer: a five-point scale: ≥4 was defined as habitual snorers; ≤3 was defined as nonhabitual snorers	Questionnaire: self-report DM or confirmed by medical records	(—)	8

OR, odds ratio; RR, risk ratio; BMI, body mass index; SBP, systolic blood pressure; CRP, C reactive protein; TC, cholesterol; BP, blood pressure; DM, diabetes mellitus; HbA1c, glycosylated hemoglobin; OGTT, oral glucose tolerance test; WHO, World Health Organization; NOS: Newcastle-Ottawa scale. Note: a means studies report OR, while b means study reports RR.

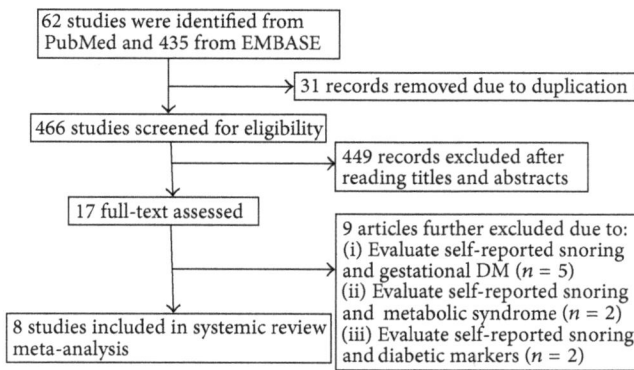

FIGURE 1: Flow chart of the literature search and study selection process.

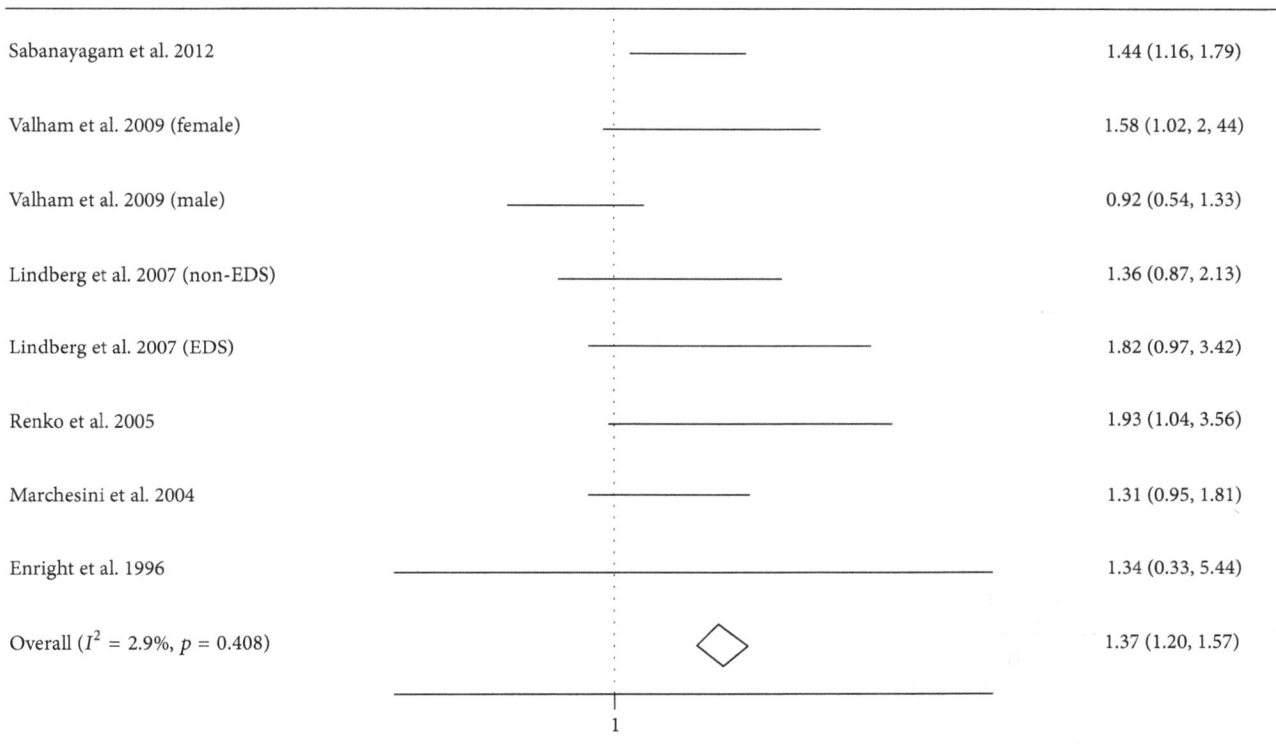

FIGURE 2: Forest plot of the association between self-reported habitual snoring and diabetes mellitus risk. Valham et al.'s study provided the data in female and male population not the whole population, and Lindberg et al.'s study provided the data in excessive daytime sleepiness (EDS) and non-EDS snorers.

and Italy [20]. All the included studies were observational and population-based; six were designed as cross-sectional studies, and the other two [1, 23] were prospective cohorts. The follow-up duration of the two prospective studies was 10 years. Three of the included studies got a high score of eight, and the other five studies scored seven in quality assessment. The detailed properties of the studies are summarized in Table 1.

3.3. Pooled and Subgroup Analysis: Snoring and Risk for DM. In this meta-analysis, we summarized the mostly adjusted

ORs and 95% CIs by pooling the six cross-sectional studies containing 28,890 subjects. Of the six studies, one study provided the data in female and male population not the whole population [18], and the other study provided the data in excessive daytime sleepiness (EDS) and non-EDS snorers [21]. The OR and 95% CI of DM in individuals with self-reported habitual snoring compared with nonsnorers were 1.37 (95% CI, 1.20–1.57, $p < 0.001$) (Figure 2). There was no heterogeneity across the included studies ($I^2 = 2.9\%$, $p = 0.408$).

In subgroup analysis of the six cross-sectional studies, only two studies stratified according to gender [18, 20], and

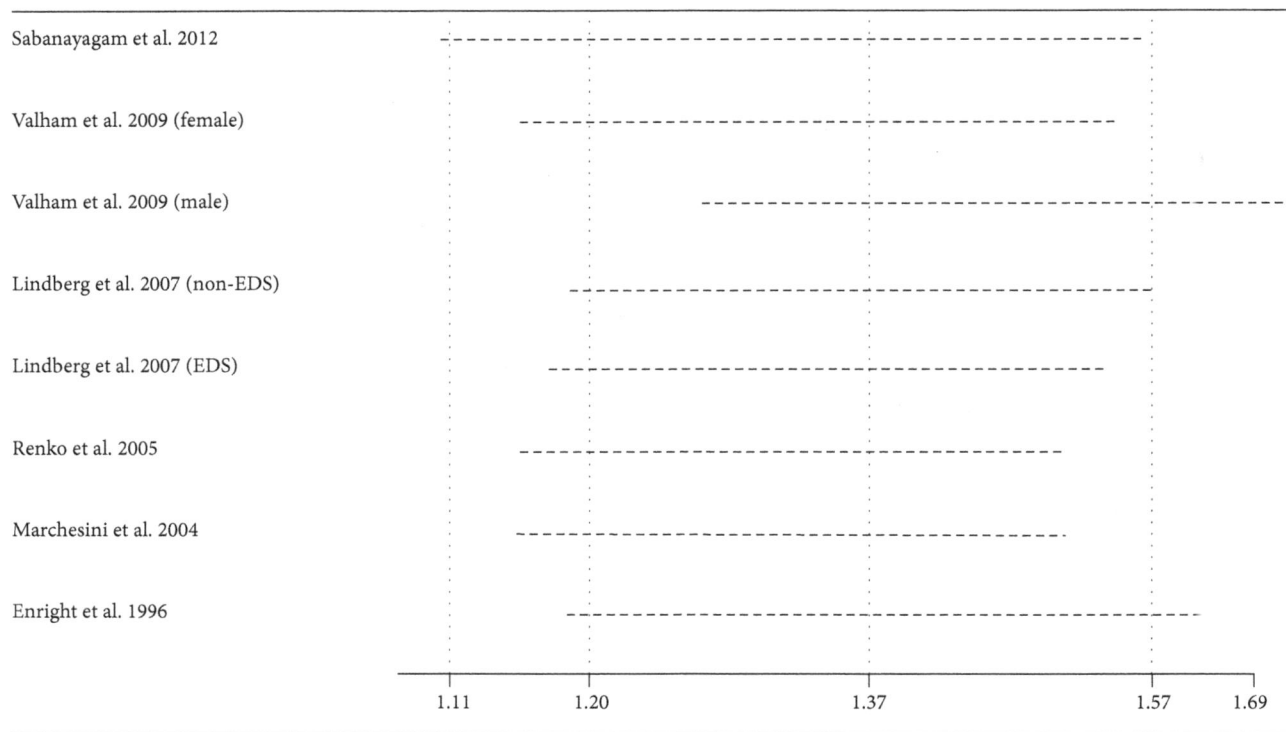

FIGURE 3: Effect of individual studies on the pooled OR for the self-reported habitual snoring and diabetes mellitus risk.

one study was conducted in a female population [21]. In the female population ($n = 12298$), the pooled OR was 1.59 (95% CI, 1.20–2.11), whereas OR = 0.89 (95% CI, 0.65–1.22) in the male population ($n = 4276$) [18, 20].

For the two prospective cohort studies, one study [23] was conducted in a female population of 69,852 subjects; the RR was 1.63 (95% CI, 1.29–2.07). The second study [1] was conducted in a male population of 2,504 subjects, and the RR was 1.06 (95% CI, 0.36–3.1) and 7.0 (95% CI, 2.9–16.9) in nonobese and obese populations, respectively. The pooled RR of the two prospective studies was 1.65 (95% CI, 1.30–2.08).

3.4. Sensitivity Analysis. Sensitivity analyses were performed to verify the robustness of the results. These separate statistical analyses were conducted by omitting one study each time. The OR (95% CI) estimates ranged from 1.42 (1.27–1.60) to 1.54 (1.37–1.74). The data suggested that no individual study affected the results in the meta-analysis (Figure 3).

3.5. Publication Bias. To assess publication bias among the included cross-sectional studies, Begg's rank correlation tests and Egger linear regression tests were performed; the p value of these two tests was 0.386 and 0.648, respectively. No asymmetrical funnel plots were found, as shown in Figure 4.

4. Discussion

This meta-analysis of six cross-sectional and two prospective cohort studies with a total of 101,246 participants revealed a statistically significant association between self-reported

habitual snoring and DM. When stratified according to gender, there was a strong association between snoring and DM in females, but not in males.

Snoring affects both genders, including 23% of middle-aged males and 10% of females [24]. Obese subjects have a higher proportion of snoring than do the nonobese general population (45% versus 35%) [25]. Interestingly, the current meta-analysis stratified the studies according to gender, which revealed that females with habitual snoring were found to be associated with DM (OR, 1.59; 95% CI, 1.20–2.11). Conversely, there was no statistical significance in males (OR, 0.89; 95% CI, 0.65–1.22). Two prospective cohort studies also revealed the same phenomenon: RR 1.63 (1.29–2.07) in females and OR 1.06 (0.36–3.1) in nonobese males [1, 23]. The reasons why females who snore habitually are more associated with DM than males are as follows: (1) the average age of women who suffer sleep disordered breathing was older than males; (2) polycystic ovary syndrome (PCOS) is a common condition in premenopausal women (7%); women who have PCOS are more likely to develop into DM and sleep apnea [18]. Other variables such as age and BMI could not be included in further subgroup analysis due to limited data in the included studies.

Currently, many snorers ignore the adverse health effects that are caused by snoring. Although the relationship between habitual snoring and DM has been established, the exact mechanisms for this association have not been elucidated completely. Snoring is a sign of compromised upper airways and OSA and is characterized by the recurrent collapse of respiratory structures during breathing while asleep

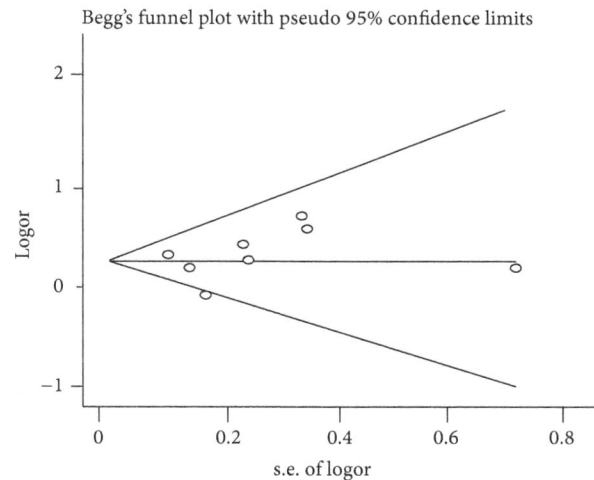

FIGURE 4: Funnel plot of the association between the self-reported habitual snoring and diabetes mellitus risk.

[26]. Nocturnal intermittent hypoxia and hypercapnia might contribute to increased sympathetic nervous activity and increased oxidative stress, which finally lead to insulin resistance [27]. The activation of proinflammatory cytokine production also plays an important role in the progression of snoring-induced DM [28]. Snoring was also closely associated with atherosclerosis and cardiovascular diseases [29], which might be prone to DM development. Due to these adverse effects, self-reported snoring might be useful as a low-cost and noninvasive indicator during the screening of persons who are prone to DM, particularly in developing countries.

Several limitations must be addressed when interpreting the results of the current meta-analysis. First, the evidence in our meta-analysis is based mostly on observational studies; therefore, no inherent causality was addressed. Second, the definition of habitual snoring and the diagnostic criteria used for DM were inconsistent among the included studies; therefore, the misclassification of snoring and DM is inevitable. Third, unmeasured confounding variables could have affected the association between snoring and DM. Although we used the most fully adjusted estimates in each study, we cannot exclude the possibility that other confounders might have affected the association. Fourth, snoring might be an early marker of unmeasured OSA. However, none of the included studies use standard method to exclude OSA. That is to say, whether snoring without OSA might be prone to DM was undetermined. Finally, most of the included studies were cross-sectional, and so additional prospective cohort studies should be performed to explore the etiology of snoring-induced DM. Despite these limitations, this is the first meta-analysis to address the association between self-reported habitual snoring and DM, there was no heterogeneity, and sensitivity analysis revealed that the results were robust.

In conclusion, the current meta-analysis pooled eight studies and revealed that habitual snoring was associated with DM. However, it remains unclear how much of the susceptibility could be attributed to OSA. Additional well-designed studies with a larger sample size are warranted to validate these findings.

Conflict of Interests

The authors declare that they have no conflict of interests.

Authors' Contribution

Xiaolu Xiong and Anyuan Zhong contributed equally to this paper.

References

[1] A. Elmasry, C. Janson, E. Lindberg, T. Gislason, M. A. Tageldin, and G. Boman, "The role of habitual snoring and obesity in the development of diabetes: a 10-year follow-up study in a male population," *Journal of Internal Medicine*, vol. 248, no. 1, pp. 13–20, 2000.

[2] D. R. Whiting, L. Guariguata, C. Weil, and J. Shaw, "IDF diabetes atlas: global estimates of the prevalence of diabetes for 2011 and 2030," *Diabetes Research and Clinical Practice*, vol. 94, no. 3, pp. 311–321, 2011.

[3] R. I. G. Holt and A. J. Mitchell, "Diabetes mellitus and severe mental illness: mechanisms and clinical implications," *Nature Reviews Endocrinology*, vol. 11, no. 2, pp. 79–89, 2015.

[4] S. E. Kahn, M. E. Cooper, and S. Del Prato, "Pathophysiology and treatment of type 2 diabetes: perspectives on the past, present, and future," *The Lancet*, vol. 383, no. 9922, pp. 1068–1083, 2014.

[5] T. Young, P. E. Peppard, and D. J. Gottlieb, "Epidemiology of obstructive sleep apnea: a population health perspective," *American Journal of Respiratory and Critical Care Medicine*, vol. 165, no. 9, pp. 1217–1239, 2002.

[6] V. Deary, J. G. Ellis, J. A. Wilson, C. Coulter, and N. L. Barclay, "Simple snoring: not quite so simple after all?" *Sleep Medicine Reviews*, vol. 18, pp. 453–462, 2014.

[7] T. Abe, Y. Komada, and Y. Inoue, "Short sleep duration, snoring and subjective sleep insufficiency are independent factors

associated with both falling asleep and feeling sleepiness while driving," *Internal Medicine*, vol. 51, no. 23, pp. 3253–3259, 2012.

[8] P. E. Brockmann, M. Schlaud, C. F. Poets, and M. S. Urschitz, "Predicting poor school performance in children suspected for sleep-disordered breathing," *Sleep Medicine*, vol. 16, no. 9, pp. 1077–1083, 2015.

[9] M. Li, K. Li, X.-W. Zhang, W. Hou, and Z. Tang, "Habitual snoring and risk of stroke: a meta-analysis of prospective studies," *International Journal of Cardiology*, vol. 185, pp. 46–49, 2015.

[10] D. Li, D. Liu, X. Wang, and D. He, "Self-reported habitual snoring and risk of cardiovascular disease and all-cause mortality," *Atherosclerosis*, vol. 235, no. 1, pp. 189–195, 2014.

[11] A. F. Cicero, M. Morbini, R. Urso et al., "Association between self-reported snoring and arterial stiffness: data from the Brisighella heart study," *Internal and Emergency Medicine*, pp. 1–7, 2015.

[12] J.-P. Baguet, P.-Y. Courand, B. Lequeux et al., "Snoring but not sleepiness is associated with increased aortic root diameter in hypertensive patients. The SLEEPART study," *International Journal of Cardiology*, vol. 202, pp. 131–132, 2016.

[13] D. F. Stroup, J. A. Berlin, S. C. Morton et al., "Meta-analysis of observational studies in epidemiology: a proposal for reporting," *The Journal of the American Medical Association*, vol. 283, no. 15, pp. 2008–2012, 2000.

[14] J. P. T. Higgins and S. G. Thompson, "Quantifying heterogeneity in a meta-analysis," *Statistics in Medicine*, vol. 21, no. 11, pp. 1539–1558, 2002.

[15] R. DerSimonian and R. Kacker, "Random-effects model for meta-analysis of clinical trials: an update," *Contemporary Clinical Trials*, vol. 28, no. 2, pp. 105–114, 2007.

[16] M. Egger, G. D. Smith, M. Schneider, and C. Minder, "Bias in meta-analysis detected by a simple, graphical test," *British Medical Journal*, vol. 315, no. 7109, pp. 629–634, 1997.

[17] C. Sabanayagam, S. Teppala, and A. Shankar, "Markers of sleep disordered breathing and diabetes mellitus in a multiethnic sample of US adults: results from the national health and nutrition examination survey (2005–2008)," *International Journal of Endocrinology*, vol. 2012, Article ID 879134, 8 pages, 2012.

[18] F. Valham, B. Stegmayr, M. Eriksson, E. Hägg, E. Lindberg, and K. A. Franklin, "Snoring and witnessed sleep apnea is related to diabetes mellitus in women," *Sleep Medicine*, vol. 10, no. 1, pp. 112–117, 2009.

[19] A.-K. Renko, L. Hiltunen, M. Laakso, U. Rajala, and S. Keinänen-Kiukaanniemi, "The relationship of glucose tolerance to sleep disorders and daytime sleepiness," *Diabetes Research and Clinical Practice*, vol. 67, no. 1, pp. 84–91, 2005.

[20] G. Marchesini, A. Pontiroli, G. Salvioli et al., "Snoring, hypertension and Type 2 diabetes in obesity. Protection by physical activity," *Journal of Endocrinological Investigation*, vol. 27, no. 2, pp. 150–157, 2004.

[21] E. Lindberg, C. Berne, K. A. Franklin, M. Svensson, and C. Janson, "Snoring and daytime sleepiness as risk factors for hypertension and diabetes in women—a population-based study," *Respiratory Medicine*, vol. 101, no. 6, pp. 1283–1290, 2007.

[22] P. L. Enright, A. B. Newman, P. W. Wahl, T. A. Manolio, E. F. Haponik, and P. J. R. Boyle, "Prevalence and correlates of snoring and observed apneas in 5,201 older adults," *Sleep*, vol. 19, no. 7, pp. 531–538, 1996.

[23] W. K. Al-Delaimy, J. E. Manson, W. C. Willett, M. J. Stampfer, and F. B. Hu, "Snoring as a risk factor for type II diabetes mellitus: a prospective study," *American Journal of Epidemiology*, vol. 155, no. 5, pp. 387–393, 2002.

[24] J. R. Stradling and J. H. Crosby, "Predictors and prevalence of obstructive sleep apnoea and snoring in 1001 middle aged men," *Thorax*, vol. 46, no. 2, pp. 85–90, 1991.

[25] B. Shahi, B. Praglowski, and M. Deitel, "Sleep-related disorders in the obese," *Obesity Surgery*, vol. 2, no. 2, pp. 157–168, 1992.

[26] N. M. Punjabi, "The epidemiology of adult obstructive sleep apnea," *Proceedings of the American Thoracic Society*, vol. 5, no. 2, pp. 136–143, 2008.

[27] N. Iiyori, L. C. Alonso, J. Li et al., "Intermittent hypoxia causes insulin resistance in lean mice independent of autonomic activity," *American Journal of Respiratory and Critical Care Medicine*, vol. 175, no. 8, pp. 851–857, 2007.

[28] I. Alam, K. Lewis, J. W. Stephens, and J. N. Baxter, "Obesity, metabolic syndrome and sleep apnoea: all pro-inflammatory states," *Obesity Reviews*, vol. 8, no. 2, pp. 119–127, 2007.

[29] S. A. Lee, T. C. Amis, K. Byth et al., "Heavy snoring as a cause of carotid artery atherosclerosis," *SLEEP*, vol. 31, no. 9, pp. 1207–1213, 2008.

8

New Diagnostic and Therapeutic Approaches for Preventing the Progression of Diabetic Retinopathy

Young Gun Park and Young-Jung Roh

Department of Ophthalmology and Visual Science, Catholic University of Korea, No. 62 Yeouido-dong, Yeongdeungpo-gu, Seoul 07345, Republic of Korea

Correspondence should be addressed to Young-Jung Roh; youngjungroh@hanmail.net

Academic Editor: Ahmed Ibrahim

Diabetic retinopathy (DR) is a severe sight-threatening complication of diabetes mellitus. Retinal laser photocoagulation, antivascular endothelial growth factors, steroid therapy, and pars plana vitrectomy are now used extensively to treat advanced stages of diabetic retinopathy. Currently, diagnostic devices like ultrawide field fundus fluorescein angiography and the improvement of optical coherence tomography have provided quicker and more precise diagnosis of early diabetic retinopathy. Thus, treatment protocols have been modified accordingly. Various types of lasers, including the subthreshold micropulse laser and RPE-targeting laser, and selective targeted photocoagulation may be future alternatives to conventional retinal photocoagulation, with fewer complications. The new developed intravitreal medications and implants have provided more therapeutic options, with promising results.

1. Introduction

Diabetic retinopathy (DR) is a sight-threatening complication of diabetes and is known to be the leading cause of blindness [1]. Twenty-eight million people in the United States have type 2 diabetes and more than 350 million people worldwide [2]. Typical ocular complications range from impaired visual acuity due to diabetic retinopathy and premature cataracts all the way to blindness or loss of an eye.

DR is characterized by gradual progressive retinal vasculopathy, leading to endothelial cell dysfunction, breakdown of the blood-retinal barrier, ischemia-induced retinal neovascularization, and expansion of the extracellular matrix, resulting in the outgrowth of fibrovascular tissue at the vitreoretinal interface [3]. In addition, recent studies indicate that chronic low-grade inflammation is involved in the pathogenesis of DR [4]. Diabetic retinopathy can be clinically classified into two stages: early stages like nonproliferative diabetic retinopathy (NPDR) and late stages like PDR [5]. Arresting of NPDR at an early level would be necessary to reduce the risk of severe visual loss. However, current treatments target late stages of DR when vision has already been significantly affected, so there is a need to stop the progression of DR earlier. Moreover, most of the treatments for advanced stages, such as conventional laser therapy, intravitreal anti-VEGF or corticosteroid injections, and vitreoretinal surgery, are expensive and invasive and have serious complications.

Earlier detection and timely treatment of sight-threatening DR have reduced the incidence and progression of visual loss [6, 7]. A multidisciplinary approach is needed to design new effective prevention strategies for the early stages of DR.

Although treatment controlling systemic risk factors including hyperglycemia and hypertension is crucial to preventing and arresting DR, here we focused on local rather than systemic treatment. In this paper, we provide an outline of current trends to treat and diagnose diabetic retinopathy in the ophthalmic field.

2. Current Ophthalmic Therapeutic Options

Current treatments target the later stage of DR, but it would be highly desirable to prevent the onset of the disease or

TABLE 1: Summary of current ophthalmic therapeutic options for diabetic macular edema.

Category	Previous treatment options	New treatments options	Benefits of new treatments
Laser photocoagulation	Pan retinal photocoagulation Focal photocoagulation	Pattern scan laser (Pascal) Subthreshold diode micropulse laser (SDM) Retinal rejuvenation therapy (2RT) Selective retina therapy (SRT)	It reduces laser-induced side effects (constriction of visual fields, reduced dark adaption, and reduced color and contrast perception)
Anti-VEGF agent	Pegaptanib (Macugen) Ranibizumab (Lucentis) Bevacizumab (Avastin) Aflibercept (Eylea)	Anti-VEGF agents plus focal/grid laser therapy	(i) Intravitreal anti-VEGF therapy is generally safer (ii) Visual acuity could be maintained with tapering the injection frequency over time
Steroid	Intravitreal triamcinolone acetonide	Dexamethasone sustained-release intravitreal implant (Ozurdex) Fluocinolone acetonide implant (Retisert)	(i) It Reduces the frequency of intravitreal anti-VEGF injections (ii) It is less associated with cataract formation and increased intraocular pressure than the previous steroid agents
Surgical treatment	Conventional 20-gauge vitrectomy	Transconjunctival sutureless 23- or 25-gauge vitrectomy	It reduced surgery times and makes rehabilitation of patients faster

arrest its progression at a stage before the appearance of overt microvascular pathology. Present ocular treatment revolves around four major strategies: retinal laser photocoagulation, anti-VEGF drugs, steroids, and surgical intervention (Table 1).

2.1. Laser Photocoagulation. Laser photocoagulation is the main treatment for established DR, and it is generally indicated in PDR or in clinically significant diabetic macular edema (CSME). This intervention prevents further deterioration of vision if applied sufficiently early in the progression of the disease but does not usually restore lost vision. The Diabetes Retinopathy Study (DRS) and Early Treatment Diabetes Retinopathy Study (ETDRS) groups developed guidelines for the laser treatment of diabetic retinopathy [8–10]. In DRS, panretinal photocoagulation (PRP) was shown to reduce the risk of severe visual loss by 60% in 2 years, especially in patients with PDR and high-risk characteristics [8]. Later, ETDRS suggested that patients with severe NPDR might also benefit from scatter photocoagulation as well [10].

The exact mechanism by which PRP aids in the regression of neovascularization is unclear. It appears to be a combined effect of multiple elements including facilitation of the transport of oxygen and nutrients into the retina from the choroid, the transport of metabolic waste out of the retina, reduction of retinal metabolic load, and reduced VEGF expression [11]. Other cytokines, such as heat shock proteins and transforming growth factor-β2, have been implicated in inflammatory responses in retinal photocoagulation as well [12, 13].

The utility of focal/grid laser therapy was studied in ETDRS, and the focal laser photocoagulation of microaneurysms and localized areas of leakage in patients with CSME was shown to reduce the incidence of moderate vision loss by 50% (from 24% to 12%) [9, 10]. Apart from the direct effect, by coagulating microaneurysms, the exact mechanisms of action

of the focal laser treatment are still poorly understood. However, they are presumed to involve stimulation of RPE, closure of leaking microaneurysms, and the induction of endothelial cell proliferation. Moreover, increased oxygenation leads to constriction of arterioles, and alterations in various cytokines and growth factors play a role in reducing macular edema [14–17].

Although PRP is often used to successfully reduce the risk of severe vision loss from the progression of DR, significant visual side effects are also associated with the treatment, such as reduced peripheral vision with narrow visual field and decreased dark adaption due to loss of rod function. These interfered functions can affect the patients' driving ability and reduce color and contrast perception [18]. To minimize these side effects, less aggressive strategies, such as pattern scan laser (Pascal), subthreshold micropulse diode laser, retinal rejuvenation therapy (2RT), and selective retinal therapy (SRT), have been developed.

2.2. Intravitreal Anti-Vascular Endothelial Growth Factor (VEGF) Agents. Until the introduction of anti-VEGF medications, focal and grid laser photocoagulation was the standard treatment for CSME. However, center-involving diffuse diabetic macular edema limits functional prognosis with grid laser photocoagulation [9]. Thus, intravitreal anti-VEGF therapy has become the primary treatment compared to the grid laser photocoagulation. VEGF is known to cause leakage and retinal edema from the breakdown of the blood-retinal barrier [19]. Intravitreal injection of anti-VEGF medication allows high concentrations in the vitreous and avoidance of high systemic exposure.

Currently, four intravitreal anti-VEGF agents—pegaptanib (Macugen; Pfizer Inc., NY, USA), ranibizumab (Lucentis; Genentech Inc., San Francisco, CA, USA), bevacizumab (Avastin; Genentech Inc.), and aflibercept (Eylea; Regeneron

Pharmaceuticals Inc., NY, USA)—have emerged as new treatments for the more advanced stages of DR. Recently, major randomized controlled clinical trials investigating the use of anti-VEGF medication for DME have been reported [20–22]. These trials have provided clear evidence that intraocular administration of anti-VEGF agents shows good results both in preserving and in improving vision for patients with DME.

In randomized controlled trials that used ranibizumab injections, a total of 345 patients with DME were enrolled and treated with 0.5 mg ranibizumab as adjunctive therapy to laser photocoagulation and/or monotherapy. Ranibizumab alone and ranibizumab plus laser significantly improved BCVA compared with laser monotherapy, showing +6.1 letters, +5.9 letters, and +0.8 letters at 12 months, respectively. Compared with laser treatment alone, ranibizumab groups showed higher proportion of gain of ≥10 and ≥15 letters (resp., 37.4% versus 15.5% and 22.6% versus 8.2%) [21].

Additionally, a recent study comparing the relative efficacy and safety of intravitreous ranibizumab, bevacizumab, and aflibercept in the treatment of DME concluded that they all improved vision, but the relative effect depended on baseline visual acuity. There was no apparent difference among the treatments when the initial visual acuity loss was mild. However, aflibercept was more effective at improving vision when initial visual acuity was worse [22].

Repeated injections of anti-VEGF medications are required in patients with center-involving diabetic macular edema. Unlike neovascular age-related macular degeneration, visual acuity in patients with DME could be maintained with tapering the injection frequency over time [23]. Recent studies indicated that the average number of treatment is reduced by the progression of time, with seven injections in the first year and four in the second one [21]. Currently, some experts favor combination focal/grid laser therapy and pharmacotherapy with intravitreal anti-VEGF agents in patients with CSME. Combination therapy was shown to reduce the frequency of injections needed to control edema [24].

Though intravitreal anti-VEGF therapy is generally safe with relatively low side effects of medication, it is an invasive procedure, which may lead to local complications such as endophthalmitis and retinal detachment. Moreover, anti-VEGF drugs, when delivered into the vitreous, can pass into the systemic circulation, which could potentially result in hypertension, proteinuria, increased cardiovascular events, and impaired wound healing. These systemic effects are rare but do occur [25].

2.3. Steroid Therapy. Intravitreal steroids have been reported to generate favorable results in the treatment of diabetic macular edema. Intravitreal triamcinolone acetonide (IVTA) has been used mainly for its anti-inflammatory activity. However, the incidence of complications with corticosteroid injection is high, with the most common being intraocular pressure elevation and cataract formation. For this reason, they are generally used in patients affected by laser-refractory DME, especially in pseudophakic eyes [26].

Moreover, a major limitation of IVTA is the recurrence of DME, which develops after a relatively short duration of action (not longer than 3 months) necessitating repeated applications of IVTA that carry risks and are inconvenient for patients. Recently, sustained-release devices have been introduced and can lengthen the intervals between retreatments [27].

Recent studies have demonstrated that the biodegradable dexamethasone (DEX) 0.7 mg sustained-release intravitreal implant (Ozurdex; Allergan Inc., Irvine, CA, USA) and a nonabsorbable implant containing 190 μg fluocinolone acetonide (Retisert; Bausch and Lomb, Rochester, NY, USA) are promising new treatment options for patients with persistent DME [28, 29]. These implants provide sustained-release low-dose delivery, limiting the frequency of intravitreal injections and possibly reducing the costs associated with intravitreal anti-VEGF therapy. In a recent randomized clinical trial, it was shown that a DEX implant achieved similar rates of visual acuity improvement to bevacizumab for DME, with superior anatomic outcomes and fewer injections [30]. Despite such advantages, these devices are associated with cataract formation, increased intraocular pressure, and surgery to lower intraocular pressure [31, 32].

2.4. Surgical Treatment. In advanced cases of proliferative DR, with vitreous hemorrhage, tractional retinal detachment, and extensive fibrous membranes, pars plana vitrectomy should be performed [33]. The procedure is also used to remove the premacular posterior hyaloid from patients with persistent diffuse macular edema [34].

The Diabetic Retinopathy Clinical Research Network evaluated vitrectomy for DME associated with vitreomacular traction [35]. At 6 months, median OCT central subfield thickness decreased by 160 microns, and visual acuity improved by ≥10 letters in 38%. Factors associated with favorable outcomes after vitrectomy for DME were removal of an epiretinal membrane, removal of internal limiting membrane, and worse baseline visual acuity [36]. However, the need for internal limiting membrane peeling is still unclear.

The improvement in visual outcome achieved about 10 years ago mainly resulted from advances in vitreoretinal surgical instrumentation and technique enabling more effective removal of complex fibrovascular membranes [37]. Transconjunctival sutureless 23- or 25-gauge vitrectomy started to replace conventional 20-gauge technique and offers comparable safety and efficacy as well as reduced surgery times and faster rehabilitation of patients [38].

However, the visual outcome after vitrectomy remains unpredictable. In addition, significant postoperative complications may occur including cataract formation, recurrent vitreous hemorrhage, rhegmatogenous retinal detachment, and neovascular glaucoma [39].

3. Recent Developments in Early Diagnosis in Diabetic Retinopathy

Early detection and treatment of progressive retinal disease are another aspect of the management of DR. Important advances in diagnostic devices such as ultrawide field fundus fluorescein angiography (UWFA) and OCT allow early diagnosis of DR in recent years. Unlike fundus fluorescein

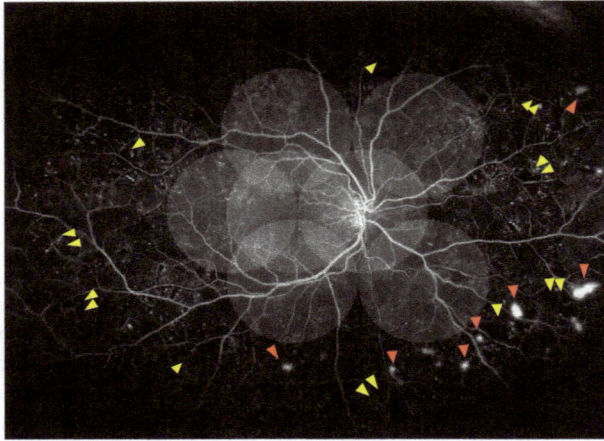

FIGURE 1: Diagram illustrating the extent of the seven standard ETDRS fields (the 75° view) on an ultrawide field fundus photo (the 200° view). Ultrawide field fundus angiography of a patient with proliferative diabetic retinopathy with extensive peripheral ischemia and extensive retinal neovascularization at the border between the perfused and nonperfused retinae.

angiography, peripheral capillary nonperfusion can also be visualized well using UWFA. OCT is another advance over the last decade that provides clear histology, including layers of retina and choroid. It provides retinal thickness to diagnose macular edema. Intraretinal cysts, vitreoretinal traction, epiretinal membranes, and other retinal macular pathologies of DR can also be diagnosed readily.

3.1. Ultrawide Field Fundus Fluorescein Angiography (UWFA).
Recently, the peripheral retina imaging has been focused in patients with DR. UWFA enables visualization of the peripheral retina up to 200° in a single frame and permits examining the peripheral capillary nonperfusion (Figure 1). One study reported that ultrawide field imaging (UWF) allowed visualization of retinal surface area 3.2 times more than the conventional ETDRS-protocol 7 standard field stereoscopic fundus photographs for the detection and management of diabetic retinopathy [40]. UWF has been increasingly used as the primary screening device for the diagnosis and monitoring of DR [41, 42]. Visualization of the peripheral retinal is improved with UWFA, and the device has provided clinical benefits and improved patient outcomes.

3.2. Optical Coherent Tomography (OCT).
OCT is a noninvasive imaging technique, and the images are presented with cross section of the retina in high resolution. Time-domain OCT (TD-OCT) shows an axial resolution of 8–10 μm by using scan rates of 400 A-scans per second [43]. Unlike TD-OCT, spectral-domain OCT (SD-OCT) can improve the resolution of the image and visualize the choroid using both image averaging and enhanced depth imaging (EDI). Using an interferometer with a high-speed spectrometer, the interference spectrum measurement of SD-OCT system detects the light echoes simultaneously. An imaging speed of 20,000 to 52,000 A-scans/sec and an axial resolution of

5–7 μm in tissue can be achieved with this technique. For diagnosing CSME, OCT is used for the gold standard test.

OCT can also demonstrate a number of microanatomical features in diabetic macular edema, as well as areas of subclinical macular edema [44]. Additionally, SD-OCT can be useful to evaluate choroidal thickness [45]. Swept-source OCT (SS-OCT) provides 3 μm resolution in tissue using scan rates of 100,000 A-scans per second and improves the visualization of the choroid [46] (Figure 2). Recently, OCT-angiography using a split-spectrum amplitude-decorrelation angiography algorithm improved the visualization of the microcirculation in the retina and choroid [47]. En face imaging in OCT-angiography may be useful to evaluate the microvascular status of the DR in detail. It was shown that the extent of the nonperfused area differed between the superficial and deep plexuses of the macula region [48] (Figure 3).

A significantly thinner choroid was observed in type 2 diabetic patients without diabetic retinopathy or early stage DR. The patients with DME also showed reduced choroidal thickness [49, 50]. Thus, choroidal thickness could be used as a marker for the risk of developing DR. OCT-angiography is expected to be helpful for evaluating the choroidal vessels. Thus, further studies are needed to confirm the relationship between DR and choroidal thickness.

4. Current Preventive Trends in Treating Progression of DR

4.1. New Concepts in Laser Therapy.
A new laser treatment was developed by modifying a diode laser in an effort to reduce unavoidable loss of the visual field from collateral damage of conventional continuous wave (CW) laser therapy. Compared with CW laser therapy, RPE-targeting lasers such as SDM, retinal rejuvenation therapy (2RT), and selective retina therapy (SRT) can cause less damage to the neural retina in DME using a short pulse duration like a microsecond or even a nanosecond [51–56]. Although the mechanism of SDM remains unknown, the laser may induce changes of cytokines in RPE and activate heat shock protein expression [13, 57]. Unlike the invisibility of SDM lesions on fundus photography and fluorescein angiography, laser spots of SRT can be visualized by fluorescein angiography due to RPE damage. However, these lesions disappeared on subsequent fluorescein angiography because the damaged area can be covered by the migration and proliferation of surrounding RPE cells [56, 58].

4.1.1. Targeted Laser for Retinal Pigment Epithelium (RPE).
Subthreshold diode micropulse laser photocoagulation (SDM) uses a diode laser with a micropulse technique and lower fluence to achieve subthreshold burns to limit the laser burns to RPE [59]. Whereas conventional laser therapy uses continuous waves of energy delivery, micropulse mode divides a single energy delivery of the laser burn with cycles of on time and off time until the full duration is delivered without a visible burn endpoint [60]. Histopathological studies have demonstrated that the micropulse diode laser affects only RPE without damaging the outer retina

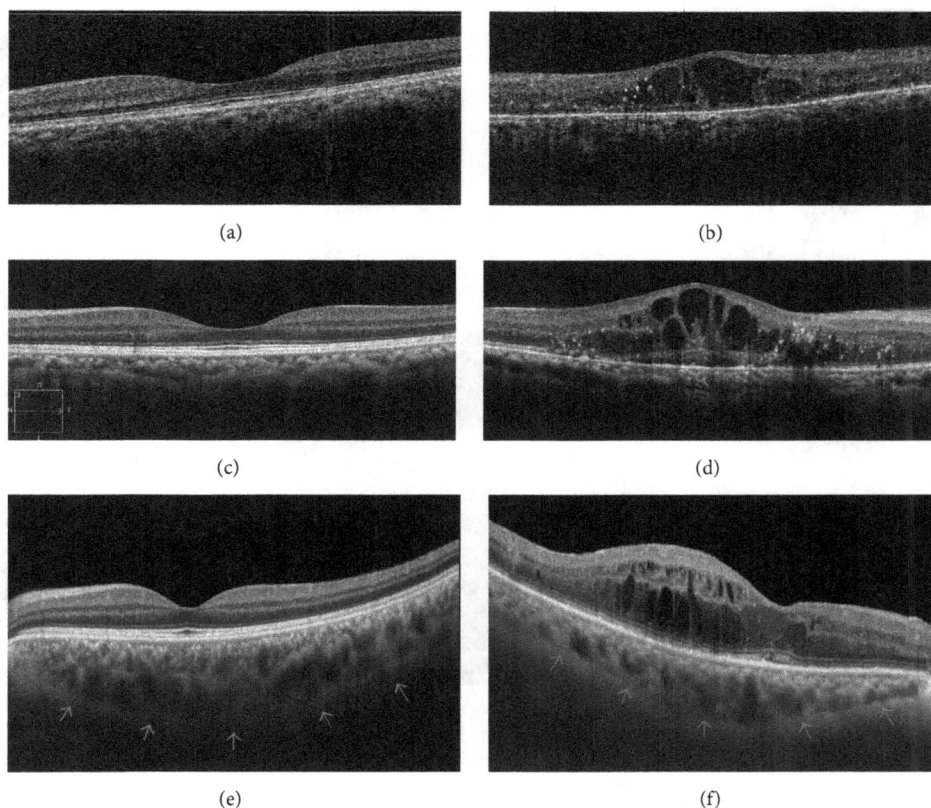

FIGURE 2: Optical coherence tomography (OCT) features of diabetic retinopathy in comparison with a normal eye. (a, b) OCT images in the normal and diabetic eyes obtained using the Cirrus HD-OCT system, respectively. (c, d) OCT images, respectively, in normal and diabetic eyes also obtained using the Cirrus HD-OCT system with the enhanced depth imaging (EDI) technique. (e, f) OCT images obtained using a swept-source OCT (SS-OCT). Note that the signal quality is improved markedly, and the vitreomacular interface and the choroid-sclera junction become clear. (e) The SS-OCT image of normal eye allows enhanced visualization of choroidal thickness (red arrows). (f) The image of a patient with DR showed reduced choroidal thickness.

[51]. Subsequently, several papers were published on the SDM in DME and found it to be equally effective as a conventional argon or threshold diode laser [51, 52]. However, there have been very few clinical studies on the RPE-targeting laser for treating progression of DR. A recent study demonstrated that pan retinal photocoagulation using SDM for DR ranging from severe nonproliferative to proliferative diabetic retinopathy showed a similar incidence of *de novo* vitreous hemorrhage and vitrectomy, compared with previous reports [61]. Additionally, SDM treatments could avoid the complications associated with conventional photocoagulation such as retinal damage, reduced vision, and reduced visual field. Because the RPE-targeting laser may induce different tissue responses depending on the degree of fundus pigmentation, our group is developing an algorithm of real time feed-back dosimetry of SRT system, which can help to deliver adequate energy for each individual person with different degrees of fundus pigmentation [56]. However, randomized long-term clinical trial is needed to confirm the efficacy of such RPE-targeting lasers for DR.

4.1.2. Targeted Laser Therapy for Ischemic Retina Areas. Targeted laser therapy is intended to selectively treat ischemic retinal areas and adjacent intermediate areas showing angiographic leakage while minimizing some of the risks and complications of conventional PRP [62]. Although DRS and ETDRS groups suggested benefits from PRP, photocoagulation can trigger complications, such as diminished visual field, reduced contrast sensitivity, and impaired night vision.

Photocoagulation targeting only ischemic retinal areas has been performed widely in Japan. It has been reported that the selective photocoagulation group (PC group) for nonperfusion areas (NPA) in preproliferative diabetic retinopathy (PPDR) is more effective in preventing the progressing of DR compared with the conventional pan retinal photocoagulation group (non-PC group). Over 3 years, PDR developed in 18 (26%) of total number of the 69 patients. This incidence was significantly higher in the non-PC group (15/37 patients, 41%) than in the PC group (3/32, 9%) [63].

UWF allows identification of peripheral areas of nonperfusion and vascular leakage, and it can perform a role as a guide for targeted retinal photocoagulation (TRP) [62]. Silva et al. suggested that these peripheral lesions have implications for diagnosing more severe DR and peripheral pathology serves as a predictor of progression in diabetic retinopathy [64]. Although a clinical trial in Japan supported the idea

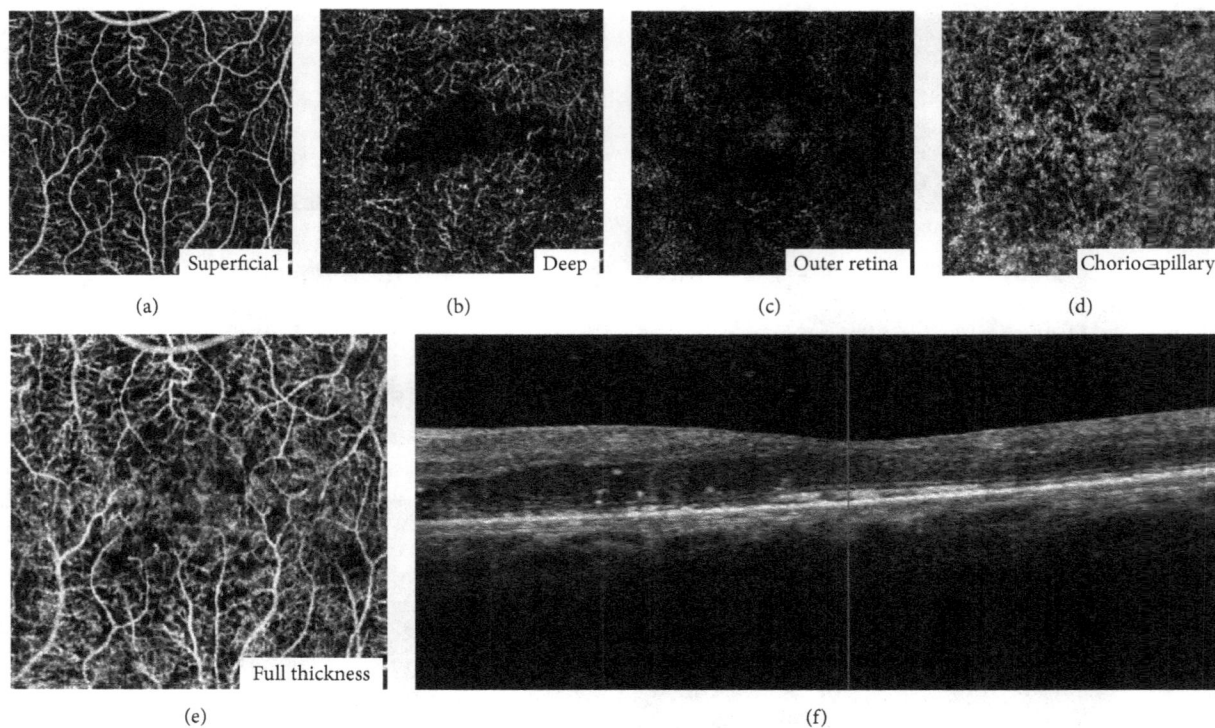

FIGURE 3: En face optical coherence tomography (OCT) angiography images of the layer segmentation and horizontal B-scan images in a patient with diabetic macular edema. (a) 3 × 3 mm OCT angiogram of the "superficial" inner retina. (b) 3 × 3 mm OCT angiogram of the "deep" inner retina. (c) 3 × 3 mm OCT angiogram of the outer retina shows absence of vasculature. The white represents noise. (d) 3 × 3 mm OCT angiogram of the choriocapillaris. There is black shadowing from the retinal vessels. (e) Full-thickness (internal limiting membrane to Bruch's membrane). (f) Highly sampled OCT b-scan image.

that selective photocoagulation (S-PC) for nonperfusion areas in preproliferative DR is effective for preventing PDR development, a further long-term clinical trial is needed to confirm the efficacy of S-PC [63].

4.2. Anti-VEGF Agent for Diabetic Retinopathy.

Although pan retinal photocoagulation was shown to reduce severe vision loss by 50% in the DRS report, no therapy reversed the progression of DR [5]. However, recent clinical studies of anti-VEGF for DME demonstrated that monthly ranibizumab for 36 months prevented the worsening of DR and induced severity scale reduction on the Early Treatment Diabetic Retinopathy Study. Patients with diabetic macular edema were randomized to monthly sham, 0.3 mg ranibizumab, or 0.5 mg ranibizumab intravitreal injections ($n = 759$). At 2 years, the percentage of participants with DR progression (worsening by 2 or 3 steps) was significantly reduced in ranibizumab-treated eyes compared with sham-treated eyes, and DR regression (improving by 2 or 3 steps) was significantly more likely. The cumulative probability of clinical progression of DR at 2 years was 33.8% of sham-treated eyes compared with 11.2% to 11.5% of ranibizumab-treated eyes. They demonstrated that intravitreal ranibizumab reduced the risk of DR progression and early intervention is important to reduce the DR severity level [19, 65]. This result supports the idea that anti-VEGF agents could be useful to control the progression of DR.

4.3. Intravitreal Corticosteroids.

There is some basis for considering the question of whether corticosteroids could reduce the risk of progression of retinopathy, including development of proliferative diabetic retinopathy. Corticosteroids have been shown experimentally to downregulate VEGF production, reduce breakdown of the blood-retinal barrier, and possibly have antiangiogenic properties [66]. Moreover, intravitreal triamcinolone acetonide has been used in the prevention of retinal neovascularization in various studies [67].

Recently, several studies of intravitreal corticosteroids for DME showed the regression of DR [68, 69]. For example, patients with diabetic retinopathy were assigned randomly to laser or intravitreal triamcinolone acetonide (1 mg or 4 mg). After 2 years, the cumulative probability of progression of retinopathy was 31% (laser), 29% (1 mg), and 21% (4 mg), compared with laser group, $P = 0.65$ in the 1 mg group and 0.005 in the 4 mg group. These differences appeared to be sustained at 3 years [69]. As a result, intravitreal triamcinolone acetonide (4 mg) appeared to reduce the risk of progression of diabetic retinopathy.

However, use of this corticosteroid treatment just to reduce the progression of DR is not useful because of the possible complications such as glaucoma and cataracts and the need for reinjection due to short duration of action. If new steroid implants avoiding or lowering these complications are developed, corticosteroids could be another treatment option for controlling the progression of DR.

5. Conclusions

Improvements in diabetes care and management have been crucial in lowering the incidence and severity of DR. Nevertheless, the effectiveness of current treatments for DR is limited, and they are currently indicated at advanced stages of the disease. Thus, a multidisciplinary approach and novel strategies to detect, prevent, and treat DR in the early stages are needed. Several therapeutic strategies in the early stages of DR are being evaluated. However, when the early stages of DR are the therapeutic target, it would be recommended that less aggressive and more prudent treatments should be used, avoiding serious adverse effects.

New technologies in both retinal imaging and functional assessments, such as UWFA or OCT, will allow the detection of early changes and designing a personalized, noninvasive treatment. These efforts will be effective in reducing the burden and improving the clinical outcome of this potentially devastating complication of diabetes.

Conflict of Interests

No author has financial or proprietary interests in any material or method mentioned.

References

[1] R. L. Thomas, F. Dunstan, S. D. Luzio et al., "Incidence of diabetic retinopathy in people with type 2 diabetes mellitus attending the diabetic retinopathy screening service for Wales: retrospective analysis," *British Medical Journal*, vol. 344, no. 7848, article e874, 2012.

[2] J. E. Shaw, R. A. Sicree, and P. Z. Zimmet, "Global estimates of the prevalence of diabetes for 2010 and 2030," *Diabetes Research and Clinical Practice*, vol. 87, no. 1, pp. 4–14, 2010.

[3] E. S. Shin, C. M. Sorenson, and N. Sheibani, "Diabetes and retinal vascular dysfunction," *Journal of Ophthalmic & Vision Research*, vol. 9, no. 3, pp. 362–373, 2014.

[4] A. M. A. El-Asrar, "Role of inflammation in the pathogenesis of diabetic retinopathy," *Middle East African Journal of Ophthalmology*, vol. 19, no. 1, pp. 70–74, 2012.

[5] The Diabetic Retinopathy Study Research Group, "Preliminary report on effects of photocoagulation therapy," *American Journal of Ophthalmology*, vol. 81, no. 4, pp. 383–396, 1976.

[6] E. Stefánsson, T. Bek, M. Porta, N. Larsen, J. K. Kristinsson, and E. Agardh, "Screening and prevention of diabetic blindness," *Acta Ophthalmologica Scandinavica*, vol. 78, no. 4, pp. 374–385, 2000.

[7] N. Cheung, P. Mitchell, and T. Y. Wong, "Diabetic retinopathy," *The Lancet*, vol. 376, no. 9735, pp. 124–136, 2010.

[8] The Diabetic Retinopathy Study Research Group, "Photocoagulation treatment of proliferative diabetic retinopathy: the second report of diabetic retinopathy study findings," *Ophthalmology*, vol. 85, no. 1, pp. 82–106, 1978.

[9] "Early photocoagulation for diabetic retinopathy—ETDRS report number 9. Early Treatment Diabetic Retinopathy Study Research Group," *Ophthalmology*, vol. 98, no. 5, supplement, pp. 766–785, 1991.

[10] Early Treatment Diabetic Retinopathy Study Research Group, "Treatment techniques and clinical guidelines for photocoagulation of diabetic macular edema. Early Treatment Diabetic Retinopathy Study Report Number 2," *Ophthalmology*, vol. 94, no. 7, pp. 761–774, 1987.

[11] M. S. Blumenkranz, "The evolution of laser therapy in ophthalmology: a perspective on the interactions between photons, patients, physicians, and physicists: the LXX Edward Jackson Memorial Lecture," *American Journal of Ophthalmology*, vol. 158, no. 1, pp. 12.e1–25.e1, 2014.

[12] M. Matsumoto, N. Yoshimura, and Y. Honda, "Increased production of transforming growth factor-β2 from cultured human retinal pigment epithelial cells by photocoagulation," *Investigative Ophthalmology and Visual Science*, vol. 35, no. 13, pp. 4245–4252, 1994.

[13] C. Sramek, M. Mackanos, R. Spitler et al., "Non-damaging retinal phototherapy: dynamic range of heat shock protein expression," *Investigative Ophthalmology and Visual Science*, vol. 52, no. 3, pp. 1780–1787, 2011.

[14] N. Bhagat, R. A. Grigorian, A. Tutela, and M. A. Zarbin, "Diabetic macular edema: pathogenesis and treatment," *Survey of Ophthalmology*, vol. 54, no. 1, pp. 1–32, 2009.

[15] Á. Arnarsson and E. Stefánsson, "Laser treatment and the mechanism of edema reduction in branch retinal vein occlusion," *Investigative Ophthalmology and Visual Science*, vol. 41, no. 3, pp. 877–879, 2000.

[16] N. Ogata, A. Ando, M. Uyama, and M. Matsumura, "Expression of cytokines and transcription factors in photocoagulated human retinal pigment epithelial cells," *Graefe's Archive for Clinical and Experimental Ophthalmology*, vol. 239, no. 2, pp. 87–95, 2001.

[17] N. Ogata, J. Tombran-Tink, N. Jo, D. Mrazek, and M. Matsumura, "Upregulation of pigment epithelium-derived factor after laser photocoagulation," *American Journal of Ophthalmology*, vol. 132, no. 3, pp. 427–429, 2001.

[18] D. S. Fong, A. Girach, and A. Boney, "Visual side effects of successful scatter laser photocoagulation surgery for proliferative diabetic retinopathy: a literature review," *Retina*, vol. 27, no. 7, pp. 816–824, 2007.

[19] T. Qaum, Q. Xu, A. M. Joussen et al., "VEGF-initiated blood-retinal barrier breakdown in early diabetes," *Investigative Ophthalmology and Visual Science*, vol. 42, no. 10, pp. 2408–2413, 2001.

[20] P. Massin, F. Bandello, J. G. Garweg et al., "Safety and efficacy of ranibizumab in diabetic macular edema (RESOLVE study): a 12-month, randomized, controlled, double-masked, multicenter phase II study," *Diabetes Care*, vol. 33, no. 11, pp. 2399–2405, 2010.

[21] P. Mitchell, F. Bandello, U. Schmidt-Erfurth et al., "The RESTORE study: ranibizumab monotherapy or combined with laser versus laser monotherapy for diabetic macular edema," *Ophthalmology*, vol. 118, no. 4, pp. 615–625, 2011.

[22] The Diabetic Retinopathy Clinical Research Network, "Aflibercept, bevacizumab, or ranibizumab for diabetic macular edema," *The New England Journal of Medicine*, vol. 372, no. 13, pp. 1193–1203, 2015.

[23] M. J. Elman, H. Qin, L. P. Aiello et al., "Intravitreal ranibizumab for diabetic macular edema with prompt versus deferred laser

treatment: three-year randomized trial results," *Ophthalmology*, vol. 119, no. 11, pp. 2312–2318, 2012.

[24] J. A. Ford, A. Elders, D. Shyangdan, P. Royle, and N. Waugh, "The relative clinical effectiveness of ranibizumab and bevacizumab in diabetic macular oedema: an indirect comparison in a systematic review," *British Medical Journal*, vol. 345, no. 7875, Article ID e5182, 2012.

[25] C. Costagliola, L. Agnifili, B. Arcidiacono et al., "Systemic thromboembolic adverse events in patients treated with intravitreal anti-VEGF drugs for neovascular age-related macular degeneration," *Expert Opinion on Biological Therapy*, vol. 12, no. 10, pp. 1299–1313, 2012.

[26] F. Bandello, C. Preziosa, G. Querques, and R. Lattanzio, "Update of intravitreal steroids for the treatment of diabetic macular edema," *Ophthalmic Research*, vol. 52, no. 2, pp. 89–96, 2014.

[27] M. M. Nentwich and M. W. Ulbig, "The therapeutic potential of intraocular depot steroid systems: developments aimed at prolonging duration of efficacy," *Deutsches Arzteblatt International*, vol. 109, no. 37, pp. 584–590, 2012.

[28] W. B. Messenger, R. M. Beardsley, and C. J. Flaxel, "Fluocinolone acetonide intravitreal implant for the treatment of diabetic macular edema," *Drug Design, Development and Therapy*, vol. 7, pp. 425–434, 2013.

[29] M. Dutra Medeiros, M. Postorino, R. Navarro, J. Garcia-Arumí, C. Mateo, and B. Corcóstegui, "Dexamethasone intravitreal implant for treatment of patients with persistent diabetic macular edema," *Ophthalmologica*, vol. 231, no. 3, pp. 141–146, 2014.

[30] W. M. Amoaku, S. Saker, and E. A. Stewart, "A review of therapies for diabetic macular oedema and rationale for combination therapy," *Eye*, vol. 29, no. 9, pp. 1115–1130, 2015.

[31] S. Guigou, S. Pommier, F. Meyer et al., "Efficacy and safety of intravitreal dexamethasone implant in patients with diabetic macular edema," *Ophthalmologica*, vol. 233, no. 3-4, pp. 169–175, 2015.

[32] P. A. Pearson, T. L. Comstock, M. Ip et al., "Fluocinolone acetonide intravitreal implant for diabetic macular edema: a 3-year multicenter, randomized, controlled clinical trial," *Ophthalmology*, vol. 118, no. 8, pp. 1580–1587, 2011.

[33] J. O. Mason III, C. T. Colagross, and R. Vail, "Diabetic vitrectomy: risks, prognosis, future trends," *Current Opinion in Ophthalmology*, vol. 17, no. 3, pp. 281–285, 2006.

[34] M. P. Simunovic, A. P. Hunyor, and I.-V. Ho, "Vitrectomy for diabetic macular edema: a systematic review and meta-analysis," *Canadian Journal of Ophthalmology*, vol. 49, no. 2, pp. 188–195, 2014.

[35] Diabetic Retinopathy Clinical Research Network Writing Committee, J. A. Haller, H. Qin et al., "Vitrectomy outcomes in eyes with diabetic macular edema and vitreomacular traction," *Ophthalmology*, vol. 117, no. 6, pp. 1087–1093.e3, 2010.

[36] C. J. Flaxel, A. R. Edwards, L. P. Aiello et al., "Factors associated with visual acuity outcomes after vitrectomy for diabetic macular edema: diabetic retinopathy clinical research network," *Retina*, vol. 30, no. 9, pp. 1488–1495, 2010.

[37] J. G. Arumi, A. Boixadera, V. Martinez-Castillo, and B. Corcóstegui, "Transconjunctival sutureless 23-gauge vitrectomy for diabetic retinopathy. Review," *Current Diabetes Reviews*, vol. 5, no. 1, pp. 63–66, 2009.

[38] D. H. Park, J. P. Shin, and S. Y. Kim, "Comparison of clinical outcomes between 23-gauge and 20-gauge vitrectomy in patients with proliferative diabetic retinopathy," *Retina*, vol. 30, no. 10, pp. 1662–1670, 2010.

[39] D. K. Newman, "Surgical management of the late complications of proliferative diabetic retinopathy," *Eye*, vol. 24, no. 3, pp. 441–449, 2010.

[40] A. Kaines, S. Oliver, S. Reddy, and S. D. Schwartz, "Ultrawide angle angiography for the detection and management of diabetic retinopathy," *International Ophthalmology Clinics*, vol. 49, no. 2, pp. 53–59, 2009.

[41] A. Manivannan, J. Plskova, A. Farrow, S. Mckay, P. F. Sharp, and J. V. Forrester, "Ultra-wide-field fluorescein angiography of the ocular fundus," *American Journal of Ophthalmology*, vol. 140, no. 3, pp. 525–527, 2005.

[42] M. M. Wessel, G. D. Aaker, G. Parlitsis, M. Cho, D. J. D'Amico, and S. Kiss, "Ultra-wide-field angiography improves the detection and classification of diabetic retinopathy," *Retina*, vol. 32, no. 4, pp. 785–791, 2012.

[43] A. C. Sull, L. N. Vuong, L. L. Price et al., "Comparison of spectral/fourier domain optical coherence tomography instruments for assessment of normal macular thickness," *Retina*, vol. 30, no. 2, pp. 235–245, 2010.

[44] B. L. Sikorski, G. Malukiewicz, J. Stafiej, H. Lesewska-Junk, and D. Raczynska, "The diagnostic function of OCT in diabetic maculopathy," *Mediators of Inflammation*, vol. 2013, Article ID 434560, 12 pages, 2013.

[45] R. F. Spaide, H. Koizumi, and M. C. Pozonni "Enhanced depth imaging spectral-domain optical coherence tomography," *American Journal of Ophthalmology*, vol. 146, no. 4, pp. 496–500, 2008.

[46] A. Unterhuber, B. Považay, B. Hermann, H. Sattmann, A. Chavez-Pirson, and W. Drexler, "In vivo retinal optical coherence tomography at 1040 nm—enhanced penetration into the choroid," *Optics Express*, vol. 13, no. 9, pp. 3252–3258, 2005.

[47] Y. Jia, O. Tan, J. Tokayer et al., "Split-spectrum amplitude-decorrelation angiography with optical coherence tomography," *Optics Express*, vol. 20, no. 4, pp. 4710–4725, 2012.

[48] A. Ishibazawa, T. Nagaoka, A. Takahashi et al., "Optical coherence tomography angiography in diabetic retinopathy: a prospective pilot study," *American Journal of Ophthalmology*, vol. 160, no. 1, pp. 35–44.e31, 2015.

[49] B. S. Gerendas, S. M. Waldstein, C. Simader et al., "Three-dimensional automated choroidal volume assessment on standard spectral-domain optical coherence tomography and correlation with the level of diabetic macular edema" *American Journal of Ophthalmology*, vol. 158, no. 5, pp. 1039–1048, 2014.

[50] C. V. Regatieri, L. Branchini, J. Carmody, J. G. Fujimoto, and J. S. Duker, "Choroidal thickness in patients with diabetic retinopathy analyzed by spectral-domain optical coherence tomography," *Retina*, vol. 32, no. 3, pp. 563–568, 2012.

[51] J. K. Luttrull and G. Dorin, "Subthreshold diode micropulse laser photocoagulation (SDM) as invisible retinal phototherapy for diabetic macular edema: a review," *Current Diabetes Reviews*, vol. 8, no. 4, pp. 274–284, 2012.

[52] J. K. Luttrull, D. C. Musch, and M. A. Mainster, "Subthreshold diode micropulse photocoagulation for the treatment of clinically significant diabetic macular oedema," *British Journal of Ophthalmology*, vol. 89, no. 1, pp. 74–80, 2005.

[53] J. K. Luttrull and S. H. Sinclair, "Safety of transfoveal subthreshold diode micropulse laser for fovea-involving diabetic macular edema in eyes with good visual acuity," *Retina*, vol. 34, no. 10, pp. 2010–2020, 2014.

[54] L. Pelosini, R. Hamilton, M. Mohamed, A. P. Hamilton, and J. Marshall, "Retina rejuvenation therapy for diabetic macular EDEMA: a pilot study," *Retina*, vol. 33, no. 3, pp. 548–558, 2013.

[55] J. Roider, S. H. M. Liew, C. Klatt et al., "Selective retina therapy (SRT) for clinically significant diabetic macular edema," *Graefe's Archive for Clinical and Experimental Ophthalmology*, vol. 248, no. 9, pp. 1263–1272, 2010.

[56] Y.-G. Park, E. Seifert, Y. J. Roh, D. Theisen-Kunde, S. Kang, and R. Brinkmann, "Tissue response of selective retina therapy by means of a feedback-controlled energy ramping mode," *Clinical and Experimental Ophthalmology*, vol. 42, no. 9, pp. 846–855, 2014.

[57] X. Gao and D. Xing, "Molecular mechanisms of cell proliferation induced by low power laser irradiation," *Journal of Biomedical Science*, vol. 16, article 4, 2009.

[58] J. Roider, N. A. Michaud, T. J. Flotte, and R. Birngruber, "Response of the retinal pigment epithelium to selective photocoagulation," *Archives of Ophthalmology*, vol. 110, no. 12, pp. 1786–1792, 1992.

[59] S. Sivaprasad, M. Elagouz, D. McHugh, O. Shona, and G. Dorin, "Micropulsed diode laser therapy: evolution and clinical applications," *Survey of Ophthalmology*, vol. 55, no. 6, pp. 516–530, 2010.

[60] G. Dorin, "Subthreshold and micropulse diode laser photocoagulation," *Seminars in Ophthalmology*, vol. 18, no. 3, pp. 147–153, 2003.

[61] J. K. Luttrull, D. C. Musch, and C. A. Spink, "Subthreshold diode micropulse panretinal photocoagulation for proliferative diabetic retinopathy," *Eye*, vol. 22, no. 5, pp. 607–612, 2008.

[62] S. Reddy, A. Hu, and S. D. Schwartz, "Ultra wide field fluorescein angiography guided Targeted Retinal Photocoagulation (TRP)," *Seminars in Ophthalmology*, vol. 24, no. 1, pp. 9–14, 2009.

[63] The Japanese Society of Ophthalmic Diabetology and Subcommittee on the Study of Diabetic Retinopathy Treatment, "Multicenter randomized clinical trial of retinal photocoagulation for preproliferative diabetic retinopathy," *Japanese Journal of Ophthalmology*, vol. 56, no. 1, pp. 52–59, 2012.

[64] P. S. Silva, J. D. Cavallerano, J. K. Sun, A. Z. Soliman, L. M. Aiello, and L. P. Aiello, "Peripheral lesions identified by mydriatic ultrawide field imaging: distribution and potential impact on diabetic retinopathy severity," *Ophthalmology*, vol. 120, no. 12, pp. 2587–2595, 2013.

[65] M. S. Ip, A. Domalpally, J. K. Sun, and J. S. Ehrlich, "Long-term effects of therapy with ranibizumab on diabetic retinopathy severity and baseline risk factors for worsening retinopathy," *Ophthalmology*, vol. 122, no. 2, pp. 367–374, 2015.

[66] L. Diaz-Flores, R. Gitoerrez, and H. Varela, "Angiogenesis: an update," *Histology and Histopathology*, vol. 9, no. 4, pp. 807–843, 1994.

[67] A. N. Antoszyk, J. L. Gottlieb, R. Machemer, and D. L. Hatchell, "The effects of intravitreal triamcinolone acetonide on experimental pre-retinal neovascularization," *Graefe's Archive for Clinical and Experimental Ophthalmology*, vol. 231, no. 1, pp. 34–40, 1993.

[68] M. J. Elman, L. P. Aiello, R. W. Beck et al., "Randomized trial evaluating ranibizumab plus prompt or deferred laser or triamcinolone plus prompt laser for diabetic macular edema," *Ophthalmology*, vol. 117, no. 6, pp. 1064.e35–1077.e35, 2010.

[69] N. M. Bressler, A. R. Edwards, R. W. Beck et al., "Exploratory analysis of diabetic retinopathy progression through 3 years in a randomized clinical trial that compares intravitreal triamcinolone acetonide with focal/grid photocoagulation," *Archives of Ophthalmology*, vol. 127, no. 12, pp. 1566–1571, 2009.

9

The Motivating Function of Healthcare Professional in eHealth and mHealth Interventions for Type 2 Diabetes Patients and the Mediating Role of Patient Engagement

Guendalina Graffigna,[1] Serena Barello,[1] Andrea Bonanomi,[2] and Julia Menichetti[1]

[1]Department of Psychology, Università Cattolica del Sacro Cuore, Largo A. Gemelli 1, 20123 Milan, Italy
[2]Department of Statistical Sciences, Università Cattolica del Sacro Cuore, Largo A. Gemelli 1, 20123 Milan, Italy

Correspondence should be addressed to Guendalina Graffigna; guendalina.graffigna@unicatt.it

Academic Editor: Bernard Portha

eHealth and mHealth interventions for type 2 diabetes are emerging as useful strategies to accomplish the goal of a high functioning integrated care system. However, mHealth and eHealth interventions in order to be successful need the clear endorsement from the healthcare professionals. This cross-sectional study included a sample of 93 Italian-speaking type 2 diabetes patients and demonstrated the role of the perceived ability of healthcare professionals to motivate patients' initiative in improving the level of their engagement and activation in type 2 diabetes self-management. The level of type 2 diabetes patients' activation resulted also in being a direct precursor of their attitude to the use of mHealth and eHealth. Furthermore, patient engagement has been demonstrated to be a mediator of the relationship between the perceived ability of healthcare professionals in motivating type 2 diabetes patients and patients' activation. Finally, type 2 diabetes patients adherence did not result in being a direct consequence of the frequency of mHealth and eHealth use. Patient adherence appeared to be directly influenced by the level of perceived healthcare professionals ability of motivating patients' autonomy. These results offer important insights into the psychosocial and organizational elements that impact on type 2 diabetes patients' activation in self-management and on their willingness to use mHealth and eHealth devices.

1. Introduction

Diabetes currently constitutes a large and growing clinical problem, and its costs for society are high and are escalating. Worldwide, estimated 387 million adults are living with diabetes, and this number is projected to increase to 592 million by 2035 [1–3]. Effective prevention strategies are, therefore, crucial to slow the diabetes tide and its burden. Nearly 9 out of 10 new diabetes cases are type 2 diabetes, characterized by a gradual increase in glycemia [1]; obesity and physical inactivity are some of the most common risk factors [2].

Since type 2 diabetes requires long-term treatment, over the past 20 years the responsibility for the care of people affected by this condition has shifted away from hospitals to primary care settings. The long-term management of chronic conditions requires a revision of classical models of care in order to guarantee positive care outcomes [4] and enhance patient's quality of life [5]. To address this requirement and to manage the patients' care, a more effective synergy between healthcare organizations and territorial services is required [6–8]. Chronic conditions, such as type 2 diabetes need long-term approach to care, which imply a higher synergy and service integration "outside" of the institutional boundaries of hospitals [9–11]. Thus healthcare organizations not only are concerned with the long-term management of type 2 diabetes patient but also are claimed to redesign their organizational models in accordance with local resources and demands of care. This requires a better integration with the resources (formal and informal; expert and lay) that are present in the territories [12, 13].

Integrated care organizational models are currently envisaged as the potential solution to improve quality and sustainability of healthcare services, particularly when the management of chronic condition (such as type 2 diabetes) is concerned. However, to achieve the goal of an integrated system of care, the role of the patient, as main actor of such a process, needs to be questioned [14]. In order to guarantee the fruitful collaboration and dialogue between the lay territory of reference for the patient and his/her reference healthcare provider, type 2 diabetes patients need to be helped in enacting an active and cocreative role along their process of care, moving from the traditional passive position of recipients of care to the one of the real engaged consumers in the design and delivery of healthcare services [15–18]. Type 2 diabetes patients' engagement is regarded as a key factor to improve the quality and the sustainability of healthcare services [15, 17, 19]. Previous studies have shown how an engaged patient is more likely keen to act improved health behaviors [20], to have better clinical outcomes [21], to perceive a better quality of life [22], and to be more satisfied with their relationship with the healthcare system [23]. Furthermore, empirical researches have demonstrated how patient engagement may contribute to a reduction of healthcare costs and to better economically sustainable organizational processes [24, 25].

In such a frame, eHealth and mHealth interventions are emerging as a useful strategy to accomplish the goal of a better integrated system of care [11, 26, 27]. As technology-based interventions are becoming regular part of the health care environment, viewing these tools in light of the skills (knowledge and behaviors) required for patients to successfully use them becomes essential if the power of eHealth and mHealth is to be leveraged to deliver health care effectively. As a consequence, promoting patient's eHealth literacy, defined as the ability to seek, find, understand, and appraise health information from electronic sources and apply the knowledge gained to addressing or solving a health problem [28], becomes a priority to enhance the continuity of care. Indeed, eHealth and mHealth offer continuous monitoring of clinical parameters, allowing the "on-demand" communication with the reference healthcare professionals, and, consequently, they are able of empowering the patient in the self-management of the disease condition and his/her therapy [29, 30]. A systematic review showed a positive impact of mHealth on patient engagement in the management of chronic diseases [31]: diabetic patients who transferred daily glucose readings to physicians using a telematics system and received telephone medication regimen feedback improved their clinical outcomes and presented a better glycemic control [32]. Likewise, the use of text message interventions, such as reminders and updates through SMS, ensured a greater adherence to prescription and improved clinical outcomes [33]. Furthermore, studies confirmed the effectiveness of mHealth interventions in modifying type 2 diabetes patients lifestyles, especially those related to dietary behaviors and physical activity, by facilitating diabetes self-management processes outside the clinical setting [34–36].

However, mHealth and eHealth interventions in order to be successful need the clear endorsement from the healthcare system. Particularly, the reference healthcare professionals are the key actors, from the patients' perspective, that can legitimize the intervention process and can motivate type 2 diabetes patients in being compliant with mHealth and

eHealth [37]. This underlines the role of healthcare organizational and professional cultures in enhancing or inhibiting the effectiveness of mHealth and eHealth interventions in managing type 2 diabetes. More attention is needed to explore how innovation through the introduction of new health technologies can be integrated in the systems of symbols, practices, and power relationships already existent in healthcare organizations [38]. Thus, the enabling role of healthcare professionals in the eHealth and mHealth interventions for type 2 diabetes needs to be further considered as a fundamental ingredient for their clinical success. Healthcare professionals should sustain type 2 diabetes patients' autonomy in care management and thus their motivation to adhere to the mHealth and eHealth intervention.

Based on these premises, the present study, carried out on a sample of Italian type 2 diabetes patients, was aimed at verifying the following hypotheses:

(1) The perceived ability of the healthcare professionals to support patients' autonomy influences the level of patients' engagement towards their care management.

(2) The perceived ability of the healthcare professionals to support patients' autonomy influences the level of patients' activation towards their care management.

(3) The levels of patients engagement mediate the association between the perceived ability of healthcare professionals to support patients' autonomy and the level of patients' activation.

(4) A higher level of activation is associated with a higher use of mHealth and eHealth technologies to seek information for managing type 2 diabetes care.

(5) A higher level of use of mHealth and eHealth technologies to seek information for managing type 2 diabetes care is associated with a higher patients' adherence to type 2 diabetes care.

2. Materials and Methods

2.1. Recruitment and Data Collection. This cross-sectional quantitative study included a sample of 93 Italian-speaking type 2 diabetes patients and was conducted on the basis of a structured questionnaire including validated measures (see Section 2.2) to assess the causal relations among the constructs under analysis (see research hypotheses stated above). Patients were recruited through the online panel provided by Research Now (http://www.researchnow.com/en-US.aspx). The panel covers a wide range of chronic conditions and counts more than 6.5 million registered subjects worldwide. Subjects belonging to the panel are carefully screened for authenticity and legitimacy via digital fingerprint and geo-IP-validation from the provider. All panelists are profiled on the basis of their sociodemographic, clinical, and lifestyle characteristics. The panel is certified to be statistically representative of all the covered populations. In our study, in order to guarantee data quality, respondents were asked to confirm their demographics (i.e., sex, date and place of birth, ethnicity, nationality, educational level, and place of residency) and clinical condition previously collected by the panel. To be included in our study, patients belonging to the panel had to be Italian, affected by type 2 diabetes, aged over 18 years, and of both genders. Patients with dementia, cognitive impairments, active psychiatric disorders, blindness, deafness, or insufficient Italian language skills to meaningfully answer the questions or without informed consent were excluded from this study. All participants gave written informed consent before being enrolled in the study. Patients completed the study questionnaire between October and December 2014. Ethic approval was attained from the Ethics Committee of the Università Cattolica del Sacro Cuore, Milan (Italy).

2.2. Measures. Patient Health Engagement Scale (PHE-S) developed by Graffigna and colleagues [39] is a measure of patient engagement that is grounded in rigorous conceptualization and appropriate psychometric methods. The scale consists of 5 ordinal items and was developed based on the authors' conceptual model of patient engagement (PHE-model), which features four positions along a continuum of engagement (i.e., blackout; arousal; adhesion; eudaimonic project). These engagement positions result from the conjoint cognitive (thinking), emotional (feeling), and conative (acting) enactment of individuals toward their health management [15].

Patient Activation Measure (PAM) developed by Hibbard and colleagues [40], the 13-item Patient Activation Measure, is an interval-level, unidimensional Guttman-like measure that contains items measuring self-assessed knowledge about chronic conditions, beliefs about illness and medical care, and self-efficacy for self-care. The PAM focused on physical conditions, and it was designed to measure activation as a broad construct. In the present study, we used the Italian validated version of the PAM [41].

Morisky Medication Adherence Scale (MMAS-4). Medication-taking behavior was assessed using the 4-item Morisky Medication Adherence Scale. This simple 4-question survey assesses the likelihood of patients taking their drug therapy as prescribed. The items measure the degree to which the patients self-report nonadherence to prescribed medication due to forgetting, carelessness, stopping the drug when feeling better or stopping the drug when feeling worse. In the present study, we used the Italian validated version of the MMAS-4 [42].

Health Care Climate Questionnaire (HCCQ). This scale assesses patients' perceptions of the ability of the healthcare professionals in supporting their autonomy (versus "controllingness") and in motivating their initiative in care management. The HCCQ consists of 15 items on a seven-point Likert scale ranging from *strongly disagree* to *strongly agree*. The scale was firstly developed and validated on the diabetic population by Williams and colleagues [43, 44].

Demographic characteristics included age (<60; ≥60); gender (male or female); education (elementary school, junior high school, high school, college education, Ph.D. degree, or M.S. degree); occupational status (employed, retired, housewife, student, unemployed, or other); marital status (never married, married, divorced, or widowed).

Frequency of mHealth/eHealth Use. An ad hoc item was developed to assess patients' behaviors concerning the use of mHealth and eHealth technologies to seek information for managing type 2 diabetes care (i.e., "*I usually use internet or mobile devices to seek information for managing my care*"). The item has 7 response options on a Likert scale (never, almost never, occasionally, sometimes, often, almost always, or always).

2.3. Data Analysis. Data analysis was conducted in four steps. In the first step of analysis, descriptive analyses were conducted, with particular reference to sociodemographic characteristics of the sample. Furthermore, descriptive statistics were provided regarding the use of mHealth and eHealth technologies to seek information for managing type 2 diabetes care.

In the second step of the analysis, the psychometric properties of the instruments were assessed in terms of reliability by using Cronbach's alpha for metric variables or ordinal alpha via Empirical Copula for ordinal variables [45]. A Cronbach or ordinal alpha higher than 0.7 was considered acceptable.

In the third step of analysis, correlations between all the considered variables were calculated. Since every instrument produces a metric score, the linear correlation coefficient r was calculated and evaluated with a significance test.

In the last step, a Structural Equation Model with observed variables using ML estimation method was implemented [46], in order to evaluate the relationships between the considered variables and to explore the theoretical hypothesized model (see the 5 hypotheses stated above). In the model we considered *HCCQ* as an exogenous variable and mediator (*PHE-S*) and dependent variables (*PAM, MMAS-4,* and *frequency of mHealth/eHealth use*) as endogenous variables. The goodness-of-fit indexes were examined through Chi square test, RMSEA, CFI, and SRMR, particularly suitable for both large and small samples. Models with acceptable fit presented nonsignificant Chi square value, RMSEA < 0.08 CFI > 0.90 and SRMR < 0.08 [47]. To improve the goodness-of-fit, modification indices were considered.

2.4. Ethical Concerns. The study received approval from the Università Cattolica del Sacro Cuore Ethics Committee. Patients consented to participate in the study, and they were allowed to withdraw from the study whenever they wanted. The data were collected anonymously and analyzed in an aggregated way.

3. Results

Overall, 93 patients were invited to participate in the study and completely answered the questionnaire for the analysis. All patients (29 females) completed the survey, mean age of 58.3 (±12.4) years with a mean disease duration of almost 11 years. Sociodemographic and psychometric characteristics are summarized in Table 1. Mean, standard deviation (unless otherwise indicated), and a suitable reliability index (Cronbach's alpha or ordinal alpha via Empirical Copula) are reported for all the psychometric measures considered. All the psychometric measures presented a good or excellent

TABLE 1: Characteristics of the sample.

Sociodemographic characteristics	
Age (years)	M = 58.3; DS = 12.4
Gender (% female)	31.2
Disease duration	M = 14.4; DS = 11.1
Marital status (%)	
Never married	7.5
Married	79.5
Divorced	10.8
Widowed	2.2
Employment (%)	
Employed	43.0
Retired	44.0
Housewife	3.2
Student	2.2
Unemployed	5.4
Other	2.2
Education (%)	
Elementary school	5.4
Junior high school	14.0
High school	50.5
College education	23.7
Ph.D. or M.S. degree	6.4
Psychometric measures	
PHE-S	Median = 3 (range 1–4); entropy = 0.89; ordinal alpha = 0.82
PAM	M = 66.8 (range 0–100); DS = 18.3; Cronbach's alpha = 0.93
MMAS-4	M = 1.3 (range 0–4); DS = 1.3; Cronbach's alpha = 0.81
HCCQ	M = 66.8 (range 13–91); DS = 15.1; Cronbach's alpha = 0.92

TABLE 2: Frequency of mHealth/eHealth use.

I usually use internet or mobile devices to seek information for managing my care (%)	
Never	14.0
Almost never	5.3
Occasionally	5.3
Sometimes	19.4
Often	17.2
Almost always	19.4
Always	19.4

reliability, with a Cronbach's or ordinal alpha ranged from 0.81 to 0.93.

Table 2 reports the distribution of the ad hoc item (*frequency of mHealth/eHealth use*), created to assess patients' behaviors concerning the use of mHealth and eHealth technologies to seek information for managing type 2 diabetes care (i.e., "*I usually use internet or mobile devices to seek information for managing my care*"). Table 2 shows that much more than 50% of our sample used regularly (i.e., often, very often, or always) mHealth or eHealth technologies to seek for information for managing their type 2 diabetes care. Only 20% of the sample did not regularly use such technologies.

In Table 3 linear correlation coefficients between the considered psychometric variables are reported.

HCCQ presented a significant correlation with all the measures: a positive correlation with *PHE-S, PAM,* and *frequency of mHealth/eHealth use* and a negative correlation with *MMAS-4* were detected. *PHE-S* showed a significant direct correlation with *HCCQ* and *PAM,* while it had no significant correlation with *MMAS-4* and *frequency of mHealth/eHealth use. PAM* had a significant direct correlation with all the measures except from *MMAS-4: PAM* and *MMAS-4* were negatively correlated. *Frequency of mHealth/eHealth use* significantly only depended on *HCCQ* and *PAM.*

Considering the five hypotheses to be tested in the study and the detected correlations between the psychometric measures and the *frequency of mHealth/eHealth use,* a Structural Equation Model was implemented.

Relationships between patients' perceptions of the ability of the healthcare professionals in supporting their autonomy (*HCCQ*), patients' engagement (*PHE-S*), patient's activation (*PAM*), medication adherence (*MMAS-4*), and the *frequency of mHealth/eHealth use* were tested. Figure 1 shows the explanatory model of the hypotheses we wanted to verify.

TABLE 3: Linear correlations coefficients between psychometric measures and frequency of mHealth/eHealth use.

	HCCQ	PHE-S	PAM	MMAS-4	mHealth/eHealth
HCCQ	—	0.356**	0.406**	−0.315**	0.292**
PHE-S		—	0.428**	−0.244*	0.034
PAM			—	−0.222*	0.373**
MMAS-4				—	−0.090
mHealth/eHealth					—

*$p < 0.05$; **$p < 0.01$.

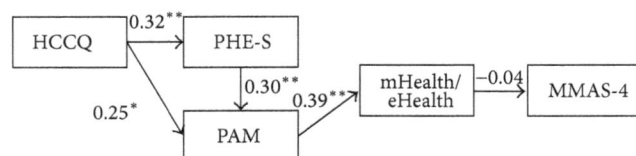

FIGURE 1: Structural Equation Model 1.

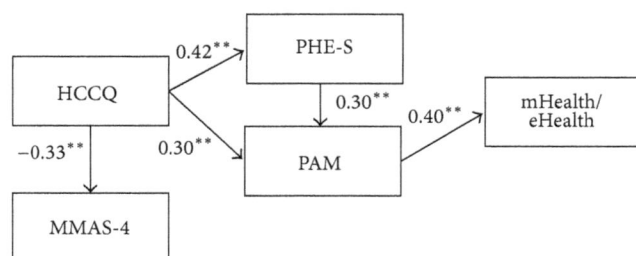

FIGURE 2: Structural Equation Model 2.

The model showed an exogenous observed variable (*HCCQ*), four endogenous observed variables (PHE-S, PAM, *frequency of mHealth/eHealth use,* and *MMAS-4*). The *PHE-S* mediates the relationship between *HCCQ* and *PAM*.

The model fit was deemed to be not acceptable ($\chi^2(5) = 15.50$, $p < 0.01$; CFI = 0.59; RMSEA = 0.15). Almost all the paths were found to be significant (**$p < 0.01$, *$p < 0.05$), except the path between *frequency of mHealth/eHealth use* and *MMAS-4* (−0.04, $p = 0.74$).

The hypotheses were only partially verified. On the basis of the evaluation of the modification indexes, the correlations, and the estimated paths, a modification of the model was hypothesized and tested. In particular modification indexes suggested to emphasize the direct relationship between *HCCQ* and *MMAS-4* and to delete the relationship between *frequency of mHealth/eHealth use* and *MMAS-4*. The *MMAS-4* resulted consequently from a high level of patients' perceptions about the ability of the healthcare system in supporting their autonomy (*HCCQ*). The *frequency of mHealth/eHealth use* resulting is strongly dependent on the level of patients' activation (*PAM*), but it did not seem to impact on patients' adherence (*MMAS-4*). Figure 2 shows the final model.

Model 2 presented an acceptable goodness-of-fit. Chi square test was not significant ($\chi^2(5) = 7.54$, $p = 0.15$). All the goodness-of-fit was satisfactory (RMSEA = 0.07, CFI = 0.90, and SRMR = 0.06). The estimated paths were

significant ($p < 0.001$). The adjusted goodness-of-fit (AGFI) was superior to 0.90 (AGFI = 0.901). Overall, model fit indices significantly increased from Model 1 to Model 2.

4. Discussion

This study aimed to verify how the perceived ability of the healthcare professionals to support type 2 diabetes patients' autonomy and motivation to self-care initiative might impact on their level of activation and engagement and, consequently, on their adoption of mHealth and eHealth technologies to seek information for managing care. Furthermore, the study aimed to test the mediating role of patient engagement in the relationship between the healthcare professional motivating role and patient activation. Finally the study explored the impact of mHealth and eHealth technologies use for health information seeking on type 2 diabetes patients' adherence.

Concerning the first two hypotheses, the study confirmed the crucial role of the healthcare professionals in influencing the level of type 2 diabetes patients' engagement and activation, according to other studies on chronic populations [17]. Furthermore, the level of type 2 diabetes patients' activation was confirmed in influencing patients' adoption of mHealth/eHealth technologies to support care management and seek health information [48, 49].

This study showed how the more clinicians are perceived by patients as able to motivate their initiatives towards self-care, the more the patients report higher level of engagement and activation in healthcare processes. Type 2 diabetes patients' perception and assessment of the healthcare professionals' ability to be aligned with their needs and expectations toward care management are, thus, demonstrated to be a crucial antecedent of the patients' ability to take an active role in their care management. The more the healthcare system is perceived as facilitating type 2 diabetes patients' autonomy, the more the patients show higher level of engagement towards their care management. To foster patients engagement in care management means to support the complex psychosocial elaboration of the illness condition and of the new medical requirements that individuals undergo when diagnosed with type 2 diabetes (and/or when new symptoms occur) [14, 50]. Consequently, the role of healthcare professionals appears pivotal in supporting type 2 diabetes patients engagement in adopting healthier lifestyles and gaining higher quality of life [29, 51].

Furthermore, as this study showed, high level of type 2 diabetes patients engagement is predictive of the patients activation in self-management: the more the type 2 diabetes patient is engaged, the more he/she appears able to feel self-confident in assuming a proactive and empowered role in the care process. The huge impact of cognitions and behaviors is well reported in literature [14, 29]. However, patients' engagement is the result of a dynamic synergy among different experiential dimensions: patient engagement, indeed, is not only dependent on knowledge and skills related to the health condition and treatment management. It also implies patients' enactment of an adaptive emotional elaboration and acceptance of the new patient identity and of its consequences on quality of life [14, 22].

The level of type 2 diabetes patients' activation in its turn resulted to be a crucial antecedent of patients' attitude towards the adoption of mHealth and eHealth technologies to seek information for care management. Patients' activation refers to the patients' ability and willingness to directly manage their own health and health care [39]. To seek health and care information through mHealth and eHealth technologies to manage care might be considered as a behavioral manifestation of the patients' willingness of taking a "starring role" in the management of their care [50].

Different studies investigated the potential role of mHealth/eHealth technologies to support patient activation and used the patient activation as a compass to personalize the intervention with promising results [35, 52]. In this sense, our study provides further evidences on a crucial antecedent of patient activation: that is patient engagement. This concept might be useful when developing and delivering technological solutions, which are aligned with the complex emotional elaboration the patient undergoes when dealing with diabetes care and allow them to communicate with their referential health professional [53].

Moreover, our results confirmed the importance of questioning the readiness of the healthcare organization and of its employees in receiving and adopting technological innovations devoted to sustaining better integrated models of care [54, 55]. Implicit values and practices rooted into the organizational culture might play the role of enhancers or inhibitors of such organizational innovation. Relational, psychological, and pragmatic implications of eHealth and mHealth should be considered when planning and delivering such interventions in order to maximize their clinical and organizational effectiveness. Healthcare professionals' education oriented to uncovering of clinicians' experiential knowledge and attitudes towards patients' engagement should be a priority in this changing scenario [56].

Finally, it is interesting to note that the last hypothesis of this study was not confirmed. The level of patients' adherence was not proved to be directly dependent on the frequency of mHealth and eHealth adoption to seek information for type 2 diabetes care management, thus demonstrating that this is still a controversial topic according to other studies [57]. In this sense, spontaneous behaviors of information seeking through mHealth and eHealth sources are not an indication of greater patients' adherence. Health information obtained through online sources has been widely debated for their inaccurate and misleading nature which can lead to ineffective self-care regimens if not properly sustained

by healthcare professionals [58]. Furthermore, the ability of mHealth or eHealth to foster type 2 diabetes patients' adherence might be dependent on the characteristics of the intervention and of the specific tools employed in it; mHealth and eHealth tools for information seeking probably need tailored and multiple strategies to promote adherence [57]. Patients' adherence resulted, on the contrary, from direct function of the healthcare professionals' perceived ability to support patients' autonomy and motivation towards their diabetes care. This result appears particularly interesting because it is a further empirical confirmation of the crucial role played by the healthcare organization and by its employees to enable the success of clinical interventions. Indeed, healthcare professionals seem to have a vicarious role in the proper use of health information and in the activation of patients towards managing their health and, consequently, in patients' adherence. Different studies confirmed that the quality of the relationship between healthcare professionals and patients is a crucial factor for improving the adherence of patients [59, 60]. Our results suggest the importance of supporting the introduction of new technological tools to innovate healthcare processes with a deep understanding of the psychosocial, relational, and pragmatic implication of such innovation: only "taking on board" the human resources implied in this organizational change, the challenge of innovating care process in an effective integrated model can be successful [61, 62]. Healthcare professionals, in particular, need to be accompanied to understand and accept the value of such tools to improve their ability to follow and treat their type 2 diabetes patients. Healthcare professionals are the enablers, from patients' perspective, of the mHealth or eHealth interventions' clinical potentials; they are perceived as the legitimators of the active role of the patient in the care process [17] and thus of the possibility to adopt new technologies within the type 2 diabetes care pathway within a shared decision making process [63].

Therefore, mHealth or eHealth initiatives for type 2 diabetes care should be designed and delivered having in mind the goal of sustaining the engagement of the different stakeholders implied in the healthcare process (i.e., the patients, their lay caregivers but also their healthcare professionals both inside and outside the hospital) [11, 14, 38]. This goal could be achieved by assuming a psychosocial and organizational view of the different level of needs and expectations towards the care process (and its innovation) carried out by the different stakeholders: to fail in this consideration may result in psychosocial and relational hindrances to the process of adoption of mHealth or eHealth and thus to their clinical effectiveness. This could also have an impact on the success of integrated care models featuring the adoption of new technologies [12].

Limitations. Although the results of our study appear interesting to cast light on the complex psychosocial and organizational dimensions implied in sustaining patient engagement and the adoption of mHealth or eHealth for seeking information for type 2 diabetes care in integrated care models, some limitations have to be considered. Firstly, the study was carried out on a fairly small sample of Italian patients.

However the sample features were enough to allow the robustness of the conducted statistical analysis. Furthermore, the sample of patients included in our study is not representative of the Italian type 2 diabetes population. However, we used it only to explore the relationships of the variables under analysis and not for an estimation of their dimensions: based on these considerations full representativeness is not necessarily required [64, 65]. Furthermore, our study was not conceived as an effectiveness evaluation of a real mHealth or eHealth intervention, but it took into account the spontaneous behaviors of patients when adopting mHealth or eHealth technologies to seek information for type 2 diabetes care management. This may be envisaged as a limitation because it does not allow the researcher to understand what technological and organizational characteristic of a mHealth or eHealth intervention may impact on patients' engagement and activation and on their adherence to treatment. Results should be interpreted with caution because of the explorative nature of this study. Furthermore, we only measured the frequency of spontaneous behaviors of mHealth and eHealth use to seek information for diabetes care instead of measuring also type of technologies adopted or type of information searched.

However, this analysis has the value of offering some precious insights into the patients' spontaneous attitudes and behaviors in a natural setting and should be considered as a "baseline" evidence of the general approach of patients to mHealth or eHealth and of the psychosocial and organizational dynamics that may impact on their effectiveness [66].

5. Conclusions

Type 2 diabetes requires a long-term approach to care and the good synergy between hospitals and primary care resources. To address this requirement, to "give back" an active role to patients in managing their health is crucial. mHealth/eHealth interventions for type 2 diabetes care are considered as an effective strategy to improve type 2 patients' empowerment and clinical outcomes. Moreover they are demonstrated to be powerful in enhancing patients-doctors communication, in fostering patients' satisfaction with care and in making healthcare cost-effective. However, in order to be effective, the introduction of such technological interventions needs to be supported by the reference healthcare professionals, who should legitimize the intervention process and sustain the autonomous initiative of the type 2 diabetes patients throughout it.

From this perspective, our study confirmed the important role of healthcare professionals' ability to foster type 2 diabetes patients' autonomy in enhancing their activation and engagement towards self-management, this being a precursor of patients' attitude to the use of mHealth/eHealth technologies. Furthermore, our study well highlighted how patient engagement, defined as a multidimensional psychosocial process resulting from the conjoint cognitive, emotional, and behavioral enactment of individuals toward their health conditions and their management [15, 17, 38], is a pivotal precursor of patient activation towards self-management and

thus towards patients' use of new technological interventions. This finding is relevant and opens insights into the psychosocial and relational antecedent of patients' activation in self-management. The function of patients' activation in guaranteeing improved clinical outcomes, better patients' satisfaction towards healthcare, and reduced costs in services delivery has been demonstrated by several studies [67–69]. However, till now, still little is known about the factors that may support the increase of patients' activation [70]. This study, by focusing on type 2 diabetes patients, offers an important theoretical and pragmatic contribution by demonstrating the role of patient engagement in determining the level of patients' behavioral activation and self-confidence in type 2 diabetes care management.

Finally, the indirect relationship that our study showed between the frequency of mHealth/eHealth use and the level of type 2 diabetes patients' adherence, although it needs further confirmation, opens the door to interesting debate about how new technologies can be effectively designed in order to improve adherence. Too often, the debate about new mHealth/eHealth interventions for sustaining patient engagement in type 2 diabetes care management has been primarily focused on the technological ("hard") features of such interventions [71]. The psychosocial and organizational ("soft") aspects may mediate the effectiveness of mHealth and eHealth interventions and, consequently, deserve an enhanced attention, as an important complement of the analysis of the "hard" determinants of such interventions effectiveness [72].

Conflict of Interests

The authors declare that there is no conflict of interests regarding the publication of this paper.

References

[1] Committee on Quality of Health Care in America IoM, *Crossing the Quality Chasm: A New Health System for the 21st Century*, National Academy Press, Washington, DC, USA, 2001.

[2] American Diabetes Association, "Standards of medical care in diabetes—2014," *Diabetes Care*, vol. 37, pp. 14–80, 2014.

[3] Ministero della Salute, *Piano sulla Malattia Diabetica*, DG Programmazione Sanitaria—Commissione Nazionale Diabete, 2012.

[4] O. Gröne and M. Garcia-Barbero, "Integrated care: a position paper of the WHO European Office for Integrated Health Care Services," *International Journal of Integrated Care*, vol. 1, article e21, 2001.

[5] L. Bellardita, G. Graffigna, S. Donegani et al., "Patient's choice of observational strategy for early-stage prostate cancer," *Neuropsychological Trends*, vol. 12, no. 1, pp. 107–116, 2012.

[6] C. M. Renders, G. D. Valk, S. J. Griffin, E. H. Wagner, J. T. M. Van Eijk, and W. J. J. Assendelft, "Interventions to improve the management of diabetes in primary care, outpatient, and community settings: a systematic review," *Diabetes Care*, vol. 24, no. 10, pp. 1821–1833, 2001.

[7] M. Ouwens, H. Wollersheim, R. Hermens, M. Hulscher, and R. Grol, "Integrated care programmes for chronically ill patients: a

review of systemic reviews," *International Journal for Quality in Health Care*, vol. 17, no. 2, pp. 141–146, 2005.

[8] N. Goodwin, J. Smith, A. Davies et al., *Integrated Care for Patients and Populations: Improving Outcomes by Working Together*, King's Fund, London, UK, 2012.

[9] J. Bousquet, J. M. Anto, P. J. Sterk et al., "Systems medicine and integrated care to combat chronic noncommunicable diseases," *Genome Medicine*, vol. 3, article 43, 12 pages, 2011.

[10] C. Bosio, G. Graffigna, and G. Scaratti, "Knowing, learning and acting in health care organizations and services: challenges and opportunities for qualitative research," *Qualitative Research in Organizations and Management: An International Journal*, vol. 7, no. 3, pp. 256–274, 2012.

[11] G. Graffigna, S. Barello, S. Triberti, B. K. Wiederhold, A. C. Bosio, and G. Riva, "Enabling eHealth as a pathway for patient engagement: a toolkit for medical practice," *Studies in Health Technology and Informatics*, vol. 199, pp. 13–21, 2014.

[12] D. L. Kodner and C. Spreeuwenberg, "Integrated care: meaning, logic, applications, and implications—a discussion paper," *International Journal of Integrated Care*, vol. 2, article e12, 2002.

[13] H. J. M. Vrijhoef, R. Berbee, E. H. Wagner, and L. M. G. Steuten, "Quality of integrated chronic care measured by patient survey: identification, selection and application of most appropriate instruments," *Health Expectations*, vol. 12, no. 4, pp. 417–429, 2009.

[14] G. Graffigna, S. Barello, G. Riva, and A. C. Bosio, "Patient engagement: the key to redesign the exchange between the demand and supply for healthcare in the era of active ageing," in *Active Ageing and Healthy Living: A Human Centered Approach in Research and Innovation as Source of Quality of Life*, vol. 203, pp. 85–95, IOS Press, 2014.

[15] G. Graffigna, S. Barello, C. Libreri, and C. A. Bosio, "How to engage type-2 diabetic patients in their own health management: implications for clinical practice," *BMC Public Health*, vol. 14, no. 1, article 648, 2014.

[16] J. E. Epping-Jordan, S. D. Pruitt, R. Bengoa, and E. H. Wagner, "Improving the quality of health care for chronic conditions," *Quality and Safety in Health Care*, vol. 13, no. 4, pp. 299–305, 2004.

[17] S. Barello, G. Graffigna, E. Vegni, M. Savarese, F. Lombardi, and A. C. Bosio, "'Engage me in taking care of my heart': a grounded theory study on patient-cardiologist relationship in the hospital management of heart failure," *BMJ Open*, vol. 5, no. 3, Article ID e005582, 2015.

[18] M. J. Crawford, D. Rutter, C. Manley et al., "Systematic review of involving patients in the planning and development of health care," *BMJ Open*, vol. 325, article 1263, 2002.

[19] K. L. Carman, P. Dardess, M. Maurer et al., "Patient and family engagement: a framework for understanding the elements and developing interventions and policies," *Health Affairs*, vol. 32, no. 2, pp. 223–231, 2013.

[20] J. H. Hibbard, E. R. Mahoney, R. Stock, and M. Tusler, "Do increases in patient activation result in improved self-management behaviors?" *Health Services Research*, vol. 42, no. 4, pp. 1443–1463, 2007.

[21] E. I. Lubetkin, W.-H. Lu, and M. R. Gold, "Levels and correlates of patient activation in health center settings: building strategies for improving health outcomes," *Journal of Health Care for the Poor and Underserved*, vol. 21, no. 3, pp. 796–808, 2010.

[22] S. Barello and G. Graffigna, "Engaging patients to recover life projectuality: an Italian cross-disease framework," *Quality of Life Research*, vol. 24, no. 5, pp. 1087–1096, 2014.

[23] M. P. Manary, W. Boulding, R. Staelin, and S. W. Glickman, "The patient experience and health outcomes," *The New England Journal of Medicine*, vol. 368, no. 3, pp. 201–203, 2013.

[24] J. H. Hibbard, J. Greene, and V. Overton, "Patients with lower activation associated with higher costs; delivery systems should know their patients' 'scores,'" *Health Affairs*, vol. 32, no. 2, pp. 216–222, 2013.

[25] E. O. Lee and E. J. Emanuel, "Shared decision making to improve care and reduce costs," *The New England Journal of Medicine*, vol. 368, no. 1, pp. 6–8, 2013.

[26] V. Weber, F. Bloom, S. Pierdon, and C. Wood, "Employing the electronic health record to improve diabetes care: a multifaceted intervention in an integrated delivery system," *Journal of General Internal Medicine*, vol. 23, no. 4, pp. 379–382, 2008.

[27] J. E. Aikens, K. Zivin, R. Trivedi, and J. D. Piette, "Diabetes self-management support using mHealth and enhanced informal caregiving," *Journal of Diabetes and its Complications*, vol. 28, no. 2, pp. 171–176, 2014.

[28] C. D. Norman and H. A. Skinner, "eHealth literacy: essential skills for consumer health in a networked world," *Journal of Medical Internet Research*, vol. 8, no. 2, article e9, 2006.

[29] J. E. Jordan, A. M. Briggs, C. A. Brand, and R. H. Osborne, "Enhancing patient engagement in chronic disease self-management support initiatives in Australia: the need for an integrated approach," *Medical Journal of Australia*, vol. 189, supplement, no. 10, pp. S9–S13, 2008.

[30] G. Castelnuovo, G. M. Manzoni, G. Pietrabissa et al., "Obesity and outpatient rehabilitation using mobile technologies: the potential mHealth approach," *Frontiers in Psychology*, vol. 5, article 559, 2014.

[31] C. K. L. Or and D. Tao, "Does the use of consumer health information technology improve outcomes in the patient self-management of diabetes? A meta-analysis and narrative review of randomized controlled trials," *International Journal of Medical Informatics*, vol. 83, no. 5, pp. 320–329, 2014.

[32] J. M. Wojcicki, P. Ladyzynski, J. Krzymien et al., "What we can really expect from telemedicine in intensive diabetes treatment: results from 3-year study on type 1 pregnant diabetic women," *Diabetes Technology & Therapeutics*, vol. 3, no. 4, pp. 581–589, 2001.

[33] A. S. Shetty, S. Chamukuttan, A. Nanditha, R. K. C. Raj, and A. Ramachandran, "Reinforcement of adherence to prescription recommendations in Asian Indian diabetes patients using short message service (SMS)—a pilot study," *Journal of Association of Physicians of India*, vol. 59, no. 11, pp. 711–714, 2011.

[34] A. P. Cotter, N. Durant, A. A. Agne, and A. L. Cherrington, "Internet interventions to support lifestyle modification for diabetes management: a systematic review of the evidence," *Journal of Diabetes and its Complications*, vol. 28, no. 2, pp. 243–251, 2013.

[35] B. Holtz and C. Lauckner, "Diabetes management via mobile phones: a systematic review," *Telemedicine and e-Health*, vol. 18, no. 3, pp. 175–184, 2012.

[36] K. Lorig, P. L. Ritter, D. D. Laurent et al., "Online diabetes self-management program: a randomized study," *Diabetes Care*, vol. 33, no. 6, pp. 1275–1281, 2010.

[37] P. Newton, K. Asimakopoulou, and S. Scambler, "A qualitative exploration of motivation to self-manage and styles of self-management amongst people living with type 2 diabetes," *Journal of Diabetes Research*, vol. 2015, Article ID 638205, 9 pages, 2015.

[38] R. E. Herzlinger, "Why innovation in health care is so hard," *Harvard Business Review*, vol. 84, no. 5, pp. 58–66, 2006.

[39] G. Graffigna, S. Barello, A. Bonanomi, and E. Lozza, "Measuring patient engagement: development and psychometric properties of the Patient Health Engagement (PHE) scale," *Frontiers in Psychology*, vol. 6, article 274, 2015.

[40] J. H. Hibbard, J. Stockard, E. R. Mahoney, and M. Tusler, "Development of the patient activation measure (PAM): conceptualizing and measuring activation in patients and consumers," *Health Services Research*, vol. 39, no. 4, pp. 1005–1026, 2004.

[41] G. Graffigna, S. Barello, A. Bonanomi, E. Lozza, and J. Hibbard, "Measuring patient activation in Italy: translation, adaptation and validation of the Italian version of the patient activation measure 13 (PAM13-I)," *BMC Medical Informatics and Decision Making*, vol. 15, no. 1, article 109, pp. 1–13, 2015.

[42] G. Fabbrini, G. Abbruzzese, P. Barone et al., "Adherence to anti-Parkinson drug therapy in the 'rEASON' sample of Italian patients with Parkinson's disease: the linguistic validation of the Italian version of the 'Morisky Medical Adherence Scale-8 Items'," *Neurological Sciences*, vol. 34, no. 11, pp. 2015–2022, 2013.

[43] G. C. Williams, V. M. Grow, Z. R. Freedman, R. M. Ryan, and E. L. Deci, "Motivational predictors of weight loss and weight-loss maintenance," *Journal of Personality and Social Psychology*, vol. 70, no. 1, pp. 115–126, 1996.

[44] G. C. Williams, Z. R. Freedman, and E. L. Deci, "Supporting autonomy to motivate patients with diabetes for glucose control," *Diabetes Care*, vol. 21, no. 10, pp. 1644–1651, 1998.

[45] A. Bonanomi, G. Cantaluppi, M. N. Ruscone, and S. A. Osmetti, "A new estimator of Zumbo's Ordinal Alpha: a copula approach," *Quality & Quantity*, vol. 49, no. 3, pp. 941–953, 2015.

[46] K. G. Jöreskog and F. Yang, "Nonlinear structural equation models: the Kenny-Judd model with interaction effects," in *Advanced Structural Equation Modeling: Issues and Techniques*, pp. 57–88, Lawrence Erlbaum Associates, 1996.

[47] P. M. Bentler, "Comparative fit indexes in structural models," *Psychological Bulletin*, vol. 107, no. 2, pp. 238–246, 1990.

[48] S. G. Smith, A. Pandit, S. R. Rush, M. S. Wolf, and C. Simon, "The association between patient activation and accessing online health information: results from a national survey of US adults," *Health Expectations*, vol. 18, no. 6, pp. 3262–3273, 2015.

[49] P. C. B. Crouch, C. D. Rose, M. Johnson, and S. L. Janson, "A pilot study to evaluate the magnitude of association of the use of electronic personal health records with patient activation and empowerment in HIV-infected veterans," *PeerJ*, vol. 3, article e852, 2015.

[50] J. Menichetti, C. Libreri, E. Lozza, and G. Graffigna, "Giving patients a starring role in their own care: a bibliometric analysis of the on-going literature debate," *Health Expectations*, 2014.

[51] E. Aung, M. Donald, J. R. Coll, and G. M. Williams, "Association between patient activation and patient-assessed quality of care in type 2 diabetes: results of a longitudinal study," *Health Expectations*, 2015.

[52] M. Solomon, S. L. Wagner, and J. Goes, "Effects of a Web-based intervention for adults with chronic conditions on patient activation: online randomized controlled trial," *Journal of Medical Internet Research*, vol. 14, no. 1, article e32, 2012.

[53] S. Barello, G. Graffigna, and E. C. Meyer, "Ethics and etiquette in neonatal intensive care: the value of parents' engagement in everyday ethics and recommendations for further advancing the field," *JAMA Pediatrics*, vol. 169, no. 2, article 190, 2015.

[54] T. Greenhalgh, G. Robert, F. Macfarlane, P. Bate, and O. Kyriakidou, "Diffusion of innovations in service organizations: systematic review and recommendations," *Milbaak Quarterly*, vol. 82, no. 4, pp. 581–629, 2004.

[55] G. M. Manzoni, F. Pagnini, S. Corti, E. Molinari, and G. Castelnuovo, "Internet-based behavioral interventions for obesity: an updated systematic review," *Clinical Practice and Epidemiology in Mental Health: CP & EMH*, vol. 7, pp. 19–28, 2011.

[56] G. Lamiani, S. Barello, D. M. Browning, E. Vegni, and E. C. Meyer, "Uncovering and validating clinicians experiential knowledge when facing difficult conversations: a cross-cultural perspective," *Patient Education and Counseling*, vol. 87, no. 3, pp. 307–312, 2012.

[57] H. Anglada-Martinez, G. Riu-Viladoms, M. Martin-Conde, M. Rovira-Illamola, J. M. Sotoca-Momblona, and C. Codina-Jane, "Does mHealth increase adherence to medication? Results of a systematic review," *International Journal of Clinical Practice*, vol. 69, no. 1, pp. 9–32, 2015.

[58] S. A. Iverson, K. B. Howard, and B. K. Penney, "Impact of internet use on health-related behaviors and the patient-physician relationship: a survey-based study and review," *Journal of the American Osteopathic Association*, vol. 108, no. 12, pp. 699–711, 2008.

[59] J. Laugesen, K. Hassanein, and Y. Yuan, "The impact of internet health information on patient compliance: a research model and an empirical study," *Journal of Medical Internet Research*, vol. 17, no. 6, article e143, 2015.

[60] M. L. Parchman, J. E. Zeber, and R. F. Palmer, "Participatory decision making, patient activation, medication adherence, and intermediate clinical outcomes in type 2 diabetes: a starnet study," *The Annals of Family Medicine*, vol. 8, no. 5, pp. 410–417, 2010.

[61] M. Sorrentino, C. Guglielmetti, S. Gilardi, and M. Marsilio, "Health care services and the coproduction puzzle filling in the blanks," *Administration & Society*, 2015.

[62] L. Moja, E. G. Liberati, L. Galuppo et al., "Barriers and facilitators to the uptake of computerized clinical decision support systems in specialty hospitals: protocol for a qualitative cross-sectional study," *Implementation Science*, vol. 9, article 105, 2014.

[63] S. Barello and G. Graffigna, "Patient engagement in healthcare: pathways for effective medical decision making," *Neuropsychological Trends*, vol. 17, pp. 53–65, 2015.

[64] P. Sturgis, "Survey and sampling," in *Research Methods in Psychology*, G. M. Breakwell, S. Hamond, C. Fife-Schaw, and J. A. Smith, Eds., Sage, London, UK, 2006.

[65] E. Lozza, C. Libreri, and A. C. Bosio, "Temporary employment, job insecurity and their extraorganizational outcomes," *Economic and Industrial Democracy*, vol. 34, no. 1, pp. 89–105, 2013.

[66] G. Graffigna, S. Barello, and S. Triberti, *Patient Engagement: A Consumer-Centered Model to Innovate Healthcare*, DeGruyter Open, Varsavia, Poland, 2015.

[67] D. M. Mosen, J. Schmittdiel, J. Hibbard, D. Sobel, C. Remmers, and J. Bellows, "Is patient activation associated with outcomes of care for adults with chronic conditions?" *The Journal of Ambulatory Care Management*, vol. 30, no. 1, pp. 21–29, 2007.

[68] J. Greene and J. H. Hibbard, "Why does patient activation matter? An examination of the relationships between patient activation and health-related outcomes," *Journal of General Internal Medicine*, vol. 27, no. 5, pp. 520–526, 2012.

[69] S. Barello, G. Graffigna, and M. Savarese, "Engaging patients in health management: towards a preliminary theoretical conceptualization," *Psicologia della Salute*, vol. 23, pp. 11–33, 2014.

[70] I. Bos-Touwen, M. Schuurmans, E. M. Monninkhof et al., "Patient and disease characteristics associated with activation for self-management in patients with diabetes, chronic obstructive pulmonary disease, chronic heart failure and chronic renal disease: a cross-sectional survey study," *PLoS ONE*, vol. 10, no. 5, Article ID e0126400, 2015.

[71] G. Graffigna, S. Barello, and G. Riva, "How to make health information technology effective: the challenge of patient engagement," *Archives of Physical Medicine and Rehabilitation*, vol. 94, no. 10, pp. 2034–2035, 2013.

[72] G. Graffigna, S. Barello, and G. Riva, "Technologies for patient engagement," *Health Affairs*, vol. 32, no. 6, article 1172, 2013.

10

Subclinical Alterations of Cardiac Mechanics Present Early in the Course of Pediatric Type 1 Diabetes Mellitus: A Prospective Blinded Speckle Tracking Stress Echocardiography Study

Kai O. Hensel, Franziska Grimmer, Markus Roskopf, Andreas C. Jenke, Stefan Wirth, and Andreas Heusch

Department of Pediatrics, HELIOS Medical Center Wuppertal, Centre for Clinical & Translational Research (CCTR), Centre for Biomedical Education & Research (ZBAF), Faculty of Health, Witten/Herdecke University, Heusnerstraße 40, 42283 Wuppertal, Germany

Correspondence should be addressed to Kai O. Hensel; kai.hensel@uni-wh.de

Academic Editor: John Skoularigis

Diabetic cardiomyopathy substantially accounts for mortality in diabetes mellitus. The pathophysiological mechanism underlying diabetes-associated nonischemic heart failure is poorly understood and clinical data on myocardial mechanics in early stages of diabetes are lacking. In this study we utilize speckle tracking echocardiography combined with physical stress testing in order to evaluate whether left ventricular (LV) myocardial performance is altered early in the course of uncomplicated type 1 diabetes mellitus (T1DM). 40 consecutive asymptomatic normotensive children and adolescents with T1DM (mean age 11.5 ± 3.1 years and mean disease duration 4.3 ± 3.5 years) and 44 age- and gender-matched healthy controls were assessed using conventional and quantitative echocardiography (strain and strain rate) during bicycle ergometer stress testing. Strikingly, T1DM patients had increased LV longitudinal ($p = 0.019$) and circumferential ($p = 0.016$) strain rate both at rest and during exercise ($p = 0.021$). This was more pronounced in T1DM patients with a longer disease duration ($p = 0.038$). T1DM patients with serum $HbA_{1c} > 9\%$ showed impaired longitudinal ($p = 0.008$) and circumferential strain ($p = 0.005$) and a reduced E/A-ratio ($p = 0.018$). In conclusion, asymptomatic T1DM patients have signs of hyperdynamic LV contractility early in the course of the disease. Moreover, poor glycemic control is associated with early subclinical LV systolic and diastolic impairment.

1. Introduction

Type 1 diabetes mellitus (T1DM) is ranging among the most common chronic disorders of childhood and adolescence [1] with increasing incidence worldwide [2, 3]. Cardiovascular disease is the most common cause of death in diabetic patients and currently one of the leading causes of death overall in the industrialized world [4]. While ischemic events range highest in the list of diabetic cardiovascular complications [5], diabetic patients also develop heart failure in the absence of arterial hypertension and myocardial ischemia [6–8]. Even though the existence of "diabetic cardiomyopathy" in humans is a current matter of ongoing scientific controversy [9, 10], there is growing evidence for the assumption that diabetes can lead to systolic and diastolic cardiac dysfunction

without other obvious causes for cardiomyopathy, such as overt ischemia, coronary artery disease, arterial hypertension, or valvular heart disease [11–16]. While there is a variety of causes contributing to diabetes-associated heart failure including impaired calcium homeostasis, enhanced fatty acid metabolism, suppressed glucose oxidation, altered intracellular signaling, and pathologic remodeling, the underlying pathophysiology of diabetic cardiomyopathy is still not well understood [8]. Whether uncomplicated diabetes mellitus already affects myocardial function in asymptomatic children at an early stage of the disease currently remains elusive [17]. Hence, children and adolescents with uncomplicated diabetes may serve as an ideal model to study the effect of diabetic metabolic conditions in the absence of potentially confounding ischemic events.

Myocardial deformation is a complex three-dimensional process influenced by heterogeneously organized heart muscle fibers. Measurements of left ventricular (LV) function are important for the evaluation, management, and estimation of prognosis in patients with various forms of cardiovascular disease [18]. However, ejection fraction (EF), the current echocardiographic gold standard for the assessment of systolic function, bears considerable limitations as a prognostic parameter [19] and does not correlate well with quantitative measures of functional capacity [20]. It uses a simplistic approach based on visual assessment of inward motion and wall thickening that underestimates the true complexity of myocardial contraction and suffers from significant inter- and intrarater variability [21]. Thus, subtle alterations in myocardial wall motion remain occult. Speckle tracking echocardiography (STE) is a quantitative diagnostic method for the assessment of myocardial deformation [22]. STE derived measurements correlate well with functional capacity [23] and feature promising inter- and intraobserver reproducibility [24]. Moreover, STE has been shown to detect subclinical systolic LV impairment in asymptomatic patients with preserved EF and arterial hypertension [25] or heart failure [26], respectively.

The aim of this study was to investigate whether STE can be used to detect subclinical alterations of LV myocardial deformation in asymptomatic pediatric patients with uncomplicated T1DM. Furthermore, we combined STE with physical stress testing in order to unmask subtle changes of cardiac contractility that might potentially be occult at rest.

2. Methods

2.1. Study Population. For this prospective diagnostic study we enrolled 40 consecutive children and adolescents with T1DM aged 6 to 17 years (mean age 11.5 ± 3.1 years; 40% female) and 44 age- and sex-matched healthy controls (mean age 11.4 ± 2.9 years; 45% female). Mandatory inclusion criteria in the study group were the diagnosis of insulin-dependent T1DM and a good general health state. Exclusion criteria were other past or present medical conditions that may affect the cardiovascular system such as congenital heart disease, systemic inflammatory disease, for example, history of Kawasaki disease, proteinuria, the use of any type of systemically acting medication (other than insulin for the study group), developmental delay, body mass index > 30 kg/m^2, submaximal effort during exercise testing, short leg length, or pathologic EKG-changes at rest or during exercise. None of the included patients suffered from sings of end-organ damage such as evidence of renal failure or retinal changes. Healthy control subjects had an entirely negative medical history with regard to the cardiovascular as well as to any other organ system. A written informed consent was obtained from each participant as well as from their legal guardian prior to inclusion in the study. Subsequently, a thorough history and physical examination as well as both resting and exercise echocardiography and EKG were obtained. The sample size was achieved by including all patients from the hospital's diabetes clinic that were willing to participate in the study. A priori study design was established dividing the diabetes population into subgroups of patients with a disease duration of less than 4 years (n = 23, 57.5%) and more than 4 years (n = 17, 42.5%) as well as a three-column stratification according to glycemic control with serum HbA$_{1c}$ < 7.5% (n = 10, 25%), HbA$_{1c}$ 7.5–9% (n = 19, 47.5%), and HbA$_{1c}$ > 9% (n = 11, 27.5%). The study was approved by the Witten/Herdecke University ethics committee and carried out in accordance with declaration of Helsinki's ethical principles for medical research involving human subjects. The study was registered to the Witten/Herdecke University Ethics and Clinical Trials Committee and assigned the trial number 113/2013.

2.2. Conventional and Doppler Echocardiography. All examinations were performed with the commercially available ultrasound device iE33 by Phillips Ultrasound Inc., USA, using a S5-1 Sector Array transducer (Sector 1–5 MHz). All images were digitally recorded and transferred to an offline workstation for analysis, using XCelera Version 3.1.1.422 by Phillips Ultrasound Inc., USA. According to echocardiography guidelines a complete standard 2D study, as well as a spectral and color flow Doppler examination, was carried out [27]. Image acquisition was performed in the parasternal long axis view, three short axis views, and the apical 4-, 3-, and 2-chamber views. M-mode images were taken at level of the aortic valve and the LV for subsequent measurement of aortic root diameter, left atrial diameter, interventricular septum, LV cavity, and LV posterior wall. Fractional shortening, LV mass, relative wall thickness, LV end-diastolic/end-systolic volume, EF, stroke volume, and cardiac output were calculated. Utilizing pw-Doppler and pw-TDI E/A-ratio, E/E$'$-ratio, mitral deceleration time, and isovolumetric relaxation time were measured for the assessment of LV diastolic function as previously described [28]. All measurements were evaluated using Z-scores [29]. During the entire examination a particular focus was set on the exclusion of any congenital heart disease as well as morphological or functional abnormalities.

2.3. Speckle Tracking Echocardiography. Myocardial deformation parameters (strain and strain rate) were measured acquiring standard 2D grayscale LV images. Circumferential strain (CS) was assessed in the standard parasternal short axis at the mitral valve plane (SAXB) and the papillary muscle plane (SAXM). Longitudinal strain (LS) was measured with standard apical 4-chamber (AP4), 3-chamber (AP3), and 2-chamber (AP2) apical views using conventional B-Mode imaging as previously described [22]. Five consecutive heart beats synchronized to a continuous EKG were recorded with frame rate set between 60 and 90 frames per second as recently suggested [30]. Caution was paid to minimize artifacts and to reduce noise for most accurate 2D strain estimation. All loops were digitally stored anonymized in the DICOM format and transferred to an offline workstation for postprocessing using the commercially available software Qlab 9. Segmental and global LS and CS were measured in 7 and 6 segments per view, respectively, by manual tracing of the endocardial contour at end-systole. The following frames were automatically analyzed by temporal tracking of acoustic speckles that are individual to each segment of the myocardial tissue. Real-time verification of adequate tracking and full thickness coverage of the myocardium including the epicardial and endocardial borders were optimized by manual readjustment of poorly tracked segments where necessary. More negative strain and strain rate values will be described as "higher" in this paper, even though mathematically it is vice versa, as more negative values represent an increased contraction of the myocardium.

Both resting and exercise echocardiographic images were additionally analyzed by a second, independent reader who was blinded to the results of the first examiner and the study group status of the respective echocardiographic image in order to determine interobserver reliability.

2.4. Quantitative Stress Echocardiography. After the general echocardiographic studies, participants pedaled in a supine position utilizing a standard cycle ergometer at approximately 60 rounds per minute against a ramp protocol with increasing resistance. Image acquisition for speckle tracking deformation analyses was carried out in the resting state and at the maximum level of physical exhaustion ($\approx$2 Watt per kilogram body weight). A standardized pattern of consecutive images was acquired at each time point in the following order: SAXB, SAXM, AP4, AP2, and AP3. A 12-channel EKG was continuously monitored and blood pressure measurements were collected at 2-minute intervals.

All echocardiographic analyses were performed by the same investigators, who were blinded to the study group status at the time of the assessment of strain and strain rate. The results were reproducible and interobserver variability was below 5.8% in our study.

In order to reduce the risk of exercise induced hypoglycemia in diabetic patients, serum glucose levels should exceed 100 mg/dL to 150 mg/dL. Patients with blood sugar levels below 100 mg/dL were provided with extra carbohydrate exchange such as candy bars or orange juice prior to physical exercise testing.

2.5. Biostatistical Analysis. Baseline demographics, clinical data, hemodynamic parameters, and echocardiographic characteristics of the two groups were described by mean and standard deviation. Clinical parameters, hemodynamic data, and echocardiographic characteristics of the two study groups were compared using the Mann-Whitney U test. Wilcoxon signed-rank test was used for the measurement of the effect of exercise within one group. p values <0.05 constituted statistical significance. Box-Whisker-Plots were used for the graphic representation of the data distribution. SPSS Statistics for Macintosh, Version 22.0. (IBM Corporation, USA), was used for all statistical analyses.

3. Results

3.1. Epidemiological Data. Baseline demographic and hemodynamic data of the study population are summarized in Table 1. There was no significant difference in age, body weight, height, bmi, or the level of exercise routine between the two groups. Blood pressure and heart rate did not differ between the two groups at rest or during stress testing except

for a slightly higher heart rate in T1DM patients at rest (84.4 ± 11.3 bpm) when compared to healthy controls (76.2 ± 9.3 bpm; $p = 0.001$). However, all baseline and hemodynamic parameters in both groups were within normal limits [31]. Mean disease duration in the study group was 4 ± 3.5 years and mean glycated hemoglobin (HbA_{1c}) was $8.3 \pm 1.2\%$. One patient was excluded from the study due to detection of a previously unknown valvular aortic stenosis.

3.2. Conventional Echocardiography. Conventional echocardiographic characteristics are outlined in Table 2. There are no significant differences of atrial/aortic diameters or LV function parameters such as fractional shortening, EF, stroke volume, and cardiac output, except for a marginally larger systolic diameter of the interventricular septum in the control group (1.17 ± 0.20 cm) when compared to T1DM patients (1.06 ± 0.22 cm). Yet all values were within the normal range evaluated by Z-scores [29]. Analysis of diastolic function showed a significantly decreased E/A-ratio in the T1DM group (1.6 ± 0.28) when compared to healthy controls (1.72 ± 0.26; $p = 0.031$). E/E'-ratio, IVRT, and mitral deceleration time as well as all other assessed parameters of diastolic function showed no significant differences between the two groups.

3.3. Speckle Tracking Stress Echocardiography. Myocardial deformation was quantitatively measured using speckle tracking echocardiography at rest and during physical stress testing on a bicycle ergometer. Results for peak LV myocardial *strain rate* are displayed in Table 3. T1DM patients were shown to have increased myocardial contractility both at rest ($p = 0.016$) and during stress ($p = 0.021$). While statistical significance was reached in 4 out of 14 comparisons, T1DM patients had higher circumferential and longitudinal *strain rate* than healthy controls in 13 out of 14 comparisons. The significance of the difference of AP2 derived longitudinal strain rate in the diabetic and control group at rest (-1.94 ± 1.14 versus $-1.54 \pm 0.25 \, s^{-1}$) is limited by the nonnormal distribution of the parameters.

The effect of disease duration on LV myocardial contractility is demonstrated in Figure 1. While T1DM patients had overall higher global LV *strain rates* at rest when compared to healthy controls, patients with a disease duration of >4 years had significantly increased LV *strain rate* at rest ($p = 0.038$) and during exercise ($p = 0.05$). Figure 2 illustrates generic speckle tracking echocardiography images of increased peak LV systolic *strain rate* in a patient with T1DM and a healthy sex- and age-matched control subject.

Overall, peak LV myocardial *strain* was not shown to be statistically different between the two groups, neither at rest, nor during physical exercise (see Table 4). However, significant differences could be demonstrated when analyzing the T1DM group stratified by glycemic control as visualized in Figure 3. T1DM patients with serum $HbA_{1c} > 9\%$ had significantly depressed peak LV CS ($p = 0.005$) and LS ($p = 0.008$) when compared to diabetic patients with better glycemic control and healthy controls, respectively.

T1DM patients showed beginning impairment of LV diastolic function (E/A-ratio) when compared to healthy

TABLE 1: Baseline clinical characteristics and hemodynamics of the study population.

	Diabetes (n = 40)	Control (n = 44)	p value
Age (years)	11.5 ± 3.1	11.4 ± 2.9	n.s.
Height (cm)	153.0 ± 18.2	154.1 ± 16.8	n.s.
Weight (kg)	46.9 ± 16.9	48.0 ± 16.3	n.s.
Body surface (m^2)	1.4 ± 0.3	1.4 ± 0.3	n.s.
Body mass index (kg/m^2)	19.3 ± 3.1	19.6 ± 3.5	n.s.
Exercise routine (1: in school; 2: <3 times/week; 3: ≥3 times/week)	1.7 ± 0.8	2.0 ± 0.7	n.s.
Duration of disease (years)	4 ± 3.5	—	—
HbA$_{1c}$ (%)	8.3 ± 1.2	—	—
Rest			
Heart rate (beats/minute)	84.4 ± 11.3	76.2 ± 9.4	0.001
BP systolic (mmHg)	105.7 ± 9.6	105.8 ± 9.2	n.s.
BP diastolic (mmHg)	58.5 ± 7.9	59.4 ± 9.2	n.s.
Low stress level			
Heart rate (beats/minute)	112.0 ± 9.3	108.6 ± 12.8	n.s.
BP systolic (mmHg)	122.3 ± 18.2	120.2 ± 16.9	n.s.
BP diastolic (mmHg)	65.2 ± 13.6	63.7 ± 11.0	n.s.
Level of resistance (W/kg body weight)	0.4 ± 0.3	0.5 ± 0.3	n.s.
High stress level			
Heart rate (beats/minute)	161.5 ± 13.1	156.8 ± 17.5	n.s.
BP systolic (mmHg)	148.1 ± 21.9	140.1 ± 22.9	n.s.
BP diastolic (mmHg)	74.9 ± 12.6	71.2 ± 13.8	n.s.
Level of resistance (W/kg body weight)	1.7 ± 0.4	1.8 ± 0.4	n.s.

p values calculated with the Man-Whitney U test, level of significance = 0.05.

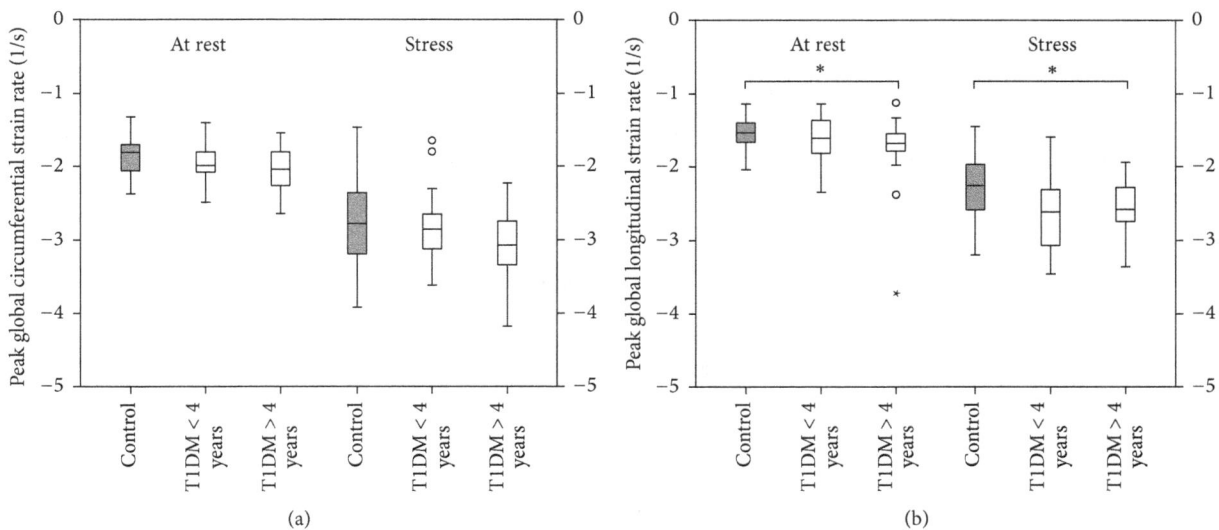

FIGURE 1: Peak systolic global left ventricular *strain rate* in relation to the duration of disease. Type 1 diabetic children ($n = 40$) have increased strain rate both at rest and during exercise when compared to healthy controls ($n = 44$). Patients with a disease duration >4 years ($n = 17$, 42.5%) exhibit higher strain rates than those with a disease duration <4 years ($n = 23$, 57.5%). (a) Peak systolic global LV circumferential *strain rate*. (b) Peak systolic global LV longitudinal *strain rate*. $^*p < 0.05$; p values were calculated with Mann-Whitney U and Wilcoxon signed-rank tests.

TABLE 2: Conventional echocardiographic parameters derived from two-dimensional and Doppler imaging.

	Diabetes (n = 40)	Control (n = 44)	p value
Aortic root (AoR) diameter (cm)	2.33 ± 0.35	2.41 ± 0.35	n.s.
Left atrial (LA) diameter (cm)	2.56 ± 0.38	2.71 ± 0.45	n.s.
LA/AoR	1.11 ± 0.16	1.13 ± 0.16	n.s.
Fractional shortening (%)	33.41 ± 4.08	34.78 ± 3.94	n.s.
Interventricular septal end-systolic diameter (cm)	1.06 ± 0.22	1.17 ± 0.20	0.011
Interventricular septal end-diastolic diameter (cm)	0.84 ± 0.18	0.89 ± 0.16	n.s.
LV end-systolic diameter (cm)	2.70 ± 0.43	2.76 ± 0.41	n.s.
LV end-diastolic diameter (cm)	4.05 ± 0.56	4.27 ± 0.46	n.s.
LV posterior wall diameter, systolic (cm)	1.23 ± 0.20	1.27 ± 0.21	n.s.
LV posterior wall diameter, diastolic (cm)	0.79 ± 0.16	0.81 ± 0.15	n.s.
LV mass (g)	102.74 ± 41.82	115.18 ± 37.56	n.s.
Relative wall thickness	0.20 ± 0.04	0.19 ± 0.03	n.s.
End-diastolic volume of the left ventricle (mL)	70.18 ± 24.66	79.63 ± 27.97	n.s.
End-systolic volume of the left ventricle (mL)	27.69 ± 9.82	31.66 ± 11.78	n.s.
Ejection fraction (%)	61.29 ± 4.77	60.16 ± 4.67	n.s.
Stroke volume (mL)	44.7 ± 14.4	49.3 ± 18.1	n.s.
Cardiac output (L/min)	3.7 ± 1.1	3.7 ± 1.3	n.s.
Mitral inflow: E-wave (cm/s)	95.36 ± 13.45	96.86 ± 14.26	n.s.
Mitral inflow: A-wave (cm/s)	60.84 ± 12.27	57.36 ± 10.41	n.s.
E-wave/A-wave	1.60 ± 0.28	1.72 ± 0.26	0.031
Mitral deceleration time (s)	0.17 ± 0.04	0.18 ± 0.04	n.s.
Isovolumetric relaxation time (s)	0.05 ± 0.01	0.05 ± 0.01	n.s.
S' (cm/s)	7.92 ± 0.97	8.17 ± 1.19	n.s.
E' (cm/s)	12.54 ± 1.81	13.03 ± 1.87	n.s.
A' (cm/s)	5.42 ± 1.20	5.51 ± 1.11	n.s.
E'/A' (cm/s)	2.44 ± 0.75	2.48 ± 0.72	n.s.
E/E' (cm/s)	7.71 ± 1.20	7.56 ± 1.42	n.s.

p values calculated with the Man-Whitney U test, level of significance = 0.05.

controls (see Table 2). This effect was statistically significant for the comparison of the entire T1DM group to healthy controls ($p = 0.031$) and more pronounced in patients with poor glycemic control represented by serum HbA_{1c} levels > 9% ($p = 0.018$) as visualized in Figure 4.

4. Discussion

4.1. Type 1 Diabetic Children Have Increased Peak Left Ventricular Strain Rate. In order to assess the effect of type 1 diabetes mellitus on LV myocardial contractility in the absence of ischemic events early in the course of the disease we performed speckle tracking echocardiography in combination with ergometer stress testing in asymptomatic normotensive pediatric patients with uncomplicated T1DM and healthy controls. Interestingly and somewhat counterintuitively, we found diabetic children to exhibit LV systolic hypercontractility represented by overall increased peak circumferential and longitudinal *strain rate* both at rest and during exercise (see Table 3 and Figures 1 and 2). The observed statistically significant increases in LV strain rate in the T1DM group such as increased global longitudinal strain rate during stress testing (-2.59 ± 0.47 versus $-2.32 \pm 0.41\,s^{-1}$) should not be overinterpreted as a single finding with direct clinical implication but rather regarded as the tip of the iceberg of the overall tendency for T1DM patients to exhibit increased peak systolic LV strain rate. At first, this may seem surprising given the fact that diabetic cardiomyopathy potentially results in a gradual decline of myocardial function with the ultimate end-point of diabetic heart failure. However, we hypothesize that diabetic cardiomyopathy may in fact feature an early subclinical phase of paradoxical LV hyperdynamics as a sign of

TABLE 3: Speckle tracking derived peak systolic LV *strain rate* at rest and during stress testing.

	Diabetes (n = 40)	Control (n = 44)	p value
Rest			
Global circumferential strain rate (s^{-1})	-1.99 ± 0.28	-1.87 ± 0.24	n.s.
Circumferential strain rate (SAXM) (s^{-1})	-2.05 ± 0.35	-1.86 ± 0.25	0.016
Circumferential strain rate (SAXB) (s^{-1})	-1.96 ± 0.29	1.90 ± 0.31	n.s.
Global longitudinal strain rate (s^{-1})	-1.70 ± 0.44	-1.55 ± 0.21	n.s.
Longitudinal strain rate (AP4) (s^{-1})	-1.58 ± 0.34	-1.52 ± 0.28	n.s.
Longitudinal strain rate (AP2) (s^{-1})	-1.94 ± 1.14	-1.54 ± 0.25	0.019
Longitudinal strain rate (AP3) (s^{-1})	-1.64 ± 0.35	-1.63 ± 0.30	n.s.
Stress			
Global circumferential strain rate (s^{-1})	-2.92 ± 0.54	-2.76 ± 0.60	n.s.
Circumferential strain rate (SAXM) (s^{-1})	-2.92 ± 0.58	-2.73 ± 0.61	n.s.
Circumferential strain rate (SAXB) (s^{-1})	-2.86 ± 0.52	-2.66 ± 0.68	n.s.
Global longitudinal strain rate (s^{-1})	-2.59 ± 0.47	-2.32 ± 0.41	0.021
Longitudinal strain rate (AP4) (s^{-1})	-2.64 ± 0.53	-2.23 ± 0.37	0.002
Longitudinal strain rate (AP2) (s^{-1})	-2.40 ± 0.47	-2.47 ± 0.45	n.s.
Longitudinal strain rate (AP3) (s^{-1})	-2.71 ± 0.72	-2.60 ± 0.75	n.s.

SAXM: parasternal short axis view at the papillary muscle plane, SAXB: parasternal short axis view at the mitral valve plane, AP4: apical four-chamber view, AP2: apical two-chamber view, and AP3: apical three-chamber view; p values calculated with Man-Whitney U test, level of significance = 0.05.

TABLE 4: Speckle tracking derived peak systolic LV *strain* at rest and during stress echocardiography.

	Diabetes (n = 40)	Control (n = 44)	p value
Rest			
Global circumferential strain rate (%)	-25.5 ± 3.3	-25.0 ± 3.4	n.s.
Circumferential strain rate (SAXM) (%)	-26.6 ± 4.7	-25.9 ± 3.9	n.s.
Circumferential strain rate (SAXB) (%)	-24.4 ± 3.2	-24.0 ± 4.4	n.s.
Global longitudinal strain rate (%)	-20.1 ± 2.3	-20.7 ± 2.5	n.s.
Longitudinal strain rate (AP4) (%)	-19.9 ± 2.5	-20.2 ± 3.0	n.s.
Longitudinal strain rate (AP2) (%)	-20.6 ± 3.2	-20.9 ± 3.1	n.s.
Longitudinal strain rate (AP3) (%)	-20.3 ± 2.3	-21.6 ± 2.8	n.s.
Stress			
Global circumferential strain rate (%)	-24.2 ± 3.9	-23.8 ± 4.1	n.s.
Circumferential strain rate (SAXM) (%)	-24.6 ± 4.0	-23.9 ± 4.6	n.s.
Circumferential strain rate (SAXB) (%)	-23.3 ± 4.1	-23.3 ± 4.3	n.s.
Global longitudinal strain rate (%)	-21.6 ± 2.9	-21.0 ± 2.7	n.s.
Longitudinal strain rate (AP4) (%)	-21.6 ± 3.1	-21.0 ± 2.3	n.s.
Longitudinal strain rate (AP2) (%)	-21.8 ± 3.7	-21.2 ± 0.5	n.s.
Longitudinal strain rate (AP3) (%)	-21.7 ± 3.7	-21.7 ± 4.4	n.s.

SAXM: parasternal short axis view at the papillary muscle plane, SAXB: parasternal short axis view at the mitral valve plane, AP4: apical four-chamber view, AP2: apical two-chamber view, and AP3: apical three-chamber view; p values calculated with Man-Whitney U test, level of significance = 0.05.

impaired mechanical efficiency long before long-term deterioration of myocardial function becomes evident. While most studies focus on intermediate or late stage disease reporting of depressed LV systolic function, there are a number of human and animal model studies in favor of our hypothesis.

Chung et al. found increased LV torsion despite preserved EF, circumferential strain, and longitudinal shortening using tagged MRI in young adult patients with tightly controlled T1DM [32]. Similarly, a stress MRI spectroscopy study revealed a reduced phosphocreatine/γ-ATP ratio as a sign of altered myocardial energetics in young adults with uncomplicated T1DM, independent of coronary microvascular function [33]. In another tagged MRI study hyperdynamic LV twist mechanics were described in coexistence with

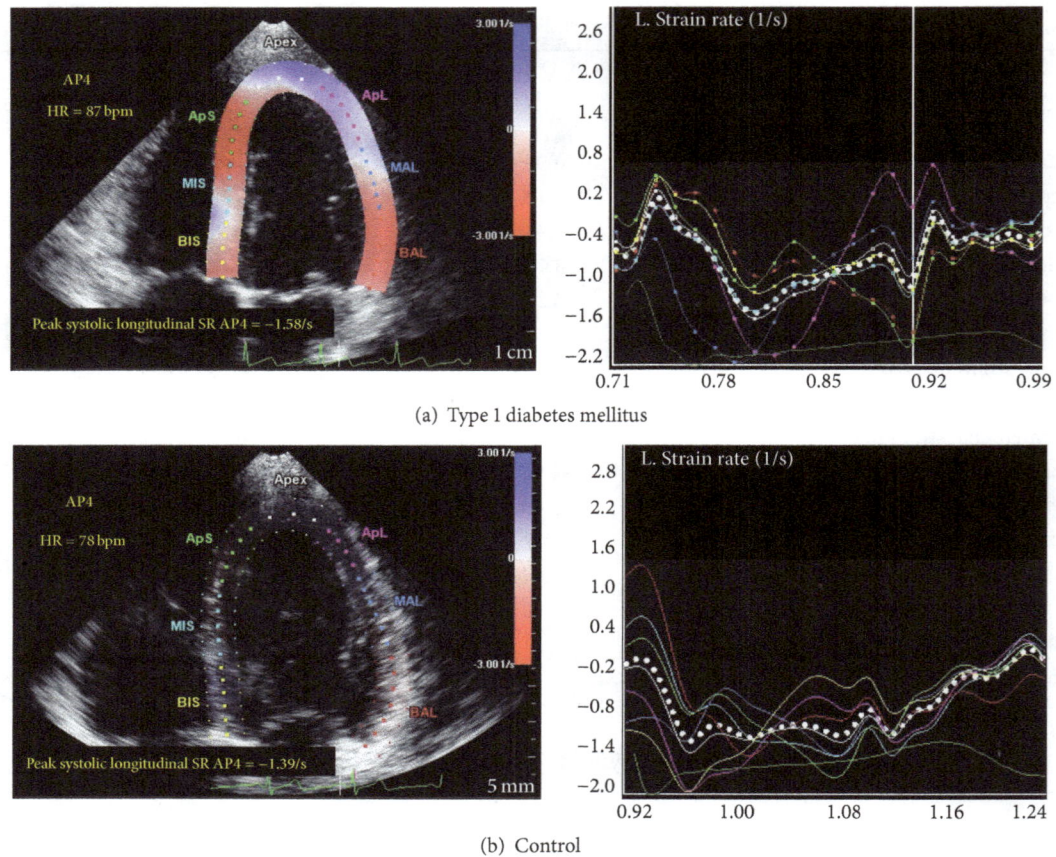

(a) Type 1 diabetes mellitus

(b) Control

FIGURE 2: Speckle tracking echocardiography at rest in the apical 4-chamber view. (a) Peak systolic global LV longitudinal *strain rate* in a pediatric patient with type 1 diabetes mellitus. (b) Peak systolic global LV longitudinal *strain rate* in a healthy control subject. Dotted white line: global longitudinal *strain rate*, the coloured lines on the right correspond to the myocardial segments indicated on the left, dark green line at the bottom: ECG. Note the increased peak early systolic strain rate in the diabetic patient.

signs of altered myocardial perfusion in young patients with uncomplicated T1DM [34]. Moreover, our results are in accordance with two conventional echocardiographic studies demonstrating increased LV contractility in diabetic children without arterial hypertension, ischemic heart disease, or nephropathy using M-mode and Doppler imaging [35, 36]. Furthermore, our finding of LV hyperdynamic contractility early in the course of diabetes mellitus is in agreement with results from animal model studies in leptin receptor-deficient mice utilizing in vivo catheterization. Buchanan et al. discovered diabetes-associated LV hypercontractility as an indication for altered myocardial substrate use and reduced myocardial efficiency in hyperglycemia. The phenomenon occurred early and slightly faded subsequently [37]. Additionally, Van den Bergh et al. described impaired mechanical efficiency and increased ventriculoarterial coupling that was associated with altered cardiac loading conditions [38]. Therefore, for the assessment of myocardial contractility in human subjects, a noninvasive measure that is least dependent on variations in LV loading must be utilized in order to minimize potential confounding.

Strain and strain rate are quantitative measures for the echocardiographic assessment of myocardial deformation [39]. Strain is an index of deformation describing a percentage change from the original dimension. Strain rate is a measure of the rate at which this change happens and is expressed as per second (s^{-1}). While most studies assessing myocardial deformation in diabetic patients mainly focus on strain, strain rate is in fact a more robust index of LV myocardial contractility as it is less dependent on confounding factors such as pre- and afterload [40–43] and it is even more closely related to contractility than the widely used EF [44]. The present study is the first clinical study demonstrating overall increased strain rate in the early stage of human T1DM.

In contrast, Di Cori and colleagues used tissue-Doppler imaging to analyze myocardial deformation in adult T1DM patients (mean age 30 ± 4.1 years and mean disease duration 8.9 ± 3.7 years) and found depressed LV myocardial strain and equivocal strain rate [45]. There are several explanations for this deviation in deformation parameters. First, Di Cori and colleagues only assessed regional segmental strain (rate) of the midposterior septum (decreased in T1DM) and midlateral wall (increased in T1DM) and not global strain (rate). Given the strong heterogeneity of myocardial fiber organization in the LV, myocardial deformation naturally exhibits regional variations [46–48]. Thus, the assessment of

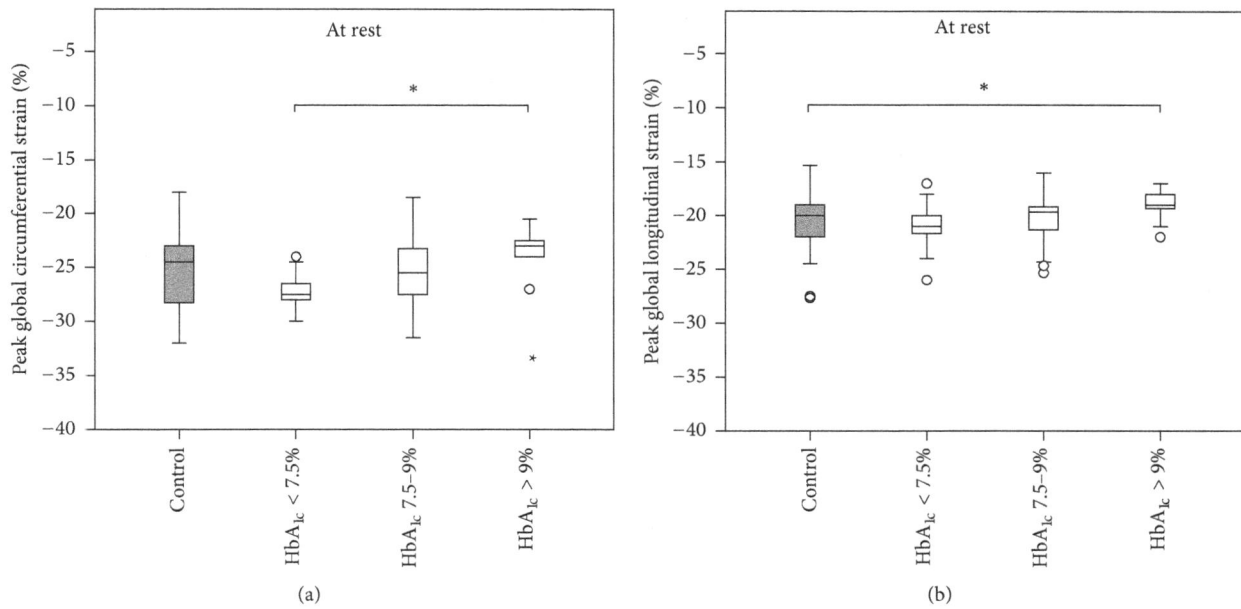

FIGURE 3: Peak systolic global left ventricular *strain* in relation to glycemic control. Type 1 diabetic children with poor glycemic control have decreased peak systolic global left ventricular *strain* when compared to healthy controls. (a) Peak systolic global LV circumferential *strain*. (b) Peak systolic global LV longitudinal *strain*. $HbA_{1c} < 7.5\%$ ($n = 10, 25\%$), HbA_{1c} 7.5–9% ($n = 19, 47.5\%$), and $HbA_{1c} > 9\%$ ($n = 11, 27.5\%$); *$p < 0.05$; p values were calculated with Mann-Whitney U and Wilcoxon signed-rank tests.

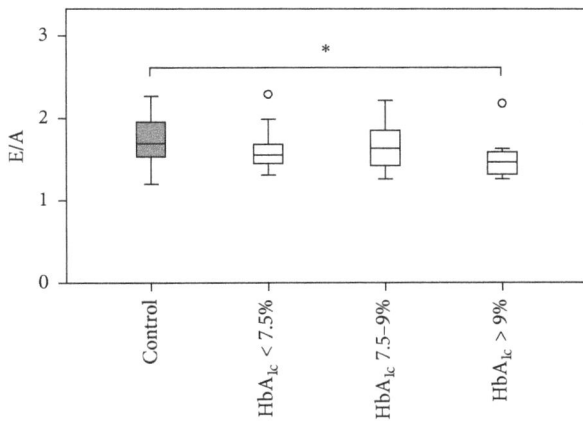

FIGURE 4: Left ventricular diastolic function (E/A-ratio) in relation to glycemic control. Type 1 diabetic children with poor glycemic control have echocardiographic evidence of impaired diastolic filling of the left ventricle in comparison to healthy control subjects.* $p < 0.05$; p values were calculated with Mann-Whitney U and Wilcoxon signed-rank tests.

only two isolated segments likely is an oversimplification of the complex mechanism underlying LV myocardial contractility. Second, tissue-Doppler echocardiography was used, a method that bears considerable limitations such as angle-dependency and interrater variability [49]. Third, Di Cori and colleagues included an older diabetic study population with a markedly longer disease duration in comparison to the present study population. In our study the mean disease duration in the T1DM group was 4 ± 3.5 years. Interestingly,

a subgroup analysis revealed that the increase in global LV peak longitudinal strain rate is statistically significant for T1DM patients with a disease duration >4 years (see Figure 1). Hence, it is well imaginable that the here described diabetes-associated cardiac changes require a certain time interval of a few years to become evident. Furthermore, the observed hypercontractility in T1DM in the present study is possibly a transient effect in the early phase of diabetic nonischemic cardiomyopathy that fades in the subsequent course of the disease, as observed by Di Cori and colleagues. Longitudinal studies are needed in order to further elucidate the natural course of diabetic cardiomyopathy throughout childhood and adulthood.

4.2. Left Ventricular Longitudinal and Circumferential Strain Is Impaired in Children with Poorly Controlled Type 1 Diabetes Mellitus. In this study there was no significant difference in overall peak LV longitudinal or circumferential strain between T1DM patients and healthy controls neither at rest nor during stress testing. This is in accordance with a Korean study of a very similar (age, disease duration, and glycemic control) T1DM population that also failed to demonstrate overall impairment of systolic strain [50]. Strain rate however was not measured in that study. While there is a considerable number of clinical studies reporting an impairment of (mainly global longitudinal) strain in diabetes mellitus type 1 [51–53] and type 2 [54], all of these studies either include adult patients and/or are confounded by longer disease duration [51, 55–57], LV structural abnormalities [51, 55, 58], impaired EF [52], obesity, arterial hypertension [51, 54, 59–61], nephropathy [51, 57, 61], heart failure [55], overt peripheral vascular disease [56], use of negatively inotropic medications [51, 54, 60], or tobacco use [51]. Furthermore, in contrast to our study design all of the abovementioned studies are considerably limited by the fact that the echocardiographic interpreter was not blinded. This is a substantial limitation because speckle tracking derived myocardial deformation parameters are extremely sensible to manual adjustments.

Recently, a blinded speckle tracking study in 1065 normotensive T1DM patients (mean age 49.5 ± 14.5 years and mean disease duration 26.1 ± 15.7 years) convincingly demonstrated that the impairment of myocardial strain in T1DM is solely driven by the presence of albuminuria [62]. There was no difference in myocardial strain between T1DM patients without albuminuria and healthy controls. Strain rate however was not assessed in that study. As our study participants were screened negative for albuminuria and disease duration was considerably shorter than in the abovementioned study, the absence of overall impaired systolic strain in the present study population is not surprising. Moreover, our findings are in concordance with two MRI studies demonstrating preserved LV strain mechanics in young adult diabetic patients [63, 64].

Subdividing our T1DM population according to the degree of glycemic control, an association of both longitudinal and circumferential strains with serum levels of HbA_{1c} became evident (see Figure 3). This is in agreement with recent 3D speckle tracking studies demonstrating a negative impact of HbA_{1c} on LV myocardial strain in adult patients with diabetes mellitus [55, 65, 66]. Furthermore, this is underlined by prospective observational studies reporting the association of poor glycemic control with the development of heart failure in large cohorts of T1DM patients [5, 67]. In addition, several animal model studies are in accordance with our observations of diabetes-associated alterations in LV myocardial contractility [68, 69]. Accountable pathologic mechanisms are diabetes-induced loss of t-tubule structure [14], formation of advanced glycosylation end products with subsequent pathologically increased collagen cross-linking [70], altered mitochondrial energetics [71], and several other metabolic imbalances [11, 72]. The finding of overall preserved myocardial strain in the entire diabetic study population and decreased strain only in those subjects with poor glycemic control can be explained by the timing of the investigation. At this early state of T1DM only subjects with poor glycemic control exhibit advanced impairment of LV strain. The majority of the included patients either do not yet suffer from impaired contractility or are still in the previously described early occurring hyperdynamic state of diabetic cardiomyopathy. Taken together, our findings demonstrate the presence of early subclinical cardiac changes in diabetes mellitus that are most probably driven by metabolic dysfunction as previously suggested [73].

4.3. Type 1 Diabetic Children Have Signs of Beginning Diastolic Dysfunction. The present study provides further evidence for the presence of diastolic dysfunction in diabetes mellitus. We found a statistically significant decrease of E/A-ratio in poorly controlled T1DM patients when compared to healthy controls (see Figure 4). This is in accordance with observations in animal models [74–76] as well as with human MRI [64] and echocardiographic studies in pediatric [53] and adult [33, 77–80] patients with diabetes mellitus type 1 [33, 53, 80] and type 2 [77, 78] demonstrating signs of (beginning) diastolic dysfunction in nonischemic diabetic cardiomyopathy. A new aspect from the present study is the fact that signs of diastolic impairment already become evident very early in the course of T1DM. This further underlines the concept of nonischemic diabetes-associated myocardial impairment as a continuous process driven by metabolic imbalances.

4.4. Study Limitations. In a recent study on premature infants Sanchez and colleagues demonstrated a link of the reliability of two-dimensional speckle tracking derived deformation parameters and adjusted frame rate during image acquisition [81]. A frame rate/heart rate ratio of 0.7 to 0.9 frames per second per bpm has been proposed for optimal myocardial speckle tracking. In our study frame rate settings meet these criteria during echocardiography at rest. However, frame rates were not adjusted during stress testing. Accordingly, strain and strain rate parameters during exercise testing in our study may in fact be somewhat underestimated in both the study and the control group. Secondly, this was a cross-sectional study in a limited number of asymptomatic patients. Thus, the final clinical outcome of the observed subclinical alterations yet remains to be established in large study populations.

5. Conclusion

The present study provides further evidence for diabetes-associated nonischemic cardiomyopathy. A paradoxical increase of LV myocardial performance may occur very early in T1DM as a sign of impaired mechanical efficiency. T1DM patients with poor glycemic control have early signs of subclinical LV systolic and diastolic dysfunction. Consequently, tight glycemic control must be a high priority therapeutic aim for diabetic patients in order to minimize the ultimate risk of heart failure. Further experimental and clinical studies are needed in order to illuminate the spatiotemporal complexity of diabetes-associated heart failure.

Conflict of Interests

The authors declare that there is no conflict of interests regarding the publication of this paper.

Authors' Contribution

Kai O. Hensel designed and supervised the study, interpreted the data, and wrote the paper. Franziska Grimmer performed the echocardiographic studies, postprocessing, and statistical analyses and prepared the figures and tables. Markus Roskopf was involved in echocardiographic image acquisition and postprocessing analyses. Andreas Heusch helped recruiting patients and performing echocardiographic examinations. Andreas Heusch, Stefan Wirth, and Andreas C. Jenke critically reviewed the paper.

Acknowledgments

The authors thank all study participants and Matthias Wisbauer for his support with regard to echocardiographic image acquisition. This study was supported with a research grant by HELIOS Research Center (HRC-ID 000416).

References

[1] D. E. Stanescu, K. Lord, and T. H. Lipman, "The epidemiology of type 1 diabetes in children," *Endocrinology and Metabolism Clinics of North America*, vol. 41, no. 4, pp. 679–694, 2012.

[2] G. Imperatore, J. P. Boyle, T. J. Thompson et al., "Projections of type 1 and type 2 diabetes burden in the U.S. population aged <20 years through 2050: dynamic modeling of incidence, mortality, and population growth," *Diabetes Care*, vol. 35, no. 12, pp. 2515–2520, 2012.

[3] D. M. Maahs, N. A. West, J. M. Lawrence, and E. J. Mayer-Davis, "Epidemiology of type 1 diabetes," *Endocrinology and Metabolism Clinics of North America*, vol. 39, no. 3, pp. 481–497, 2010.

[4] N. Poulter, "Global risk of cardiovascular disease," *Heart*, vol. 89, supplement 2, pp. ii2–ii37, 2003.

[5] I. M. Stratton, A. I. Adler, H. A. W. Neil et al., "Association of glycaemia with macrovascular and microvascular complications of type 2 diabetes (UKPDS 35): prospective observational study," *British Medical Journal*, vol. 321, no. 7258, pp. 405–412, 2000.

[6] G. de Simone, R. B. Devereux, M. Chinali et al., "Diabetes and incident heart failure in hypertensive and normotensive participants of the Strong Heart study," *Journal of Hypertension*, vol. 28, no. 2, pp. 353–360, 2010.

[7] L. Ernande and G. Derumeaux, "Diabetic cardiomyopathy: myth or reality?" *Archives of Cardiovascular Diseases*, vol. 105, no. 4, pp. 218–225, 2012.

[8] T. Miki, S. Yuda, H. Kouzu, and T. Miura, "Diabetic cardiomyopathy: pathophysiology and clinical features," *Heart Failure Reviews*, vol. 18, no. 2, pp. 149–166, 2013.

[9] S. E. Litwin, "Diabetes and the heart: is there objective evidence of a human diabetic cardiomyopathy?" *Diabetes*, vol. 62, no. 10, pp. 3329–3330, 2013.

[10] S. M. Genuth, J.-Y. C. Backlund, M. Bayless et al., "Effects of prior intensive versus conventional therapy and history of glycemia on cardiac function in type 1 diabetes in the DCCT/EDIC," *Diabetes*, vol. 62, no. 10, pp. 3561–3569, 2013.

[11] J. D. Schilling and D. L. Mann, "Diabetic cardiomyopathy: bench to bedside," *Heart Failure Clinics*, vol. 8, no. 4, pp. 619–63, 2012.

[12] A. Aneja, W. H. W. Tang, S. Bansilal, M. J. Garcia, and M. E. Farkouh, "Diabetic cardiomyopathy: insights into pathogenesis, diagnostic challenges, and therapeutic options," *The American Journal of Medicine*, vol. 121, no. 9, pp. 748–757, 2008.

[13] S. Boudina and E. D. Abel, "Diabetic cardiomyopathy, causes and effects," *Reviews in Endocrine & Metabolic Disorders*, vol. 11, no. 1, pp. 31–39, 2010.

[14] M. L. Ward and D. J. Crossman, "Mechanisms underlying the impaired contractility of diabetic cardiomyopathy," *World Journal of Cardiology*, vol. 6, no. 7, pp. 577–584, 2014.

[15] R. Tarquini, C. Lazzeri, L. Pala, C. M. Rotella, and G. F. Gensini, "The diabetic cardiomyopathy," *Acta Diabetologica*, vol. 48, no. 3, pp. 173–181, 2011.

[16] C. H. Mandavia, A. R. Aroor, V. G. Demarco, and J. R. Sowers, "Molecular and metabolic mechanisms of cardiac dysfunction in diabetes," *Life Sciences*, vol. 92, no. 11, pp. 601–608, 2013.

[17] S. D. de Ferranti, I. H. de Boer, V. Fonseca et al., "Type 1 diabetes mellitus and cardiovascular disease: a scientific statement from the American Heart Association and American Diabetes Association," *Diabetes Care*, vol. 37, no. 10, pp. 2843–2863, 2014.

[18] S. D. Solomon, N. Anavekar, H. Skali et al., "Influence of ejection fraction on cardiovascular outcomes in a broad spectrum of heart failure patients," *Circulation*, vol. 112, no. 24, pp. 3738–3744, 2005.

[19] R. S. Bhatia, J. V. Tu, D. S. Lee et al., "Outcome of heart failure with preserved ejection fraction in a population-based study," *The New England Journal of Medicine*, vol. 355, no. 3, pp. 260–269, 2006.

[20] E. S. Carell, S. Murali, D. S. Schulman, T. Estrada-Quintero, and B. F. Uretsky, "Maximal exercise tolerance in chronic congestive heart failure: relationship to resting left ventricular function," *Chest*, vol. 106, no. 6, pp. 1746–1752, 1994.

[21] R. Hoffmann, H. Lethen, T. Marwick et al., "Analysis of interinstitutional observer agreement in interpretation of dobutamine stress echocardiograms," *Journal of the American College of Cardiology*, vol. 27, no. 2, pp. 330–336, 1996.

[22] H. Geyer, G. Caracciolo, H. Abe et al., "Assessment of myocardial mechanics using speckle tracking echocardiography: fundamentals and clinical applications," *Journal of the American Society of Echocardiography*, vol. 23, no. 4, pp. 351–369, 2010.

[23] J. W. Petersen, T. F. Nazir, L. Lee, C. S. Garvan, and A. Karimi, "Speckle tracking echocardiography-determined measures of global and regional left ventricular function correlate with functional capacity in patients with and without preserved ejection fraction," *Cardiovascular Ultrasound*, vol. 11, article 20, 2013.

[24] R. Leischik, B. Dworrak, and K. Hensel, "Intraobserver and interobserver reproducibility for radial, circumferential and longitudinal strain echocardiography," *The Open Cardiovascular Medicine Journal*, vol. 8, no. 1, pp. 102–109, 2014.

[25] K. O. Hensel, A. Jenke, and R. Leischik, "Speckle-tracking and tissue-doppler stress echocardiography in arterial hypertension: a sensitive tool for detection of subclinical LV impairment," *BioMed Research International*, vol. 2014, Article ID 472562, 9 pages, 2014.

[26] Y. T. Tan, F. Wenzelburger, E. Lee et al., "The pathophysiology of heart failure with normal ejection fraction: exercise echocardiography reveals complex abnormalities of both systolic and diastolic ventricular function involving torsion, untwist, and longitudinal motion," *Journal of the American College of Cardiology*, vol. 54, no. 1, pp. 36–46, 2009.

[27] L. Lopez, S. D. Colan, P. C. Frommelt et al., "Recommendations for quantification methods during the performance of a pediatric echocardiogram: a report from the Pediatric Measurements Writing Group of the American Society of Echocardiography Pediatric and Congenital Heart Disease Council," *Journal of the American Society of Echocardiography*, vol. 23, no. 5, pp. 465–495, 2010.

[28] S. F. Nagueh, C. P. Appleton, T. C. Gillebert et al., "Recommendations for the evaluation of left ventricular diastolic function by echocardiography," *Journal of the American Society of Echocardiography*, vol. 22, no. 2, pp. 107–133, 2009.

[29] H. Chubb and J. M. Simpson, "The use of Z-scores in paediatric cardiology," *Annals of Pediatric Cardiology*, vol. 5, no. 2, pp. 179–184, 2012.

[30] A. Rösner, D. Barbosa, E. Aarsæther, D. Kjønås, H. Schirmer, and J. D'hooge, "The influence of frame rate on two-dimensional speckle-tracking strain measurements: a study on silico-simulated models and images recorded in patients," *European*

Heart Journal—Cardiovascular Imaging, vol. 16, no. 10, pp. 1137–1147, 2015.

[31] S. Fleming, M. Thompson, R. Stevens et al., "Normal ranges of heart rate and respiratory rate in children from birth to 18 years of age: a systematic review of observational studies," *The Lancet*, vol. 377, no. 9770, pp. 1011–1018, 2011.

[32] J. Chung, P. Abraszewski, X. Yu et al., "Paradoxical increase in ventricular torsion and systolic torsion rate in type I diabetic patients under tight glycemic control," *Journal of the American College of Cardiology*, vol. 47, no. 2, pp. 384–390, 2006.

[33] G. N. Shivu, T. T. Phan, K. Abozguia et al., "Relationship between coronary microvascular dysfunction and cardiac energetics impairment in type 1 diabetes mellitus," *Circulation*, vol. 121, no. 10, pp. 1209–1215, 2010.

[34] G. N. Shivu, K. Abozguia, T. T. Phan et al., "Increased left ventricular torsion in uncomplicated type 1 diabetic patients: the role of coronary microvascular function," *Diabetes Care*, vol. 32, no. 9, pp. 1710–1712, 2009.

[35] O. Gotzsche, K. Sorensen, B. McIntyre, and P. Henningsen, "Reduced left ventricular afterload and increased contractility in children with insulin-dependent diabetes mellitus: an M-mode and Doppler-echocardiographic evaluation of left ventricular diastolic and systolic function," *Pediatric Cardiology*, vol. 12, no. 2, pp. 69–73, 1991.

[36] O. Gøtzsche, A. Darwish, L. Gøtzsche, L. P. Hansen, and K. E. Sørensen, "Incipient cardiomyopathy in young insulin-dependent diabetic patients: a seven-year prospective Doppler echocardiographic study," *Diabetic Medicine*, vol. 13, no. 9, pp. 834–840, 1996.

[37] J. Buchanan, P. K. Mazumder, P. Hu et al., "Reduced cardiac efficiency and altered substrate metabolism precedes the onset of hyperglycemia and contractile dysfunction in two mouse models of insulin resistance and obesity," *Endocrinology*, vol. 146, no. 12, pp. 5341–5349, 2005.

[38] A. Van den Bergh, W. Flameng, and P. Herijgers, "Type II diabetic mice exhibit contractile dysfunction but maintain cardiac output by favourable loading conditions," *European Journal of Heart Failure*, vol. 8, no. 8, pp. 777–783, 2006.

[39] F. Weidemann, B. Eyskens, F. Jamal et al., "Quantification of regional left and right ventricular radial and longitudinal function in healthy children using ultrasound-based strain rate and strain imaging," *Journal of the American Society of Echocardiography*, vol. 15, no. 1, pp. 20–28, 2002.

[40] V. Ferferieva, A. Van Den Bergh, P. Claus et al., "The relative value of strain and strain rate for defining intrinsic myocardial function," *American Journal of Physiology—Heart and Circulatory Physiology*, vol. 302, no. 1, pp. H188–H195, 2012.

[41] N. L. Greenberg, M. S. Firstenberg, P. L. Castro et al., "Doppler-derived myocardial systolic strain rate is a strong index of left ventricular contractility," *Circulation*, vol. 105, no. 1, pp. 99–105, 2002.

[42] S. Urheim, T. Edvardsen, H. Torp, B. Angelsen, and O. A. Smiseth, "Myocardial strain by Doppler echocardiography. Validation of a new method to quantify regional myocardial function," *Circulation*, vol. 102, no. 10, pp. 1158–1164, 2000.

[43] V. Mor-Avi, R. M. Lang, L. P. Badano et al., "Current and evolving echocardiographic techniques for the quantitative evaluation of cardiac mechanics: ASE/EAE consensus statement on methodology and indications endorsed by the Japanese society of echocardiography," *European Journal of Echocardiography*, vol. 12, no. 3, pp. 167–205, 2011.

[44] A. Stoylen, A. Heimdal, K. Bjornstad, H. G. Torp, and T. Skjaerpe, "Strain rate imaging by ultrasound in the diagnosis of regional dysfunction of the left ventricle," *Echocardiography*, vol. 16, no. 4, pp. 321–329, 1999.

[45] A. Di Cori, V. Di Bello, R. Miccoli et al., "Left ventricular function in normotensive young adults with well-controlled type 1 diabetes mellitus," *American Journal of Cardiology*, vol. 99, no. 1, pp. 84–90, 2007.

[46] W. Y. W. Lew and M. M. LeWinter, "Regional comparison of midwall segment and area shortening in the canine left ventricle," *Circulation Research*, vol. 58, no. 5, pp. 678–691, 1986.

[47] M. K. Heng, R. F. Janz, and J. Jobin, "Estimation of regional stress in the left ventricular septum and free wall an echocardiographic study suggesting a mechanism for asymmetric septal hypertrophy," *American Heart Journal*, vol. 110, no. 1, part 1, pp. 84–90, 1985.

[48] A. DeAnda Jr., M. Komeda, M. R. Moon et al., "Estimation of regional left ventricular wall stresses in intact canine hearts," *American Journal of Physiology—Heart and Circulatory Physiology*, vol. 275, no. 5, pp. H1879–H1885, 1998.

[49] J. D'Hooge, A. Heimdal, F. Jamal et al., "Regional strain and strain rate measurements by cardiac ultrasound: principles, implementation and limitations," *European Journal of Echocardiography*, vol. 1, no. 3, pp. 154–170, 2000.

[50] E. H. Kim and Y. H. Kim, "Left ventricular function in children and adolescents with type 1 diabetes mellitus," *Korean Circulation Journal*, vol. 40, no. 3, pp. 125–130, 2010.

[51] H. Nakai, M. Takeuchi, T. Nishikage, R. M. Lang, and Y. Otsuji, "Subclinical left ventricular dysfunction in asymptomatic diabetic patients assessed by two-dimensional speckle tracking echocardiography: correlation with diabetic duration," *European Journal of Echocardiography*, vol. 10, no. 8, pp. 926–932, 2009.

[52] Z. Abdel-Salam, M. Khalifa, A. Ayoub, A. Hamdy, and W. Nammas, "Early changes in longitudinal deformation indices in young asymptomatic patients with type 1 diabetes mellitus: assessment by speckle-tracking echocardiography," *Minerva Cardioangiologica*, In press.

[53] F. Labombarda, M. Leport, R. Morello et al., "Longitudinal left ventricular strain impairment in type 1 diabetes children and adolescents: a 2D speckle strain imaging study," *Diabetes and Metabolism*, vol. 40, no. 4, pp. 292–298, 2014.

[54] A. C. T. Ng, V. Delgado, M. Bertini et al., "Findings from left ventricular strain and strain rate imaging in asymptomatic patients with type 2 diabetes mellitus," *American Journal of Cardiology*, vol. 104, no. 10, pp. 1398–1401, 2009.

[55] Q. Wang, Y. Gao, K. Tan, and P. Li, "Subclinical impairment of left ventricular function in diabetic patients with or without obesity: a study based on three-dimensional speckle tracking echocardiography," *Herz*, vol. 40, no. 3, pp. 260–268, 2015.

[56] T. Cognet, P.-L. Vervueren, L. Dercle et al., "New concept of myocardial longitudinal strain reserve assessed by a dipyridamole infusion using 2D-strain echocardiography: the impact of diabetes and age, and the prognostic value," *Cardiovascular Diabetology*, vol. 12, no. 1, article 84, 2013.

[57] Y. Mochizuki, H. Tanaka, K. Matsumoto et al., "Clinical features of subclinical left ventricular systolic dysfunction in patients with diabetes mellitus," *Cardiovascular Diabetology*, vol. 14, no. 1, article 37, 2015.

[58] A. Karagöz, T. Bezgin, I. Kutlutürk et al., "Subclinical left ventricular systolic dysfunction in diabetic patients and its association with retinopathy: a 2D speckle tracking echocardiography study," *Herz*, vol. 40, no. S3, pp. 240–246, 2015.

[59] Z. Y. Fang, S. Yuda, V. Anderson, L. Short, C. Case, and T. H. Marwick, "Echocardiographic detection of early diabetic myocardial disease," *Journal of the American College of Cardiology*, vol. 41, no. 4, pp. 611–617, 2003.

[60] A. Zoroufian, T. Razmi, M. Taghavi-Shavazi, M. Lotfi-Tokaldany, and A. Jalali, "Evaluation of subclinical left ventricular dysfunction in diabetic patients: longitudinal strain velocities and left ventricular dyssynchrony by two-dimensional speckle tracking echocardiography study," *Echocardiography*, vol. 31, no. 4, pp. 456–463, 2014.

[61] R. Guo, K. Wang, W. Song et al., "Myocardial dysfunction in early diabetes patients with microalbuminuria: a 2-dimensional speckle tracking strain study," *Cell Biochemistry and Biophysics*, vol. 70, no. 1, pp. 573–578, 2014.

[62] M. T. Jensen, P. Sogaard, H. U. Andersen et al., "Global longitudinal strain is not impaired in type 1 diabetes patients without albuminuria: the thousand & 1 study," *JACC: Cardiovascular Imaging*, vol. 8, no. 4, pp. 400–410, 2015.

[63] J. N. Khan, E. G. Wilmot, M. Leggate et al., "Subclinical diastolic dysfunction in young adults with type 2 diabetes mellitus: a multiparametric contrast-enhanced cardiovascular magnetic resonance pilot study assessing potential mechanisms," *European Heart Journal—Cardiovascular Imaging*, vol. 15, no. 11, pp. 1263–1269, 2014.

[64] E. G. Wilmot, M. Leggate, J. N. Khan et al., "Type 2 diabetes mellitus and obesity in young adults: the extreme phenotype with early cardiovascular dysfunction," *Diabetic Medicine*, vol. 31, no. 7, pp. 794–798, 2014.

[65] X. Zhang, X. Wei, Y. Liang, M. Liu, C. Li, and H. Tang, "Differential changes of left ventricular myocardial deformation in diabetic patients with controlled and uncontrolled blood glucose: a three-dimensional speckle-tracking echocardiography-based study," *Journal of the American Society of Echocardiography*, vol. 26, no. 5, pp. 499–506, 2013.

[66] M. Tadic, S. Ilic, C. Cuspidi et al., "Left ventricular mechanics in untreated normotensive patients with type 2 diabetes mellitus: a two- and three-dimensional speckle tracking study," *Echocardiography*, vol. 32, no. 6, pp. 947–955, 2015.

[67] M. Lind, I. Bounias, M. Olsson, S. Gudbjörnsdottir, A.-M. Svensson, and A. Rosengren, "Glycaemic control and incidence of heart failure in 20 985 patients with type 1 diabetes: an observational study," *The Lancet*, vol. 378, no. 9786, pp. 140–146, 2011.

[68] P. M. Kralik, G. Ye, N. S. Metreveli, X. Shem, and P. N. Epstein, "Cardiomyocyte dysfunction in models of type 1 and type 2 diabetes," *Cardiovascular Toxicology*, vol. 5, no. 3, pp. 285–292, 2005.

[69] S. U. Trost, D. D. Belke, W. F. Bluhm, M. Meyer, E. Swanson, and W. H. Dillmann, "Overexpression of the sarcoplasmic reticulum Ca^{2+}-ATPase improves myocardial contractility in diabetic cardiomyopathy," *Diabetes*, vol. 51, no. 4, pp. 1166–1171, 2002.

[70] G. R. Norton, G. Candy, and A. J. Woodiwiss, "Aminoguanidine prevents the decreased myocardial compliance produced by streptozotocin-induced diabetes mellitus in rats," *Circulation*, vol. 93, no. 10, pp. 1905–1912, 1996.

[71] H. Bugger, S. Boudina, X. X. Hu et al., "Type 1 diabetic akita mouse hearts are insulin sensitive but manifest structurally abnormal mitochondria that remain coupled despite increased uncoupling protein 3," *Diabetes*, vol. 57, no. 11, pp. 2924–2932, 2008.

[72] H. Bugger and E. D. Abel, "Molecular mechanisms of diabetic cardiomyopathy," *Diabetologia*, vol. 57, no. 4, pp. 660–671, 2014.

[73] S. Boudina and E. D. Abel, "Diabetic cardiomyopathy revisited," *Circulation*, vol. 115, no. 25, pp. 3213–3223, 2007.

[74] L. M. Semeniuk, A. J. Kryski, and D. L. Severson, "Echocardiographic assessment of cardiac function in diabetic *db/db* and transgenic *db/db*-hGLUT$_4$ mice," *American Journal of Physiology: Heart and Circulatory Physiology*, vol. 283, no. 3, pp. H976–H982, 2002.

[75] T. L. Broderick and A. K. Hutchison, "Cardiac dysfunction in the euglycemic diabetic-prone BB Wor rat," *Metabolism: Clinical and Experimental*, vol. 53, no. 11, pp. 1391–1394, 2004.

[76] R. Basu, G. Y. Oudit, X. Wang et al., "Type 1 diabetic cardiomyopathy in the Akita ($Ins2^{WT/C96Y}$) mouse model is characterized by lipotoxicity and diastolic dysfunction with preserved systolic function," *The American Journal of Physiology: Heart and Circulatory Physiology*, vol. 297, no. 6, pp. H2096–H2108, 2009.

[77] P. Poirier, P. Bogaty, C. Garneau, L. Marois, and J.-G. Dumesnil, "Diastolic dysfunction in normotensive men with well-controlled type 2 diabetes: importance of maneuvers in echocardiographic screening for preclinical diabetic cardiomyopathy," *Diabetes Care*, vol. 24, no. 1, pp. 5–10, 2001.

[78] J. E. Liu, V. Palmieri, M. J. Roman et al., "The impact of diabetes on left ventricular filling pattern in normotensive and hypertensive adults: the strong heart study," *Journal of the American College of Cardiology*, vol. 37, no. 7, pp. 1943–1949, 2001.

[79] P. Pacher, L. Liaudet, F. G. Soriano, J. G. Mabley, É. Szabó, and C. Szabó, "The role of poly(ADP-ribose) polymerase activation in the development of myocardial and endothelial dysfunction in diabetes," *Diabetes*, vol. 51, no. 2, pp. 514–521, 2002.

[80] K. Gul, A. S. Celebi, F. Kacmaz et al., "Tissue Doppler imaging must be performed to detect early left ventricular dysfunction in patients with type 1 diabetes mellitus," *European Journal of Echocardiography*, vol. 10, no. 7, pp. 841–846, 2009.

[81] A. A. Sanchez, P. T. Levy, T. J. Sekarski, A. Hamvas, M. R. Holland, and G. K. Singh, "Effects of frame rate on two-dimensional speckle tracking-derived measurements of myocardial deformation in premature infants," *Echocardiography*, vol. 32, no. 5, pp. 839–847, 2015.

11

Vitamin B6 Prevents Endothelial Dysfunction, Insulin Resistance, and Hepatic Lipid Accumulation in $Apoe^{-/-}$ Mice Fed with High-Fat Diet

Zhan Liu,[1] Peng Li,[2] Zhi-Hong Zhao,[1] Yu Zhang,[1] Zhi-Min Ma,[3] and Shuang-Xi Wang[2,4]

[1]*Department of Clinical Nutrition and Gastroenterology, The First Affiliated Hospital (People's Hospital of Hunan Province), Hunan Normal University, Changsha 430070, China*
[2]*College of Pharmacy, Xinxiang Medical University, Xinxiang 453003, China*
[3]*Division of Endocrinology, The Second Affiliated Hospital, Soochow University, Suzhou 215000, China*
[4]*The Key Laboratory of Cardiovascular Remodeling and Function Research, Chinese Ministry of Education and Chinese Ministry of Health, Qilu Hospital, School of Medicine, Shandong University, Jinan 250012, China*

Correspondence should be addressed to Shuang-Xi Wang; shuangxiwang@sdu.edu.cn

Academic Editor: Hiroshi Okamoto

Backgrounds. VitB6 deficiency has been associated with a number of adverse health effects. However, the effects of VitB6 in metabolic syndrome are poorly understood. *Methods.* VitB6 (50 mg/kg/day) was given to $Apoe^{-/-}$ mice with hkdigh-fat diet (HFD) for 8 weeks. Endothelial dysfunction, insulin resistance, and hepatic lipid contents were determined. *Results.* VitB6 administration remarkably increased acetylcholine-induced endothelium-dependent relaxation and decreased random blood glucose level in $Apoe^{-/-}$ mice fed with HFD. In addition, VitB6 improved the tolerance of glucose and insulin, normalized the histopathology of liver, and reduced hepatic lipid accumulation but did not affect the liver functions. Clinical and biochemical analysis indicated that the levels of VitB6 were decreased in patients with fatty liver. *Conclusions.* Vitamin B6 prevents endothelial dysfunction, insulin resistance, and hepatic lipid accumulation in $Apoe^{-/-}$ mice fed with HFD. Supplementation of VitB6 should be considered to prevent metabolic syndrome.

1. Introduction

Vitamin B6 (VitB6) includes pyridoxal, pyridoxine, and pyridoxamine, which function as essential cofactors for enzymes involved in various metabolic activities, which include amino acid, fat, and glucose metabolism [1]. The phosphate ester derivative pyridoxal $5'$-phosphate (PLP) is the biologically active form of this vitamin and reflects long-term body storage [2]. Studies have shown that low plasma PLP concentrations are associated with increased risk of cardiovascular disease (CVD) [3, 4].

Nutrient overload is associated with high incidence of chronic metabolic diseases, including obesity, insulin resistance, and type 2 diabetes [5]. Prolonged exposure to high concentrations of saturated fatty acids leads to oxidative stress and endoplasmic reticulum stress, which may impair insulin signaling [6]. Moreover, supplementation of a high-fat diet (HFD) with branched-chain amino acids caused insulin resistance, as a part of metabolic syndrome [7]. Metabolic syndrome is associated with a risk of CVD and is a common early abnormality in the development of type 2 diabetes. In patients with nonalcoholic fatty liver disease (NAFLD), metabolic abnormalities have been reported in 33% to 100% of cases [8]. Patients presenting with NAFLD need to be examined for the presence of the components of the metabolic syndrome and their complications [9]. We also previously reported that apoptosis of liver cells contributes to liver dysfunction [10].

The identification of the link between VitB6 and metabolic syndrome including insulin and NAFLD might help to define novel nutritional and pharmacological approaches for the treatment of diabetes, obesity, and insulin resistance. Here, we reported that administration of VitB6 prevents endothelial dysfunction, insulin resistance, and hepatic lipid accumulation in $Apoe^{-/-}$ mice fed with high-fat diet. Clinically, deficiency of VitB6 should be considered as a high risk factor of NAFLD.

2. Materials and Methods

2.1. Materials. Human recombinant insulin was purchased from Sigma-Aldrich (St. Louis, MO). Antibodies against Akt (pAkt), GLUT4, glycogen synthase kinase-3β (GSK3), forkhead box protein O (FOXO), and GAPDH were purchased from Santa Cruz Biotechnology (Dallas, TX). The secondary antibodies were obtained from Jackson ImmunoResearch Laboratories (West Grove, PA). VitB6, acetylcholine (ACh), sodium nitroprusside (SNP), and phenylephrine were from Sigma-Aldrich Company. All drug concentrations are expressed as final working concentrations in the buffer.

2.2. Animals and Experimental Protocols. Male $Apoe^{-/-}$ mice were purchased from Hua-Fu-Kang Animal Company (Beijing, China). All animals were housed in temperature-controlled cages with a 12-hour light-dark cycle and given free access to water and normal chow. This study was carried out in strict accordance with the recommendations in the *Guide for the Care and Use of Laboratory Animals* of the National Institutes of Health.

Model of hyperlipidemia was induced by feeding mice with HFD containing 0.21% cholesterol and 21% fat (Research Diets Inc., D12079B). This diet was administered at 6 weeks of age and continued for 8 consecutive weeks. At 6 weeks of age, VitB6 (50 mg/kg/day) was also added to the drinking water for 8 weeks. The animal protocol was reviewed and approved by the Animal Care and Use Committee of Hunan Normal University.

2.3. Determinations of Serum Lipid Profiles and Liver Functions. Blood was sampled from mice for determination of total bilirubin (TB), aspartate aminotransferase (AST), alanine aminotransferase (ALT), alkaline phosphatase (ALP), and albumin (ALB). Serum levels of TB, AST, ALT, AP, and ALB were determined by commercial kits (Nanjing Jiancheng Biology Company, Nanjing, China).

2.4. Organ Chamber. In vivo or ex vivo organ chamber study was performed as described previously [11]. Mice were sacrificed under anesthesia by intravenous injection with pentobarbital sodium (30 mg/kg). The descending aorta isolated by removing the adhering perivascular tissue carefully was cut into rings (2-3 mm in length). Aortic rings were suspended and mounted to organ chamber by using two stainless hooks. The rings were placed in organ baths filled with Krebs buffer of the following compositions (in mM): NaCl, 118.3; KCl, 4.7; MgSO$_4$, 0.6; KH$_2$PO$_4$, 1.2; CaCl$_2$, 2.5; NaHCO$_3$, 25.0;

EDTA, 0.026; pH 7.4 at 37°C; and they were gassed with 95% O$_2$ plus 5% CO$_2$, under tension of 1.0 g, for 90-minute equilibration period. During this period, the Krebs solution was changed every 15 min. After the equilibration, aortic rings were challenged with 60 mM KCl. After washing and another 30-minute equilibration period, contractile response was elicited by phenylephrine (1 μM). At the plateau of contraction, accumulative ACh (0.01, 0.03, 0.1, 0.3, 1, and 3 μM) or SNP (0.01, 0.03, 0.1, 0.3, 1, 3, and 10 μM) was added to induce the relaxation.

2.5. Glucose Tolerance Test (GTT) and Insulin Tolerance Test (ITT). As described previously [12], glucose (2.0 g/kg) was given to mice (i.p.) after an overnight fast. Blood glucose (BG) levels were then measured at indicated times with a portable glucose meter (LifeScan, Milpitas, CA) after tail snipping. For ITT, mice were injected with insulin (0.55 IU/kg, i.p.) after 6-hour fast. BG levels were measured at indicated times with a portable glucose meter (LifeScan, Milpitas, CA) after tail snipping.

2.6. HE or Oil Red O Staining. Histological specimens were taken at the end of the study period for all mouse groups as described previously [13]. For each mouse, liver segments were fixed in 4% buffered formaldehyde and embedded in paraffin for histological analysis. Sections (5 μm) were stained with either hematoxylin or eosin. Degree of severity of liver fibrosis was derived from blind analysis of each of the animals in each group. To determine hepatic lipid accumulation, frozen liver sections were stained with 0.5% Oil Red O for 10 min, washed, and counterstained with Mayer's hematoxylin for 45 sec. Data for Oil Red O staining were presented as the mean percentage of stained area to a total hepatic region in 10 fields from each liver section. Quantitative analysis was performed using analySIS-FIVE program (Olympus Soft Imaging System, Münster, Germany).

2.7. Western Blotting. The protocol for western blot was described as previously with some modifications [14]. Liver tissues were homogenized and the protein content in supernatant was assayed by BCA protein assay reagent (Pierce, USA). 20 μg proteins were loaded to SDS-PAGE and then transferred to membrane. Membrane was incubated with 1 : 1000 dilution of primary antibody, followed by 1 : 2000 dilution of horseradish peroxides-conjugated secondary antibody. Protein bands were visualized by ECL (GE Healthcare, USA). The intensity (area × density) of the individual bands on western blots was measured by densitometry (model GS-700, Imaging Densitometer; Bio-Rad). The background was subtracted from the calculated area. The average of density for the bands in control group is considered as 100%.

2.8. Measurement of Cholesterol and Triglyceride Contents in Liver. Lipids in mouse liver were extracted as described by Folch et al. [15, 16]. Cholesterol and triglyceride levels in extracted lipids were measured enzymatically using the reagents from Cayman Chemical (Ann Arbor, MI) according to the manufacturer's instruction.

(a)

(b)

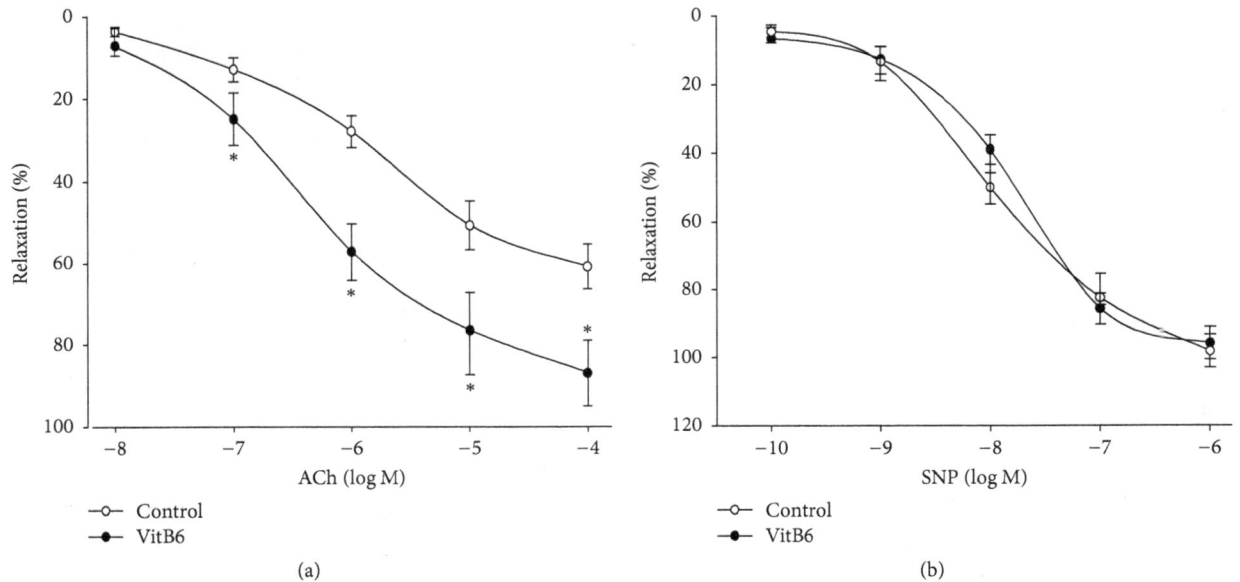

FIGURE 1: Administration of VitB6 prevents endothelial dysfunction in $Apoe^{-/-}$ mice fed with high-fat diet. Male $Apoe^{-/-}$ mice at the age of 6 weeks received high-fat diet and VitB6 (50 mg/kg/day) administration in drinking water for 8 weeks. At the end of experiments, mice were sacrificed under anaesthesia. The descending aortas were isolated and cut into rings. (a) ACh-induced endothelium-dependent relaxation and (b) SNP-induced endothelium-independent relaxation were determined by organ chamber as described in Section 2. All data were expressed as mean ± SEM. N is 10–15 in each group. $^{*}P < 0.05$ versus control.

2.9. Statistical Analysis. The results were expressed as mean ± SEM. One-way ANOVA followed by t-test was used for two groups' comparison. $P < 0.05$ was considered significant.

3. Results

3.1. VitB6 Prevents Endothelial Dysfunction in $Apoe^{-/-}$ Mice Fed with HFD. Endothelial dysfunction has been identified as an early hallmark of CVD, such as atherosclerosis and hypertension [17–20]. We firstly determined whether VitB6 prevents endothelial dysfunction in mice with metabolic syndromes. The hyperlipidemia model was induced by feeding $Apoe^{-/-}$ mice with HFD [21]. As indicated in Table 1, HFD in $Apoe^{-/-}$ mice dramatically increased serum levels of triglyceride, cholesterol, and LDL, indicating that the model is successfully established. Importantly, the random level of blood sugar was also increased in $Apoe^{-/-}$ mice fed with HFD. However, treatment of these mice with VitB6 did not alter the levels of triglyceride, cholesterol, and LDL, except for random level of blood glucose.

The endothelial function was determined by using ACh. As shown in Figure 1(a), ACh-induced vasorelaxation was significantly improved by VitB6. The SNP-induced vasorelaxation was not affected by VitB6 (Figure 1(b)), demonstrating that the protective effects of VitB6 on vascular function are limited to endothelium.

3.2. VitB6 Enhances Insulin Sensitivity in $Apoe^{-/-}$ Mice Fed with HFD. Insulin resistance is a high risk factor of endothelial dysfunction in CVD [22]. We next examined whether

TABLE 1: Serum sugar and lipid levels in $Apoe^{-/-}$ mice.

| | WT | | $Apoe^{-/-}$ | |
	ND	ND	HFD	HFD + VitB6
Glucose (mM)	6.5 ± 1.3	8.2 ± 1.3	13.5 ± 0.8	10.2 ± 0.9*
Cholesterol (mM)	3.7 ± 0.5	10.5 ± 2.1	28.4 ± 5.3	26.4 ± 4.9
Triglyceride (mM)	0.7 ± 0.2	0.8 ± 0.2	1.6 ± 0.3	1.5 ± 0.5
HDL-C (mg/L)	128 ± 15	252 ± 30	267 ± 38	257 ± 39
LDL-C (mg/L)	109 ± 14	249 ± 23	417 ± 53	435 ± 67

After 8-week administration of VitB6 in $Apoe^{-/-}$ mice fed with high-fat diet, serum sugar levels and lipid levels were determined. WT: wild-type; ND: normal diet; HFD: high-fat diet; HDL: high density lipoprotein; LDL: low density lipoprotein. All data were expressed as mean ± SEM. N is 10–15 in each group. $^{*}P < 0.05$ versus $Apoe^{-/-}$ mice fed with HFD.

VitB6 improves insulin sensitivity in HFD-fed $Apoe^{-/-}$ mice. As shown in Figure 2(a), injection of D-glucose dramatically increased the levels of blood glucose (BG) in HFD-fed $Apoe^{-/-}$ mice. The peak level of BG was about 500 mg/dL after 30 minutes. The level of BG was back to the basal level after 90 minutes. However, administration of VitB6 delayed and lowered the peak levels of BG (470 mg/dL). After 90 minutes of glucose injection, the level of BG was also back to the basal level. These data indicate that VitB6 increases the tolerance of glucose.

The protective effect of VitB6 on glucose metabolism was further confirmed by measuring the sensitivity of insulin (Figure 2(b)). By injecting exogenous insulin into HFD-fed $Apoe^{-/-}$ mice, the levels of BG were reduced to 40% of basal level at the 60th minute and then went back to 80% of basal

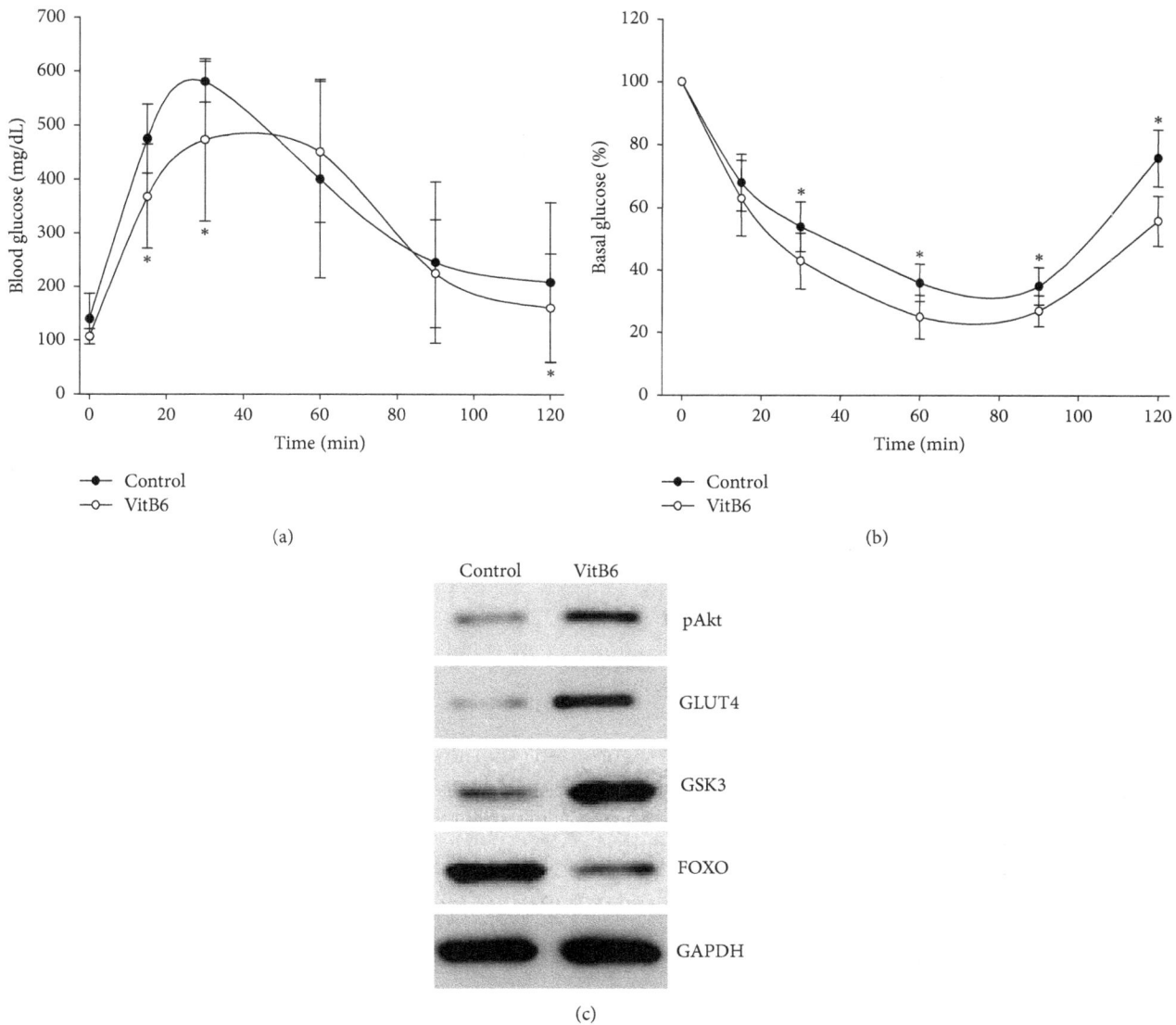

(a)

(b)

(c)

FIGURE 2: VitB6 improves insulin resistance in $Apoe^{-/-}$ mice fed with high-fat diet. Male $Apoe^{-/-}$ mice at the age of 6 weeks received high-fat diet and VitB6 (50 mg/kg/day) administration in drinking water. At the 8th weekend after VitB6 treatment, (a) GTT and (b) ITT were evaluated as described in Section 2. All data were expressed as mean ± SEM. N is 10–15 in each group. $^{*}P < 0.05$ versus control. (c) Homogenates of liver tissues were subjected to perform western blotting analysis to assay the levels of pAKt, GLUT4, GSK3, and FOXO. The picture is a representative blot from 10–15 mice.

level at the 120th minute. However, VitB6 further reduced the level of BG at the 90th minute to 25%. After the 120th minute, the level of BG was 55% of the basal level. Collectively, this suggests that VitB6 enhances insulin sensitivity in mice.

3.3. Increased Hepatic Levels of pAkt, GSK3, and GLUT4 Proteins and Decreased FOXO Protein Expression in VitB6-Treated $Apoe^{-/-}$ Mice.
The beneficial effects of VitB6 on insulin resistance were further examined by assaying the hepatic levels of pAkt, GSK3, GLUT4, and FOXO, which are proteins related to glucose metabolism [23]. As depicted in Figure 2(c), compared to HFD-fed $Apoe^{-/-}$ mice, the levels

of pAkt, GSK3, GLUT4, and BG were increased and the level of FOXO was reduced in HFD-fed $Apoe^{-/-}$ mice with VitB6, further supporting the notion that VitB6 improves insulin resistance in mice.

3.4. VitB6 Treatment Prevents Hepatic Lipid Accumulation in Mice.
NAFLD is characterized by insulin resistance [24]. Thus, we detected the liver function in these mice. In Table 2, the markers of liver function, such as ALB, ALP, ALT, AST, and TB, were comparable in HFD-fed $Apoe^{-/-}$ mice with or without VitB6 treatment. Histological analysis of HE staining in liver sections from mice at the end of the experiment

TABLE 2: The indexes for liver function in mice.

	Control	VitB6
AST (IU/L)	132.2 ± 27.9	157.4 ± 31.8
ALT (IU/L)	186.7 ± 21.3	195.7 ± 28.6
TB (mg/dL)	0.13 ± 0.07	0.15 ± 0.09
ALP (IU/L)	255.5 ± 32.8	279.8 ± 35.8
ALB (g/L)	17.2 ± 1.4	20.6 ± 16.8

After 8-week administration of VitB6 in $Apoe^{-/-}$ mice fed with high-fat diet, serum levels of AST, ALT, TB, ALP, and ALB were determined. All data were expressed as mean ± SEM. N is 10–15 in each group.

TABLE 3: The levels of serum VitB6, homocysteine, folate, and VitB12 in patients with fatty liver.

	Control (57)	Patients (49)
VitB6 (PLP, nM)	55.8 ± 10.7	23.9 ± 8.1[*]
VitB12 (pg/mL)	686.7 ± 21.3	518.7 ± 28.6[*]
folic acid (ng/mL)	8.3 ± 0.7	7.7 ± 0.9
Homocysteine (nM)	15.8 ± 2.8	22.8 ± 5.4[*]

Serum levels of VitB6, VitB12, folic acid, and homocysteine were determined in patients with fatty liver and control subjects. All data were expressed as mean ± SEM. [*]$P < 0.05$ versus control.

(Figure 3(a)) revealed that HFD caused marked neurosis and fibrosis, which was reversed by VitB6 treatment, suggesting that VitB6 is effective to protect the liver.

The typical feature of NAFLD is the elevated hepatic lipid accumulation [25, 26]. We next investigated whether VitB6 prevents hepatic lipid accumulation in hyperlipidemia mice by Oil Red O staining (Figure 3(a)). Compared to control HFD-fed $Apoe^{-/-}$ mice, the contents of liver triglycerides (Figure 3(b)) and cholesterol (Figure 3(c)) were decreased, demonstrating that VitB6 prevents hepatic lipid accumulation in mice and is potentially considered to serve as prevention of NAFLD.

3.5. Plasmatic Lower Levels of VitB6 in Patients with Fatty Liver. Finally, in order to establish the clinical association between VitB6 deficiency and NAFLD, we performed clinical and biochemical analysis. As described in Table 3, fifty-seven healthy humans and forty-nine patients had a clinical and biochemical analysis completed in the study. Compared to the healthy human subjects, the levels of folic acid were similar in patients with fatty liver. The levels of VitB12 were lightly increased. However, the levels of homocysteine in NAFLD patients were significantly increased, consistent with other reports [27, 28]. Most importantly, we found that the levels of VitB6 were lower in NAFLD than control healthy humans. These results indicate that deficiency of VitB6 might be a risk factor of NAFLD clinically.

4. Discussion

In the present study, we provide the first evidence that administration of VitB6 prevents endothelial dysfunction, insulin resistance, and hepatic lipid accumulation in $Apoe^{-/-}$ mice fed with HFD *in vivo*. Clinically, the serum level of VitB6 is low in patients with NAFLD. Our data not only indicate that VitB6 protects endothelial function and improves insulin resistance, but also imply that low VitB6 status might be a risk factor of NAFLD, as a component of metabolic syndrome.

The major discovery in the present study is that VitB6 produces several beneficial effects to prevent metabolic syndrome, such as insulin resistance and NAFLD. Traditionally, VitB6, in the form of PLP, is the coenzyme of 5 enzymes in these metabolic pathways: cystathionine-β-synthase (CBS), cystathionine-γ-lyase (CGL), cytoplasmic and mitochondrial serine hydroxymethyltransferase (cSHMT and mSHMT), and glycine decarboxylase (GDC) in the mitochondria [29]. In this way, VitB6 regulates the transsulfuration pathway which contributes to homocysteine regulation and provides cysteine synthesis and consists of sequential reactions catalyzed by CBS and CGL. CBS catalyzes the condensation of homocysteine and serine to form cystathionine in a reaction that is subject to positive allosteric regulation by S-adenosylmethionine (SAM), whereas CGL catalyzes the cleavage of cystathionine to yield α-ketobutyrate, ammonia, and cysteine. Because both CBS and CGL require PLP as a coenzyme, inadequate VitB6 status might lead to impaired regulation of cellular homocysteine concentration. High levels of homocysteine impair endothelial function and cause metabolic syndrome including insulin resistance and lipid accumulation in liver. HHCY might play a role in the pathogenesis of vascular disorders and is considered as an independent risk factor for atherosclerosis [30]. From our observations, supplementation of VitB6 should be a helpful therapy to improve endothelial dysfunction and metabolic syndrome. Of course, the mechanism of VitB6 in prevention of metabolic syndrome needs further investigations.

We also identified VitB6 deficiency as a new risk factor of NAFLD. Obesity, metabolic syndrome, and type 2 diabetes mellitus are strictly related and are key pathogenetic factors of NAFLD, the most frequent liver disease worldwide. NAFLD is a clinicopathological syndrome including a wide spectrum of liver damage instances, ranging from hepatic steatosis to nonalcoholic steatohepatitis (NASH) to cirrhosis [31]. Epidemiologic studies showed that low VitB6 nutritional status is associated with increased risk of CVD, venous thrombosis, stroke, and possibly colon cancer [32]. Although a connection between VitB6 status and lipid metabolism has appeared periodically for more than 80 years, there is no evidence to support the role of PLP in NAFLD. To our knowledge, this is the first study to investigate whether marginal VitB6 deficiency affects hepatic lipid accumulation in human adults. We observed a significant decrease of plasma PLP concentration in patients with NAFLD. A potential mechanism responsible for the observations of lower plasma VitB6 level linking to NAFLD is impairment of PUFA interconversion because it has been reported that marginal VitB6 deficiency decreases plasma (n-3) and (n-6) PUFA concentrations in healthy men and women [33]. Further investigation should focus on the direct target of VitB6 on regulation of lipid metabolism in liver.

A limitation of this study is that $Apoe^{-/-}$ mouse is suitable for studying atherosclerosis resulting from hypercholesterolemia. Additionally, this mouse has several intriguing

(a)

(b)

(c)

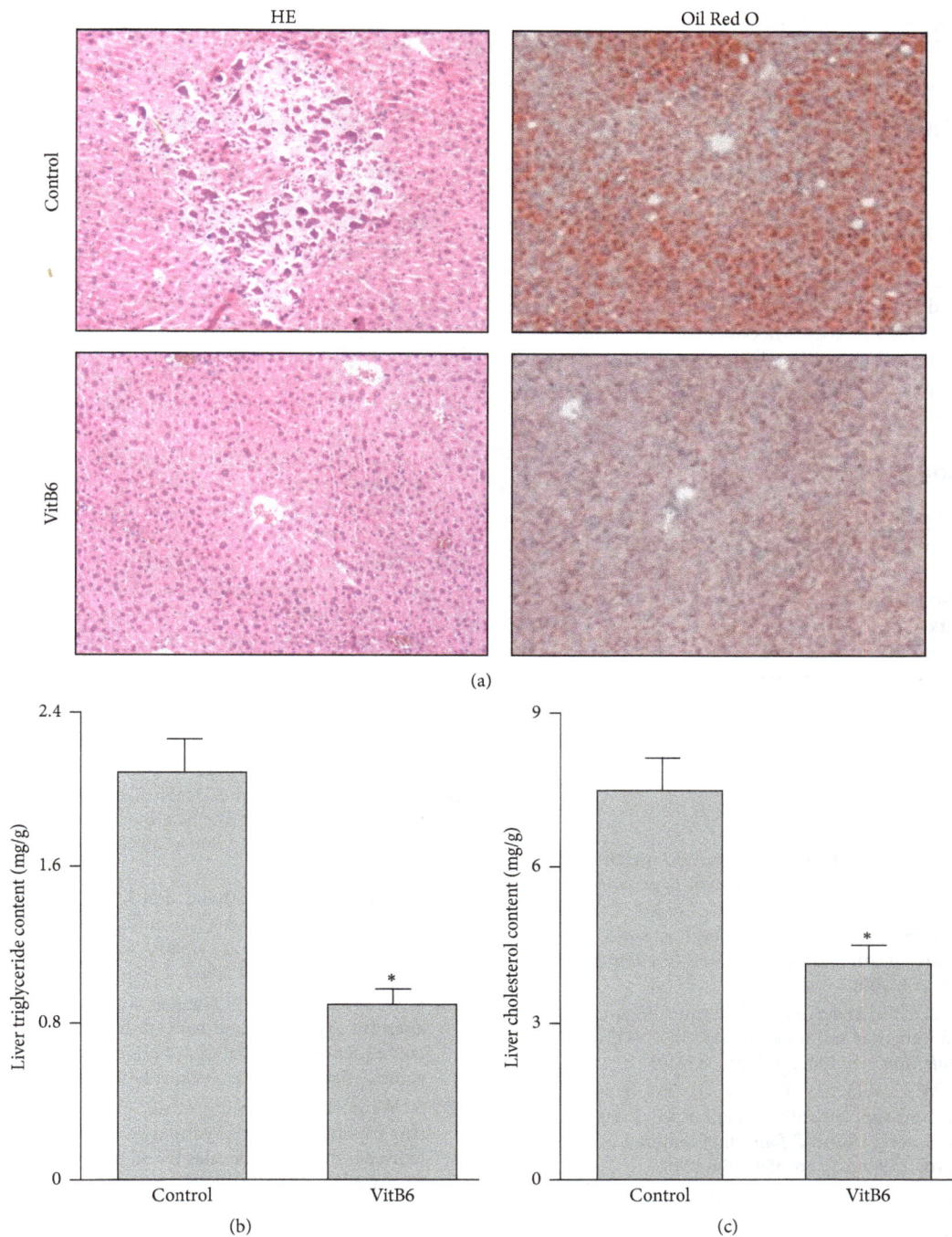

FIGURE 3: VitB6 reduces hepatic lipid accumulation in $Apoe^{-/-}$ mice fed with high-fat diet. Male $Apoe^{-/-}$ mice at the age of 6 weeks received high-fat diet and VitB6 (50 mg/kg/day) administration in drinking water. At the end of experiments, mice were sacrificed under anaesthesia. (a) Histological analysis of liver tissue by HE or Oil Red O staining. (b and c) Liver lipids were extracted and hepatic triglyceride and cholesterol levels were assayed using a commercial kit. The quantitative data were expressed as mean ± SEM. N is 10–15 in each group. $^{*}P < 0.05$ versus Control.

characteristics. First, $Apoe^{-/-}$ mice show obesity-resistant phenotype, resulting in remarkable insulin sensitivity. Second, this mouse has hepatic steatosis due to impairment of VLDL secretion from liver. Third, this mouse basically possesses endothelial dysfunction damaged from excess beta lipoprotein. It would be better to investigate the metabolic effects of vitamin B6 on wild-type mice with diet-induced metabolic disorders, such as C57B16 strain.

In summary, the results of this study have shown that low VitB6 status has substantial effects on metabolism including glucose and fatty acid. The results of this study also demonstrate that the deficiency of VitB6 might be a risk factor of NAFLD.

Conflict of Interests

The authors confirm that there is no conflict of interests.

Authors' Contribution

Zhan Liu and Peng Li designed and performed all experiments, analyzed the data, and wrote the paper. Zhi-Hong Zhao, Yu Zhang, and Zhi-Min Ma collected the clinical samples. Zhan Liu and Shuang-Xi Wang conceived the project and wrote the paper. Zhan Liu and Peng Li contributed equally to this work.

Acknowledgments

This work was supported by National 973 Basic Research Program of China (2013CB530700) and National Natural Science Foundation of China (81570723, 81470591, and 81370411). This project was also sponsored by Program for New Century Excellent Talents in University (NCET-13-0351), the Scientific Research Foundation for the Returned Overseas Chinese Scholars, State Education Ministry, and Program of Clinical Investigation (Nanshan Group), Qilu Hospital, Shandong University (2014QLKY15). Shuang-Xi Wang is a recipient of Qilu Professional Scholar of Shandong University.

References

[1] D. B. Coursin, "Present status of vitamin B6 metabolism," *The American Journal of Clinical Nutrition*, vol. 9, pp. 304–314, 1961.

[2] X. Jouven, M.-A. Charles, M. Desnos, and P. Ducimetière, "Circulating nonesterified fatty acid level as a predictive risk factor for sudden death in the population," *Circulation*, vol. 104, no. 7, pp. 756–761, 2001.

[3] V. Lotto, S.-W. Choi, and S. Friso, "Vitamin B6: a challenging link between nutrition and inflammation in CVD," *The British Journal of Nutrition*, vol. 106, no. 2, pp. 183–195, 2011.

[4] E. B. Rimm, W. C. Willett, F. B. Hu et al., "Folate and vitamin B6 from diet and supplements in relation to risk of coronary heart disease among women," *Journal of the American Medical Association*, vol. 279, no. 5, pp. 359–364, 1998.

[5] L. Lionetti, M. P. Mollica, A. Lombardi, G. Cavaliere, G. Gifuni, and A. Barletta, "From chronic overnutrition to insulin resistance: the role of fat-storing capacity and inflammation," *Nutrition, Metabolism and Cardiovascular Diseases*, vol. 19, no. 2, pp. 146–152, 2009.

[6] M. Cnop, "Fatty acids and glucolipotoxicity in the pathogenesis of Type 2 diabetes," *Biochemical Society Transactions*, vol. 36, no. 3, pp. 348–352, 2008.

[7] C. B. Newgard, J. An, J. R. Bain et al., "A branched-chain amino acid-related metabolic signature that differentiates obese and lean humans and contributes to insulin resistance," *Cell Metabolism*, vol. 9, no. 4, pp. 311–326, 2009.

[8] N. Alkhouri, C. Carter-Kent, and A. E. Feldstein, "Apoptosis in nonalcoholic fatty liver disease: diagnostic and therapeutic implications," *Expert Review of Gastroenterology and Hepatology*, vol. 5, no. 2, pp. 201–212, 2011.

[9] M. Li, C. M. Reynolds, S. A. Segovia, C. Gray, and M. H. Vickers, "Developmental programming of nonalcoholic fatty liver disease: the effect of early life nutrition on susceptibility and disease severity in later life," *BioMed Research International*, vol. 2015, Article ID 437107, 12 pages, 2015.

[10] Z. Liu, S. Wang, H. Zhou, Y. Yang, and M. Zhang, "Na$^+$/H$^+$ exchanger mediates TNF-α-induced hepatocyte apoptosis via the calpain-dependent degradation of Bcl-xL," *Journal of Gastroenterology and Hepatology*, vol. 24, no. 5, pp. 879–885, 2009.

[11] X.-H. Yang, P. Li, Y.-L. Yin et al., "Rosiglitazone via PPARγ-dependent suppression of oxidative stress attenuates endothelial dysfunction in rats fed homocysteine thiolactone," *Journal of Cellular and Molecular Medicine*, vol. 19, pp. 826–835, 2015.

[12] T.-Y. Xu, L.-L. Guo, P. Wang et al., "Chronic exposure to nicotine enhances insulin sensitivity through α7 nicotinic acetylcholine receptor-STAT3 pathway," *PLoS ONE*, vol. 7, no. 12, Article ID e51217, 2012.

[13] S. Wang, C. Zhang, M. Zhang et al., "Activation of AMP-activated protein kinase alpha2 by nicotine instigates formation of abdominal aortic aneurysms in mice in vivo," *Nature Medicine*, vol. 18, no. 6, pp. 902–910, 2012.

[14] S. Wang, B. Liang, B. Viollet, and M.-H. Zou, "Inhibition of the AMP-activated protein kinase-α2 accentuates agonist-induced vascular smooth muscle contraction and high blood pressure in mice," *Hypertension*, vol. 57, no. 5, pp. 1010–1017, 2011.

[15] H. Li, Q. Min, C. Ouyang et al., "AMPK activation prevents excess nutrient-induced hepatic lipid accumulation by inhibiting mTORC1 signaling and endoplasmic reticulum stress response," *Biochimica et Biophysica Acta—Molecular Basis of Disease*, vol. 1842, no. 9, pp. 1844–1854, 2014.

[16] J. Folch, M. Lees, and G. H. Sloane Stanley, "A simple method for the isolation and purification of total lipides from animal tissues," *The Journal of Biological Chemistry*, vol. 226, no. 1, pp. 497–509, 1957.

[17] S. Wang, Q. Peng, J. Zhang, and L. Liu, "Na$^+$/H$^+$ exchanger is required for hyperglycaemia-induced endothelial dysfunction via calcium-dependent calpain," *Cardiovascular Research*, vol. 80, no. 2, pp. 255–262, 2008.

[18] S. Wang, M. Zhang, B. Liang et al., "AMPKα2 Deletion causes aberrant expression and activation of NAD(P)H Oxidase and consequent endothelial dysfunction in vivo: role of 26S proteasomes," *Circulation Research*, vol. 106, no. 6, pp. 1117–1128, 2010.

[19] S. Wang, J. Xu, P. Song et al., "Acute inhibition of guanosine triphosphate cyclohydrolase 1 uncouples endothelial nitric oxide synthase and elevates blood pressure," *Hypertension*, vol. 52, no. 3, pp. 484–490, 2008.

[20] S. Wang, J. Xu, P. Song, B. Viollet, and M.-H. Zou, "In vivo activation of AMP-activated protein kinase attenuates diabetes-enhanced degradation of GTP cyclohydrolase I," *Diabetes*, vol. 58, no. 8, pp. 1893–1901, 2009.

[21] A. K. Leamy, R. A. Egnatchik, and J. D. Young, "Molecular mechanisms and the role of saturated fatty acids in the progression of non-alcoholic fatty liver disease," *Progress in Lipid Research*, vol. 52, no. 1, pp. 165–174, 2013.

[22] M. Iantorno, U. Campia, N. Di Daniele et al., "Obesity, inflammation and endothelial dysfunction," *Journal of Biological Regulators and Homeostatic Agents*, vol. 28, no. 2, pp. 169–176, 2014.

[23] M. Yuan, E. Pino, L. Wu, M. Kacergis, and A. A. Soukas, "Identification of Akt-independent regulation of hepatic lipogenesis by mammalian target of rapamycin (mTOR) complex 2," *The*

Journal of Biological Chemistry, vol. 287, no. 35, pp. 29579–29588, 2012.

[24] T. Khoury, A. Ben Ya'acov, Y. Shabat, L. Zolotarovya, R. Snir, and Y. Ilan, "Altered distribution of regulatory lymphocytes by oral administration of soy-extracts exerts a hepatoprotective effect alleviating immune mediated liver injury, non-alcoholic steatohepatitis and insulin resistance," *World Journal of Gastroenterology*, vol. 21, no. 24, pp. 7443–7456, 2015.

[25] H. Malhi and G. J. Gores, "Molecular mechanisms of lipotoxicity in nonalcoholic fatty liver disease," *Seminars in Liver Disease*, vol. 28, no. 4, pp. 360–369, 2008.

[26] J. Wang, C. Zhang, Z. Zhang et al., "BL153 partially prevents high-fat diet induced liver damage probably via inhibition of lipid accumulation, inflammation, and oxidative stress," *Oxidative Medicine and Cellular Longevity*, vol. 2014, Article ID 674690, 10 pages, 2014.

[27] S. C. R. de Carvalho, M. T. C. Muniz, M. D. V. Siqueira et al., "Plasmatic higher levels of homocysteine in non-alcoholic fatty liver disease (NAFLD)," *Nutrition Journal*, vol. 12, article 37, 2013.

[28] E. Bravo, S. Palleschi, P. Aspichueta et al., "High fat diet-induced non alcoholic fatty liver disease in rats is associated with hyperhomocysteinemia caused by down regulation of the transsulphuration pathway," *Lipids in Health and Disease*, vol. 10, article 60, 2011.

[29] H. F. Nijhout, J. F. Gregory, C. Fitzpatrick et al., "A mathematical model gives insights into the effects of vitamin B-6 deficiency on 1-carbon and glutathione metabolism," *Journal of Nutrition*, vol. 139, no. 4, pp. 784–791, 2009.

[30] K. S. McCully, "Vascular pathology of homocysteinemia: implications for the pathogenesis of arteriosclerosis," *The American Journal of Pathology*, vol. 56, no. 1, pp. 111–128, 1969.

[31] H. Azzam and S. Malnick, "Non-alcoholic fatty liver disease—the heart of the matter," *World Journal of Hepatology*, vol. 7, pp. 1369–1376, 2015.

[32] C. P. Lima, S. R. Davis, A. D. Mackey, J. B. Scheer, J. Williamson, and J. F. Gregory III, "Vitamin B-6 deficiency suppresses the hepatic transsulfuration pathway but increases glutathione concentration in rats fed AIN-76A or AIN-93G diets," *The Journal of Nutrition*, vol. 136, no. 8, pp. 2141–2147, 2006.

[33] M. Zhao, Y. Lamers, M. A. Ralat et al., "Marginal vitamin B-6 deficiency decreases plasma (n-3) and (n-6) PUFA concentrations in healthy men and women," *The Journal of Nutrition*, vol. 142, no. 10, pp. 1791–1797, 2012.

12

Breaking the Taboo: Illicit Drug Use among Adolescents with Type 1 Diabetes Mellitus

Anna M. Hogendorf,[1] **Wojciech Fendler,**[1] **Janusz Sieroslawski,**[2] **Katarzyna Bobeff,**[3] **Krzysztof Wegrewicz,**[3] **Kamila I. Malewska,**[3] **Maciej W. Przudzik,**[3] **Malgorzata Szmigiero-Kawko,**[4] **Beata Sztangierska,**[4] **Malgorzata Mysliwiec,**[4] **Agnieszka Szadkowska,**[1] **and Wojciech Mlynarski**[1]

[1]*Department of Pediatrics, Oncology, Hematology and Diabetology, Medical University of Lodz, 91-738 Lodz, Poland*
[2]*Department of Studies on Alcoholism and Other Dependencies, Institute of Psychiatry and Neurology, 02-957 Warsaw, Poland*
[3]*Students' Scientific Circle at the Department of Pediatrics, Oncology, Hematology and Diabetology, Medical University of Lodz, 91-738 Lodz, Poland*
[4]*Department of Pediatrics, Diabetology and Endocrinology, Medical University of Gdańsk, 80-211 Gdańsk, Poland*

Correspondence should be addressed to Anna M. Hogendorf; anna.hogendorf@gmail.com

Academic Editor: Andrea Scaramuzza

Background. The aim of the study was to explore the prevalence of illicit drug use in a group of Polish adolescents with type 1 diabetes (DM1) in comparison with a national cohort of their healthy peers. *Methods.* Two hundred and nine adolescents with DM1, aged 15–18 years, were studied in 2013 with an anonymous questionnaire prepared for the European School Survey Project on Alcohol and Other Drugs (ESPAD). The control group was a representative sample of 12114 students at the same age who took part in ESPAD in 2011. Metabolic control was regarded as good if self-reported HbA1c was <8% or poor if HbA1c was ≥8%. *Results.* Lifetime prevalence of illicit drug use was lower among adolescents with DM1 than in the control group [58 (28%) versus 5524 (46%), $p = 10^{-5}$]. Cannabis preparations were the most frequently used substances [38 (18.3%) versus 3976 (33.1%), $p = 10^{-5}$], followed by tranquilizers, sedatives, and amphetamine. Lifetime and last 12-month use of cannabis were associated with poorer glycemic control (HbA1c ≥ 8%), $p < 0.01$ and 0.02, respectively. *Conclusions.* Adolescents with DM1 report using illicit drugs to a lesser extent than their healthy peers. The use of cannabis is associated with a poorer metabolic control in teens with DM1.

1. Introduction

Experimental behaviors are a characteristic feature of adolescence. Growing evidence suggests that adolescents with chronic conditions, including type 1 diabetes mellitus (DM1), are likely to engage in risky behavior to at least similar, if not greater, extent than their healthy peers [1, 2]. However, drug abuse or even single experimental use of recreational drugs may be especially dangerous in patients with DM1, due to inability to self-manage diabetes [3]. This may contribute to increased morbidity, mortality, and healthcare costs associated with acute diabetes-related events [4–8].

Despite the medical and social importance of the problem, it seems that the topic remains a taboo in families and is underrecognized or easily neglected in complex medical management [9]. Current medical literature contains little data on the prevalence of drug use and abuse in type 1 diabetes, as only a few case reports and a small number of methodologically varying and incomparable analyses are available [2, 3, 10–14]. The problems with conducting such surveys are collecting a proper sample size and an appropriate reference group recruited from the community, over- or underreporting, and the use of self-report questionnaires that are less reliable in clinically recruited samples.

We aimed to evaluate the prevalence of illicit drug use among Polish adolescents with DM1 and to compare it with the habits of healthy peers from a large national cohort, participating in the European School Survey Project on Alcohol and Other Drugs (ESPAD).

2. Patients and Methods

2.1. DM1 Group. Adolescents with DM1 were studied in May and June 2013 in three diabetes centers: Department of Pediatrics, Oncology, Hematology, and Diabetology, Medical University of Lodz, Department of Pediatrics, Diabetology, and Endocrinology, Medical University of Gdańsk, and Diabetes Outpatient Clinics in Sanok area. The study comprised patients scheduled for a routine visit in each of the above sites during the study period (May-June 2013), born between 1994–1997, and with at least one-year history of diabetes. To ensure complete anonymity, the patients were recruited by medical students, not involved in diabetes management. The subjects and their parents had been informed about the aim of the study, its anonymous, and voluntary character and were allowed to ask questions. Written informed consent was obtained before the inclusion in the study. Confidentiality and anonymity were warranted by asking the patients to fill in the questionnaires in separate rooms, without the presence and supervision of their parents or diabetic team members. After completing the questionnaires, the patients were asked to deposit closed envelops with their response sheets into a box which remained closed until the end of the study.

The questionnaire contained initial questions regarding the course of diabetes, and the main standardized questionnaire used in the Polish edition of ESPAD, conducted in May and June 2011. The ESPAD is a collaborative effort of independent research teams in more than forty European countries and the largest cross-national research project on adolescent substance use in the world. The program was launched in 1995 and the surveys are repeated every four years. The aim of ESPAD is to collect comparable data on substance use among 15-16- (and in some countries also 17-18-) year-old students in as many European countries as possible. Poland has been collecting ESPAD data since 1995. The methodology of the survey, including the questionnaire, is described in detail elsewhere [15]. Briefly, the surveys are conducted with common group-administered questionnaires. The students answer the questionnaires anonymously in the classroom with teachers or research assistants functioning as survey leaders. The 2011 Polish sample of classes was nationally representative. To avoid seasonal variability, data was collected in spring (in May and June). Participants were divided into two subgroups, depending on their age (15-16- and 17-18-year-olds, resp.).

We retrieved and analyzed only these questions from the ESPAD questionnaire which regarded lifetime use of illicit drugs, such as cannabis (marijuana and hashish), ecstasy, amphetamines, cocaine, crack, LSD or other hallucinogens, heroin, gamma hydroxybutyrate (GHB), tranquillizers or sedatives without a doctor's prescription, inhalants, magic mushrooms, anabolic steroids, and Polish heroine (a crude preparation of heroin made from poppy straw intended for injection). Because some adolescents tend to pretend to have used drugs, the nonexistent dummy drug *"Relevin"* was included among real drugs in the questionnaire in order to test the validity of the survey.

Metabolic control was assessed by asking the patients to indicate the interval (6–8%, 8–10%, 10–12%, and >12%) in which the mean value of their last three HbA1c measurements was found. It was regarded as good if HbA1c <8% or as poor if ≥8%.

2.2. Control Group. The control group was a representative sample of 12144 Polish students, aged 15–18 years, born in 1992–1995, who participated in the fifth data collection of ESPAD in May and June 2011. The survey was performed as a written questionnaire during school time, according to the ESPAD Protocol [15].

Our study was approved by the Bioethics Committee of the Medical University of Lodz.

2.3. Statistical Analysis. Differences in the prevalence of illicit drug use were evaluated using Pearson's Chi-square test. Odds ratios with a 95% Confidence Intervals were also calculated where appropriate. Differences between DM1 and control groups for continuous variables were assessed using Mann-Whitney U test. Comparisons with p values lower than 0.05 were considered as statistically significant.

3. Results

3.1. Participants. In the three participating centers there were 400 patients treated for type 1 diabetes, aged 15–18 years. However, out of these 400 adolescents, 175 were not scheduled for a visit in the clinic between May and June 2013 and could not be included in the study. 16 of remaining 225 eligible patients refused to participate, which was reportedly motivated by the lack of time to complete the questionnaire. The acceptance of participating amounted to 92.9% and so 209 patients returned the questionnaires. Characteristics of teenagers with DM1 and the control group are shown in Table 1.

The DM1 and the control groups had similar gender and age distribution. The mean ages of the DM1 and the control groups members were 16.5 ± 1.0 and 16.9 ± 0.9 years, respectively ($p = 0.4$).

The mean duration of diabetes was 6.5 years ± 4.4. Half of the DM1 patients (53%) had HbA1c level above 8%.

Lifetime prevalence of illicit drug use was significantly lower among adolescents with DM1 than in the control ESPAD group: 58 (28%) versus 5524 (46%); $p < 10^{-5}$; odd ratio OR (95% CI) = 0.46 (0.34–0.62). This held true for all drugs in the ESPAD survey (Table 2). Moreover, some adolescents tried several illicit substances over the course of their adolescent years. Cannabis was the most commonly used illicit drugs among adolescents in both groups: 38 (18.3%) versus 3976 (33.1%), $p = 10^{-5}$. A much smaller percentage reported using amphetamine: 8 (3.9%), LSD and other hallucinogens were mentioned by 3 (1.4%), cocaine was mentioned by 3 (1.4%), and magic mushrooms was

TABLE 1: Clinical characteristics of patients with diabetes and controls.

	Diabetic patients ($n = 209$)	Healthy controls ($n = 12144$)	p level
Female (%) versus male (%)	102 (48.8) versus 107 (51.2)	5982 (50.6) versus 6132 (49.3)	$p = 0.6$
Age (year) Mean ± SD	16.5 ± 1.0	16.9 ± 0.9	$p = 0.4$
15-16 years (%)	98 (47.1)	6050 (49.9)	
17-18 years (%)	110 (52.8)	5055 (50.0)	
Diabetes duration (year) Median (interquartile range)	6 (3–10)	—	
HbA1c (%)*		—	
6–8%	89 (47)		
8–10%	62 (33)		
10–12%	30 (16)		
>12%	8 (4)		
Insulin (units/day) Median (interquartile range)	50 (30–65)	—	
Insulin pump therapy (%)**	79/183 (43)	—	

*Response rate of 189/209; **response rate of 183/209.

mentioned by 3 (1.4%) of the DM1 patients, and the rates for ecstasy 1 (0.5%), crack 1 (0.5%), heroin 1 (0.5%), and gamma hydroxybutyrate (GHB) 1 (0.5%) were even lower. Interestingly, tranquilizers and sedatives without medical supervision were used by 20 (9.6%) of teens with DM1 versus 1911 (15.9%) of controls ($p = 0.01$), more frequently by girls than boys. The use of nonexisting "*Relevin*" was reported by 0 (0%) of the patients versus 157 (1.3%) of the students, $p = 0.17$.

Sex differences were evident in the DM1 group. Male adolescents, as shown, were more likely than their female counterparts to use illicit drugs (30.5% versus 25.7%). Girls with DM1 reported the use of cannabis, amphetamine, and tranquillizers only.

The median age at first consumption of cannabis, tranquillizers, amphetamine, ecstasy, and inhalants was similar in both groups (Table 3). Similarly as in the general population group, inhalants were the first tried psychoactive substances used in the DM1 group.

There were no statistical differences between the level of HbA1c in patients who admitted or denied lifetime experimenting/using any of the drugs, $p = 0.1438$.

However, lifetime and last 12-month use of marijuana were associated with poorer glycemic control (HbA1c ≥ 8%), $p < 0.01$ and 0.02, respectively. The proportion of patients who tried or did not try marijuana, according to HbA1c levels, is shown in Figure 1.

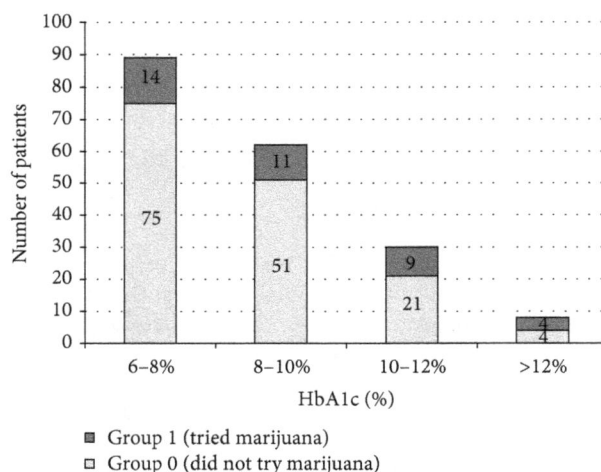

■ Group 1 (tried marijuana)
□ Group 0 (did not try marijuana)

FIGURE 1: The proportion of patients who tried or did not try marijuana, according to HbA1c levels, $p = 0.03$; response rate to that question was 189/209.

No significant associations were found for duration of diabetes and use of any drugs or marijuana in particular, even after adjusting for patients' age and sex ($p = 0.22$).

4. Discussion

Illicit drugs have acute detrimental effects that are often fatal in healthy young people [16]. In patients with type 1 diabetes, their use may thoroughly disrupt diabetes management and precipitate acute and chronic complications. Stimulants are also likely to cause or mask many mental disorders that are more often encountered in DM1 patients than in general population [16–19].

Some of recreational drugs have a direct influence on glucose metabolism. Amphetamine, ecstasy, or cocaine increases the release of catecholamines, cortisol and other contraregulatory hormones that enhance gluconeogenesis, glycogenolysis, and lipolysis and are associated with reported episodes of diabetic ketoacidosis (DKA) [20–22]. Cocaine and heroin abuse has been reported to cause hyperglycaemic hyperosmolar state [23] and to be the strongest independent risk factor for recurrent DKA [21, 22, 24]. Androgenic-anabolic steroids (AS), taken orally or by injection at doses much higher than would be prescribed, increase the risk of early heart attacks, strokes, liver tumors, kidney failure, serious psychiatric problems, and long-term effects [25]. Regular use of GHB may lead to Cushing's syndrome [26, 27]. The health-related harms of cannabinoids use differ from those of other drugs in that they contribute little to mortality. However, cannabinoids impair judgment and cause food cravings or loss of appetite which are likely to have a negative effect on self-management behaviors (e.g., carbohydrate counting). Chronic use of cannabis may reduce motivation to maintain good metabolic control [23] and may increase the risk of neurologic or psychiatric disorders [29, 30].

In our study, the prevalence of illicit drug use was only half as high among adolescents with diabetes than in

TABLE 2: Lifetime prevalence of illicit drugs use in 209 teenage patients with T1D compared with their healthy peers ($n = 12114$).

Stimulant	Subjects	Lifetime prevalence		p
		DM1 n (%)	C n (%)	
Illicit drugs	All	58 (28.2)	5524 (46.1)	$p < 10^{-5}$
	15-16 years	22 (23.0)	2436 (40.7)	$p = 0.0004$
	17-18 years	36 (33.0)	3085 (51.4)	$p = 0.0001$
	Boys	32 (30.5)	2893 (49.0)	$p = 0.0002$
	Girls	26 (25.7)	2631 (43.3)	$p = 0.0004$
Marijuana/hashish	All	38 (18.4)	3976 (33.1)	$p = 10^{-5}$
	15-16 years	12 (12.4)	1587 (26.5)	$p = 0.0018$
	17-18 years	26 (23.9)	2387 (39.8)	$p = 0.0007$
	Boys	24 (22.6)	2396 (40.5)	$p = 0.0002$
	Girls	14 (13.9)	1580 (26)	$p = 0.006$
Amphetamine	All	8 (3.9)	814 (6.8)	$p = 0.127$
	15-16 years	3 (3.1)	295 (4.9)	$p = 0.546$
	17-18 years	5 (4.6)	518 (8.6)	$p = 0.188$
	Boys	7 (6.5)	484 (8.2)	$p = 0.669$
	Girls	1 (1.0)	330 (5.4)	$p = 0.083$
LSD and hallucinogens	All	3 (1.4)	473 (3.9)	$p = 0.097$
	15-16 years	1 (1.0)	212 (3.5)	$p = 0.287$
	17-18 years	2 (1.8)	260 (4.3)	$p = 0.301$
	Boys	3 (2.8)	289 (4.9)	$p = 0.446$
	Girls	0 (0.0)	184 (3.0)	$p = 0.140$
Ecstasy	All	1 (0.5)	486 (4.0)	$p = 0.015$
	15-16 years	0 (0.0)	209 (3.5)	$p = 0.110$
	17-18 years	1 (0.9)	276 (4.6)	$p = 0.111$
	Boys	1 (0.9)	305 (5.1)	$p = 0.081$
	Girls	0 (0.0)	181 (3.0)	$p = 0.145$
Magic mushrooms	All	3 (1.4)	428 (3.6)	$p = 0.147$
	15-16 years	0 (0.0)	185 (3.1)	$p = 0.142$
	17-18 years	3 (2.8)	242 (4.0)	$p = 0.671$
	Boys	3 (2.8)	301 (5.1)	$p = 0.399$
	Girls	0 (0.0)	127 (2.1)	$p = 0.267$
Tranquillizers and sedatives	All	20 (9.6)	1911 (15.9)	$p = 0.014$
	15-16 years	8 (8.2)	906 (15.1)	$p = 0.079$
	17-18 years	12 (11.0)	1004 (16.7)	$p = 0.114$
	Boys	7 (6.5)	632 (10.6)	$p = 0.227$
	Girls	13 (12.9)	1279 (21.0)	$p = 0.062$
Crack	All	1 (0.5)	237 (2.0)	$p = 0.199$
	15-16 years	1 (0.9)	118 (2.0)	$p = 0.763$
	17-18 years	0 (0.0)	118 (2.3)	$p = 0.263$
	Boys	1 (0.9)	161 (2.7)	$p = 0.414$
	Girls	0 (0.0)	76 (1.3)	$p = 0.500$
Cocaine	All	3 (1.4)	439 (3.7)	$p = 0.133$
	15-16 years	2 (2.0)	196 (3.3)	$p = 0.698$
	17-18 years	1 (0.9)	242 (4.0)	$p = 0.161$
	Boys	3 (1.4)	247 (4.2)	$p = 0.649$
	Girls	0 (0.0)	192 (3.1)	$p = 0.128$
Heroine	All	1 (0.5)	275 (2.3)	$p = 0.133$
	15-16 years	1 (0.9)	150 (2.5)	$p = 0.545$
	17-18 years	0 (0.0)	124 (2.1)	$p = 0.241$
	Boys	1 (0.9)	166 (2.8)	$p = 0.385$
	Girls	0 (0.0)	109 (1.8)	$p = 0.330$

TABLE 2: Continued.

| Stimulant | Subjects | Lifetime prevalence | | p |
		DM1 n (%)	C n (%)	
Drugs by injection with needle	All	1 (0.5)	212 (1.8)	$p = 0.257$
	15-16 years	1 (0.9)	98 (1.6)	$p = 0.841$
	17-18 years	0 (0.0)	113 (1.9)	$p = 0.321$
	Boys	1 (0.9)	142 (2.4)	$p = 0.507$
	Girls	0 (0.0)	70 (1.2)	$p = 0.543$
GHB	All	1 (0.5)	154 (1.3)	$p = 0.481$
	15-16 years	1 (0.9)	79 (1.3)	$p = 0.837$
	17-18 years	0 (0.0)	74 (1.2)	$p = 0.469$
	Boys	1 (0.9)	142 (2.4)	$p = 0.769$
	Girls	0 (0.0)	70 (1.2)	$p = 0.759$
Anabolic steroids	All	2 (1.0)	328 (2.7)	$p = 0.179$
	15-16 years	0 (0.0)	143 (2.4)	$p = 0.226$
	17-18 years	2 (1.8)	184 (3.1)	$p = 0.271$
	Boys	2 (1.8)	271 (4.6)	$p = 0.271$
	Girls	0 (0.0)	57 (0.9)	$p = 0.651$
Relevin	All	0 (0.0)	157 (1.3)	$p = 0.178$
	15-16 years	0 (0.0)	79 (1.3)	$p = 0.489$
	17-18 years	0 (0.0)	77 (1.3)	$p = 0.449$
	Boys	0 (0.0)	111 (1.9)	$p = 0.287$
	Girls	0 (0.0)	46 (0.8)	$p = 0.770$

TABLE 3: Initiation time of illicit drugs use in years of age.

Substance	DM1 (n)	Mean	Median	Q25–75%	Control (n)	Mean	Median	Q25–75%	p level
Marijuana/hashish	33	15.21	15.00	15.00–16.00	4084	15.32	15.00	15.00–16.00	0.6657
Tranquilizers	18	14.22	14.00	14.00–15.00	1894	14.58	15.00	14.00–16.00	0.1879
Amphetamine	6	15.50	15.00	14.00–17.00	864	15.16	16.00	14.00–17.00	0.9993
Ecstasy	1	14.00	14.00	14.00–14.00	498	14.76	15.00	14.00–16.00	1.0000
Inhalants	4	12.50	13.00	10.50–14.50	687	13.59	14.00	12.00–15.00	0.3810

the healthy controls. This proportion held true for both age groups: 15-16- and 17-18-year-olds, which may indicate a better health awareness in the group of DM1 patients and/or a better parental control.

Teenagers with DM1 confessed using a wide range of illicit drugs, including those taken intravenously. Like in the general population and as shown in other studies, the most popular was marijuana. Male adolescents were more likely to use illicit drugs compared to their female counterparts. Girls with DM1 reported the use of only cannabis, amphetamine, and tranquilizers or sedatives. None of the DM1 girls admitted experimenting with "hard" drugs. However, it is notable that more girls than boys with DM1 reported the use of tranquillizers or sedatives for nonmedicinal purposes but still fewer than the healthy controls. Tranquilizers or sedatives are a widely used group of prescription medication; however, these drugs may also be used for the purpose of "getting high" rather than for medical reasons. In the ESPAD survey nearly half of the examined students in Poland (48%) admitted that both tranquilizers and sedatives were easily available.

Our study had several strong sides, including the use of a validated questionnaire, proven in the ESPAD surveys

since 1995, and a large national control group of 12114 healthy students. The investigated substance use habits of Polish students turned out to be similar to those of the European average in students who participated in the ESPAD survey in 2011. One may argue, however, that, due to the unwillingness of adolescent patients to confess a risky behavior, self-reported data might underestimate the problem and limit the validity of the survey. We found it crucial to diminish the risk of underreporting by giving the patients a feeling of complete anonymity. Therefore, the questionnaires were collected by medical students not involved in the diabetes patients management. Owing to that, the participation and response rates were very high, as only 16 out of 225 patients refused to take part in our study. When it comes to validity measures, the use of the nonexistent dummy drug was reported by none of the patients, making the survey reliable.

The study, however, did have some limitations. The first was a relatively small sample size in comparison with the large control group, which may have influenced its statistical power. To avoid bias caused by different patterns of substance use by DM1 adolescent patients throughout the school year, we were able to enroll only the patients scheduled for

TABLE 4: Prevalence of illicit drug use in young people with type 1 diabetes.

Authors [reference]	Year of publication	Country	Subjects (age)	Prevalence of drug use (%)	Methodology
Gold and Gladstein [11]	1993	USA	79 (11-12)	9%	Anonymous self-administered questionnaire, summer camps
Glasgow et al. [10]	1991	USA	101 (12–20)	25%	Anonymous self-administered questionnaire with verification by urine drug screening
Frey et al. [14]	1997	USA	155 (10–20)	10%	A descriptive cross-sectional design, self-report on routine clinic visit
Martínez-Aguayo et al. [12]	2007	Chile	193 (13–20)	10%	Anonymous self-administered questionnaire, diabetes summer camps
Ng et al. [13]	2004	UK	158 (16–30)	29%	Anonymous self-reported postal questionnaire
Lee et al. [3]	2012	Australia	506 (13–44)	77%	Radio broadcast/hospital advertising
Scaramuzza et al. [2]	2010	Italy	215 (12–16)	39,5% cannabis, 3,25% other drugs	Anonymous self-administered questionnaire, diabetes camps

the outpatient clinical visit in May and June (209 out of 400), according to the Polish ESPAD Protocol. However, in spite of the strict inclusion criteria, the study group contained over 50% of DM1 teens in the three study sites (from around 2000 pediatric patients), that is, 12–14% of all Polish pediatric patients with type 1 diabetes.

The second constraint was the metabolic control, performed only with the patient-reported mean value of the last three HbA1c measurements and no DKA-related questions were added. This, however, gave the participants an enhanced sense of anonymity. Moreover, due to our observations that adolescent people seldom remembered their last HbA1c, the patients were asked to indicate the interval (6–8%, 8–10%, 10–12%, and >12%) in which the mean value of their last three HbA1c measurements was found. Therefore, the metabolic control was regarded as good if HbA1c <8% or as poor if ≥8%, a value close to the limit of good metabolic recommended by ISPAD and ADA (HbA1c < 7.5%). Nevertheless, possibly due to the lack of exact HbA1c values, we were able to show the association of worse glycaemic control with lifetime and 30-day use of marihuana only. Other authors observed clearer association between overall drug use, worse glycaemic control, and a higher risk of diabetic ketoacidosis [3, 20].

Our results are more encouraging than the ones obtained in other countries (Table 4). In an Italian study, the overall drug use was shown to be slightly higher in T1D group. Female adolescents with DM1 exhibited even a higher rate of consumption of all illicit drugs studied than the healthy peers, while in male patients the rate was similar to the controls [2].

A survey conducted by Martínez-Aguayo et al. showed that lifetime illicit drug use by older DM1 students (in the 11th through 12th grades) approached the Chile national average. Lower rates (9.6% versus 22%) were observed only in younger students (in 8th through 10th grades) [12]. In a British postal questionnaire study, 29% of young diabetic patients (16–30 years of age) reported using street drugs, and 68% of them used them more than once a month [13].

Lifetime prevalence of illicit drugs among young Australians with DM1 was 77%, and 47% of them admitted using them within the last year. Recreational drug use was the most common among persons under 20 years (80%). Among those who used drugs, 24% reported daily use and 68% were polydrug users [3].

The observed inconsistency of results from various studies on illicit drug use among adolescents with type 1 diabetes mellitus is mostly due to methodological differences as well as different time of performing them. It is difficult to compare the results from the present study with those obtained 10–30 years ago [10, 11]. Variations may also result from the overall discrepancy of the prevalence of drug use in different countries. For example, according to ESPAD, countries like Czech Republic, France, and Monaco have the highest prevalence in Europe while in many Balkan countries and Norway the problem is less frequent [31].

Although the initiation time of drug use, as shown in our study, was similar in the clinical and control groups, the data indicate that better preventive strategies should be introduced as early as possible (even in children under 10 as the first use of inhalants starts at 10.5 years). The high rate of unawareness (up to 72%) of the adverse effects of illicit drugs on diabetes among young patients with DM has been reported in literature [13]. Therefore, proper education and the early introduction of prevention programs are necessary. Adolescents with diabetes should be regularly encouraged to refrain from drugs and be given this information through a friendly dialog at each visit. Because only a small number of patients inform health professionals about drug use [13], doctors should be able to recognize signs of recreational use or addiction and organize regular screening, especially in those with poor glycemic control and those who experience recurrent ketoacidosis.

5. Conclusions

This study showed that adolescents with T1D use recreational drugs less frequently than their healthy peers. The use of cannabis is associated with a poorer metabolic control in teens with DM1. Illicit drug use prevention must be an integral part of medical care for teenagers with DM1 and intervention introduced as early as possible.

Conflict of Interests

The authors declare that there is no conflict of interests regarding the publication of this paper.

Acknowledgments

The study was supported by Medical University of Lodz Grant no. 503/1-090-01/503-01. The Polish ESPAD 2011 edition was financed by The National Bureau for Drug Prevention and The State Agency for the Prevention of Alcohol-Related Problems (PARPA).

References

[1] J.-C. Suris and N. Parera, "Sex, drugs and chronic illness: health behaviours among chronically ill youth," European Journal of Public Health, vol. 15, no. 5, pp. 484–488, 2005.

[2] A. E. Scaramuzza, C. De Palma, C. Mameli, D. Spiri, L. Santoro, and G. V. Zuccotti, "Adolescents with type 1 diabetes and risky behaviour," Acta Paediatrica, vol. 99, no. 8, pp. 1237–1241, 2010.

[3] P. Lee, J. R. Greenfield, K. Gilbert, and L. V. Campbell, "Recreational drug use in type 1 diabetes: an invisible accomplice to poor glycaemic control?" Internal Medicine Journal, vol. 42, no. 2, pp. 198–202, 2012.

[4] S. P. Laing, M. E. Jones, A. J. Swerdlow, A. C. Burden, and W. Gatling, "Psychosocial and socioeconomic risk factors for premature death in young people with type 1 diabetes," Diabetes Care, vol. 28, no. 7, pp. 1618–1623, 2005.

[5] R. T. Webb, P. Lichtenstein, M. Dahlin, N. Kapur, J. F. Ludvigsson, and B. Runeson, "Unnatural deaths in a national cohort of people diagnosed with diabetes," Diabetes Care, vol. 37, no. 8, pp. 2276–2283, 2014.

[6] L. Wibell, L. Nyström, J. Östman et al., "Increased mortality in diabetes during the first 10 years of the disease. A population-based study (DISS) in Swedish adults 15–34 years old at diagnosis," Journal of Internal Medicine, vol. 249, no. 3, pp. 263–270, 2001.

[7] S. A. Saunders, J. Democratis, J. Martin, and I. A. Macfarlane, "Intravenous drug abuse and Type 1 diabetes: financial and healthcare implications," Diabetic Medicine, vol. 21, no. 12, pp. 1269–1273, 2004.

[8] M. L. Isidro and S. Jorge, "Recreational drug abuse in patients hospitalized for diabetic ketosis or diabetic ketoacidosis," Acta Diabetologica, vol. 50, no. 2, pp. 183–187, 2013.

[9] P. Lee, A. J. Nicoll, M. McDonough, and P. G. Colman, "Substance abuse in young patients with type I diabetes: easily neglected in complex medical management," Internal Medicine Journal, vol. 35, no. 6, pp. 359–361, 2005.

[10] A. M. Glasgow, D. Tynan, R. Schwartz et al., "Alcohol and drug use in teenagers with diabetes mellitus," Journal of Adolescent Health Care, vol. 12, no. 1, pp. 11–14, 1991.

[11] M. A. Gold and J. Gladstein, "Substance use among adolescents with diabetes mellitus: preliminary findings," Journal of Adolescent Health, vol. 14, no. 2, pp. 80–84, 1993.

[12] A. Martínez-Aguayo, J. C. Araneda, D. Fernandez, A. Gleisner, V. Perez, and E. Codner, "Tobacco, alcohol, and illicit drug use in adolescents with diabetes mellitus," Pediatric Diabetes, vol. 8, no. 5, pp. 265–271, 2007.

[13] R. S. H. Ng, D. A. Darko, and R. M. Hillson, "Street drug use among young patients with Type 1 diabetes in the UK," Diabetic Medicine, vol. 21, no. 3, pp. 295–296, 2004.

[14] M. A. Frey, B. Guthrie, C. Loveland-Cherry, P. S. Park, and C. M. Foster, "Risky behavior and risk in adolescents with IDDM," Journal of Adolescent Health, vol. 20, no. 1, pp. 38–45, 1997.

[15] European School Survey Project on Alcohol and Other Drugs, http://www.espad.org/en/Reports-Documents/ESPAD-Documents/.

[16] C. Michael White, "How MDMA's pharmacology and pharmacokinetics drive desired effects and harms," Journal of Clinical Pharmacology, vol. 54, no. 3, pp. 245–252, 2014.

[17] M. Kovacs, D. Goldston, D. S. Obrosky, and L. K. Bonar, "Psychiatric disorders in youths with IDDM: rates and risk factors," Diabetes Care, vol. 20, no. 1, pp. 36–44, 1997.

[18] A. Butwicka, L. Frisén, C. Almqvist, B. Zethelius, and P. Lichtenstein, "Risks of psychiatric disorders and suicide attempts in children and adolescents with type 1 diabetes: a population-based cohort study," Diabetes Care, vol. 38, no. 3, pp. 453–459, 2015.

[19] B. Johnson, C. Eiser, V. Young, S. Brierley, and S. Heller, "Prevalence of depression among young people with Type 1 diabetes: a systematic review," Diabetic Medicine, vol. 30, no. 2, pp. 199–208, 2013.

[20] P. Lee and L. V. Campbell, "Diabetic ketoacidosis: the usual villain or a scapegoat? A novel cause of severe metabolic acidosis in type 1 diabetes," Diabetes Care, vol. 31, no. 3, article e13, 2008.

[21] E. A. Warner, G. S. Greene, M. S. Buchsbaum, D. S. Cooper, and B. E. Robinson, "Diabetic ketoacidosis associated with cocaine use," Archives of Internal Medicine, vol. 158, no. 16, pp. 1799–1802, 1998.

[22] E. A. Nyenwe, R. S. Loganathan, S. Blum et al., "Active use of cocaine: an independent risk factor for recurrent diabetic ketoacidosis in a city hospital," Endocrine Practice, vol. 13, no. 1, pp. 22–29, 2007.

[23] M. R. Abraham and R. Khardori, "Hyperglycemic hyperosmolar nonketotic syndrome as initial presentation of type 2 diabetes in a young cocaine abuser," Diabetes Care, vol. 22, no. 8, pp. 1380–1381, 1999.

[24] M. P. Gama, B. de Souza, A. Ossowski, and R. Perraro, "Diabetic ketoacidosis complicated by the use of ecstasy: a case report," *Journal of Medical Case Reports*, vol. 4, no. 1, article 240, 2010.

[25] P. Vanberg and D. Atar, "Androgenic anabolic steroid abuse and the cardiovascular system," *Handbook of Experimental Pharmacology*, vol. 195, pp. 411–457, 2010.

[26] A. Gonzalez and D. J. Nutt, "Gamma hydroxy butyrate abuse and dependency," *Journal of Psychopharmacology*, vol. 19, no. 2, pp. 195–204, 2005.

[27] A. J. Razenberg, J. W. F. Elte, A. P. Rietveld, H. C. T. van Zaanen, and M. C. Cabezas, "A 'smart' type of Cushing's syndrome," *European Journal of Endocrinology*, vol. 157, no. 6, pp. 779–781, 2007.

[28] M. A. Permutt, D. W. Goodwin, R. Schwin, and S. Y. Hill, "The effect of marijuana on carbohydrate metabolism," *The American Journal of Psychiatry*, vol. 133, no. 2, pp. 220–224, 1976.

[29] W. Hall and L. Degenhardt, "Adverse health effects of non-medical cannabis use," *The Lancet*, vol. 374, no. 9698, pp. 1383–1391, 2009.

[30] R. Radhakrishnan, S. T. Wilkinson, and D. C. D'Souza, "Gone to pot—a review of the association between cannabis and psychosis," *Frontiers in Psychiatry*, vol. 5, article 54, 2014.

[31] European School Survey Project on Alcohol and Other Drugs, http://www.espad.org/en/Keyresult-Generator.

13

Clinical Trial Assessing the Efficacy of Gabapentin Plus B Complex (B1/B12) versus Pregabalin for Treating Painful Diabetic Neuropathy

Alberto Mimenza Alvarado and Sara Aguilar Navarro

Geriatrics Department, National Institute of Medical Sciences and Nutrition Salvador Zubirán, Vasco de Quiroga No. 15, Colonia Section XVI, Delegación Tlalpan, 14000 Mexico, DF, Mexico

Correspondence should be addressed to Alberto Mimenza Alvarado; a.mimenza@hotmail.com

Academic Editor: Dan Ziegler

Introduction. Painful diabetic neuropathy (PDN) is a prevalent and impairing disorder. The objective of this study was to show the efficacy and safety of gabapentin (GBP) plus complex B vitamins: thiamine (B1) and cyanocobalamine (B12) compared to pregabalin in patients with moderate to severe intensity PDN. *Method.* Multicenter, randomized, blind study. Two hundred and seventy patients were evaluated, 147 with GBP/B1/B12 and 123 with PGB, with a 7/10 pain intensity on the Visual Analog Scale (VAS). Five visits (12 weeks) were scheduled. The GBP/B1 (100 mg)/B12 (20 mg) group started with 300 mg at visit 1 to 3600 mg at visit 5. The PGB group started with 75 mg/d at visit 1 to 600 mg/d at visit 5. Different safety and efficacy scales were applied, as well as adverse event assessment. *Results.* Both drugs showed reduction of pain intensity, without significant statistical difference ($P = 0.900$). In the GBP/B1/B12 group, an improvement of at least 30% on VAS correlated to a 900 mg/d dose, compared with PGB 300 mg/d. Likewise, occurrence of vertigo was lower in the GBP/B1-B12 group, with a significant statistical difference, $P = 0.014$. *Conclusions.* Our study shows that GPB/B1-B12 combination is as effective as PGB. Nonetheless, pain intensity reduction is achieved with 50% of the minimum required gabapentin dose alone (800 to 1600 mg/d) in classic NDD trials. Less vertigo and dizziness occurrence was also observed in the GBP/B1/B12 group. This trial is registered with ClinicalTrials.gov NCT01364298.

1. Introduction

The most common cause of neuropathy worldwide is diabetes mellitus [1]. A neuropathy prevalence of 30% is reported in diabetic patients, estimating more than 50% could suffer from it during the course of the disease [2].

Painful diabetic neuropathy (PDN) is one of the most common causes of chronic pain. Chronic pain affects 30% of the United States (US) population and has high treatment costs, estimated approximately to be 650 billion dollars [3].

Chronic pain treatment requires a multidisciplinary intervention and, sometimes, use of multimodal treatments [3]. This situation has required using combination drugs as a treatment alternative, towards improving the patient prognosis.

There is evidence suggesting that more than half of chronic pain patients receive two or more analgesics, although evidence supporting most of these combinations is limited [4].

Even when efforts for developing new drugs have allowed new treatment options, searching for further alternatives, effective and safe, is necessary. Therefore, it is possible, through synergy between drugs with different mechanisms of action, to provide greater pain killing effects with less adverse events.

Treatment of painful diabetic neuropathy (PDN) includes using of antidepressants, anticonvulsants (calcium channel blockers), and opioid drugs, among others. One of the main problems when using these drugs is adverse events (AE), occasionally limiting the possibility to use drugs recommended in clinical trials [5].

Complex B vitamins, specifically thiamine (B1) and cyanocobalamin (B12), have been shown to be of clinical use in some painful diseases, derived from their effects on the central nervous system, synthesis, and secretion of serotonin in several brain areas [6], blocking metabolic pathways related to oxidative stress [7], as well as their effects on the nitric oxide/guanosine monophosphate cyclic (NO/GMPc) pathway [8], among other mechanisms. Synergy of these vitamins with other drugs, for example, gabapentin, allows for reducing recommended doses of these vitamins as monotherapy, achieving greater reduction effects on pain intensity with less AE occurrence. Gabapentin (GBP), a calcium channel a2δ ligand, has proven useful in the treatment of neuropathic pain, with effective results on a daily dosage interval of 1800–3600 mg, although this doses are related to a higher AE rate (nausea, vomit, dizziness, and somnolence of 20–50%) [9]. Pregabalin (PGB), another calcium channel a2δ ligand, has also shown benefit in the treatment of neuropathic pain, although such benefits are related to high doses, which are evidently associated with AE occurrence, including dizziness, somnolence, and peripheral edema[10].

Our study objective was to determine the efficacy of gabapentin/vitamins B1 and B12 (GBP/B1/B12) versus pregabalin (PGB) for painful diabetic neuropathy (PDN) during 12 weeks of treatment.

2. Materials and Methods

Phase IV, multicenter, randomized, open-label, parallel group, noninferiority study was conducted in Mexico City.

Patients enrolled had the following characteristics:

  (i) Low to moderate intensity PDN.

  (ii) Diagnosed by Leeds Assessment of Neuropathic Symptoms and Signs (LANSS).

  (iii) ≥1 year of evolution.

  (iv) Less than 5 years of being diagnosed.

  (v) Stable hypoglycemic treatment (≥6 weeks).

  (vi) In stable condition (HbA1c ≤ 10% at selection visit).

  (vii) >40 mm score in the Visual Analog Scale (VAS).

  (viii) Numeric Pain Intensity (NPI) Scale (at least 4 days a week) completed on a daily basis during the week previous to randomization.

      (a) Daily average score of at least 4, during the 7 days prior to randomization.

Subject eligibility was initially assessed in a preselection period of 4–7 days. The selection period was planned to last at least 4 days, to a maximum of 7 days; in this stage, inclusion and exclusion criteria of every subject were assessed according to protocol specifications. At this stage, patients entered a wash-out period equivalent to 3 mean lives of the drug or a maximum of 7 days (whatever happened first) and randomized to either one of the study groups.

The treatment and follow-up stage comprise 6 visits (visit 0 to visit 5), from day 0 to day 84, and a total duration of 12 weeks.

The primary efficacy endpoint was mean change score in VAS. We compared two treatment groups and used a design capable of detecting 0.1-point differences, with a type I error of 0.05 and a power of 0.90, considering a standard deviation (SD) of 26 mm. According to calculation, 286 patients were needed. In order to consider a dropout rate of 25%, a total of 360 patients were considered, 180 in each group.

We used randomization envelopes to control treatment allocation. The randomization list was generated by a statistical program. Randomization was controlled in blocks of 6 patients to achieve a 1 : 1 proportion in the two arms.

We used an ANCOVA analysis with treatment in the model and baseline mean NPI score, as covariates. Differences between treatment groups were assessed each visit, based on adjusted treatment means. The same analysis was done for the VAS. Parametric (paired t-tests) and nonparametric (Wilcoxon) statistical methods were applied to compare each visit with baseline and each consecutive visit. Responses of 30% and 50% were analyzed through Pearson chi-squared, on the case of NPI and VAS. Response to the PGIC and CGIC and the time it took the patients to fall asleep were analyzed through a nonparametric method, Gamma statistics.

For other secondary scores resulting from adding several items, as subjective well-being items and profile of mood states factors, comparison between treatments was done by Mann-Whitney tests. We also obtained adjusted ANCOVA means, by baseline measures, of profile of mood states factors, as well as total scores, and tested differences in means. Descriptive statistics of measures were obtained by visit and treatment in general. The analysis considered a last observation carried forward (LOCF) imputation and a type I error of 0.05.

The study was conducted in 270 subjects, 18 to 65 years old, with diabetes mellitus type 1 or 2, and documented diagnosis of sensory motor PDN, moderate to severe, in accordance with LANSS scale [11], and fulfilling the following criteria:

  (i) Neuropathic pain present during at least a year before the study.

  (ii) >40 mm score in the Visual Analog Scale (VAS) [12] (at screening and baseline visit).

  (iii) Stable hypoglycemic treatment for at least 6 weeks before randomization.

  (iv) HbA1c < 8.5% at screening visit.

One group ($n = 147$) received oral gabapentin tablets, 300 mg/thiamine 100 mg/cyanocobalamin 0.20 mg, starting with 300 mg/day (day 1), followed by 900 mg/day on visit 1, 1800 mg/day on visit 2, 2700 mg/day on visit 3, and 3600 mg/day on visits 4 and 5. Other group ($n = 123$) received oral pregabalin capsules, 75 mg/day every 12 h, followed by 300 mg/day every 12 h on visit 2, and followed by 600 mg/day on visits 3, 4, and 5.

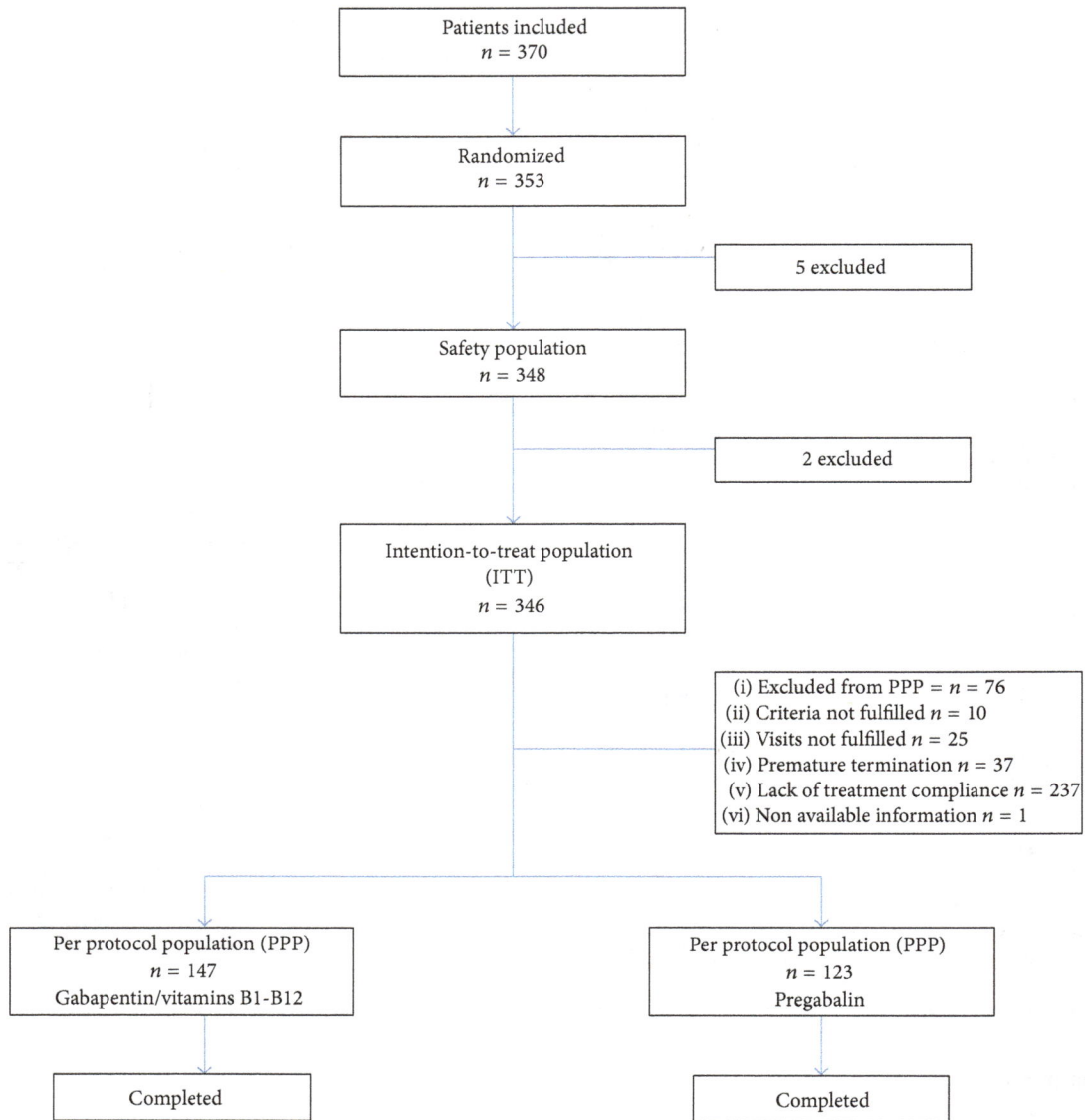

FIGURE 1: Study design.

In case of patient intolerance upon dose increase in the corresponding visit, patients were kept for the rest of the study with the previous tolerated dose.

We used VAS, Clinical Global Impression (CGI) [13], and Patients' Global Impression of Change (PGIC) [14], at baseline and end of study, to assess pain improvement. Information about sleeping hours overnight was obtained and question 4 of the sleep questionnaire (Mexican population) [15] was analyzed, consisting of 10 questions.

We established 5 visits; total study duration was 15 weeks (1 for prescreening, 1 for screening, and 12 weeks of randomized treatment) (see Figure 1).

For the statistical analysis, we assessed homogeneity between groups, applying chi-square for categorical variables and Student's t-test for continuous variables. For analyzing changes in baseline and postbaseline changes, as well as between visits, Student's t-test was used for matched samples and the Mantel-Haenszel test for safety measures between visits. All statistics tests have a significance level of 0.05 and 95% confidence intervals (CI). We used SPSS software for Windows (SPSS Inc., Chicago, IL, 18,0 version).

All related and nonrelated adverse events (AE) were recorded, as well as changes in physical examination (weight and size) and laboratory analysis (including glycated hemoglobin).

The protocol was submitted to and approved by an Independent Ethics Committee in Mexico City, fulfilling all ethics regulations, in accordance with the World Medical Association Declaration of Helsinki of 1975 (Ethical principles for medical research involving human subjects) and 2000 revision. All patients included in the study signed an informed consent to participate in the study.

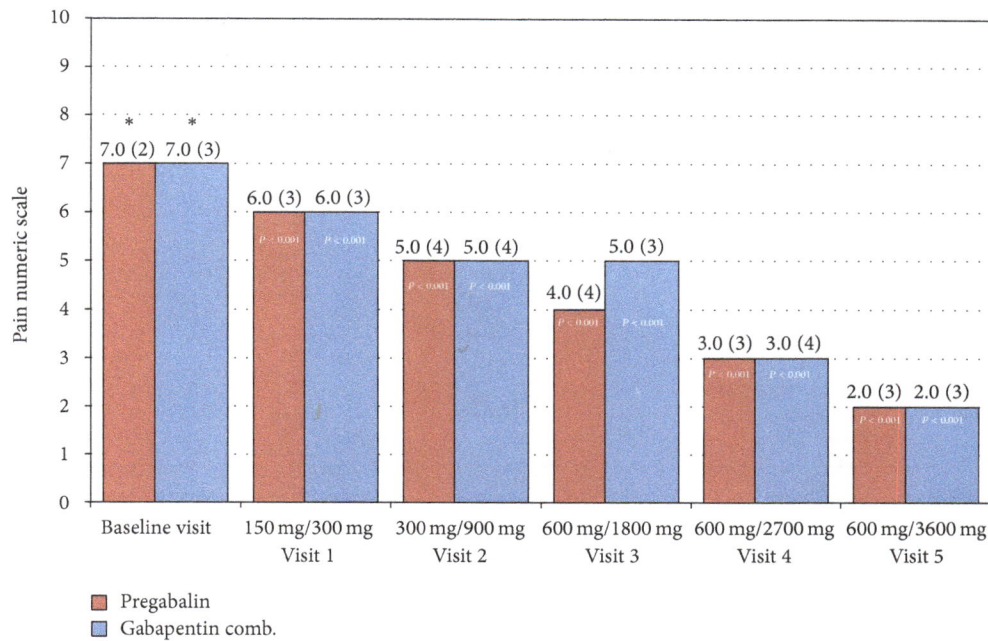

FIGURE 2: Median comparison per visit, between gabapentin-B complex and pregabalin, in pain intensity reduction, per visit and dose. Pain Visual Analog Scale (VAS), median (interquartile range) per visit, per protocol population. *Statistically significant change from baseline visit, $P < 0.05$. HbA1c: glycated hemoglobin, BMI: body mass index.

3. Results

Four hundred and fifty nine subjects were selected, 353 of which were randomized; 346 constituted the intention-to-treat population. Five patients had type 1 diabetes (2 in the group of GBP and two in the group of PGB). They were divided in parallel groups: 173 patients treated with GBP/B1/B12 and 173 patients treated with PGB. Two patients were discontinued from the study due to missing information after their initial visit (one of each group), remaining 346 (intention-to-treat population, ITT). Seventy-two patients were discontinued from the study due to several reasons, remaining 270 patients, as per protocol population (PPP) (see Figure 1).

4. Sociodemographic Characteristics

Sixty-eight percent of GBP/B1-B12 and 74% of PGB groups were female; average age was 54 (± 9.4 years old) in the PGB group and 53 (± 10.5 years old) in the GBP/B1-B12 group. No significant statistical differences were observed between both groups regarding comorbidity, body mass index (BMI), and glycated hemoglobin (HbA1c) levels; 115 (78) patients in the GBP/B complex used metformin, and 95 (77%) used metformin in the pregabalin group. Diabetes duration, PDN, and treatment used for controlling the disease, as well as other comorbidities, are shown in Table 1.

4.1. Efficacy (VAS). Pain intensity at baseline visit was 7 (SD ± 1.5), measured by VAS, in the GBP/B1-B12 group, and 7.1 (SD ± 1.7) in the PGB group. By analyzing pain intensity reduction

through VAS, expressed as median, by visit and dose, both drugs equally decreased pain, without a significant statistical difference between both treatment groups, $P > 0.05$. However, pain intensity showed a statistically significant reduction from baseline by visit in both treatment groups, $P \leq 0.001$ (see Figure 2).

Pain intensity reduction (at least 30%) was 78% for the GBP/B1-B12 group and 85% for PGB, without statistical difference ($P = 0.133$). For a decrease of at least 50%, no significant statistical difference was observed.

4.2. Effects on Sleeping. Analysis on improvement of sleep patterns was measured by sleep questionnaire, showing that both drugs improved sleeping hours toward the end of the study, from baseline visit (7.2 h for PGB, $P = 0.0002$, and 7.0 h for GBP, $P < 0.001$). Regarding the sleep questionnaire question, "have you slept all you needed?," an average change for visit 5 of −0.57 was observed for the GBP/B1-B12 ($P = 0.0015$) group and −0.37 for the PGB ($P = 0.049$) group.

4.3. Patients' Global Impression of Change (IGCP). Analysis of PGIC scale showed a significant reduction over time by visit and dose, in both treatment groups, $P \leq 0.0001$. Regarding the question of visit 5 "From study start, my health has improved a lot or a lot more" no difference was observed between both treatment groups (see Figure 3).

4.4. Adverse Events. Adverse events (AE) occurred in 44% of patients with pregabalin and 43% of patients with gabapentin/B1-B12. With PGB, the most common AE were dizziness

TABLE 1: Demographics characteristics and per group treatment characteristics ($n = 270$).

Demographics characteristics and per group treatment baselines, per protocol population					
	Pregabalin		Combined gabapentin		P value
	$n = 123$	%	$n = 147$	%	
Gender					
Female	74	60.2 95% CI (51.4–68.9)	100	68.0 95% CI (60.4–75.7)	0.179
Male	49	39.8 95% CI (31.1–48.6)	47	32.0 95% CI (24.3–39.6)	
Age (years)					
Average	53.6		52.5		
Std. deviation	9.4		10.5		0.344
Minimum–maximum	25.0–71.0		19.0–70.0		
Risk factors					
Smoking					
Yes	8	6.5 95% CI (2.1–10.9)	13	8.8 95% CI (4.2–13.5)	0.475
Arterial hypertension					
History	42	34.1 95% CI (25.6–42.6)	58	39.4 95% CI (31.5–47.4)	0.369
Hypothyroidism					
History	1	0.8 95% CI (0.0–2.4)	1	0.7 95% CI (0.0–2.0)	0.900
Cholesterol (baseline measure)					
Average	198.3		195.2		
Std. deviation	47.5		38.3		0.560
Minimum–maximum	101.0–542.0		71.0–366.0		
Triglycerides (baseline measure)					
Average	207.7		189.9		
Std. deviation	183.4		116.3		0.352
Minimum–maximum	53.0–1390.0		63.0–952.0		
BMI (Kg/m^2)					
Average	28.2		27.9		
Std. deviation	3.9		4.1		0.610
Minimum–maximum	18.4–39.4		17.4–39.4		
Diabetes duration					
Average	9.8		9.5		
Std. deviation	5.9		6.5		0.765
Minimum–maximum	1.5–25.5		1.4–32.0		
With diabetic neuropathic					
Average	2.9		2.8		
Std. deviation	1.1		1.1		0.603
Minimum–maximum	0.6–5.9		1.0–5.9		
Diabetes treatment					
Oral	100	81.3 95% CI (74.3–88.3)	112	76.2 95% CI (69.2–83.2)	
Insulin	3	2.4 95% CI (0.0–5.2)	5	3.4 95% CI (0.4–6.2)	0.333
Both	20	16.3 95% CI (9.7–22.9)	30	20.4 95% CI (13.8–27.0)	

TABLE 1: Continued.

	Demographics characteristics and per group treatment baselines, per protocol population				
	Pregabalin		Combined gabapentin		P value
	n = 123	%	n = 147	%	
Glucose (baseline)					
Average	126.9		128.9		
Std. deviation	53.0		51.2		0.603
Minimum–maximum	44.0–410.0		64.0–325.0		
HbA1c					
Average	7.4		7.4		
Std. deviation	1.3		1.4		0.603
Minimum–maximum	5.2–10.2		4.9–10.0		

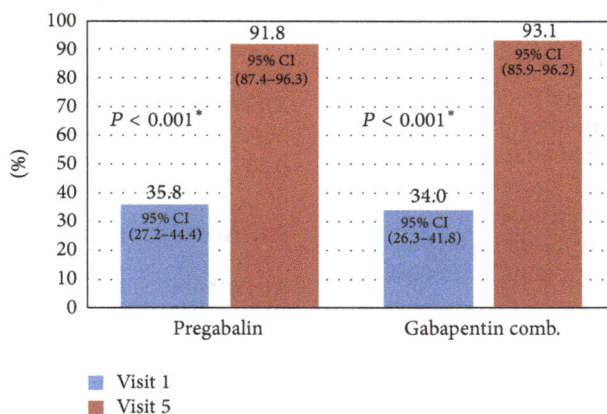

FIGURE 3: Patients' Global Impression of Change (PGIC) between baseline and visit 5, specifically the question: "From study start, my health is much improved or very much improved." Patient Global Impression of Change (IGCP) at visit 1 (baseline) and visit 5 (Day 84). From study start, my health is much improved or very much improved. *Statistically significant change from the baseline by visit in both treatment groups.

(24%), somnolence (23%), headache (3%), and vertigo (4%); for the GBP/B1/B12 group they were dizziness (17%), somnolence (27%), light-headedness (24.1%), headache (7.5%), and vertigo (3.2%). Vertigo was less common in the GBP/B1-B12 group, with a statistically significant difference ($P = 0.014$). Comparing adverse events by dose used, 11% presented dizziness in the PGB group (300 mg/d) and 3% in the GBP group, with doses of 1800 mg/d, and a statistically significant difference ($P = 0.0206$).

5. Discussion

Our results show that the GBP plus vitamins B1-B12 combination is as effective as PGB for pain treatment. Pain intensity reduction was achieved with a 300 to 1800 mg/day dose of GBP/B1/B12 and in the same proportion as PGB 600 mg (maximum dose). Gorson et al. showed in a crossover study that GBP 900 mg per day is ineffective or minimally effective for PDN treatment [16]. Gómez-Pérez et al., in a parallel group trial, concluded that gabapentin doses greater than 1200 mg caused pain reduction in more than 50% [17] and Backonja and Glanzman showed, in a systematic review, that

GBP doses (1800–3600 mg/d) are effective and safe for treating neuropathic pain [18]. It is possible that adding vitamins B1-B12 to GBP creates a synergistic effect, due to their antiallodynic and antihyperalgesic effect. The use of B vitamins for the treatment of PDN is controversial. Ang et al. reported in a meta-analysis that there is no sufficient evidence to recommend or disqualify the use of B complex vitamins when treating diabetic neuropathy, due to study heterogeneity [19].

Several mechanisms of action have been proposed to explain the effect of thiamine (B1) and cyanocobalamin (B12) when treating pain. Reyes-García et al. showed the synergy of GBP/B1-B12 as consequence of multiple effects of these vitamins at a metabolic level [6]. These effects can be divided into two categories, those decreasing damage mechanisms on nervous fibers and those with antihyperalgesic and antinociceptive effects [5].

Vitamin B1 decreases formation of protein glycation final products, which is a powerful generator of free radicals and oxidative stress [20]. Another effect is through inhibition of the diacylglycerol (DAG) pathway, which decreases protein kinase C (PKC) activation, thus decreasing damage to vascular endothelium. Likewise, it also reduces the activity of the hexosamine pathway; and it is through alternative pathways of the latter that metabolism improves via the pentose-phosphate pathway. B1 (thiamine diphosphate) works as coenzyme for erythrocyte transketolase, an essential enzyme for the metabolism of carbohydrates [21].

Clinical trials showed that 17–79% of type 1 and type 2 diabetics have thiamine deficiency, due to its participation in carbohydrate metabolism, with both euglycemic and hyperglycemic status [21]. The principal action of these effects is reducing nervous fiber damage, which is undoubtedly one of the factors contributing to the development of painful diabetic neuropathy.

B complex vitamins also act directly on pain control, since they have antiallodynic, antinociceptive, and antihyperalgesic effects [6]. Through the Nitric Oxide-Cyclic Guanosine Monophosphate pathway (NO-cGMP pathway), it potentiates soluble guanylyl cyclase and generates cGMP, while activating a type-G protein kinase (PGK), subsequently hyperpolarizing nociceptor potassium channels [22]. Likewise, it also increases nociceptive inhibitory control in afferent neurons of the spinal cord and reduces thalamic neuron response to nociceptive stimulation [23]. Another effect explaining its antihyperalgesic action is through an increase in serotonin and GABA synthesis, decreasing glutamate levels in several brain areas [24]. Therefore, the sum of all effects on carbohydrate metabolism and pain pathways explains its effectiveness in painful diabetic neuropathy.

Our study, through an improvement analysis measuring Patients' Global Impression of Change (PGIC), showed that both drugs improve pain. Backonja et al. showed, in clinical trials with PDN patients, efficacy of gabapentin in treating PDN with a moderate improvement of 60% in PGIC [9].

Both drugs increased sleep time from baseline visit. Backonja et al. showed doses of 1800 mg/d improved measurements in sleep interference scales [9, 18]. Lo et al. reported that GBP increases slow-wave sleep in primary insomnia patients, improving sleep quality (by increasing its efficiency and decreasing spontaneous awakening) [25].

Use of neuromodulators is associated with appearance of adverse events, particularly dizziness, vertigo, and somnolence, which in occasions limit use of greater doses and frequently cause treatment discontinuation. Freeman et al. showed, in a meta-analysis, that adverse events related to pregabalin use are dose-related, dizziness being the most common AE (28%), with 600 mg/d, followed by peripheral edema (16%) and somnolence (13%) [10]. The most frequently reported AE with GBP was dizziness (24%), somnolence (23%), and headache (11%) [9]. A safety and tolerability trial in 336 PDN patients showed reduced dizziness and vertigo frequency in the GBP/B1-B12 group versus pregabalin ($P = 0.012$ and $P = 0.006$, resp.) [5].

Decreased vertigo was observed with GBP/B1/B12 (GBP: 300 to 1800 mg, B1: 100 to 600 mg, and B12: 0.20 mg to 0.120 mg per day), compared to PGB (75–600 mg per day), $P = 0.014$, possibly related to the smaller GBP dose used in the study. The latter, in addition to the synergistic effect of vitamins B1 and B12, allowed for reduction of GBP dose needed to decrease pain intensity, achieving a greater safety and tolerability margin. Through a per dose analysis, less dizziness (3.4%) was observed with a 1800 mg dose in the GBP/B1-B12 group, compared to PGB 300 mg (11%), with a statistically significant difference, $P = 0.0206$.

6. Conclusion

One of this trial's strengths is that it shows that vitamins B1 and B12 have a synergistic effect in combination with gabapentin in PDN treatment, since pain intensity reduction was obtained with 50% of the GBP dose required as monotherapy. Likewise, regarding GBP dose reduction, there are less adverse events (vertigo). Nonetheless, it is necessary to confirm the role of vitamins, isolated and versus placebo, to prove the absolute and potential benefit of this combination.

Conflict of Interests

Development of the study, as well as fees for publishing the paper, was sponsored by Merck S.A. de C.V laboratories. Dr. Alberto Mimenza Alvarado declares to have received payment from Merck S.A. de C.V. for creating the paper. Dr. Sara Aguilar Navarro declares no conflict of interests.

Authors' Contribution

All authors read and approved the final version of the paper. Alberto Mimenza Alvarado and Sara Aguilar Navarro created and designed the investigation protocol. Alberto Mimenza Alvarado wrote the introduction and discussion of the paper, as well as the methodology and results of the study. Sara Aguilar Navarro participated in the methodology, results analysis, and table and figure design, as well as introduction and discussion of the paper.

Acknowledgments

The authors thank OME Statistics, Catalina Palme- Arrache, and Javier Pérez García for the statistical analysis. The authors also thank Dr. Melchor Alpizar Salazar, Dr. Roberto Olivares Santos, Dr. Graciela Villalpando Ramos, and Dr. Maria del Lourdes Rosas Heredia for their participation in the clinical trial as investigators.

References

[1] L. Johannsen, T. Smith, A. M. Havasger et al., "Evaluation of patients with symptoms suggestive of chronic polyneuropathy," *Journal of Clinical Neuromuscular Disease*, vol. 3, no. 2, pp. 47–52, 2001.

[2] R. E. Maser, A. R. Steenkiste, J. S. Dorman et al., "Epidemiological correlates of diabetic neuropathy. Report from Pittsburgh Epidemiology of Diabetes Complications Study," *Diabetes*, vol. 38, no. 11, pp. 1456–1461, 1989.

[3] I. Gilron, T. S. Jensen, and A. H. Dickenson, "Combination pharmacotherapy for management of chronic pain: From bench to bedside," *The Lancet Neurology*, vol. 12, no. 11, pp. 1084–1095, 2013.

[4] A. Berger, A. Sadosky, E. Dukes, J. Edelsberg, and G. Oster, "Clinical characteristics and patterns of healthcare utilization in patients with painful neuropathic disorders in UK general

practice: a retrospective cohort study," *BMC Neurology*, vol. 12, article 8, 2012.

[5] A. Mimenza and S. Aguilar, "Comparative clinical trial of safety and tolerability of gabapentin plus vitamin B1/B12 versus pregabalin in the treatment of painful peripheral diabetic neuropathy," *Journal of Pain & Relief*, vol. 3, pp. 1–6, 2014.

[6] G. Reyes-García, N. L. Caram-Salas, R. Medina-Santillán, and V. Granados-Soto, "Oral administration of B vitamins increases the antiallodynic effect of gabapentin in the rat," *Proceedings of the Western Pharmacology Society*, vol. 47, pp. 76–79, 2004.

[7] T. Várkonyi and P. Kempler, "Diabetic neuropathy: new strategies for treatment," *Diabetes, Obesity and Metabolism*, vol. 10, no. 2, pp. 99–108, 2008.

[8] D. L. Vesely, "B complex vitamins activate rat guanylate cyclase and increase cyclic GMP levels," *European Journal of Clinical Investigation*, vol. 15, no. 5, pp. 258–262, 1985.

[9] M. Backonja, A. Beydoun, K. R. Edwards et al., "Gabapentin for the symptomatic treatment of painful neuropathy in patients with diabetes mellitus: a randomized controlled trial," *The Journal of the American Medical Association*, vol. 280, no. 21, pp. 1831–1836, 1998.

[10] R. Freeman, E. Durso-DeCruz, and B. Emir, "Efficacy, safety, and tolerability of pregabalin treatment for painful diabetic peripheral neuropathy: findings from seven randomized, controlled trials across a range of doses," *Diabetes Care*, vol. 31, no. 7, pp. 1448–1454, 2008.

[11] M. Bennett, "The LANSS pain scale: the Leeds assessment of neuropathic symptoms and signs," *Pain*, vol. 92, no. 1-2, pp. 147–157, 2001.

[12] E. C. Huskisson, "Measurement of pain," *The Lancet*, vol. 304, no. 7889, pp. 1127–1131, 1974.

[13] W. Guy, *ECDEU Assessment Manual for Psychopharmacology*, Psychopharmacology Research Branch, Division of Extramural Research Programs, US Department of Health, Education, and Welfare, Public Health Service, Alcohol, Drug Abuse, and Mental Health Administration, National Institute of Mental Health, Rockville, Md, USA, 1976.

[14] H. Hurst and J. Bolton, "Assessing the clinical significance of change scores recorded on subjective outcome measures," *Journal of Manipulative and Physiological Therapeutics*, vol. 27, no. 1, pp. 26–35, 2004.

[15] M. W. Johns, "A new method for measuring daytime sleepiness: the Epworth sleepiness scale," *Sleep*, vol. 14, no. 6, pp. 540–545, 1991.

[16] K. C. Gorson, C. Schott, R. Herman, A. H. Ropper, and W. M. Rand, "Gabapentin in the treatment of painful diabetic neuropathy: a placebo controlled, double blind, crossover trial," *Journal of Neurology, Neurosurgery & Psychiatry*, vol. 66, no. 2, pp. 251–252, 1999.

[17] F. J. Gómez-Pérez, A. Perez-Monteverde, O. Nascimento et al., "Gabapentin for the treatment of painful diabetic neuropathy: dosing to achieve optimal clinical response," *British Journal of Diabetes and Vascular Disease*, vol. 4, no. 3, pp. 173–178, 2004.

[18] M. Backonja and R. L. Glanzman, "Gabapentin dosing for neuropathic pain: evidence from randomized, placebo-controlled clinical trials," *Clinical Therapeutics*, vol. 25, no. 1, pp. 81–104, 2003.

[19] C. D. Ang, M. J. M. Alviar, A. L. Dans, and et al, "Vitamin B for treating peripheral neuropathy," *Cochrane Database of Systematic Reviews*, no. 3, Article ID CD004573, 2008.

[20] T. Mixcoatl-Zecuatl, G. N. Quiñónez-Bastidas, N. L. Caram-Salas et al., "Synergistic antiallodynic interaction between gabapentin or carbamazepine and either benfotiamine or cyanocobalamin in neuropathic rats," *Methods and Findings in Experimental and Clinical Pharmacology*, vol. 30, no. 6, pp. 431–441, 2008.

[21] G. Jermendy, "Evaluating thiamine deficiency in patients with diabetes," *Diabetes and Vascular Disease Research*, vol. 3, no. 2, pp. 120–121, 2006.

[22] G. Reyes-García, R. Medina-Santillán, H. I. Rocha-González, and V. Granados-Soto, "Synergistic interaction between spinal gabapentin and oral B vitamins in a neuropathic pain model," *Proceedings of the Western Pharmacology Society*, vol. 46, pp. 91–94, 2003.

[23] Z.-B. Wang, Q. Gan, R. L. Rupert, Y.-M. Zeng, and X.-J. Song, "Thiamine, pyridoxine, cyanocobalamin and their combination inhibit thermal, but not mechanical hyperalgesia in rats with primary sensory neuron injury," *Pain*, vol. 114, no. 1-2, pp. 266–277, 2005.

[24] M. J. M. Cohen, L. A. Menefee, K. Doghramji, W. R. Anderson, and E. D. Frank, "Sleep in chronic pain: problems and treatments," *International Review of Psychiatry*, vol. 12, no. 2, pp. 115–116, 2000.

[25] H.-S. Lo, C.-M. Yang, H. G. Lo, C.-Y. Lee, H. Ting, and B.-S. Tzang, "Treatment effects of gabapentin for primary insomnia," *Clinical Neuropharmacology*, vol. 33, no. 2, pp. 84–90, 2010.

14

Diabetic Retinopathy: Animal Models, Therapies, and Perspectives

Xue Cai[1] and James F. McGinnis[1,2,3]

[1]*Department of Ophthalmology, Dean McGee Eye Institute, Oklahoma University Health Sciences Center, Oklahoma City, OK 73104, USA*
[2]*Department of Cell Biology, Oklahoma University Health Sciences Center, Oklahoma City, OK 73104, USA*
[3]*Oklahoma Center for Neuroscience, Oklahoma University Health Sciences Center, Oklahoma City, OK 73104, USA*

Correspondence should be addressed to Xue Cai; xue-cai@ouhsc.edu and James F. McGinnis; james-mcginnis@ouhsc.edu

Academic Editor: Shuang-Xi Wang

Diabetic retinopathy (DR) is one of the major complications of diabetes. Although great efforts have been made to uncover the mechanisms underlying the pathology of DR, the exact causes of DR remain largely unknown. Because of multifactor involvement in DR etiology, currently no effective therapeutic treatments for DR are available. In this paper, we review the pathology of DR, commonly used animal models, and novel therapeutic approaches. Perspectives and future directions for DR treatment are discussed.

1. Introduction

Diabetic retinopathy (DR) is one of the major complications of diabetes and is the leading cause of blindness among working people in developed countries. The symptoms are elevated blood sugar levels, blurred vision, dark spots or flashing lights, and sudden loss of vision. The development of DR can be divided into nonproliferative DR (NPDR; subdivided into mild, moderate, and severe stages) with microaneurysms, hard exudates, hemorrhages, and venous abnormalities [1, 2] and proliferative DR (PDR; advanced stage) with neovascularization, preretinal or vitreous hemorrhages, and fibrovascular proliferation [1, 2]. Development of glaucoma, retinal detachment, and vision loss may also happen at this stage. DR may cause macular edema when blood and fluid leak into the retina caused by swelling of the central retina [3]. DR is not easily diagnosed at early stages but is more readily noticed with the advanced stages or with edema. Multiple techniques have been used for detection, diagnosis, and evaluation of this disease including fundoscopic photography, fluorescence angiography, B-scan ultrasonography, and optical coherence tomography (OCT) [4].

2. Pathology and Molecular Mechanism of DR

Initially, DR was considered a microvascular complication of endothelial dysfunction, as it is characterized by capillary basement membrane (BM) thickening, pericyte and endothelial cell loss, blood-retinal barrier (BRB) breakdown and leakage, acellular capillaries, and neovascularization [5, 6]. However, it is currently acknowledged that before the typical features of DR occur and can be clinically diagnosed, cellular, molecular, and functional changes are evidenced in the retina [7, 8], where all types of retinal cells are affected including ganglion cells [5, 6, 9]. Also, thinning of the inner nuclear layer (INL), reduction in synapse numbers and synaptic proteins, changes in dendrite morphology, and retinal pigment epithelium (RPE) dysfunction occur in DR and result in the gradual loss of retinal function [9]. In addition, glia activation and innate immunity/sterile inflammation [5, 6] occur early in DR. Therefore, DR is not only a vascular disease but also a neurodegenerative disease.

DR shares numerous similarities in its etiology and pathology with other neovascular diseases which have been documented to be associated with chronic inflammation, including increased vascular permeability, edema, inflammatory cell infiltration, tissue destruction, neovascularization, proinflammatory cytokines, and chemokines in the retina [3, 10]. Some of the potential risk factors leading to the pathology of other neovascular diseases also contribute to the pathology of DR.

Diabetes is the number one risk factor for the development of DR. Type 1 diabetes (juvenile diabetes, in which no insulin is made) is more likely to develop vision loss than type 2 diabetes (adult onset diabetes with insufficient insulin synthesis). In addition, race (Hispanic and African Americans), smoking, hyperglycemia (high blood sugar), hypertension (high blood pressure), and hyperlipidemia (high cholesterol) or dyslipidemia are also high risk factors [11, 12]. Vascular endothelial growth factor (VEGF) elevation induces a decrease in the tight-junction proteins and breakdown of the BRB [13], an increase of leukostasis within retinal vessels [14], inflammation [15, 16], upregulation of ICAM-1 (intercellular adhesion molecule-1) expression, an increase in all NOS (nitric oxide synthase) isoforms [17], and a metabolic imbalance in inorganic phosphate [18], all of which have been reported to contribute to DR pathology. Multiple interconnecting biochemical pathways, including an increased polyol pathway, elevated hexosamine biosynthesis pathway (HBP), activation of protein kinase C (PKC), hemodynamic changes, and advanced glycation end product (AGE) formation [5, 6, 14, 19], have also been found to play key roles in development of DR. RhoA is a small guanosine-$5'$-triphosphate-binding protein and acts as a GTPase. The RhoA/mDia-1 (mammalian diaphanous homolog-1)/profiling-1 [20] or RhoA/ROCK1 (Rho-associated coiled-coil-containing protein kinase 1) [21] pathways have been shown to be involved in the pathology of DR via triggering microvascular endothelial dysfunction. Activation of these pathways leads to the increase of growth factors such as VEGF and insulin-like growth factor-1 (IGF-1), activation of the renin-angiotensin-aldosterone system (RAAS), subclinical inflammation, and capillary occlusion [14]. Also increased endoplasmic reticulum (ER) stress and oxidative stress [22] resulting from deregulation of ER and mitochondrial quality control by autophagy/mitophagy, RPE dysfunction, genetic variants, and epigenetic changes in chromatin, such as DNA methylation, histone posttranslational modifications affecting gene transcription, and regulation by noncoding RNAs [23–26], have also been shown to be associated with DR. Interestingly, deletion of transforming growth factor-β (TGF-β) signaling results in undifferentiated pericytes that cause retinal changes in structure and function which mimic those of DR [27]. Loss of other gene functions such as BMP2 (bone morphogenetic protein 2) [28] and Toll-like receptor 4 [29] has been implicated in the pathogenesis of DR. Activation of the P2X7 receptor, a member of ligand-gated membrane ion channels, resulted in the formation of large plasma membrane pores that exacerbate the development of DR through induction of inflammation [30]. Recently, a prooxidant and proapoptotic thioredoxin interacting protein (TXNIP) was shown to be highly upregulated in DR and by high glucose (HG) in retinal cells in culture. TXNIP binds to thioredoxin (Trx) inhibiting its oxidant scavenging and thiol-reducing capacity. Hence, prolonged overexpression of TXNIP causes ROS/RNS stress, mitochondrial dysfunction, inflammation, and premature cell death in DR [31]. Collectively, hyperglycemia-induced vascular dysfunction and subsequent tissue damage have been proposed to act through the following four main pathways [32, 33]: (1) increased polyol pathway flux, in which cytosolic redox imbalance occurs with an increased NADH/NAD$^+$ ratio via the sorbitol pathway resulting in a decrease in cytosolic NADPH and cellular functions, (2) increased AGE formation, in which nonenzymatic glycosylation of proteins and production of AGEs alter gene expression and AGEs also induce the synthesis of numerous inflammatory cytokines, (3) activation of PKC via the formation of intracellular diacylglycerol (DAG) and AGEs, which contributes to the generation of ROS which induces VEGF and multiple other growth factors and transcription factors, and (4) increased hexosamine pathway flux, in which fructose-6-phosphate is converted to glucosamine-6-phosphate and finally to uridine diphosphate N-acetyl glucosamine. This modification results in changes in gene expression and protein function. However, each of the four major pathways is linked by overproduction of superoxide and increased generation of ROS [33], which provides a common target for potential treatment.

3. Animal Models

At present, most animal models of DR are rodents, mice, and rats. Based on the experimental approaches to induce DR, these models can be classified as chemically induced, spontaneous, and genetically created. However, knowledge of the molecular mechanisms underlying the initiation and development of DR is insufficient and largely unknown because there are no reliable and appropriate good animal models of spontaneous diabetes in which phenotypic characteristics exactly mimic the pathogenesis of clinical DR. Although various traditionally used animal models of DR present a number of pathological changes similar to those of human DR, several pathological characteristics of human DR, such as retinal neovascularization, cannot yet be fully mimicked in any existing animal model of DR [34].

3.1. Chemically Induced Model. The commonly used streptozotocin (STZ) or alloxan induced DR animal models (rats or mice) exhibit rapid onset of hyperglycemia (3 days after treatment) and some of the symptoms of early DR (type I diabetes), such as loss of retinal pericytes and capillaries, thickening of the vascular basement membrane, vascular occlusion, and increased vascular permeability [3, 34, 35]. However, variability of pathological characteristics, such as loss of retinal capillaries, ganglion cell death, and reduction of retinal function, has been reported among different species and even within the same species [3, 34, 35].

3.2. Akita Mice. The Akita (Ins2$^{Akita+/-}$) mouse, a spontaneous diabetes model for early stage of DR (type I diabetes), is caused by a missense mutation in the diabetogenic *Insulin 2* gene (*Ins2*) and is characterized by a rapid onset of hyperglycemia and hypoinsulinemia and marked reduction of insulin secretion by 4 weeks of age [36]. Significant increases in vascular permeability were seen when measured at 12 weeks after hyperglycemia. The thickness of the inner plexiform layer (IPL) and INL in the peripheral region was decreased and the number of ganglion cells was significantly reduced when measured at 22 weeks after hyperglycemia [37]. Recently, Hombrebueno et al. reported that the Akita mice exhibit progressive thinning of the retina and cone loss from 3 months onwards, severe impairment of synaptic connectivity at the outer plexiform layer (OPL), and significant reduction in the number of amacrine and ganglion cells [38, 39]. ER stress associated proteins were upregulated in this mouse model [40]. The transportation of proinsulin from the endoplasmic reticulum (ER) to the Golgi apparatus is blocked, and instead the mutant proinsulin is accumulated in the ER forming complexes with BiP (binding immunoglobulin protein) which are eventually degraded [41].

3.3. Kimba Mice. The Kimba mice were generated by microinjection of human VEGF$_{165}$ isoform driven by a photoreceptor-specific promoter (rhodopsin). Pathological changes in the retinal vasculature, focal fluorescein leakage, relatively mild degree, and slow onset of neovascularization were shown at 3-4 weeks of age and stable retinopathy persisted for 3 months, which resembles NPDR and early stage of PDR [1]. A thinner outer nuclear layer (ONL) and INL, severe and extensive outer and inner retinal neovascularization, hemorrhage, retinal detachment [1], microaneurysm, leaky capillaries, capillary dropout [42], leaky blood vessels, and BRB loss [42, 43] were presented in this mouse model. However, the mice overexpressing photoreceptor-specific hVEGF are not on a hyperglycemic background and do not induce choroidal neovascularization [1, 42].

3.4. Akimba Mice. The Akimba (Ins2^{Akita}VEGF$^{+/-}$) mouse, generated from the Kimba (VEGF$^{+/-}$) (trVEGF029) and the Akita (Ins2^{Akita}) mice, is a model for advanced DR [42]. This model retains the parental retinal neovascularization with hyperglycemia and displays the majority of signs of advanced clinical DR including more diffuse vascular leakage (compared to the more focal leakage in Kimba mice) and the BRB disruption, which was linked to decreased expression of endothelial junction proteins, pericyte dropout, and vessel loss [42, 43]. With aging, Akimba mice exhibit enhanced photoreceptor loss, thinning of the retina, more severe and progressive retinal vascular pathology, capillary nonperfusion, much higher prevalence and persistence of edema, and retinal detachment [42]. Plasmalemma vesicle associated protein (PLVAP) is an endothelial cell specific protein which is absent in intact BRB but is significantly increased in Akimba mice (and also in Kimba mice). Therefore PLVAP plays an important role in the regulation of BRB permeability [43].

3.5. db/db Mice. The db/db (*lepr^{db}*) mouse, a spontaneous diabetic model of type 2 diabetes [44, 45], is caused by a mutation in the leptin receptor gene. It exhibits high glial activation, progressive loss of ganglion cells, and significant reduction of neuroretinal thickness. Significant abnormal retinal function is pronounced at 16 weeks of age. In addition, significantly higher levels of glial fibrillary acidic protein (GFAP, a marker for glial cells) expression, increases in accumulation of glutamate, and downregulation of abundant neurotransmission genes were found at 8 weeks of age [44]. Also, breakdown of the BRB is a hallmark of the db/db mice [46] and RPE dysfunction is concomitant with sustained hyperglycemia [45]. Proteomic analysis of 10-week-old retinas from db/db and wild type mice showed that 98 membrane proteins, out of a total of 844, were significantly differentially abundant in db/db versus wild type mice, in which 80 were downregulated and 18 were upregulated in the db/db retinas [47]. The major proteins decreased are synaptic transmission proteins, especially the vesicular glutamate transporter 1 (VGLUT1) [47], which is responsible for the loading of glutamate into synaptic vesicles and is expressed at the ribbon synapses in the photoreceptors and "ON" bipolar cells [48].

3.6. New Animal Models. In recent years, two new animal models were reported. One is a transgenic mouse overexpressing insulin-like growth factor-1 (IGF-1), which develops the most retinal alteration seen in human diabetic eyes on a nonhyperglycemic background [49] and exhibits progressive development of vascular alteration (from NPDR to PDR), increased VEGF level, BRB breakdown, vascular permeability, and glial alteration with age (3 months and older) [49, 50]. Retinal neurodegeneration was seen at 6 months of age with the number of bipolar and ganglion cells reduced and a 40% reduction of ONL and INL thickness was observed in 7.5-month-old mice. Microarray analysis on 4-month-old retinas, with evidence of NPDR and gliosis [50], revealed upregulation of genes associated with retinal stress, gliosis, and angiogenesis. Increased GFAP immunostaining was seen at 1.5 months of age and was maintained throughout the entire life. Activation of ERK signaling was detected at 3 months and was more pronounced at 7.5 months. In addition, expression of oxidative stress markers was increased; in particular a striking upregulation of all three subunits of NADPH oxidase, impaired glutamate recycling, and significantly higher levels of TNF-α and MCP-1 were seen at 7.5 months [51]. The other model is the hyperhexosemic marmosets (*Callithrix jacchus*) which, with a 30% galactose- (gal-) rich diet for two years, develops significantly high blood glucose levels, vascular permeability, macular edema, increased number of acellular capillaries, pericyte loss, vascular BM thickening, increased vessel tortuosity in the retinas, and microaneurysms. High-speed spectral domain OCT (SD-OCT) scan reveals significant thickening of the foveal and the juxtafoveal area resulting from intraretinal fluid accumulation. Also there are potential break in the RPE and discontinuous photoreceptor layers in the macular area starting at 15 months of galactose feeding. All these characteristics have striking similarities to the human DR [52].

4. Current Therapies

During the nonproliferative stages, treatment is usually not recommended because normal visual function is not disturbed at these stages. However, at the advanced stages, the

PDR, treatment has to be undertaken. Traditional approaches for treatment of DR and associated microvasculature and neovascularization include laser treatment, optimizing blood glucose level, and controlling blood pressure. Currently, laser treatment (photocoagulation) to stop the leakage and scattered laser burns to shrink abnormal blood vessels and prevent retinal detachment are effective and are widely employed and are the primary treatment strategy. Surgical treatment to remove the vitreous (vitrectomy) is usually taken for advanced PDR in type I diabetes if persistent vitreous hemorrhage or severe tractional retinal detachment occurs. Intravitreal injection of anti-VEGF (Avastin, Lucentis, and Eylea) and corticosteroids to prevent abnormal blood vessel growth are effective and are also beneficial treatments for PDR [2, 19, 53].

Clinical trial (ClinicalTrials.gov number: NCT01627249) phase III study (660 adults) with intravitreal injection of Aflibercept, Bevacizumab, or Ranibizumab for diabetic macular edema (DME) showed that visual acuity was improved, and Aflibercept is more effective when the initial visual acuity is worse [54]. A five-year clinical trial study reported that intravitreal injection of 0.5 mg Ranibizumab with prompt (124 patients) or deferred (111 patients) focal/grid laser treatment for diabetic macular edema resulted in the maintenance of vision gains obtained by the first year through 5 years in most of the eyes [55]. However, another clinical trial study (322 of 582 eyes) showed that repeated intravitreal Ranibizumab injections for DME may increase the risk of sustained elevation of intraocular pressure or the need for ocular hypotensive treatment [56] and a risk of stroke [2]. Another clinical trial, phase I/II study, evaluating the safety and bioactivity of intravitreal injection of a designed ankyrin repeat protein (MP0112) for specific and high-affinity binding to VEGF in patients with DME, showed reduction of edema and improvement of visual acuity, although several patients showed inflammation [57]. An ongoing clinical trial eliminates the source of inflammation from a new preparation [57].

DR associated pathological factors, molecular signaling pathways, and other mechanisms underlying the pathology of DR, as well as the direct pathological defects (retinal degeneration, synaptic connection impairment and cell loss, accumulation of glutamate, etc.), provide a broad spectrum of potential new therapeutic targets for the treatment of DR. Therapeutic treatment strategies targeting these molecules, components, or defects, including various factors, hyperglycemia- and glutamate-triggered pathways, and microvascular impairment and angiogenesis, have been shown to produce an effective outcome [11, 58, 59]. Chinese traditional medicine HF (He-Ying-Qing-Re formula), in which chlorogenic acid, ferulic acid, and arctin were identified as major components, was shown to have anti-DR effects, although hyperglycemia was not significantly inhibited. Its action on suppression of activation of AGEs and endothelial dysfunction occurs by inactivation of AGEs receptor and their downstream Akt signaling pathway [60]. Deletion of placental growth factor prevents DR by inactivation of Akt and inhibition of the HIF1α-VEGF pathway [11, 61]. Recently, angiopoietin-like 4 (ANGPTL 4) was identified

as a potential angiogenic factor which was upregulated in the PDR patients and was shown to be independent of VEGF levels and localized in the area of retinal neovascularization. Neutralizing ANGPTL4 antibody can inhibit the angiogenic effect in PDR patients with low VEGF levels or produce an additive effect with anti-VEGF treatment for inhibition of VEGF expression [62].

Preclinical therapies targeting other factors have been reported. A single intravitreal injection of a vector expressing insulin-like growth factor binding protein-3 (IGFBP-3) into diabetic rat retina after 2 months of diabetes restores normal insulin signal transduction via regulation of the insulin receptor/TNF-α (tumor necrosis factor-alpha) pathway and leads to the reduction of proapoptotic markers or increases of antiapoptotic markers and the restoration of retinal function [63]. Blockage of TNF-α by intravitreal and intraperitoneal delivery of anti-TNF-α antibody in STZ-induced mice and Akita mice resulted in a dose-dependent prevention of increased retinal leukostasis, acellular capillary, BRB breakdown, and cell death [64]. Intraperitoneal injection of anti-VEGFR1 antibody (MF1) prevents vascular leakage and inhibits inflammation associated gene expression and abnormal distribution of tight-junction proteins in STZ-induced mice and Akita mice [65].

Fenofibrate is a peroxisome proliferator-activated receptor-α (PPAR-α) agonist and is known for clinical treatment for dyslipidemia. Recently, it was shown to significantly ameliorate retinal vascular leakage and leukostasis in DR of STZ-induced diabetic rats and Akita mice through downregulation of ICAM-1, MCP-1 (monocyte chemoattractant protein-1), and NF-κB (nuclear factor-kappa B) signaling [66]. Clinical studies demonstrated that Fenofibrate has protective effects on progression of proliferative DR in type 2 diabetic patients [67, 68]. Now, the use of this medication for DR is approved [69].

Omega-3 polyunsaturated fatty acid (ω-3PUFA) has been shown to be decreased in STZ-induced diabetic rat retina [70]. ω-3PUFA rich diets enhanced glucose homeostasis and preserved retinal function in db/db/mice, but the effect is independent of preservation of retinal vasculature integrity, inflammatory modulation, and retinal neuroprotection [71].

5. Novel Potential Therapeutic Targets

Because of the complicated etiology of DR, drugs such as inhibitors for signaling pathways and growth factors have been shown to be effective for the treatment of DR but have limitations. Currently, intravitreal injection of anti-VEGF and corticosteroids are popular therapeutics, but a high proportion of patients (~40%) do not respond to these therapies [58, 72]. This implies that other factors or pathways, independent of VEGF, are involved in the development of microvasculature and neovascularization. Therefore, there is an urgent need for finding potential target candidates and for the development of new treatment strategies for DR therapy.

Epigenetic chromatin modifications (DNA methylation, histone posttranslational modifications, and regulation by noncoding RNAs), acting on both cis- and trans-chromatin structural elements, can be regulated by TXNIP [25]. Aberrant epigenetic modifications have been identified in DR and implicated in the progression of DR [25, 26]. MicroRNAs (miRNAs) are a group of noncoding RNA sequences which are short and highly conservative and can posttranscriptionally control gene expression by degradation or repression of target mRNAs. They are implicated in a variety of biological activities including modulation of glucose, angiogenesis, and inflammatory responses, as well as pathogenesis of diabetes and related complications such as DR [10]. However, conflicting data were seen with different miRNAs. It has been shown that retinal miRNA expression was altered in early DR rats induced by STZ, in which miRNAs were differentially regulated compared to the controls without DR [73]. Downregulation of miR-200b has been shown to increase VEGF expression, and polycomb repressive complex 2 (PRC2) (histone methyltransferase complex) represses miR-200b through its histone H3 lysine-27 trimethylation. Thus inhibition of PRC2 through histone methylation of miR-200b increases miR-200b and reduces VEGF in STZ-induced diabetic rats [74]. The $3'$-untranslated region ($3'$-UTR) of mRNA sequence contains regulatory regions including binding sites for miRNAs to repress translation and degrade mRNA transcripts. In DR rats, miRNA-195 was significantly upregulated after one month of diabetes, and the antioxidant enzyme MnSOD level was reduced. *In situ* hybridization indicated that miR-195 was overexpressed in the cells of INL and ONL and ganglion cell layers, but sirtuin 1 (SIRT1) was downregulated. SIRT1 is involved in many biological processes including cell survival and metabolism and miR-195 binds to the $3'$-UTR of SIRT1 to regulate its expression. Intravitreal injection of miR-195 antagomir leads to downregulation of SIRT1, thus preventing DR damage caused by SIRT1-mediated downregulation of MnSOD [75]. Collectively, increasing amounts of data demonstrate the active involvement and critical role of miRNAs in development of DR, although the exact mechanisms by which miRNA or miRNAs act are not known. Increased knowledge of how miRNAs function as therapeutic agents will lead to their effective use in the treatment of DR.

Reactive oxygen species (ROS), the primary causative factor for a variety of diseases, have been shown to play an important role in promoting DR [12, 58, 76]. As a treatment target, evidence from preclinical and clinical studies indicates that antioxidant therapies which directly target ROS-producing enzymes are beneficial, although the outcome of large clinical trials has been less promising [76]. However, nuclear factor erythroid 2-related factor 2 (Nrf2), the regulator of phase II enzymes system and the network of cytoprotective genes [77, 78], is still attractive. Its activators have been proven effective in prevention of the development and progression of DR [79]. Here, we specifically point out that nanomedicine attracts more attention in the past several years because it has been beneficial in a variety of medical applications including its promising effects on disease therapy [80, 81]. We have been using cerium oxide nanoparticles (nanoceria) to treat several animal models for ocular diseases and demonstrated their nontoxic and long-lasting effectiveness in delaying retinal degeneration in *tubby* mice [82] and

inhibiting retinal and choroidal neovascularization [83]. Due to their unique physicochemical features, nanoceria themselves exhibit superoxide dismutase and catalase activities under redox conditions and can upregulate phase II enzymes [84] and regulate the common antioxidant gene network downstream of Trx [85]. Nanoceria have an atom-comparable size which enables them to freely cross the cellular and nuclear membrane barriers. In addition, they do not need repeat dosing as is required by other antioxidants. Thus one single dose produces sustained protective effects [82–84] which suggests their great potential to be excellent agents for the treatment of DR.

Stem cells emerged as a regenerative therapeutic strategy for treatment of a variety of diseases because they are undifferentiated and retain their stem cell characteristics and possess the potential to differentiate into many different cell types under certain biological conditions [86, 87]. Stem cells have been obtained from multiple sources and have been shown to have a great potential for tissue repair and ocular disease treatment [87, 88]. Human embryonic stem cells (hESCs) can differentiate into more than 99% pure RPE cells and integrate into the host RPE layer and become matured. Phase I/II clinical trials for assessing the tolerability and safety of subretinal transplantation of hESC-derived RPE cells in patients with Stargardt's macular dystrophy (ClinicalTrials.gov number: NCT01345006) and advanced dry AMD (ClinicalTrials.gov number: NCT01344993) have shown that hESCs improve visual acuity [89]. Assessment of their medium- and long-term safety, graft, and survival in patients is ongoing [90]. Mesenchymal stromal cells (MSCs) have been shown to have multiple effects including tissue repair, secretion of neuroprotective growth factors, suppression of host immune response, and lowering glucose levels [91, 92]. Bone marrow derived MSCs have been reported to be differentiated into retinal cells and rescue retinal degeneration in several animal models [91]. Clinical trial phase I assessing their effects on visual acuity in patients with retinitis pigmentosa (RP) (ClinicalTrials.gov number: NCT01068561) has been completed and phase I/II in patients with AMD and Stargardt (ClinicalTrials.gov number: NCT01518127) will be completed in December 2015 (also see review [92]). However, no clinical study of therapeutic effects of MSCs in DR has been reported. Progress has also been made in using several classes of stem cells (EPCs, endothelial progenitor cells; ASCs, adipose stromal cells; PSCs, pluripotent stem cells) to stimulate both neuroregeneration and vascular regeneration in the diabetic retina [92]. EPCs are circulating cells and can be recruited to the sites of vessel damage and tissue ischemia and promote vascular healing and reperfusion [93]. Clinical studies have shown that altered numbers of EPCs were found in patients of type I and type II diabetes with NPDR and PDR, suggesting that EPCs are potential biomarkers for DME and PDR and may be used as therapeutic modalities to treat DR [72]. Preclinical study of STZ-induced diabetic rats receiving a single intravitreal injection of human derived ASCs at two months after diabetes onset showed significant decreases in vascular leakage and apoptotic cells and downregulation of inflammatory gene expression and improved rod b-wave amplitude within one week after injection [94]. Furthermore, mouse ASCs (mASCs) were intravitreally injected into 5-week-old Akimba mice, and the mASCs integrated and associated with retinal microvasculature. Injection of TGF-β1-preconditioned mASCs into P9 Akimba pups resulted in a great decrease in capillary dropout areas and avascular areas [95]. These results suggest that regenerative medicine could be a permanent solution for fighting diabetes and associated complications.

Nevertheless, as we previously mentioned, DR has a complicated etiology and involves many factors. Among these causative factors, genetic background seems to contribute most heavily and current approaches for the treatment of DR can only delay the disease progression and do not provide a complete treatment or cure for DR. Correction of the defective gene(s) appears to be potentially the most effective way for DR treatment (see below). In the clinic, the challenge faced is the lack of detection methods for as yet unknown early clinical symptoms which would enable immediate and proper treatment for inhibition of the progression of NPDR to PDR.

6. Perspective and Future Direction for DR Treatment

With wide exploration of the etiology of the diseases using modern molecular techniques, one finds that almost all the diseases are linked with mutation(s) of a specific gene or multiple genes. Current effective gene therapy methods involve gene replacement therapy in which the defective copy of the gene is replaced by the wild type allele to compliment the defect; or knockdown of the defective gene by RNA interference (RNAi) silences the effects of the mutated gene; or introduces a gene to produce a product causing cell apoptosis (http://www.ghr.nlm.nih.gov/handbook). None of the above mentioned strategies can completely eliminate the products or effects of the defective genes indicating that the diseases cannot be completely cured. CRISPR/Cas9-mediated genome editing, which emerged as a new therapeutic strategy for defective gene repairing, has attracted significant attention in recent years. Indeed, at the 2015 annual ARVO (the association for research in vision and ophthalmology) meeting, several laboratories reported their progress in using this approach to correct (or repair) mutant gene sequences from patient-derived induced pluripotent stem cells (iPSCs) for treatment of inherited ocular diseases such as retinitis pigmentosa, AMD, and other retinal diseases [96–99]. Considering the similarity in the pathogenesis of AMD and DR, CRISPR/Cas9-mediated selective engineering of genes associated with DR or angiogenesis is expected to produce positive and effective treatment of DR.

Conflict of Interests

The authors declare that there is no conflict of interests regarding the publication of this paper.

Acknowledgments

This work was supported in part by NIH NEI P30EY021725, R01EY018724, and R01EY022111 and unrestricted funds from PHF and RPB.

References

[1] C.-M. Lai, S. A. Dunlop, L. A. May et al., "Generation of transgenic mice with mild and severe retinal neovascularisation," *British Journal of Ophthalmology*, vol. 89, no. 7, pp. 911–916, 2005.

[2] N. Cheung, P. Mitchell, and T. Y. Wong, "Diabetic retinopathy," *The Lancet*, vol. 376, no. 9735, pp. 124–136, 2010.

[3] R. Robinson, V. A. Barathi, S. S. Chaurasia, T. Y. Wong, and T. S. Kern, "Update on animal models of diabetic retinopathy: from molecular approaches to mice and higher mammals," *Disease Models and Mechanisms*, vol. 5, no. 4, pp. 444–456, 2012.

[4] D. A. Salz and A. J. Witkin, "Imaging in diabetic retinopathy," *Middle East African Journal of Ophthalmology*, vol. 22, no. 2, pp. 145–150, 2015.

[5] A. M. Abu El-Asrar, L. Dralands, L. Missotten, I. A. Al-Jadaan, and K. Geboes, "Expression of apoptosis markers in the retinas of human subjects with diabetes," *Investigative Ophthalmology and Visual Science*, vol. 45, no. 8, pp. 2760–2766, 2004.

[6] A. J. Barber, E. Lieth, S. A. Khin, D. A. Antonetti, A. G. Buchanan, and T. W. Gardner, "Neural apoptosis in the retina during experimental and human diabetes. Early onset and effect of insulin," *The Journal of Clinical Investigation*, vol. 102, no. 4, pp. 783–791, 1998.

[7] M. S. Ola and A. S. Alhomida, "Neurodegeneration in diabetic retina and its potential drug targets," *Current Neuropharmacology*, vol. 12, no. 4, pp. 380–386, 2014.

[8] J. S. Ng, M. A. Bearse Jr., M. E. Schneck, S. Barez, and A. J. Adams, "Local diabetic retinopathy prediction by multifocal ERG delays over 3 years," *Investigative Ophthalmology and Visual Science*, vol. 49, no. 4, pp. 1622–1628, 2008.

[9] A. J. Barber, "Diabetic retinopathy: recent advances towards understanding neurodegeneration and vision loss," *Science China Life Sciences*, vol. 58, no. 6, pp. 541–549, 2015.

[10] R. Mastropasqua, L. Toto, F. Cipollone, D. Santovito, P. Carpineto, and L. Mastropasqua, "Role of microRNAs in the modulation of diabetic retinopathy," *Progress in Retinal and Eye Research*, vol. 43, pp. 92–107, 2014.

[11] A. Das, P. G. McGuire, and S. Rangasamy, "Diabetic macular edema: pathophysiology and novel therapeutic targets," *Ophthalmology*, vol. 122, no. 7, pp. 1375–1394, 2015.

[12] H.-P. Hammes, Y. Feng, F. Pfister, and M. Brownlee, "Diabetic retinopathy: targeting vasoregression," *Diabetes*, vol. 60, no. 1, pp. 9–16, 2011.

[13] D. A. Antonetti, A. J. Barber, S. Khin, E. Lieth, J. M. Tarbell, and T. W. Gardner, "Vascular permeability in experimental diabetes is associated with reduced endothelial occludin content: vascular endothelial growth factor decreases occludin in retinal endothelial cells. Penn State Retina Research Group," *Diabetes*, vol. 47, no. 12, pp. 1953–1959, 1998.

[14] J. M. Tarr, K. Kaul, M. Chopra, E. M. Kohner, and R. Chibber, "Pathophysiology of diabetic retinopathy," *ISRN Ophthalmology*, vol. 2013, Article ID 343560, 13 pages, 2013.

[15] A. M. Joussen, V. Poulaki, M. L. Le et al., "A central role for inflammation in the pathogenesis of diabetic retinopathy," *The FASEB Journal*, vol. 18, no. 12, pp. 1450–1452, 2004.

[16] F. Semeraro, A. Cancarini, R. dell'Omo, S. Rezzola, M. R. Romano, and C. Costagliola, "Diabetic retinopathy: vascular and inflammatory disease," *Journal of Diabetes Research*, vol. 2015, Article ID 582060, 16 pages, 2015.

[17] E. C. Leal, A. Manivannan, K.-I. Hosoya et al., "Inducible nitric oxide synthase isoform is a key mediator of leukostasis and blood-retinal barrier breakdown in diabetic retinopathy," *Investigative Ophthalmology and Visual Science*, vol. 48, no. 11, pp. 5257–5265, 2007.

[18] H. Vorum and J. Ditzel, "Disturbance of inorganic phosphate metabolism in diabetes mellitus: its relevance to the pathogenesis of diabetic retinopathy," *Journal of Ophthalmology*, vol. 2014, Article ID 135287, 8 pages, 2014.

[19] A. Das, S. Stroud, A. Mehta, and S. Rangasamy, "New treatments for diabetic retinopathy," *Diabetes, Obesity and Metabolism*, vol. 17, no. 3, pp. 219–230, 2015.

[20] Q. Lu, L. Lu, W. Chen, H. Chen, X. Xu, and Z. Zheng, "RhoA/mDia-1/profilin-1 signaling targets microvascular endothelial dysfunction in diabetic retinopathy," *Graefe's Archive for Clinical and Experimental Ophthalmology*, vol. 253, no. 5, pp. 669–680, 2015.

[21] Q. Y. Lu, W. Chen, L. Lu et al., "Involvement of RhoA/ROCK1 signaling pathway in hyperglycemia-induced microvascular endothelial dysfunction in diabetic retinopathy," *International Journal of Clinical and Experimental Pathology*, vol. 7, no. 10, pp. 7268–7277, 2014.

[22] T. Oshitari, N. Hata, and S. Yamamoto, "Endoplasmic reticulum stress and diabetic retinopathy," *Vascular Health and Risk Management*, vol. 4, no. 1, pp. 115–122, 2008.

[23] Z. H. Tang, L. Wang, F. Zeng, and K. Zhang, "Human genetics of diabetic retinopathy," *Journal of Endocrinological Investigation*, vol. 37, no. 12, pp. 1165–1174, 2014.

[24] M. A. Reddy, E. Zhang, and R. Natarajan, "Epigenetic mechanisms in diabetic complications and metabolic memory," *Diabetologia*, vol. 58, no. 3, pp. 443–455, 2015.

[25] L. Perrone, C. Matrone, and L. P. Singh, "Epigenetic modifications and potential new treatment targets in diabetic retinopathy," *Journal of Ophthalmology*, vol. 2014, Article ID 789120, 10 pages, 2014.

[26] F. A. A. Kwa and T. R. Thrimawithana, "Epigenetic modifications as potential therapeutic targets in age-related macular degeneration and diabetic retinopathy," *Drug Discovery Today*, vol. 19, no. 9, pp. 1387–1393, 2014.

[27] B. M. Braunger, S. V. Leimbeck, A. Schlecht, C. Volz, H. Jägle, and E. R. Tamm, "Deletion of ocular transforming growth factor β signaling mimics essential characteristics of diabetic retinopathy," *The American Journal of Pathology*, vol. 185, no. 6, pp. 1749–1768, 2015.

[28] K. A. Hussein, K. Choksi, S. Akeel et al., "Bone morphogenetic protein 2: a potential new player in the pathogenesis of diabetic retinopathy," *Experimental Eye Research*, vol. 125, pp. 79–88, 2014.

[29] H. Wang, H. Shi, J. Zhang et al., "Toll-like receptor 4 in bone marrow-derived cells contributes to the progression of diabetic retinopathy," *Mediators of Inflammation*, vol. 2014, Article ID 858763, 7 pages, 2014.

[30] T. Sugiyama, "Role of P2X7 receptors in the development of diabetic retinopathy," *World Journal of Diabetes*, vol. 5, no. 2, pp. 141–145, 2014.

[31] L. P. Singh, "Thioredoxin interacting protein (TXNIP) and pathogenesis of diabetic retinopathy," *Journal of Clinical & Experimental Ophthalmology*, vol. 4, 2013.

[32] C. D. A. Stehouwer, J. Lambert, A. J. M. Donker, and V. W. M. Van Hinsbergh, "Endothelial dysfunction and pathogenesis of diabetic angiopathy," *Cardiovascular Research*, vol. 34, no. 1, pp. 55–68, 1997.

[33] M. Brownlee, "Biochemistry and molecular cell biology of diabetic complications," *Nature*, vol. 414, no. 6865, pp. 813–820, 2001.

[34] X. Jiang, L. Yang, and Y. Luo, "Animal models of diabetic retinopathy," *Current Eye Research*, vol. 40, no. 8, pp. 761–771, 2015.

[35] A. K. W. Lai and A. C. Y. Lo, "Animal models of diabetic retinopathy: summary and comparison," *Journal of Diabetes Research*, vol. 2013, Article ID 106594, 29 pages, 2013.

[36] M. Yoshioka, T. Kayo, T. Ikeda, and A. Koizumi, "A novel locus, Mody4, distal to D7Mit189 on chromosome 7 determines early-onset NIDDM in nonobese C57BL/6 (Akita) mutant mice," *Diabetes*, vol. 46, no. 5, pp. 887–894, 1997.

[37] A. J. Barber, D. A. Antonetti, T. S. Kern et al., "The Ins2Akita mouse as a model of early retinal complications in diabetes," *Investigative Ophthalmology & Visual Science*, vol. 46, no. 6, pp. 2210–2218, 2005.

[38] M. J. Gastinger, A. R. Kunselman, E. E. Conboy, S. K. Bronson, and A. J. Barber, "Dendrite remodeling and other abnormalities in the retinal ganglion cells of Ins2Akita diabetic mice," *Investigative Ophthalmology and Visual Science*, vol. 49, no. 6, pp. 2635–2642, 2008.

[39] J. R. Hombrebueno, M. Chen, R. G. Penalva, and H. Xu, "Loss of synaptic connectivity, particularly in second order neurons is a key feature of diabetic retinal neuropathy in the Ins2Akita mouse," *PLoS ONE*, vol. 9, no. 5, Article ID e97970, 2014.

[40] Y. Ha, Y. Dun, M. Thangaraju et al., "Sigma receptor 1 modulates endoplasmic reticulum stress in retinal neurons," *Investigative Ophthalmology and Visual Science*, vol. 52, no. 1, pp. 527–540, 2011.

[41] J. Wang, T. Takeuchi, S. Tanaka et al., "A mutation in the insulin 2 gene induces diabetes with severe pancreatic β-cell dysfunction in the Mody mouse," *The Journal of Clinical Investigation*, vol. 103, no. 1, pp. 27–37, 1999.

[42] E. P. Rakoczy, I. S. Ali Rahman, N. Binz et al., "Characterization of a mouse model of hyperglycemia and retinal neovascularization," *The American Journal of Pathology*, vol. 177, no. 5, pp. 2659–2670, 2010.

[43] J. Wisniewska-Kruk, I. Klaassen, I. M. C. Vogels et al., "Molecular analysis of blood-retinal barrier loss in the Akimba mouse, a model of advanced diabetic retinopathy," *Experimental Eye Research*, vol. 122, pp. 123–131, 2014.

[44] P. Bogdanov, L. Corraliza, J. A. Villena et al., "The db/db mouse: a useful model for the study of diabetic retinal neurodegeneration," *PLoS ONE*, vol. 9, no. 5, Article ID e97302, 2014.

[45] I. S. Samuels, B. A. Bell, A. Pereira, J. Saxon, and N. S. Peachey, "Early retinal pigment epithelium dysfunction is concomitant with hyperglycemia in mouse models of type 1 and type 2 diabetes," *Journal of Neurophysiology*, vol. 113, no. 4, pp. 1085–1099, 2015.

[46] A. K. H. Cheung, M. K. L. Fung, A. C. Y. Lo et al., "Aldose reductase deficiency prevents diabetes-induced blood-retinal barrier breakdown, apoptosis, and glial reactivation in the retina of db/db mice," *Diabetes*, vol. 54, no. 11, pp. 3119–3125, 2005.

[47] A. Ly, M. F. Scheerer, S. Zukunft et al., "Retina proteome alterations in a mouse model of type 2 diabetes," *Diabetologia*, vol. 57, no. 1, pp. 192–203, 2014.

[48] D. M. Sherry, M. M. Wang, J. Bates, and L. J. Frishman, "Expression of vesicular glutamate transporter 1 in the mouse retina reveals temporal ordering in development of rod vs. cone and ON vs. OFF circuits," *Journal of Comparative Neurology*, vol. 465, no. 4, pp. 480–498, 2003.

[49] P. Villacampa, V. Haurigot, and F. Bosch, "Proliferative retinopathies: animal models and therapeutic opportunities," *Current Neurovascular Research*, vol. 12, no. 2, pp. 189–198, 2015.

[50] J. Ruberte, E. Ayuso, M. Navarro et al., "Increased ocular levels of IGF-1 in transgenic mice lead to diabetes-like eye disease," *The Journal of Clinical Investigation*, vol. 113, no. 8, pp. 1149–1157, 2004.

[51] P. Villacampa, A. Ribera, S. Motas et al., "Insulin-like growth factor I (IGF-I)-induced chronic gliosis and retinal stress lead to neurodegeneration in a mouse model of retinopathy," *The Journal of Biological Chemistry*, vol. 288, no. 24, pp. 17631–17642, 2013.

[52] A. Chronopoulos, S. Roy, E. Beglova, K. Mansfield, L. Wachtman, and S. Roy, "Hyperhexosemia-induced retinal vascular pathology in a novel primate model of diabetic retinopathy," *Diabetes*, vol. 64, no. 7, pp. 2603–2608, 2015.

[53] P. Osaadon, X. J. Fagan, T. Lifshitz, and J. Levy, "A review of anti-VEGF agents for proliferative diabetic retinopathy," *Eye*, vol. 28, no. 5, pp. 510–520, 2014.

[54] J. A. Wells, A. R. Glassman, A. R. Ayala et al., "Aflibercept, bevacizumab, or ranibizumab for diabetic macular edema," *The New England Journal of Medicine*, vol. 372, no. 13, pp. 1193–1203, 2015.

[55] M. J. Elman, A. Ayala, N. M. Bressler et al., "Intravitreal Ranibizumab for diabetic macular edema with prompt versus deferred laser treatment: 5-year randomized trial results," *Ophthalmology*, vol. 122, no. 2, pp. 375–381, 2015.

[56] S. B. Bressler, T. Almukhtar, A. Bhorade et al., "Repeated intravitreous ranibizumab injections for diabetic macular edema and the risk of sustained elevation of intraocular pressure or the need for ocular hypotensive treatment," *JAMA Ophthalmology*, vol. 133, no. 5, pp. 589–597, 2015.

[57] P. A. Campochiaro, R. Channa, B. B. Berger et al., "Treatment of diabetic macular edema with a designed ankyrin repeat protein that binds vascular endothelial growth factor: a phase I/II study," *American Journal of Ophthalmology*, vol. 155, no. 4, pp. 697–e2, 2013.

[58] R. Simo and C. Hernandez, "Novel approaches for treating diabetic retinopathy based on recent pathogenic evidence," *Progress in Retinal and Eye Research*, vol. 48, pp. 160–180, 2015.

[59] M. I. Nawaz, M. Abouammoh, H. A. Khan, A. S. Alhomida, M. F. Alfaran, and M. S. Ola, "Novel drugs and their targets in the potential treatment of diabetic retinopathy," *Medical Science Monitor*, vol. 19, no. 1, pp. 300–308, 2013.

[60] L. Wang, N. Wang, H. Tan, Y. Zhang, and Y. Feng, "Protective effect of a Chinese Medicine formula He-Ying-Qing-Re Formula on diabetic retinopathy," *Journal of Ethnopharmacology*, vol. 169, pp. 295–304, 2015.

[61] H. Huang, J. He, D. Johnson et al., "Deletion of placental growth factor prevents diabetic retinopathy and is associated with akt activation and HIF1α-VEGF pathway inhibition," *Diabetes*, vol. 64, no. 1, pp. 200–212, 2015.

[62] S. Babapoor-Farrokhran, K. Jee, B. Puchner et al., "Angiopoietin-like 4 is a potent angiogenic factor and a novel therapeutic target for patients with proliferative diabetic retinopathy," *Proceedings of the National Academy of Sciences of the United States*, vol. 112, no. 23, pp. E3030–E3039, 2015.

[63] Y. Jiang, Q. Zhang, and J. J. Steinle, "Intravitreal injection of IGFBP-3 restores normal insulin signaling in diabetic rat retina," *PLoS ONE*, vol. 9, no. 4, Article ID e93788, 2014.

[64] H. Huang, W. Li, J. He, P. Barnabie, D. Shealy, and S. A. Vinores, "Blockade of tumor necrosis factor alpha prevents complications of diabetic retinopathy," *Journal of Clinical& Experimental Ophthalmology*, vol. 5, no. 6, article 384, 2014.

[65] J. He, H. Wang, Y. Liu, W. Li, D. Kim, and H. Huang, "Blockade of vascular endothelial growth factor receptor 1 prevents inflammation and vascular leakage in diabetic retinopathy," *Journal of Ophthalmology*, vol. 2015, Article ID 605946, 11 pages, 2015.

[66] Y. Chen, Y. Hu, M. Lin et al., "Therapeutic effects of PPARα agonists on diabetic retinopathy in type 1 diabetes models," *Diabetes*, vol. 62, no. 1, pp. 261–272, 2013.

[67] A. C. Keech, P. Mitchell, P. A. Summanen et al., "Effect of fenofibrate on the need for laser treatment for diabetic retinopathy (FIELD study): a randomised controlled trial," *The Lancet*, vol. 370, no. 9600, pp. 1687–1697, 2007.

[68] R. Simó and C. Hernández, "Fenofibrate for diabetic retinopathy," *The Lancet*, vol. 370, no. 9600, pp. 1667–1668, 2007.

[69] N. Sharma, J. L. Ooi, J. Ong et al., "The use of fenofibrate in the management of patients with diabetic retinopathy: an evidence-based review," *Australian Family Physician*, vol. 44, no. 6, pp. 367–370, 2015.

[70] M. Tikhonenko, T. A. Lydic, Y. Wang et al., "Remodeling of retinal fatty acids in an animal model of diabetes: a decrease in long-chain polyunsaturated fatty acids is associated with a decrease in fatty acid elongases Elovl2 and Elovl4," *Diabetes*, vol. 59, no. 1, pp. 219–227, 2010.

[71] P. Sapieha, J. Chen, A. Stahl et al., "Omega-3 polyunsaturated fatty acids preserve retinal function in type 2 diabetic mice," *Nutrition and Diabetes*, vol. 2, article e36, 2012.

[72] N. Lois, R. V. McCarter, C. O'Neill, R. J. Medina, and A. W. Stitt, "Endothelial progenitor cells in diabetic retinopath," *Frontiers in Endocrinology*, vol. 5, article 44, 2014.

[73] F. Xiong, X. Du, J. Hu, T. Li, S. Du, and Q. Wu, "Altered retinal microRNA expression profiles in early diabetic retinopathy: an in silico analysis," *Current Eye Research*, vol. 39, no. 7, pp. 720–729, 2014.

[74] M. A. Ruiz, B. Feng, and S. Chakrabarti, "Polycomb repressive complex 2 regulates MiR-200b in retinal endothelial cells: potential relevance in diabetic retinopathy," *PLoS ONE*, vol. 10, no. 4, Article ID e0123987, 2015.

[75] R. Mortuza, B. Feng, and S. Chakrabarti, "miR-195 regulates SIRT1-mediated changes in diabetic retinopathy," *Diabetologia*, vol. 57, no. 5, pp. 1037–1046, 2014.

[76] E. Di Marco, J. C. Jha, A. Sharma, J. L. Wilkinson-Berka, K. A. Jandeleit-Dahm, and J. B. de Haan, "Are reactive oxygen species still the basis for diabetic complications?" *Clinical Science*, vol. 129, no. 2, pp. 199–216, 2015.

[77] M. Zhang, C. An, Y. Gao, R. K. Leak, J. Chen, and F. Zhang, "Emerging roles of Nrf2 and phase II antioxidant enzymes in neuroprotection," *Progress in Neurobiology*, vol. 100, no. 1, pp. 30–47, 2013.

[78] R. C. Taylor, G. Acquaah-Mensah, M. Singhal, D. Malhotra, and S. Biswal, "Network inference algorithms elucidate Nrf2 regulation of mouse lung oxidative stress," *PLoS Computational Biology*, vol. 4, no. 8, Article ID e1000166, 2008.

[79] S. M. Tan and J. B. de Haan, "Combating oxidative stress in diabetic complications with Nrf2 activators: how much is too much?" *Redox Report*, vol. 19, no. 3, pp. 107–117, 2014.

[80] J. Jeevanandam, M. K. Danquah, S. Debnath, V. S. Meka, and Y. S. Chan, "Opportunities for nano-formulations in type 2 diabetes mellitus treatments," *Current Pharmaceutical Biotechnology*, vol. 16, no. 10, pp. 853–870, 2015.

[81] D. Yohan and B. D. Chithrani, "Applications of nanoparticles in nanomedicine," *Journal of Biomedical Nanotechnology*, vol. 10, no. 9, pp. 2371–2392, 2014.

[82] X. Cai, S. A. Sezate, S. Seal, and J. F. McGinnis, "Sustained protection against photoreceptor degeneration in tubby mice by intravitreal injection of nanoceria," *Biomaterials*, vol. 33, no. 34, pp. 8771–8781, 2012.

[83] X. Cai, S. Seal, and J. F. McGinnis, "Sustained inhibition of neovascularization in vldlr-/- mice following intravitreal injection of cerium oxide nanoparticles and the role of the ASK1-P38/JNK-NF-κB pathway," *Biomaterials*, vol. 35, no. 1, pp. 249–258, 2014.

[84] L. Kong, X. Cai, X. Zhou et al., "Nanoceria extend photoreceptor cell lifespan in tubby mice by modulation of apoptosis/survival signaling pathways," *Neurobiology of Disease*, vol. 42, no. 3, pp. 514–523, 2011.

[85] X. Cai, J. Yodoi, S. Seal, and J. F. McGinnis, "Nanoceria and thioredoxin regulate a common antioxidative gene network in tubby mice," *Advances in Experimental Medicine and Biology*, vol. 801, pp. 829–836, 2014.

[86] A. Liew and T. O'Brien, "The potential of cell-based therapy for diabetes and diabetes-related vascular complications," *Current Diabetes Reports*, vol. 14, no. 3, article 469, 2014.

[87] V. Marchetti, T. U. Krohne, D. F. Friedlander, and M. Friedlander, "Stemming vision loss with stem cells," *The Journal of Clinical Investigation*, vol. 120, no. 9, pp. 3012–3021, 2010.

[88] Y. Huang, V. Enzmann, and S. T. Ildstad, "Stem cell-based therapeutic applications in retinal degenerative diseases," *Stem Cell Reviews and Reports*, vol. 7, no. 2, pp. 434–445, 2011.

[89] S. D. Schwartz, J.-P. Hubschman, G. Heilwell et al., "Embryonic stem cell trials for macular degeneration: a preliminary report," *The Lancet*, vol. 379, no. 9817, pp. 713–720, 2012.

[90] S. D. Schwartz, C. D. Regillo, B. L. Lam et al., "Human embryonic stem cell-derived retinal pigment epithelium in patients with age-related macular degeneration and Stargardt's macular dystrophy: follow-up of two open-label phase 1/2 studies," *The Lancet*, vol. 385, no. 9967, pp. 509–516, 2015.

[91] G. C. Davey, S. B. Patil, A. O'Loughlin, and T. O'Brien, "Mesenchymal stem cell-based treatment for microvascular and secondary complications of diabetes mellitus," *Frontiers in Endocrinology*, vol. 5, article 86, 2014.

[92] R. Megaw and B. Dhillon, "Stem cell therapies in the management of diabetic retinopathy," *Current Diabetes Reports*, vol. 14, no. 7, article 498, 2014.

[93] T. Asahara, T. Murohara, A. Sullivan et al., "Isolation of putative progenitor endothelial cells for angiogenesis," *Science*, vol. 275, no. 5302, pp. 964–967, 1997.

[94] G. Rajashekhar, A. Ramadan, C. Abburi et al., "Regenerative therapeutic potential of adipose stromal cells in early stage diabetic retinopathy," *PLoS ONE*, vol. 9, no. 1, Article ID e84671, 2014.

[95] T. A. Mendel, E. B. D. Clabough, D. S. Kao et al., "Pericytes derived from adipose-derived stem cells protect against retinal vasculopathy," *PLoS ONE*, vol. 8, no. 5, Article ID e65691, 2013.

[96] E. R. Burnight, P. D. Hsu, D. Ochoa et al., "Using RNA-mediated genome editing to create an animal model of retinal dystrophy for analysis of in vivo CRISPR/CAS9 treatment efficacy," *Investigative Ophthalmology & Visual Science*, vol. 56, abstract 3589, 2015, The ARVO Annual Meeting.

[97] E. M. Stone, "Gene editing for gene- and cell based treatment of inherited retinal disease," *Investigative Ophthalmology & Visual Science*, abstract 7, 2015, The ARVO Annual Meeting.

[98] S. H. Tsang, "Personalized medicine: patient specific stem cells, mouse models and therapy for retinal degenerations," The ARVO Annual Meeting, Denver, Colo, USA, abstract 8, May 2015.

[99] K. J. Wahlin, C. Kim, J. Maruotti et al., "Gene-edited human pluripotent stem cell derived 3D retinas for modeling photoreceptor development and disease," *Investigative Ophthalmology & Visual Science*, vol. 56, abstract 3596, 2015, The ARVO Annual Meeting.

15

Metabolic Health Has Greater Impact on Diabetes than Simple Overweight/Obesity in Mexican Americans

Shenghui Wu,[1] **Susan P. Fisher-Hoch,**[2] **Belinda Reninger,**[2]
Kristina Vatcheva,[2] **and Joseph B. McCormick**[2]

[1]*Department of Epidemiology & Biostatistics, University of Texas Health Science Center at San Antonio, Laredo Campus, Laredo, TX 78045, USA*
[2]*Division of Epidemiology, School of Public Health, University of Texas Health Science Center at Houston, Brownsville Campus, Brownsville, TX 78520, USA*

Academic Editor: Ed Randell

Purpose. To compare the risk for diabetes in each of 4 categories of metabolic health and BMI. *Methods.* Participants were drawn from the Cameron County Hispanic Cohort, a randomly selected Mexican American cohort in Texas on the US-Mexico border. Subjects were divided into 4 phenotypes according to metabolic health and BMI: metabolically healthy normal weight, metabolically healthy overweight/obese, metabolically unhealthy normal weight, and metabolically unhealthy overweight/obese. Metabolic health was defined as having less than 2 metabolic abnormalities. Overweight/obese status was assessed by BMI higher than $25\,kg/m^2$. Diabetes was defined by the 2010 ADA definition or by being on a diabetic medication. *Results.* The odds ratio for diabetes risk was 2.25 in the metabolically healthy overweight/obese phenotype (95% CI 1.34, 3.79), 3.78 (1.57, 9.09) in the metabolically unhealthy normal weight phenotype, and 5.39 (3.16, 9.20) in metabolically unhealthy overweight/obese phenotype after adjusting for confounding factors compared with the metabolically healthy normal weight phenotype. *Conclusions.* Metabolic health had a greater effect on the increased risk for diabetes than overweight/obesity. Greater focus on metabolic health might be a more effective target for prevention and control of diabetes than emphasis on weight loss alone.

1. Introduction

The proportion of overweight/obese adults in the US increased between 1980 and 2013 from 28.8% to 36.9% in men and from 29.8% to 38.0% in women [1]. Overweight/obesity increases the risk for type 2 diabetes mellitus [2, 3]. However, being metabolically unhealthy also increases the risk for type 2 diabetes [4–6]. Though these findings suggest that the risk for type 2 diabetes associated with overweight/obesity is influenced by the coexistence of metabolic abnormalities, the independent impact of these two conditions is unclear. Metabolically unhealthy normal weight (MUHNW) subjects are individuals with normal weight but with metabolic abnormalities [7, 8], but the phenotype is ill-defined. Among normal weight individuals aged 20 years or older in the Third National Health and Nutrition Examination Survey, 4.6% of men and 6.2% of women had three or more metabolic

abnormalities [9]. Because MUHNW subjects are not overweight or obese, they may not be aware of their risks and may be missed and therefore may not benefit from adequate prevention. Nevertheless, MUHNW carries a significant risk for cardiovascular diseases [10, 11] and mortality [12]. The findings from several studies have shown the increased risk of diabetes in MUHNW individuals [4–6] compared with metabolically healthy normal weight (MHNW) individuals in different ethnicities, but only one study was conducted in Mexican Americans [6].

There is no consensus on the risk presented by the metabolically healthy overweight/obese (MHOW) phenotype [4, 5]. Evidence regarding the risk of diabetes associated with the MHOW phenotype is also uncertain. It has been reported that MHOW individuals may be more likely to develop incident diabetes compared with normal weight individuals [4–6]; however data from Kangbuk Samsung Health

Study of more than 6 thousand individuals did not show a significant association with diabetes [5] and data in Mexican Americans is in any event limited [6]. Although metabolically unhealthy overweight/obese (MUHOW) subjects showed a higher risk of diabetes than MHNW phenotype [4–6, 13], only a few studies compared the diabetes risk between MUHOW, MUHNW, MHOW, and MHNW phenotypes [4–6] and only one was conducted in Mexican Americans [6].

Mexican Americans have higher prevalence of diabetes, overweight/obesity, and metabolic disturbances than non-Hispanic Whites [14–16]. The objective of this study was to compare the risk for diabetes among the 4 phenotypes divided by metabolic health and overweight/obesity status in a randomly selected cohort of Mexican American subjects.

2. Materials and Methods

2.1. Study Participants. This study was approved by the Committee for the Protection of Human Subjects of the UT Health, Houston and the Institutional Review Board of the University of the Texas Health Science Center, San Antonio. All study participants gave written informed consent. This cross-sectional analysis used data from the Cameron County Hispanic Cohort (CCHC), a homogenous community-dwelling Mexican American ongoing cohort study [17, 18]. Study subjects were recruited from randomly selected blocks according to the 2000 Census as described previously [17, 18]. At the baseline survey conducted between 2003 and 2014, 3,257 participants aged 18 years or older were recruited from their households in predominantly Mexican American cities along the Rio Grande border with Mexico. To reduce the effect of type I diabetes on the results, the participants who had diabetes before 18 years were excluded ($n = 10$).

All subjects responded to a detailed baseline survey of demographic characteristics, lifestyle including diet, physical activity, family, and medical history, and other exposures. Participants were asked to fast for at least 10 hours overnight before a clinic visit at the clinical research unit. Anthropometric measurements, including current weight, height, and circumferences of the waist and hip, were also taken [17, 18].

Weight was measured to the nearest tenth of a kilogram and height to the nearest tenth of a centimeter. Body mass index (BMI) was calculated as weight in kilograms divided by height squared in meters (kg/m^2). Waist circumference (WC) was measured at the level of the umbilicus and hip circumference (HC) at the level of maximum width of the buttocks with participants in a standing position and breathing normally, to the nearest 0.2 cm. Waist-to-hip ratio (WHR) was calculated as WC divided by HC [17]. Body fat percentage was estimated using the resistance values from the Quantum X bioelectric body composition analyzer with the sex-specific equations from Sun et al. [19]. The average of 3 blood pressure (BP) measurements taken 5 minutes apart were used.

All participants completed a detailed baseline survey that collected information on demographic characteristics, lifestyle and dietary histories, medical history, and other exposures. Physical activity was assessed using the International Physical Activity Questionnaire (IPAQ) short form [20]; reported minutes of physical activity per week were weighted by a metabolic equivalent (MET, multiples of resting energy expenditure) resulting in a physical activity estimate expressed as MET-minutes per week [20]. Physical activity energy expenditure was estimated using standard metabolic equivalent (MET) values [20].

2.2. Laboratory Measurements. All participants donated a blood sample at baseline. After collection, samples were placed on ice and centrifuged within 30 minutes of collection. Following processing and aliquoting, all samples were stored at $-80°C$ until laboratory analyses were conducted. Laboratory studies performed included fasting lipid panel, hemoglobin (Hb) A1c, fasting plasma glucose, and fasting serum insulin. Homeostasis model assessment insulin resistance index (HOMA-IR) was calculated as fasting glucose (mg/dL)/18 × fasting insulin (mU/L)/22.5 [21]. High sensitivity C-reactive protein (CRP) levels were measured using Quantikine ELISA kit (R & D Systems, Inc., Minneapolis, USA).

2.3. Identification of the Overweight/Obese and Metabolic Health. Participants were categorized as overweight/obese or with normal weight using a BMI cutoff of 25.0 kg/m^2 [1] and then were further categorized as metabolically healthy or unhealthy. Metabolic health was defined as having <2 of the following metabolic abnormalities: systolic BP (SBP) $\geq$ 130 mmHg and/or diastolic BP (DBP) $\geq$ 85 mmHg or on antihypertensive medication; triglyceride $\geq$ 150 mg/dL; high-density lipoprotein cholesterol < 40 mg/dL in men or <50 mg/dL in women; or HOMA-IR value > 90th percentile [22, 23]. Waist circumference was not included due to its high correlation with BMI [22]. To avoid bias we did not use blood glucose levels nor diabetes medication in the definition of metabolic health so as to compare the risk for diabetes in 4 phenotypes of metabolic health and BMI.

According to the above criteria, participants were divided into four phenotypes:

(1) MHNW: metabolically healthy, normal weight: BMI < 25 kg/m^2 and <2 metabolic risk factor;

(2) MHOW: metabolically healthy, overweight/obese: BMI $\geq$ 25 kg/m^2 and <2 metabolic risk factor;

(3) MUHNW: metabolically unhealthy, normal weight: BMI < 25 kg/m^2 and $\geq$2 metabolic risk factor;

(4) MUHOW: metabolically unhealthy, overweight/obese: BMI $\geq$ 25 kg/m^2 and $\geq$2 metabolic risk factor.

2.4. Identification of Diabetes. Diabetes was identified by the 2010 definition of diabetes of the American Diabetes Association [24] or the participants reporting being told by a health care provider that they had diabetes or if they were taking hypoglycemic medication.

2.5. *Statistical Analysis.* Descriptive results and the models reported in this paper were adjusted for the probability of sampling using weights taking into consideration clustering effects arising from the census block and household [17]. Log-transformation was conducted to normalize the distribution of the biomarkers studied as appropriate. Survey-weighted linear regression was used to obtain the t-test statistics to compare phenotypes and to be used for multiple pairwise mean comparisons for continuous data. Survey-weighted chi-square test was used to obtain Rao-Scott F adjusted chi-square statistic to compare phenotypes for categorical data. Survey-weighted logistic regression modeling was performed to estimate the odds ratios (ORs) for diabetes risk and their 95% confidence intervals (CIs) by the metabolic health and overweight/obese phenotype phenotypes adjusting for other covariates. Initially, a multivariable survey-weighted logistic regression model was created to identify independent factors associated with diabetes, among variables including the overweight/obese phenotypes, age, gender, education, reported minutes of physical activity per week, servings of fruits and vegetables per day, and alcohol drinking and cigarette smoking status. Variables that were not significant and were not confounders were excluded from the final model. The interaction effects between the independent variables were tested. The analysis involved in physical activity and dietary data was conducted in 2,044 participants because the interview was only administered in these subjects.

To compare the risk of diabetes in different metabolic health and overweight/obese phenotypes, we also used a restricted cubic spline logistic regression analysis [25] to evaluate the risk of diabetes with age (P < 0.0001 for all participants) stratified by metabolic health and over-weight/obese phenotypes. Knots were placed at the 5th, 50th, and 95th percentiles of the distribution of age at enrollment. We excluded participants whose age at enrollment was below 20 or above 70 from the restricted cubic spline model to minimize the influence of outliers.

Sensitivity analyses were performed including fasting glucose > 100 mg/dL or on hypoglycemic medication as a component for the definition of metabolic health (metabolically healthy, 0 metabolic abnormalities; metabolically unhealthy, ≥2 metabolic abnormalities) [22, 23]. Participants were categorized as overweight (25–29.9 kg/m^2) or obese (≥30 kg/m^2) using BMI cutoffs of 25.0 and 30 kg/m^2 [1] and separate analyses by overweight and obesity were also conducted. Statistical analyses were carried out by using SAS version 9.3 (SAS Institute, Cary, NC). All statistical tests were based on two-sided probability.

3. Results

At the time of this study a total of 3,257 individuals were enrolled in the CCHC, 2,893 participants from Brownsville and 242 participants from Harlingen (Lower Rio Grande Valley) and 138 participants from Laredo (Webb County), Texas. Among 3,247 remaining participants after excluding 10 subjects who developed diabetes before 18 years of age (to minimize potential type I diabetes), 475 subjects (14.6%) were classified as MHNW, 1,594 (49.1%) as MHOW, 72 (2.2%) as MUHNW, and 1,106 (34.1%) as MUHOW (Table 1). Mean age of this subset was 46 years; 34% were male. A total of 36.3% (n = 1,178) were classified as metabolically unhealthy. Detailed characteristics by overweight, obesity, and metabolic health were shown in Supplemental Table 1 (see Supplementary Material available online at http://dx.doi.org/10.1155/2016/4094876).

Metabolically unhealthy phenotypes showed significantly elevated mean values of total cholesterol, triglycerides, high-density lipid cholesterol (HDLC), fasting glucose and insulin, HOMA IR, HbA1c, CRP, and blood pressure compared with metabolically healthy phenotypes. They were more likely to be older, cigarette smokers and unemployed, less well educated, and less likely to meet the recommended guidelines for physical activity of more than 600 MET-minutes/week. They had lower household income but more frequent family history of diabetes (all Ps < 0.05). There was no difference in gender between metabolically unhealthy and healthy phenotypes (Table 1).

Overweight/obese phenotypes were also more likely to be older, less well educated, and cigarette smoking, had lower incomes but more frequent family history of diabetes, and showed significantly elevated mean values of total cholesterol, triglycerides, HDLC, fasting glucose and insulin, HOMA IR, HbA1c, CRP, blood pressure, BMI, WC, WHR, and body fat percentage compared with normal weight phenotypes (all Ps < 0.05). There was no difference in gender, employment status, and physical activity between overweight/obese and normal weight phenotypes (Table 1).

Seventy-two participants of the cohort (2.2%) were classified as metabolically unhealthy, normal weight. Compared with other three phenotypes, MUHNW subjects were more likely to be older, unemployed, and cigarette smoking, were least likely to meet the recommended guidelines for physical activity of more than 600 MET-minutes/week, and had least income and worst mean values in total cholesterol, SBP, and HbA1c (all Ps < 0.05) (Table 1).

A total of 878 (27.04%) participants had diabetes (Table 2). Among the four phenotypes the MHNW phenotype had the lowest rates of diabetes (12%) and the MUHOW phenotype had the highest (40.3%) (P < 0.0001) (Figure 1). Metabolically unhealthy subjects showed significantly higher diabetes prevalence than metabolically healthy subjects (40.3% versus 19.6%; P < 0.0001). Overweight/obese phenotypes showed significantly higher diabetes prevalence than normal weight phenotypes (29.4% versus 15.2%; P < 0.0001).

Overweight/obese individuals showed an OR of having diabetes of 2.06 (95% CI: 1.33–3.21) after adjusting for age and metabolic health. Poor metabolic health was positively related to the increased risk of diabetes (OR = 2.46; 95% CI: 1.88–3.21) after adjusting for age and overweight/obesity, suggesting that being metabolically unhealthy carried a higher risk for diabetes than being overweight/obese (2.46 versus 2.06). The risk of diabetes by categories of BMI and metabolic status is shown in Table 2. In a multivariable adjusted logistic regression model with diabetes as the dependent variable, MHOW subjects showed an OR of having diabetes of 2.25 (95% CI 1.34–3.79), MUNW individuals showed an OR of

TABLE 1: Cohort demographics and metabolic characteristics stratified by overweight/obese type and metabolic health status: Cameron County Health Cohort Study (2003–2014)[1,2].

Variable	Total (n = 3247)	Metabolically healthy		Metabolically unhealthy		P value
		Normal weight (n = 475, 14.63%)	Overweight/obese (n = 1594, 49.09%)	Normal weight (n = 72, 2.22%)	Overweight/obese (n = 1106, 34.06%)	
Categorical variables, n (%)						
Men	1108 (34.11)	139 (28.64)	544 (38.09)	25 (33.75)	400 (33.63)	0.054
Employed	1618 (49.83)	242 (50.95)	822 (51.57)	25 (34.72)	529 (47.83)	0.03
Education, below high school	1693 (52.14)	195 (41.05)	813 (51.00)	37 (51.39)	648 (58.59)	<0.0001
Met minimum recommendations for physical activity of ≥ 600 MET-minutes/week	337 (10.38)	48 (10.11)	192 (12.05)	1 (1.39)	96 (8.68)	0.02
Met recommendations of ≥ 5 servings of fruit and vegetables per day	113 (3.48)	9 (1.89)	67 (4.20)	4 (5.56)	33 (2.98)	0.32
Current smokers	495 (15.24)	64 (13.47)	222 (13.93)	14 (19.44)	195 (17.63)	0.02
Ever smokers	984 (30.3)	119 (25.05)	478 (29.99)	21 (29.17)	366 (33.09)	0.0003
Ever alcohol drinkers	1230 (37.88)	186 (39.16)	601 (37.70)	20 (27.78)	423 (38.25)	0.79
Family history of diabetes	1749 (53.87)	165 (34.74)	876 (54.96)	41 (56.94)	667 (60.31)	<0.0001
Continuous variables, mean (SE)						
Age at enrollment (years)	46.00 (0.68)	40.59 (1.90)	44.57 (0.78)	53.96 (3.04)	49.80 (1.27)	<0.0001
Annual household income (US dollars)	22360 (872.29)	19617 (1724.54)	24563 (1284.32)	14043 (1351.98)	20561 (1084.07)	<0.0001
Years of education	10.41 (0.15)	11.58 (0.39)	10.71 (0.17)	10.24 (0.69)	9.56 (0.25)	<0.0001
MET minutes/wk. of all activity	1913.02 (384.71)	1393.1 (445.87)	2384.2 (646.06)	167.15 (107.01)	1447.24 (591.89)	0.0002
MET minutes/wk. of moderate and vigorous activity	1217.83 (154.52)	1115.31 (261.88)	1572.37 (274.14)	67.47 (48.29)	768.36 (151.68)	<0.0001
Total cholesterol (mg/dL)	183.58 (1.14)	176.41 (2.62)	182.76 (1.67)	188.24 (7.55)	187.66 (1.85)	<0.0001
Triglycerides (mg/dL)	162.37 (3.62)	98.8 (3.25)	124.83 (3.51)	195.41 (13.61)	238.58 (7.11)	<0.0001
HDL cholesterol (mg/dL)	46.45 (0.38)	53.73 (1.06)	49.41 (0.44)	42.67 (1.32)	39.64 (0.45)	<0.0001
LDL cholesterol (mg/dL)	107.38 (1.00)	103.14 (2.28)	109.86 (1.49)	108.64 (6.82)	105.83 (1.72)	0.06
Body mass index (kg/m^2)	30.99 (0.21)	22.44 (0.16)	31.56 (0.24)	22.53 (0.47)	34.08 (0.32)	<0.0001
Waist circumference (cm)	102.87 (0.47)	84.69 (0.91)	103.35 (0.52)	86.98 (0.91)	110.3 (0.67)	<0.0001
Waist-to-hip ratio	0.93 (0.002)	0.88 (0.01)	0.93 (0.003)	0.89 (0.01)	0.96 (0.003)	<0.0001
Body fat (%)	35.59 (0.47)	25.80 (0.88)	36.51 (0.65)	27.69 (3.39)	38.33 (0.76)	<0.0001
C-reactive protein (mg/L)	3.90 (1.04)	1.48 (1.08)	2.18 (1.09)	2.77 (1.27)	5.75 (1.05)	<0.0001
Systolic blood pressure (mmHg)	116.92 (0.55)	107.53 (1.38)	113.3 (0.54)	126.04 (3.38)	125.42 (0.99)	<0.0001
Diastolic blood pressure (mmHg)	71.19 (0.32)	66.24 (1.18)	70.07 (0.35)	71.89 (1.51)	74.83 (0.57)	<0.0001
Insulin (mg/dL)[3]	12.55 (1.02)	7.69 (1.06)	11.47 (1.02)	9.12 (1.14)	17.29 (1.03)	<0.0001
Fasting blood glucose (mg/dL)[3]	105.64 (1.01)	93.69 (1.01)	101.49 (1.01)	111.05 (1.06)	119.10 (1.02)	<0.0001
HOMA IR[3]	3.29 (1.02)	1.82 (1.07)	2.89 (1.02)	2.53 (1.17)	5.05 (1.03)	<0.0001
HbA1c (%)[3]	5.53 (1.01)	5.05 (1.02)	5.31 (1.01)	6.23 (1.04)	5.93 (1.02)	<0.0001

[1] LDL: low-density lipoprotein; Hb: hemoglobin; HDL: high-density lipoprotein; HOMA IR: homeostatic model assessment insulin resistance; MET: metabolic equivalent.

[2] All descriptive results and the models were adjusted for the probability of sampling using weights taking into consideration clustering effects arising from the same census block and household. Linear regression models were used for continuous variables and Rao-Scott F adjusted chi-square statistic for categorical variables.

[3] Geometric concentrations.

TABLE 2: Diabetes by overweight/obese type and metabolic health status.

Diabetes	Metabolically healthy		Metabolically unhealthy		P value
	Normal weight (n = 475)	Overweight/obese (n = 1594)	Normal weight (n = 72)	Overweight/obese (n = 1106)	
Primary analysis					
Frequency					
Yes [n, (%)]	57 (12.00)	349 (21.89)	26 (36.11)	446 (40.33)	<0.0001[1]
No [n, (%)]	401 (84.42)	1208 (75.78)	42 (58.33)	641 (57.96)	
Weighted OR (95% CI)					
Unadjusted model	Reference	2.30 (1.47, 3.60)	5.20 (2.41, 11.19)	6.23 (3.94, 9.85)	<0.0001[2]
Multivariable adjusted model 1[3]	Reference	2.25 (1.34, 3.79)	3.78 (1.57, 9.09)	5.39 (3.16, 9.20)	<0.0001[2]
Multivariable adjusted model 2[4]	Reference	2.14 (1.07, 4.28)	3.18 (1.02, 9.92)	5.01 (2.43, 10.34)	<0.0001[2]
Sensitivity analysis[5]					
Frequency					
Yes [n, (%)]	41 (9.53)	145 (12.49)	42 (35.90)	650 (42.24)	<0.0001[1]
No [n, (%)]	375 (87.21)	982 (84.58)	68 (58.12)	867 (56.34)	
Weighted OR (95% CI)					
Unadjusted model	Reference	1.48 (0.87, 2.54)	4.25 (1.74, 10.37)	7.81 (4.56, 13.37)	<0.0001[2]
Multivariable adjusted model 1[3]	Reference	1.47 (0.83, 2.61)	2.93 (1.04, 8.23)	6.25 (3.54, 11.02)	<0.0001[2]
Multivariable adjusted model 2[4]	Reference	1.36 (0.59, 3.13)	3.23 (1.08, 10.01)	6.57 (2.81, 15.36)	<0.0001[2]

[1] F approximation of Rao-Scott design adjusted chi-square test P value.
[2] P values from Wald chi-square test for the effect of overweight/obese phenotype.
[3] Adjusted for age at enrollment. Other covariates were not significant and not included in the final model. The models were adjusted for the probability of sampling using weights taking into consideration clustering effects arising from the same census block and household.
[4] Adjusted for age at enrollment and family history of diabetes. Restricted to the participants who had data for family history of diabetes (n = 2,234, 68%).
[5] The definition of metabolically health included glucose component.

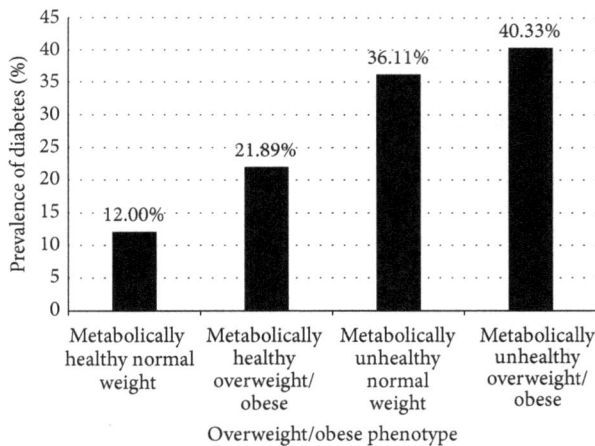

FIGURE 1: Prevalence of diabetes among Mexican Americans within each overweight/obese phenotype. Black bars indicate prevalence rate. Diabetes prevalence was different by overweight/obese phenotype (P < 0.0001).

3.78 (95% CI 1.57–9.09), and MUHOW subjects showed an OR of 5.39 (95% CI 3.16–9.20) after adjusting for confounding factors with the MHNW phenotype as the reference (Table 2). The biggest effect comes from being metabolically unhealthy and normal weight: the adjusted odds ratio for this group compared to the metabolically healthy and normal weight one is 3.8, while the OR for metabolically unhealthy and normal weight compared to metabolically healthy and normal weight is just over 2 (Table 2). The addition of metabolically unhealthy phenotypes to obesity increases the OR for diabetes to over 5-fold (Table 2). The ORs for the risk of diabetes were greater than 1 for the metabolically unhealthy phenotype and were much higher than the ORs for MHNW and MHOW phenotypes: the difference of ORs between MUHNW and MHNW phenotypes was 278%; and the difference of ORs between MUHOW and MHOW phenotypes was 140%, while the difference of ORs between MHOW and MHNW phenotypes was 125%, and the difference of ORs between MUHNW and MUHOW phenotypes was 43%. These comparisons suggested that the risk of diabetes in metabolically unhealthy phenotype was higher than healthy phenotype in any category of BMI, and the metabolic health is more important than simple overweight/obesity. Restricted to the participants who had available data for family history of diabetes (68%), the ORs in each phenotype were not materially changed. When fasting blood glucose > 100 mg/dL or being on hypoglycemic medication was included as a component for the definition of metabolic health in the sensitivity analysis, the correlation was not significant for the MHOW phenotype, the correlation for the MUHNW phenotype remained similar, and the correlation for the MUHOW phenotype became slightly stronger. The sensitivity analysis results further suggested that the metabolic health is more important than simple overweight/obesity. Supplemental Table 2 further showed the risk of diabetes by overweight, obese, and metabolic status. Similar patterns as

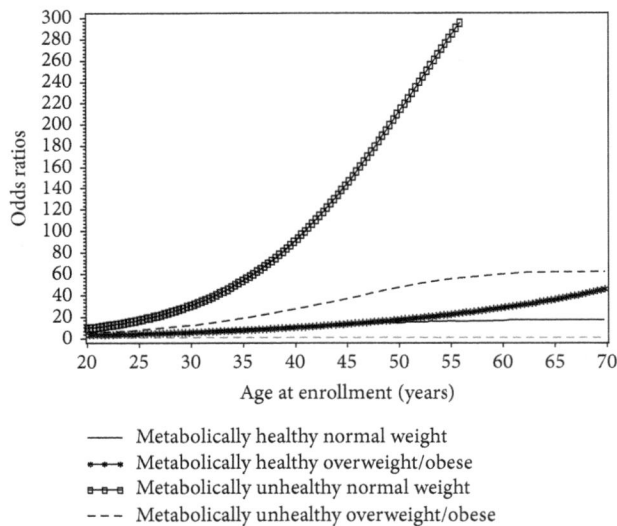

FIGURE 2: Smoothed plot for odds ratios (ORs) of the diabetes risk according to age at enrollment. Subjects were divided into four phenotypes according to overweight/obese phenotype and metabolic health status. The ORs were estimated by using the restricted cubic spline logistic regression models with knots placed at the 5th, 50th, and 95th percentiles of age at enrollment. The models were adjusted for the probability of sampling using weights taking into consideration clustering effects arising from the same census block and household. The linear correlation between age at enrollment and the risk of diabetes in each phenotype was significant (P = 0.02, 0.0001, 0.04, and <0.0001 for phenotypes with metabolically healthy normal weight, metabolically healthy overweight/obesity, metabolically unhealthy normal weight, and metabolically unhealthy overweight/obesity, resp.).

in Table 2 indicated that the risk of diabetes in metabolically unhealthy phenotype was higher than healthy phenotype, and the metabolic health is more important than simple overweight or obesity.

Figure 2 visually depicts the shape of the correlation between age and diabetes risk in four phenotypes after adjusting for potential confounding variables in a restricted cubic spline model. Age was positively and approximately linearly associated with the risk for diabetes in each phenotype (all Ps < 0.05). Metabolically unhealthy phenotypes had higher ORs than their corresponding counterparts in any category of BMI, and MUHNW phenotype had the highest ORs in the four phenotypes. MHOW subjects had higher ORs than MHNW subjects, and the latter had the lowest ORs in the four phenotypes.

4. Discussion

In a Mexican American cohort metabolically unhealthy subjects showed significantly increased risk for diabetes compared with metabolically healthy subjects in any category of BMI. Compared with the metabolically healthy normal weight participants (MHNW), the metabolically unhealthy, regardless of their BMI (MUHNW and MUHOW), and the metabolically healthy obese (MHOW) phenotypes had

significantly increased risk of diabetes. MUHNW individuals had a fourfold increased risk and MUHOW individuals had a fivefold increased risk for diabetes compared with the MHNW phenotype. Cubic spline interpolation showed that the risk of diabetes with age was higher in metabolically unhealthy phenotype than metabolically healthy phenotype in any category of BMI. The significance of these observations is that poor metabolic health puts the individual at greater risk of diabetes than obesity alone.

A high proportion of the Mexican Americans in our population are metabolically unhealthy (36.3%) but over half (59.9%) if the definition of metabolic health includes a glucose component. Because we wanted to examine the relationship of diabetes, a disease of glucose metabolism, we excluded that from our criteria for metabolic abnormalities, yet metabolic abnormalities remain the major association with diabetes. Others have shown a high prevalence of metabolically unhealthy Mexican Americans (30%) [6]. In general, Mexican Americans also have high prevalence of diabetes, overweight/obesity, and metabolic abnormalities compared to non-Hispanic Whites [14–16]. Using both logistic regression and cubic spline models, being metabolically unhealthy posed a significantly higher risk for diabetes than being overweight. Similar observations have been made in a prospective cohort study in 6,748 Koreans [5], although the results were not all statistically significant among different overweight/obese and metabolic health phenotypes [5]. Furthermore, we found that metabolically unhealthy overweight/obese individuals were more likely to develop incident diabetes compared with their normal weight counterparts which was consistent with other findings [4–6]. An important element here is the identification of those with metabolic risk factors but who are not obese since they are at high risk for diabetes but less likely to be identified early and provided prevention education. These individuals may well be overlooked in screening programs.

It is not surprising that poor metabolic health puts the individual at a higher risk of diabetes than overweight/obesity alone. In our study, metabolically unhealthy phenotype tended to do less exercise and had lower education and less income level but had increased cigarette smoking compared with metabolically healthy phenotypes. In particular, the MUHNW phenotype showed the lowest proportion of subjects who met minimum recommendations for physical activity of ≥600 MET-minutes/week despite their normal weight, although physical activity was not significant in multivariable analysis for the risk of diabetes. Because physical activity was not correlated with diabetes risk (P = 0.18) and metabolic health (P = 0.07) in logistic regression models and it was not statistically significant in the multivariable adjusted model (P = 0.46), it was not adjusted for in the final model.

Metabolically unhealthy phenotype had higher markers of inflammation which may be the key underlying pathology. Metabolically unhealthy subjects showed significantly higher levels of CRP compared with their metabolically healthy counterparts, consistent with the known role of systemic inflammation in the risk of diabetes. Several conditions that are driven by inflammatory processes are also associated with diabetes, including rheumatoid arthritis, gout, psoriasis, and Crohn's disease, and various anti-inflammatory drugs have been approved or are in late stages of development for the treatment of these conditions [26]. Another important difference between metabolically healthy and unhealthy phenotypes was markedly higher dyslipidemia, measured as hypertriglyceridemia and low HDL-C, fasting glucose, high blood pressure, or insulin resistance observed in the metabolically unhealthy phenotype. These results suggest the importance of lifestyle modification and control of systemic inflammation in maintaining metabolic health and normoglycemia, not the simple reduction in body weight, although physical activity was not significant in multivariable analysis for the risk of diabetes.

Our study found a positive dose-response with approximately linear relationship between age and the risk of diabetes in each phenotype, stratified by overweight/obesity and metabolic health. Metabolically unhealthy phenotypes had higher risk than their corresponding counterparts in any category of BMI, and MUHNW phenotype had the highest ORs in the four phenotypes. To our knowledge, this is the first study to find the risk of diabetes with age higher in metabolically unhealthy phenotypes than in metabolically healthy phenotypes in any category of BMI. The Korean Healthy Twin Study ($n = 2,687$) reported that the risk of diabetes was 4.4-fold higher in MUHNW individuals than in MHNW individuals and 3.3-fold higher in MUHOW subjects than in MHNW subjects [27]. Despite a normal weight identical to the MHNW subjects, MUHNW subjects in our study presented an increased fasting serum insulin and blood glucose, HOMA IR, and HbA1c. This phenomenon may be associated with impaired insulin sensitivity (euglycemic hyperinsulinemic clamp or oral glucose tolerance test) [11, 28]. Although the mechanism is still not clear, at least we are now aware that the MUHNW individuals are a target population in which to identify and to prevent diabetes [27].

Previous studies have suggested that metabolic healthy overweight/obesity was not a benign condition [4–6]. MHOW individuals may be more likely to have diabetes compared with metabolically healthy normal weight peers [4, 6]. Our study found that MHOW subjects had a significant 2.14-fold elevated risk of diabetes (Table 2) and they were more likely to do this before 50 years of age compared with their MHNW counterparts (Figure 1). However, in our sensitivity analysis including fasting glucose as a component for the definition of metabolic health, the risk of diabetes was not significant for the MHOW phenotype. Clearly, the risk of diabetes in MHOW populations needs to be further investigated.

Although a small proportion of the subjects (2.22%) were classified as metabolically unhealthy normal weight phenotype, their risk for diabetes was higher than MHNW and MHOW (Table 2) and they had the highest ORs for the correlation between age and diabetes risk in the four phenotypes (Figure 2). The proportion might be increased if there is no effort to protect this population, because these subjects are not overweight or obese and they may escape detection and therefore not benefit from adequate treatment or prevention measures. Furthermore, the interventions to boost metabolic health involved changes in lifestyles such as diet, exercise, and behavior (smoking and others) which may not be related to overweight/obesity [29]. Therefore, it is very important to make efforts on improving metabolic health in any categories of BMI. The MUHNW phenotype needs to be included within the scope of prevention and control, but should not be ignored.

There are some methodological limitations in our research. The study was cross-sectional in design; thus, only association but not causal relationship may be inferred. Prospective studies are needed to further investigate whether metabolic health is more important than overweight/obesity alone. Our longitudinal data currently being collected will provide that opportunity. We could not completely rule out the possibility of residual confounding due to unmeasured or inadequately measured covariates such as the missing values with some variables.

This study had several strengths. First, this is a general population-based randomly selected Mexican American cohort, thus avoiding bias inherent in studies drawn from clinic populations or other nonrandomly selected populations with established disease or mixed ethnicity. Second, detailed information on a wide range of factors related to diabetes was available, allowing us to get a relatively comprehensive analysis of the affecting factors. Third, cubic spline interpolation was used to compare the dose-response correlation between age and the diabetes risk in different metabolic health and overweight/obese phenotypes and suggested the importance of metabolic health compared to overweight/obesity for the risk of diabetes associated with age. Finally, published studies generally only compared the disease status between obesity (BMI $\geq 30 \, \text{kg/m}^2$) and normal weight phenotypes stratified by the metabolic health status, while the risk of diseases for the phenotype with BMI 25–30 kg/m^2 was neglected [6, 30]. However, previous studies [2, 3] and our study found that overweight/obese individuals (BMI $\geq 25 \, \text{kg/m}^2$) were at a higher risk of diabetes compared with normal weight individuals.

In conclusion, in our cohort those who had more than two markers indicating unhealthy metabolism had statistically higher prevalence and odds of having diabetes compared to those with healthy metabolism suggesting a higher risk of diabetes adjusting for age, gender or BMI, and overweight/obese. Therefore, being metabolically unhealthy is likely more important for the risk of diabetes than simply being overweight/obese. Efforts need to be focused on improving metabolic health in all categories of BMI. Early lifestyle intervention in these populations is likely to be more effective than simple weight loss.

Conflict of Interests

The authors declare that there is no conflict of interests regarding the publication of this paper.

Authors' Contribution

The authors' responsibilities were as follows: Joseph B. McCormick and Susan P. Fisher-Hoch designed research;

Joseph B. McCormick, Susan P. Fisher-Hoch, and Belinda Reninger conducted research; Shenghui Wu analyzed data; Kristina Vatcheva provided statistical support; Shenghui Wu, Joseph B. McCormick, and Susan P. Fisher-Hoch wrote the paper. All authors read and approved the final paper.

Acknowledgments

The authors thank their cohort team, particularly, Rocio Uribe (Brownsville), Becky Erazo (Laredo), Ariana Garza (Harlingen), and their teams, who recruited and documented the participants. The authors also thank Marcela Morris and other laboratory staff for their contributions and Christina Villarreal for administrative support. The authors thank Valley Baptist Medical Center, Brownsville, Texas, for providing them space for their Center for Clinical and Translational Science Clinical Research Unit. The authors also thank the community of Brownsville, Laredo, and Harlingen and the participants who so willingly participated in this study in their city. This work was supported by MD000170 P20 funded by the National Center on Minority Health and Health Disparities, the Centers for Translational Science Award 1U54RR023417-01 from the National Center, and the Centers for Disease Control Award RO1 DP000210-01 for Research Resources.

References

[1] M. Ng, T. Fleming, M. Robinson et al., "Global, regional, and national prevalence of overweight and obesity in children and adults during 1980–2013: a systematic analysis for the Global Burden of Disease Study 2013," The Lancet, vol. 384, no. 9945, pp. 766–781, 2014.

[2] G. Whitlock, S. Lewington, P. Sherliker et al., "Body-mass index and cause-specific mortality in 900 000 adults: collaborative analyses of 57 prospective studies," The Lancet, vol. 373, no. 9669, pp. 1083–1096, 2009.

[3] J. A. Bell, M. Kivimaki, and M. Hamer, "Metabolically healthy obesity and risk of incident type 2 diabetes: a meta-analysis of prospective cohort studies," Obesity Reviews, vol. 15, no. 6, pp. 504–515, 2014.

[4] Y. Heianza, K. Kato, S. Kodama et al., "Risk of the development of Type 2 diabetes in relation to overall obesity, abdominal obesity and the clustering of metabolic abnormalities in Japanese individuals: does metabolically healthy overweight really exist? The Niigata Wellness study," Diabetic Medicine, vol. 32, no. 5, pp. 665–672, 2015.

[5] E. Rhee, M. K. Lee, J. D. Kim et al., "Metabolic health is a more important determinant for diabetes development than simple obesity: a 4-year retrospective longitudinal study," PLoS ONE, vol. 9, no. 5, Article ID e98369, 2014.

[6] K. Aung, C. Lorenzo, M. A. Hinojosa, and S. M. Haffner, "Risk of developing diabetes and cardiovascular disease in metabolically unhealthy normal-weight and metabolically healthy obese individuals," Journal of Clinical Endocrinology and Metabolism, vol. 99, no. 2, pp. 462–468, 2014.

[7] N. Ruderman, D. Chisholm, X. Pi-Sunyer, and S. Schneider, "The metabolically obese, normal-weight individual revisited," Diabetes, vol. 47, no. 5, pp. 699–713, 1998.

[8] N. B. Ruderman, S. H. Schneider, and P. Berchtold, "The 'metabolically-obese,' normal-weight individual," American Journal of Clinical Nutrition, vol. 34, no. 8, pp. 1617–1621, 1981.

[9] Y.-W. Park, S. Zhu, L. Palaniappan, S. Heshka, M. R. Carnethon, and S. B. Heymsfield, "The metabolic syndrome: prevalence and associated risk factor findings in the US population from the Third National Health and Nutrition Examination Survey, 1988–1994," Archives of Internal Medicine, vol. 163, no. 4, pp. 427–436, 2003.

[10] S. T. Laing, B. Smulevitz, K. P. Vatcheva et al., "Subclinical atherosclerosis and obesity phenotypes among Mexican Americans," Journal of the American Heart Association, vol. 4, no. 3, Article ID e001540, 2015.

[11] F. Conus, R. Rabasa-Lhoret, and F. Péronnet, "Characteristics of metabolically obese normal-weight (MONW) subjects," Applied Physiology, Nutrition, and Metabolism, vol. 32, no. 1, pp. 4–12, 2007.

[12] K. M. Choi, H. J. Cho, H. Y. Choi et al., "Higher mortality in metabolically obese normal-weight people than in metabolically healthy obese subjects in elderly Koreans," Clinical Endocrinology, vol. 79, no. 3, pp. 364–370, 2013.

[13] E. S. Ford, C. Li, and N. Sattar, "Metabolic syndrome and incident diabetes: current state of the evidence," Diabetes Care, vol. 31, no. 9, pp. 1898–1904, 2008.

[14] M. I. Harris, K. M. Flegal, C. C. Cowie et al., "Prevalence of diabetes, impaired fasting glucose, and impaired glucose tolerance in U.S. Adults: the Third National Health and Nutrition Examination Survey, 1988–1994," Diabetes Care, vol. 21, no. 4, pp. 518–524, 1998.

[15] K. M. Flegal, C. L. Ogden, and M. D. Carroll, "Prevalence and trends in overweight in Mexican-American adults and children," Nutrition Reviews, vol. 62, supplement 2, no. 7, pp. S144–S148, 2004.

[16] L. Razzouk and P. Muntner, "Ethnic, gender, and age-related differences in patients with the metabolic syndrome," Current Hypertension Reports, vol. 11, no. 2, pp. 127–132, 2009.

[17] S. P. Fisher-Hoch, A. R. Rentfro, J. J. Salinas et al., "Socioeconomic status and prevalence of obesity and diabetes in a Mexican American community, Cameron County, Texas, 2004—2007," Preventing chronic disease, vol. 7, no. 3, article A53, 2010.

[18] S. P. Fisher-Hoch, K. P. Vatcheva, S. T. Laing et al., "Missed opportunities for diagnosis and treatment of diabetes, hypertension, and hypercholesterolemia in a Mexican American population, Cameron County Hispanic Cohort, 2003–2008," Preventing Chronic Disease, vol. 9, Article ID 110298, 2012.

[19] S. S. Sun, W. C. Chumlea, S. B. Heymsfield et al., "Development of bioelectrical impedance analysis prediction equations for body composition with the use of a multicomponent model for use in epidemiologic surveys," The American Journal of Clinical Nutrition, vol. 77, no. 2, pp. 331–340, 2003.

[20] C. L. Craig, A. L. Marshall, M. Sjostrom et al., "International physical activity questionnaire: 12-country reliability and validity," Medicine & Science in Sports & Exercise, vol. 35, no. 8, pp. 1381–1395, 2003.

[21] D. R. Matthews, J. P. Hosker, A. S. Rudenski, B. A. Naylor, D. F. Treacher, and R. C. Turner, "Homeostasis model assessment: insulin resistance and β-cell function from fasting plasma glucose and insulin concentrations in man," Diabetologia, vol. 28, no. 7, pp. 412–419, 1985.

[22] S. M. Grundy, J. I. Cleeman, S. R. Daniels et al., "Diagnosis and management of the metabolic syndrome: an American Heart

Association/National Heart, Lung, and Blood Institute scientific statement," *Circulation*, vol. 112, no. 17, pp. 2735–2752, 2005.

[23] R. P. Wildman, P. Muntner, K. Reynolds et al., "The obese without cardiometabolic risk factor clustering and the normal weight with cardiometabolic risk factor clustering: prevalence and correlates of 2 phenotypes among the US population (NHANES 1999–2004)," *Archives of Internal Medicine*, vol. 168, no. 15, pp. 1617–1624, 2008.

[24] American Diabetes Association, "Standards of medical care in diabetes—2010," *Diabetes Care*, vol. 33, supplement 1, pp. S11–S61, 2010.

[25] F. J. Harrell Jr., *Regression Modeling Strategies: With Applications to Linear Models, Logistic Regression, and Survival Analysis*, Springer, New York, NY, USA, 2001.

[26] M. Y. Donath, "Targeting inflammation in the treatment of type 2 diabetes: time to start," *Nature Reviews Drug Discovery*, vol. 13, no. 6, pp. 465–476, 2014.

[27] Y.-M. Song, J. Sung, and K. Lee, "Genetic and environmental relationships of metabolic and weight phenotypes to metabolic syndrome and diabetes: the Healthy Twin Study," *Metabolic Syndrome and Related Disorders*, vol. 13, no. 1, pp. 36–44, 2015.

[28] R. V. Dvorak, W. F. DeNino, P. A. Ades, and E. T. Poehlman, "Phenotypic characteristics associated with insulin resistance in metabolically obese but normal-weight young women," *Diabetes*, vol. 48, no. 11, pp. 2210–2214, 1999.

[29] N. Bassi, I. Karagodin, S. Wang et al., "Lifestyle modification for metabolic syndrome: a systematic review," *The American Journal of Medicine*, vol. 127, no. 12, pp. 1242.e1–1242.e10, 2014.

[30] S. L. Appleton, C. J. Seaborn, R. Visvanathan et al., "Diabetes and cardiovascular disease outcomes in the metabolically healthy obese phenotype: a cohort study," *Diabetes Care*, vol. 36, no. 8, pp. 2388–2394, 2013.

16

Cost-Effectiveness of a Short Message Service Intervention to Prevent Type 2 Diabetes from Impaired Glucose Tolerance

Carlos K. H. Wong,[1] Fang-Fang Jiao,[1] Shing-Chung Siu,[2] Colman S. C. Fung,[1] Daniel Y. T. Fong,[3] Ka-Wai Wong,[2] Esther Y. T. Yu,[1] Yvonne Y. C. Lo,[1] and Cindy L. K. Lam[1]

[1]Department of Family Medicine and Primary Care, The University of Hong Kong, Ap Lei Chau, Hong Kong
[2]Department of Medicine and Rehabilitation, Tung Wah Eastern Hospital, Causeway Bay, Hong Kong
[3]School of Nursing, The University of Hong Kong, Pokfulam, Hong Kong

Correspondence should be addressed to Carlos K. H. Wong; carlosho@hku.hk

Academic Editor: Li-Wei Cho

Aims. To investigate the costs and cost-effectiveness of a short message service (SMS) intervention to prevent the onset of type 2 diabetes mellitus (T2DM) in subjects with impaired glucose tolerance (IGT). *Methods.* A Markov model was developed to simulate the cost and effectiveness outcomes of the SMS intervention and usual clinical practice from the health provider's perspective. The direct programme costs and the two-year SMS intervention costs were evaluated in subjects with IGT. All costs were expressed in 2011 US dollars. The incremental cost-effectiveness ratio was calculated as cost per T2DM onset prevented, cost per life year gained, and cost per quality adjusted life year (QALY) gained. *Results.* Within the two-year trial period, the net intervention cost of the SMS group was $42.03 per subject. The SMS intervention managed to reduce 5.05% onset of diabetes, resulting in saving $118.39 per subject over two years. In the lifetime model, the SMS intervention dominated the control by gaining an additional 0.071 QALY and saving $1020.35 per person. The SMS intervention remained dominant in all sensitivity analyses. *Conclusions.* The SMS intervention for IGT subjects had the superiority of lower monetary cost and a considerable improvement in preventing or delaying the T2DM onset. This trial is registered with ClinicalTrials.gov NCT01556880.

1. Introduction

Prevention of diabetes mellitus (DM) is becoming an increasing urgent public health concern all over the world. It is estimated that there are 382 million diabetic subjects by 2013 in the world, and the number will increase to 592 million by 2035 [1]. The rising prevalence of DM and its devastating complications [2] poses a huge threat to human health and places enormous economic burden to the society [3, 4]. Studies indicated that prediabetes is a major factor leading to diabetes [5], and people with prediabetes have increased risk of cardiovascular disease (CVD) and mortality [6–8].

Given the potentially immerse disease burden caused by prediabetes, it is impending to implement cost-effective interventions to delay diabetes among subjects with prediabetes and even reverse the prediabetes status. Delivery of short message service (SMS) is part of mobile-based interventions that has bridged an effective communication channel to endeavor behavioral change, enhance disease-specific knowledge, and subsequently improve health outcomes in the field of preventive medicine and chronic disease self-management. Over the past decade, self-management education or support by mobile-based applications has been launched to target the blood glucose and HbA1C levels control in patients with type 2 diabetes mellitus (T2DM) [9]. Mobile-based applications are evident to modify the individual behavior to quit smoking [10], but they are rarely applied in diabetes prevention. A randomized controlled trial was conducted recently to evaluate the efficacy of the SMS intervention and it showed encouraging results in reducing T2DM onset among patients with impaired glucose tolerance (IGT) [11].

Regarding the cost-effectiveness analyses for add-on interventions conventionally applied to prediabetes, the prediabetic screening [12] and lifestyle modification [13–16] have been demonstrated to be highly cost-effective strategies in comparison with usual clinical practice. To determine whether a lifestyle modification is cost-effective, it depends on how preventive the specific strategy is and how much it costs. Although previous cost-effective strategies of lifestyle intervention have different combinations of interventions, they achieve cost-effectiveness outcomes by decreasing the incidence of T2DM and its complications through slowing the progression to T2DM and early detection of undiagnosed abnormal glucose tolerance [16–19].

In view of the significant effectiveness of the SMS intervention in preventing T2DM among prediabetes subjects and its relative low cost, it is tempting to assume that the SMS intervention is cost-effective. However, it is unethical and infeasible to wait until perfect lifetime data are available to validate the cost-effectiveness of any intervention. Decision modelling is proved to be an effective method to conduct economic evaluation of clinical interventions over lifetime. This technique compares the intervention of interest with the alternative options by incorporating all appropriate evidence of costs and effectiveness, simulating disease paths over longer time span, and reflecting uncertainty in evidence [20].

Using data from relevant epidemiological studies and clinical trials, we constructed a Markov model to compare the strategy of delivering the SMS intervention programme as an additional support to usual clinical practice and usual clinical practice alone in managing subjects with IGT. Depending upon the strategy applied, subjects in SMS intervention group had lower T2DM onset rate compared to the usual care, resulting in lower cost of managing T2DM and longer life years, which might compensate the additional cost of delivering the SMS intervention.

2. Method

2.1. Markov Model. A decision analytic model with a state-transition Markov process [21] was developed to simulate long-term effects of cost and clinical effectiveness of interventions in a cohort of prediabetes under two main strategies, which were (1) SMS intervention in addition to usual clinical practice and (2) usual clinical practice. The TreeAge Pro 2013 software (TreeAge Software, Inc., Williamstown, MA, USA) was used for the modelling. Long-term modelling referred to time horizon over a 50-year period beyond the two-year intervention. The natural history referred to previous economic evaluation of diabetes prevention [15, 22–24]. The one-year transition cycle moved from one health state to another amongst four Markov states: normal glucose tolerance (NGT), IGT, T2DM, and death (Figure 1). An individual had the likelihood to transit from current health state to a different health state or remain in their current health state at the end of one-year cycle in this Markov process [21]. Compared to the usual practice group, the SMS intervention led to different transition probabilities among these four disease states, resulting in extra cost in addition to usual care. For patients who transit to diabetes were assumed to

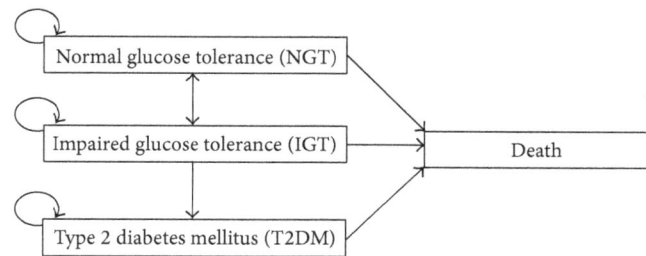

FIGURE 1: Annual transition diagram of Markov model.

stop receiving SMS intervention, therefore, the management of T2DM in these two groups was assumed to follow the same routine clinical practice in primary care setting. In other words, the costs and health effects of T2DM were the same for all subjects, regardless of which group they belonged to. An annual discount rate of 3% was undertaken in both the cost and health outcomes as per the Panel on Cost-Effectiveness in Health and Medicine recommended [25].

2.2. Transition Probability. As shown in Table 2, the annual transition probabilities between health states were taken from several data sources, including epidemiological studies and estimation from cost-effectiveness models. The annual transition probability from IGT to T2DM in the usual practice group in the first three years was adopted from the results of the placebo arm in Diabetes Prevention Program (DPP) [27], whereas the Diabetes Prevention Program Outcome Study (DPPOS) [28] provided this transition probability for the fourth year onwards. Subjects with IGT had about double risk for T2DM during the first three years compared to that in the fourth year onwards [27, 28]. The effect of SMS on the transition from IGT to T2DM was reflected in the relative risk of T2DM onset for SMS intervention against control groups, which was reported by a randomized control trial (Clinical Trials Registry Number: NCT01556880) among a sample of Chinese professional drivers with IGT [11, 29–31]. We adopted the relative risks for complete case analysis reported. This trial also reveals the drop-out rates of SMS intervention during the first year and second year, which were 38.9% and 30.3%, respectively. The proportion of subjects who regressed to normal glucose regulation was taken from the Caro et al. study [22] which was used to derive the annual transition probabilities from DPP. Subjects with diagnosed T2DM would either stay in that state or be absorbed into the death state in the next year. All-cause mortality rates for NGT were adopted from the Hong Kong Life Table 2011 [32]. The relative risks of mortality in IGT and T2DM were 1.50 (95% CI 1.10–2.00) and 2.30 (95% CI 1.60–3.20), respectively, which were used to adjust the age-specific death rate for subjects with IGT or T2DM [23]. The incidence and mortality rates reported in literature were converted to annual transition probabilities using mathematical formula [33]: $p = 1 - \exp(-rt)$, where p is the transition probability, r is the rate, and t is the unit of time. Although subjects with diabetic complication had a higher risk of mortality, our model did not differentiate different complications related to diabetes and therefore applied the average mortality of DM for all diabetic subjects.

2.3. Costs. Costs were estimated from the perspective of health service provider. No clinical health service was deployed to routinely screen or treat patients with prediabetes in Hong Kong, and thus there were no costs assigned to patients with NGT or prediabetes in the usual practice group. The cost of a SMS intervention was the sum of two components: the delivery cost of a total of 66 text messages package via online programme platform and the staff cost of sending those text messages to each subject. The delivery cost of text messages per subject was $4.15 in first year and $0.92 in second year, in total of $5.08, while the staff cost of sending text messages was estimated as $36.95 based on an estimate of 5 minutes for delivering one SMS online and a median hourly wage of $6.72 in 2011 [26]. The total intervention cost per subject was $42.03. All costs were calculated in 2011 Hong Kong dollars and converted to US dollars at a pegged rate of US$1 = HKD$7.8. The annual total medical costs attributed to each patient with type 2 diabetes were $1492.05 in 2004 year price [3], and those costs incurred in the usual clinical practice were inflated to $1,729.90 in 2011 using the medical services price index taken from Hong Kong Census and Statistics Department [26]. The medical costs associated with diabetes management were assumed to be the same for all the years in this state. All costs data are summarized in Table 1.

2.4. Utilities. To calculate the quality adjusted life years (QALYs) accumulated in the lifetime model, we adopted the utility scores for each health state from literature. We applied the same utility scores for subjects with NGT and IGT. The utility scores for NGT/IGT and T2DM were 0.76 and 0.72, respectively [23].

2.5. Cost-Effectiveness Outcomes. The main outcomes of the cost-effectiveness analysis in this study were the incremental cost-effectiveness ratios (ICER), in terms of cost per event (T2DM onset) prevented, cost per life year gained, and cost per QALY gained. The SMS intervention dominated control group if the control group was more expensive and less effective.

2.6. Sensitivity Analysis. Sensitivity analysis was performed to explore the uncertainty on the clinical and interventional parameters of model. Sensitivity analysis for the ICER of the SMS intervention compared with usual clinical practice was conducted on the transition probabilities with ranges suggested by previous literature and experts in family medicine and endocrine (Table 2). In addition, annual discount rate with limits bounded by 0% (undiscounted) and 5% was included in the analysis. Threshold analysis was undertaken to capture the threshold values of model interventional parameters at which the 50-year cumulative costs of SMS group were equivalent to those of control group. For instance, threshold values of intervention costs guided decision making on the level of intervention subsidy from the health service provider.

3. Results

3.1. Base-Case Scenario. The base-case scenario was based on the SMS intervention and T2DM costs from Table 1 and previously reported clinical parameters values from Table 2. Results of base-case scenario are shown in Table 3. During the two-year SMS intervention, compared to the usual practice group, each subject in SMS group costs $118.39 less and the SMS group reduced 5.05% of T2DM onset. Over the 50-year period of time horizon, the cumulative costs of the SMS intervention group per subject were substantially lower than the control group. Given the 0.063 life years and 0.071 QALYs gained in SMS group, the SMS intervention was a less costly but more effective strategy than control group. As a result, the SMS intervention was beneficial for effectiveness and cost-saving compared with the usual clinical practice in both short and long time horizons.

3.2. Sensitivity Analysis. Sensitivity analysis was performed by varying clinical and interventional parameters to test the robustness of model conclusion. Table 4 presents the results of sensitivity analysis which assessed the model robustness of base-case scenario. The determinant status of SMS group stayed unchanged when we varied various key parameters including SMS drop-out rates, annual transition probabilities between health states, and discount rate. Increased drop-out rate at first year from base-case value to 100% led to the zero increment cost, remaining dominant. Despite variation in drop-out rates, the SMS intervention dominated control group. When the annual transition probability from IGT to T2DM at the first year of SMS intervention was increased from 3.53% to 11.57%, which is equal to that in the control group, the SMS group still cost $76.21 less, remaining dominant. The threshold analysis, as shown in Table 5, indicated that SMS group reached the equivalent amount of total costs of control groups when the first year intervention cost was increased to $1,704.04 per person from original cost of $34.38. When the first year intervention cost was fixed at $34.38, to reach the same total cost as control group, the SMS intervention cost in the second year should have increased from $7.64 to $3,093.78. The annual transition probability from IGT to T2DM in first year in SMS group had to rise from 3.53% to 12.22% before the SMS group became no cheaper than control group. Similarly, only if the annual probability from IGT to T2DM in second year enrolled in SMS increased to 22.60% or higher, three times as base-case scenario, would their total medical cost be higher than the subjects in control group.

4. Discussion

This study found that, compared to usual clinical practice only, it was cost-saving to add the nonpharmacological SMS intervention in both the short and long time horizon. Given the high drop-out rate in the SMS group from the previous study, we assumed that the SMS intervention was provided only in the first two years. Within the two-year span, the SMS intervention led to a reduction of 5.05% of diabetes onset in comparison with the usual practice. Although it

TABLE 1: Unit costs (US$, year 2011 values) for the SMS intervention.

Resource component	Unit cost	Reference
SMS intervention		
First year		
Delivery charges of SMS via online platform*	$4.15	[11]
Staff wage for SMS delivery†	$30.23	[26]
Second year		
Delivery charges of SMS via online platform*	$0.92	[11]
Staff wage for SMS delivery†	$6.72	[26]
Annual cost of T2DM‡	$1,727.90	[3]

Note. *A total of 66 short text messages' package is sent to each subject. †An estimate of 5 minutes was spent for each SMS delivery and in total 330 minutes was used for each subject, assuming the median hourly wage of $6.72. ‡Annual cost in 2004 year price was inflated to 2011 year price using the medical services price index taken from Hong Kong Census Department.

TABLE 2: Clinical parameter value in base-case scenario and range used in sensitivity analysis.

Parameter	Base-case	Sensitivity analysis		Reference
		Minimum	Maximum	
SMS intervention				
Drop-out rate at year 1	38.89%	0%	100%	[11]
Drop-out rate at year 2	30.30%	0%	100%	[11]
Relative risk of T2DM at year 1 from IGT	0.34	0.10	1.00	[11]
Relative risk of T2DM at year 2 from IGT	0.60	0.10	1.00	[11]
Annual transition probability from IGT to NGT				
At all years	16.20%	5%	25%	[22]
Annual transition probability from NGT to IGT				
At all years	16.30%	5%	25%	[22]
Incidence rate (cases per 100 person-years) of T2DM from IGT				
Control at years 1–3	11.0	9.8	12.3	[27]
Control at year 4+	5.6	4.8	6.5	[28]
Relative risk of mortality				
IGT	1.5	1.1	2	[23]
T2DM	2.3	1.6	3.2	[23]
Utility				
NGT	0.76	NA		[23]
IGT	0.76	NA		[23]
T2DM	0.72	NA		[23]
Discount rate	3%	0%	5%	[25]

Note: NGT = normal glucose tolerance; IGT = impaired glucose tolerance; T2DM = type 2 diabetes mellitus; NA = not applicable.

TABLE 3: Results of base-case scenario.

Base-case scenario	SMS	Control	Incremental
2-year period			
Mean cost (in USD) accrued per patient	342.94	461.33	−118.39
T2DM onset	12.55%	17.60%	−5.05%
Cost per T2DM onset prevented			Dominance
50-year period			
Mean cost (in USD) accrued per patient	12107.40	12958.17	−850.77
LYs per patient	19.24	19.08	0.063
QALYs per patient	14.248	14.177	0.071
Cost per LY gained			Dominance
Cost per QALYs gained			Dominance

Note: T2DM = type 2 diabetes; LYs = life years; QALY = quality adjusted life year.

TABLE 4: Results of sensitivity analyses.

Parameters	Base-case	Range for sensitivity analysis	Range for incremental cost (USD)	Range for cost per LYs gained
SMS drop-out rate at year 1	38.89%	0.00%–100.00%	−1669.66 to 0.00	Dominance
SMS drop-out rate at year 2	30.30%	0.00%–100.00%	−1131.28 to −765.21	Dominance
Annual transition probability				
From IGT to T2DM, control at year 1–3	10.42%	9.34%–11.57%	−950.73 to −761.82	Dominance
From IGT to T2DM, SMS at year 1	3.53%	0.93%–11.57%	−1324.36 to −76.21	Dominance
From IGT to T2DM, SMS at year 2	6.25%	0.93%–11.57%	−1352.05 to −688.20	Dominance
From IGT to NGT	16.20%	5.00%–25.00%	− 922.28 to −1063.06	Dominance
From NGT to IGT	16.30%	5.00%–25.00%	−1117.45 to −979.19	Dominance
RR of mortality in IGT	1.5	1.1–2.0	−1015.49 to −1026.04	Dominance
RR of mortality in T2DM	2.3	1.6–3.2	−1087.30 to −953.95	Dominance
Discount rate	3.00%	0.00%–5.00%	−1450.41 to −836.95	Dominance

Note: NGT = normal glucose tolerance; IGT = impaired glucose tolerance; T2DM = type 2 diabetes mellitus; RR = relative risk.

TABLE 5: Threshold analysis of parameters at which the costs of SMS intervention and control became equivalent over a 50-year period.

Parameters	Base-case	Threshold
SMS intervention cost at year 1	$34.38	$1,704.04
SMS intervention cost at year 2	$7.64	$3,093.78
Annual transition probability		
From IGT to T2DM, SMS at year 1	3.53%	12.22%
From IGT to T2DM, SMS at year 2	6.25%	22.60%

Note: IGT = impaired glucose tolerance; T2DM = type 2 diabetes mellitus.

costs a total of $42.03 per subject to conduct the SMS intervention for two years, the money saved by treating less diabetic cases overcompensated the cost of SMS intervention. As a result, the SMS group cost $118.39 less per subject and prevented 5.05% of diabetes onset. When projecting the effects of the discrepancy in DM onset between the two groups to the lifetime span, we found that the SMS intervention accrued more life years gained (incremental effectiveness: 0.071 QALY) and less cost (incremental cost: −$1,020.35) than the control group. The robustness of the lifetime model was verified by sensitivity analysis through varying the transition probabilities and drop-out within wide ranges. The threshold analysis showed that only when the cost of SMS intervention climbed to about $2000 or more to reach the break-even point with the control group.

While the SMS intervention has been shown to be cost-saving in prediabetic population, the ICER values were not available as the incremental cost is negative. Using the empirical DPP/DPPOS data [16], the 10-year cost-effectiveness analysis estimated that metformin overwhelmed the control group with direct medical cost of care, and the ICER for lifestyle intervention compared to control group was $10,037 per QALYs gained. Complementary results were reported in Australian study modelling from a third-party payer perspective [23], indicating that the intensive lifestyle modification dominated the control group but the ICER for the metformin versus control group was $10,142 in Australian

dollars per QALYs gained. Lifestyle interventions in IGT were found cost-effective in other contexts as well, while most of these studies also adopted the effectiveness data from the DPP/DPPOS cohort [22, 34, 35]. Some studies on the CEA of interventions in prediabetes have established more sophisticated models, which involve development of complications after subjects developed diabetes. These studies adopted the Framingham or UKPDS risk functions to differentiate the risks of diabetic complications in long term based on the changes of clinical parameters (i.e., HbA1c, lipid profile, systolic blood pressure, etc.) observed in the trials. The incremental effectiveness in these studies is more prominent than the finding in our study that 0.14 to 0.50 life years were gained by lifestyle intervention compared to no intervention over the lifetime [14, 18]. Although the incremental life years and QALYs found in our model were smaller, it is noteworthy that we made a rather conservative estimation, as we assumed the two intervention groups have the same utilities after they developed diabetes. Moreover, we found that the SMS intervention is cost-saving over both short term and long term, which is favouring results for policy makers.

The main strength of this cost-effectiveness analysis model was that the sources of interventional parameter were the valid estimate reported in a randomized controlled trial. Additionally, our model estimated the short-term as well as long-term outcomes of cost-effectiveness. This is important as the initial setup cost invested to SMS group was shortly balanced out within two years, and the incremental cost was proportionally magnified between the two groups over a 50-year period. As the threshold analysis supported the increased costs of SMS in first and second year, there is potential area to set the patients' out-of-pocket charges of SMS intervention implemented in health service. Subsidy given by health service provider or government may be an alternative approach to deal with financing of the SMS implementation. Threshold analysis further offered cautionary advice on the termination of SMS intervention when the annual transition probabilities from IGT to T2DM in first and second year of

SMS group exceeded 12.22% and 22.60%, respectively. The scenarios implied that the SMS intervention was no longer supported by the nature of cost-saving. The feasibility and sustainability of SMS intervention are another concern due to about one-third of drop-out rates in first and second year. Owing to the high levels of drop-out, the effects of SMS intervention on ICER were considerably diluted. In a scenario of 100% drop-out in second year participation as illustrated in sensitivity analysis, the incremental cost ($765.21) of one-year intervention was smaller than that in base-case scenario.

Several drawbacks were noted in this study. Firstly, the effectiveness of SMS intervention was based on a RCT in Hong Kong Chinese population, but some clinical and epidemiological data were adopted from DPP and DPPOS, which are the US population-based studies. Due to lack of Hong Kong local data, we assumed that data from other sources were applicable in our model. It is likely that there may be substantial differences in the clinical and epidemiological data between the Hong Kong and the US populations; however, the values of these parameters were applied the same in both SMS group and control group, which will not affect the relative effectiveness in the model. Secondly, the interventional parameters were derived from randomized controlled trial on the pilot basis with 104 IGT subjects participating. Although the intervention has been shown to be effective in pilot data, the effect of SMS on the reduction of T2DM onset over time may be diluted in population-based setting. This study reflects the reasonable need for undertaking the SMS intervention on mass population with prediabetes. Thirdly, the model was built based on some simplified assumptions. For example, annual cost of T2DM was uniform regardless of gender, complication experienced, and insulin treated. Given the more diabetic complications experienced, direct medical costs associated with a T2DM subject increased sharply [36]. Furthermore, the model did not account for the health states representing the presence of diabetic complications as no evidence available shows that the SMS intervention in prediabetes has impacts on the incidence of diabetic complications.

5. Conclusions

This cost-effectiveness analysis reveals that the SMS intervention for subjects with prediabetes had the superiority of lower cost and a considerable improvement in preventing or delaying the T2DM onset. Encouraging efforts of clinical and cost-effectiveness outcomes were diluted due to the loss of participation over the 2-year intervention. This study indicated that it was cost-saving to prevent T2DM through implementing nonpharmacological SMS intervention among prediabetics.

The Significant Findings of the Study

The SMS intervention was a low-cost and effective programme for type 2 diabetes mellitus prevention in subjects with impaired glucose tolerance, resulting in cost-saving to health service provider regardless of 2-year trial and 50-year lifetime periods.

What This Study Adds

This trial-based cost-effectiveness analysis showed that the SMS may be an add-on intervention applied to impaired glucose tolerance management in routine clinical practice in primary care setting.

Abbreviations

SMS: Short message service
T2DM: Type 2 diabetes mellitus
IGT: Impaired glucose tolerance
QALY: Quality adjusted life year
DPP: Diabetes Prevention Program
DPPOS: Diabetes Prevention Program Outcome Study
ICER: Incremental cost-effectiveness ratios.

Conflict of Interests

The authors declare that they have no competing interests.

Authors' Contribution

Carlos K. H. Wong and Fang-Fang Jiao provided direct input into the design and execution of the study. Carlos K. H. Wong, Fang-Fang Jiao, and Daniel Y. T. Fong undertook statistical analysis and generated the results. Carlos K. H. Wong, Shing-Chung Siu, Fang-Fang Jiao, Daniel Y. T. Fong, Ka-Wai Wong, Esther Y. T. Yu, and Yvonne Y. C. Lo provided input to data interpretation. Carlos K. H. Wong drafted the paper. All authors contributed to its editing. All authors read and approved the final paper.

Acknowledgment

The earlier work that provided the interventional parameters of this model was kindly supported by the Board of the Tung Wah Group of Hospitals, Hong Kong. The article processing charge of this paper was supported by Tung Wah Eastern Hospital.

References

[1] L. Guariguata, D. R. Whiting, I. Hambleton, J. Beagley, U. Linnenkamp, and J. E. Shaw, "Global estimates of diabetes prevalence for 2013 and projections for 2035," *Diabetes Research and Clinical Practice*, vol. 103, no. 2, pp. 137–149, 2014.

[2] UK Prospective Diabetes Study (UKPDS) Group, "Intensive blood-glucose control with sulphonylureas or insulin compared with conventional treatment and risk of complications in patients with type 2 diabetes (UKPDS 33)," *The Lancet*, vol. 352, no. 9131, pp. 837–853, 1998.

[3] B. S. W. Chan, M. W. Tsang, V. W. Y. Lee, and K. K. C. Lee, "Cost of type 2 diabetes mellitus in Hong Kong Chinese," *International Journal of Clinical Pharmacology and Therapeutics*, vol. 45, no. 8, pp. 455–468, 2007.

[4] American Diabetes Association, "Economic costs of diabetes in the U.S. in 2012," *Diabetes Care*, vol. 36, pp. 1033–1046, 2013.

[5] D. Noble, R. Mathur, T. Dent, C. Meads, and T. Greenhalgh, "Risk models and scores for type 2 diabetes: systematic review," *British Medical Journal*, vol. 343, Article ID d7163, 2011.

[6] Y. S. Levitzky, M. J. Pencina, R. B. D'Agostino et al., "Impact of impaired fasting glucose on cardiovascular disease: the framingham heart study," *Journal of the American College of Cardiology*, vol. 51, no. 3, pp. 264–270, 2008.

[7] E. Selvin, M. W. Steffes, H. Zhu et al., "Glycated hemoglobin, diabetes, and cardiovascular risk in nondiabetic adults," *The New England Journal of Medicine*, vol. 362, no. 9, pp. 800–811, 2010.

[8] S. Seshasai, S. Kaptoge, A. Thompson et al., "Diabetes mellitus, fasting glucose, and risk of cause-specific death," *The New England Journal of Medicine*, vol. 364, no. 9, pp. 829–841, 2011.

[9] S. Krishna and S. A. Boren, "Diabetes self-management care via cell phone: a systematic review," *Journal of Diabetes Science and Technology*, vol. 2, no. 3, pp. 509–517, 2008.

[10] C. Free, R. Knight, S. Robertson et al., "Smoking cessation support delivered via mobile phone text messaging (txt2stop): a single-blind, randomised trial," *The Lancet*, vol. 378, no. 9785, pp. 49–55, 2011.

[11] C. K. H. Wong, C. S. C. Fung, S. C. Siu et al., "A short message service (SMS) intervention to prevent diabetes in Chinese professional drivers with pre-diabetes: a pilot single-blinded randomized controlled trial," *Diabetes Research and Clinical Practice*, vol. 102, no. 3, pp. 158–166, 2013.

[12] R. Chatterjee, K. M. V. Narayan, J. Lipscomb, and L. S. Phillips, "Screening adults for pre-diabetes and diabetes may be cost-saving," *Diabetes Care*, vol. 33, no. 7, pp. 1484–1490, 2010.

[13] M. K. Eriksson, L. Hagberg, L. Lindholm, E.-B. Malmgren-Olsson, J. Österlind, and M. Eliasson, "Quality of life and cost-effectiveness of a 3-year trial of lifestyle intervention in primary health care," *Archives of Internal Medicine*, vol. 170, no. 16, pp. 1470–1479, 2010.

[14] P. Lindgren, J. Lindström, J. Tuomilehto et al., "Lifestyle intervention to prevent diabetes in men and women with impaired glucose tolerance is cost-effective," *International Journal of Technology Assessment in Health Care*, vol. 23, no. 2, pp. 177–183, 2007.

[15] A. Neumann, P. Schwarz, and L. Lindholm, "Estimating the cost-effectiveness of lifestyle intervention programmes to prevent diabetes based on an example from Germany: Markov modelling," *Cost Effectiveness and Resource Allocation*, vol. 9, article 17, 2011.

[16] Diabetes Prevention Program Research Group, "The 10-year cost-effectiveness of lifestyle intervention or metformin for diabetes prevention: an intent-to-treat analysis of the DPP/DPPOS," *Diabetes Care*, vol. 35, no. 4, pp. 723–730, 2012.

[17] C. L. Gillies, P. C. Lambert, K. R. Abrams et al., "Different strategies for screening and prevention of type 2 diabetes in adults: cost effectiveness analysis," *The BMJ*, vol. 336, no. 7654, pp. 1180–1184, 2008.

[18] W. H. Herman, T. J. Hoerger, M. Brandle et al., "The cost-effectiveness of lifestyle modification or metformin in preventing type 2 diabetes in adults with impaired glucose tolerance," *Annals of Internal Medicine*, vol. 142, no. 5, pp. 323–332, 2005.

[19] T. J. Hoerger, K. A. Hicks, S. W. Sorensen et al., "Cost-effectiveness of screening for pre-diabetes among overweight and obese U.S. Adults," *Diabetes Care*, vol. 30, no. 11, pp. 2874–2879, 2007.

[20] A. Briggs, K. Claxton, and M. Sculpher, *Decision Modelling for Health Economic Evaluation*, Oxford University Press, Oxford, UK, 2006.

[21] F. A. Sonnenberg and J. R. Beck, "Markov models in medical decision making: a practical guide," *Medical Decision Making*, vol. 13, no. 4, pp. 322–338, 1993.

[22] J. J. Caro, D. Getsios, I. Caro, W. S. Klittich, and J. A. O'Brien, "Economic evaluation of therapeutic interventions to prevent type 2 diabetes in Canada," *Diabetic Medicine*, vol. 21, no. 11, pp. 1229–1236, 2004.

[23] A. J. Palmer and D. M. D. Tucker, "Cost and clinical implications of diabetes prevention in an Australian setting: a long-term modeling analysis," *Primary Care Diabetes*, vol. 6, no. 2, pp. 109–121, 2012.

[24] K. Dalziel and L. Segal, "Time to give nutrition interventions a higher profile: cost-effectiveness of 10 nutrition interventions," *Health Promotion International*, vol. 22, no. 4, pp. 271–283, 2007.

[25] J. E. Siegel, M. C. Weinstein, L. B. Russell, and M. R. Gold, "Recommendations for reporting cost-effectiveness analyses," *Journal of the American Medical Association*, vol. 276, no. 16, pp. 1339–1341, 1996.

[26] Census and Statistics Department. Hong Kong Special Administrative Region, *Hong Kong Annual Digest of Statistics 2012*, 2012.

[27] W. C. Knowler, E. Barrett-Connor, S. E. Fowler et al., "Reduction in the incidence of type 2 diabetes with lifestyle intervention or metformin," *The New England Journal of Medicine*, vol. 346, no. 6, pp. 393–403, 2002.

[28] Diabetes Prevention Program Research Group, "10-year follow-up of diabetes incidence and weight loss in the Diabetes Prevention Program Outcomes Study," *The Lancet*, vol. 374, no. 9702, pp. 1677–1686, 2009.

[29] S. C. Siu, K. W. Wong, K. F. Lee et al., "Prevalence of undiagnosed diabetes mellitus and cardiovascular risk factors in Hong Kong professional drivers," *Diabetes Research and Clinical Practice*, vol. 96, no. 1, pp. 60–67, 2012.

[30] C. K. H. Wong, C. S. C. Fung, S.-C. Siu et al., "The impact of work nature, lifestyle, and obesity on health-related quality of life in Chinese professional drivers," *Journal of Occupational and Environmental Medicine*, vol. 54, no. 8, pp. 989–994, 2012.

[31] C. K. Wong, S. C. Siu, E. Y. Wan et al., "Simple non-laboratory- and laboratory-based risk assessment algorithms and nomogram for detecting undiagnosed diabetes mellitus," *Journal of Diabetes*, 2015.

[32] Census and Statistics Department, *Hong Kong Special Administrative Region. Hong Kong Life Tables 2006–2014*, 2012.

[33] R. L. Fleurence and C. S. Hollenbeak, "Rates and probabilities in economic modelling: transformation, translation and appropriate application," *PharmacoEconomics*, vol. 25, no. 1, pp. 3–6, 2007.

[34] P. Watson, L. Preston, H. Squires, J. Chilcott, and A. Brennan, "Modelling the economics of type 2 diabetes mellitus prevention: a literature review of methods," *Applied Health Economics and Health Policy*, vol. 12, no. 3, pp. 239–253, 2014.

[35] A. J. Palmer, S. Roze, W. J. Valentine, G. A. Spinas, J. E. Shaw, and P. Z. Zimmet, "Intensive lifestyle changes or metformin in patients with impaired glucose tolerance: modeling the long-term health economic implications of the diabetes prevention program in Australia, France, Germany, Switzerland, and the United Kingdom," *Clinical Therapeutics*, vol. 26, no. 2, pp. 304–321, 2004.

[36] M. Brandle, H. Zhou, B. R. K. Smith et al., "The direct medical cost of type 2 diabetes," *Diabetes Care*, vol. 26, no. 8, pp. 2300–2304, 2003.

17

Incretin-Based Therapy for Prevention of Diabetic Vascular Complications

Akira Mima

Department of Nephrology, Nara Hospital, Kindai University Faculty of Medicine, Nara 630-0293, Japan

Correspondence should be addressed to Akira Mima; amima@nara.med.kindai.ac.jp

Academic Editor: Pedro M. Geraldes

Diabetic vascular complications are the most common cause of mortality and morbidity worldwide, with numbers of affected individuals steadily increasing. Diabetic vascular complications can be divided into two categories: macrovascular and microvascular complications. Macrovascular complications include coronary artery disease and cerebrovascular disease, while microvascular complications include retinopathy and chronic kidney disease. These complications result from metabolic abnormalities, including hyperglycemia, elevated levels of free fatty acids, and insulin resistance. Multiple mechanisms have been proposed to mediate the adverse effects of these metabolic disorders on vascular tissues, including stimulation of protein kinase C signaling and activation of the polyol pathway by oxidative stress and inflammation. Additionally, the loss of tissue-specific insulin signaling induced by hyperglycemia and toxic metabolites can induce cellular dysfunction and both macro- and microvascular complications characteristic of diabetes. Despite these insights, few therapeutic methods are available for the management of diabetic complications. Recently, incretin-based therapeutic agents, such as glucagon-like peptide-1 and dipeptidyl peptidase-4 inhibitors, have been reported to elicit vasotropic actions, suggesting a potential for effecting an actual reduction in diabetic vascular complications. The present review will summarize the relationship between multiple adverse biological mechanisms in diabetes and putative incretin-based therapeutic interventions intended to prevent diabetic vascular complications.

1. Introduction

The number of patients suffering from diabetes worldwide is rapidly increasing. A recent report prepared by the international diabetes foundation (IDF) estimates the global number of patients with diabetes to have risen to 380 million, with the total number of patients predicted to reach 590 million by 2035. Furthermore, the majority of new diabetic patients come from Southeast Asia and west Pacific regions (http://www.idf.org/). Diabetes-induced macro- and microvascular complications and their pathologies are the major contributors to morbidity and mortality. Macrovascular complications of diabetes involve large vessel obstructions, including peripheral artery disease, coronary artery disease, atherosclerosis, and cerebrovascular disease, while microvascular pathologies include retinopathy, neuropathy, and nephropathy. Abnormal metabolites formed

in hyperglycemic state are major systemic risk factors for these diabetic complications. The Diabetes Control and Complications Trial (DCCT) performed in type 1 diabetic patients and United Kingdom Prospective Diabetes Study (UKPDS) in type 2 diabetic patients clearly showed that intensive glycemic control could delay the onset of diabetes and retard the occurrence of diabetic complications [1, 2]. Furthermore, the follow-up of both DCCT and UKPDS trials showed that such intensive glycemic control could decrease diabetic macrovascular complications [3, 4]. Hyperglycemia could therefore be a major factor for initiation and progression of diabetic complications. However, hyperglycemia alone is not enough to induce such vascular complications; multiple potential biochemical pathways have been proposed to underlie the adverse effects of diabetes-induced vascular complications. Activation of diacylglycerol- (DAG-) protein kinase C (PKC) signaling, increased oxidative stress and inflammation, enhanced polyol pathway, activation of the hexosamine pathway, and overproduction of advanced glycation end products (AGEs) have all been proposed as potential intra- and extracellular changes which lead to alterations in the signaling pathways associated with vascular complications in diabetes [5–7]. While a study by Coca et al. has demonstrated that intensive glycemic control reduces albuminuria, there is currently no evidence that would suggest that intensive glycemic control reduces the risk of renal outcomes [8]. Additionally, findings of other groups suggest that hypoglycemia exacerbates both macrovascular and microvascular complications of diabetes and increases the risk of morbidity and mortality [9]. On the basis of these published findings, intensive lowering of blood glucose may be less beneficial for diabetes-induced vascular complications.

Incretins are a family of gut hormones which includes glucose-dependent insulinotropic polypeptide (GIP) and glucagon-like peptide-1 (GLP-1) [10]. Furthermore, a number of recent studies indicate that GLP-1 and dipeptidyl peptidase-4 (DPP-4) inhibitors exhibit potent pleiotropic protective effects on diabetic vascular complications, beyond their effects on glycemic control [11, 12]. One specific feature of incretin hormone-related drugs is a reduced danger of hypoglycemia [13]. Therefore, incretin-based therapeutic agents could prevent and slow the progression of diabetic vascular complications.

To elucidate these concepts, we will briefly review the multiple biochemical pathways and novel knowledge gathered about incretins, selecting the literature describing incretin-related pathways as therapeutic targets for the management of diabetic vascular complications.

2. Inflammation, Oxidative Stress, and PKC Activation in Diabetic Vascular Complications

Increasing the formation of aggressive T cells and altering the Th1/Th2 cell ratio towards the proinflammatory status have been reported to lead to the initiation and progression to overt diabetes [14]. In spite of C-reactive protein (CRP) levels in patients with recent-onset type 1 diabetes being the same as those measured in the control group, elevated CRP levels have been observed in long-term type 1 diabetes patients [15]. High glucose levels increase interleukin- (IL-) 12 production in macrophages and interferon-γ production in CD4$^+$ T cells [16]. Additionally, hyperglycemia-induced activation of nuclear factor-κ (NF-κ) B increases the levels of endothelin-1 (ET-1), vascular cell adhesion molecule- (VCAM-) 1, intercellular adhesion molecule- (ICAM-) 1, IL-6, and tumor necrosis factor- (TNF-) α [11, 17]. Furthermore, a positive relationship has been demonstrated between plasma interferon- (IFN-) γ, estimated glomerular filtration rate (eGFR), and proteinuria [18]. Therefore, anti-inflammatory drugs could provide useful new approaches for the management of diabetic vascular complications. Despite favorable results reported in rodent models, it is still unclear whether anti-inflammatory drugs, including adiponectin, NF-κB inhibitors, COX2 inhibitors,

and inhibitors of chemokine C-X-C motif ligand 2 (CXCL2), can elicit significant effects against diabetic vascular complications in humans.

Activation of DAG-PKC signal transduction pathway was shown to be related to diabetic microvascular diseases, with increases in PKC activity known to induce extracellular matrix (ECM) accumulation, epithelial cell apoptosis, monocyte adhesion, and cytokine activation [19]. PKC induces oxidative stress by activating the mitochondrial NADPH oxidase [20, 21]. Additionally, there is evidence that oxidants and AGEs can increase DAG levels and activate PKC [5]. Altered levels of reactive oxygen species (ROS) have been reported in the kidneys and retina of both animal models of diabetes and in patients [17, 22–25]. Also, increased plasma levels of 8-hydroxydeoxyguanosine (8-OHdG) and lipid peroxides have been reported to result from abnormal metabolism of glucose and free fatty acids [26–28].

In a phase II clinical trial in US, ruboxistaurin (RBX), a PKCβ isoform selective inhibitor, decreased albuminuria significantly and did not show increases of urinary TGF-β. Furthermore, RBX-treated patients maintained a stable eGFR over 1 year [29]. Administration of antioxidant agents, including vitamins C and E, has been evaluated in murine models of diabetes. In most studies, administration of these drugs was shown to effectively ameliorate the pathological changes in murine models of diabetic nephropathy [30–32]. Additionally, other studies have demonstrated the effectiveness of vitamin E administration in normalizing oxidative stress markers and decreasing PKC-induced diabetic vascular complications. Despite the favorable results observed in animal studies, in the Heart Outcomes Prevention Evaluation (HOPE) study evaluating a large cohort of patients with diabetes, administration of vitamin E did not reduce the risk of cardiovascular complications [30]. It is possible that the plasma levels of these vitamins might not reflect those at the tissue levels. Lastly, bardoxolone methyl, a new antioxidant drug, interacts with the cysteine residues on Keap1 to cause the translocation of nuclear factor erythroid 2-related factor 2 (Nrf2) to the nucleus, increasing its anti-inflammatory effects [33–35]. This drug was expected to ameliorate diabetic nephropathy on the basis of beneficial effects observed in recent placebo-controlled clinical trials [36, 37]. However, due to high mortality observed in the treated group, this phase 3 trial was suspended. The effectiveness of antioxidant therapies in management of diabetes therefore remains unknown.

3. Incretin: A New Class of Antidiabetic Drugs

Incretins are a family of gut hormones and released from the gut in response to ingestions of various nutrients [38]. GIP and GLP-1 could induce biological effects through the GIP receptors (GIPR) and GLP-1 receptors (GLP-1R). GLP-1 binds to GLP-1R in the vascular endothelial cells [39–41]. GLP-1 also binds to GLP-1R in intestinal mucosa and the portal vein to induce insulin secretion using the nervous system [42]. GLP-1 suppresses inflammatory markers, such as CD68, CXCL2, and plasminogen activator inhibitor- (PAI-) 1, and this effect could be involved in the cAMP/protein kinase A (PKA) pathway. Like GLP-1, GIP could inhibit production of reactive oxygen species (ROS) as well as PAI-1 via the cAMP pathway [43]. In addition to its effect on insulin and glucagon, GLP-1 exhibits a number of vasotropic actions beyond glycemic control; it increases insulin sensitivity in peripheral tissues, improves endothelial function, and decreases inflammation in some organs [41, 44]. Both GIP and GLP-1 are easily degraded by DPP-4, terminating biological effects. Inhibition of DPP-4 increases circulating GLP-1 levels and was shown to be a useful intervention in type 2 diabetic patients [13, 45, 46]. DPP-4 inhibitors could also reduce inflammation, with decreased levels of MCP-1 reported following administration of DPP-4 inhibitors [47]. Like GLP-1, DPP-4 inhibitors also elicit vasotropic effects and can potentially be used for the amelioration of diabetic nephropathy [48, 49].

4. The Effects of Incretin on Inflammation and Oxidative Stress

Anti-inflammatory and antioxidative stress effects of incretin have been described previously. In endothelial cells, GLP-1 reduces TNF-α expression and ROS production, inhibiting the adhesion and activation of macrophages [50]. Exenatide, a GLP-1R agonist, has been reported to significantly attenuate mRNA levels of MCP-1 and TNF-α, decreasing atherosclerosis [51]. Additionally, we have reported that administration of GLP-1 decreases diabetes-induced inflammation and oxidative stress in the glomerulus [11].

5. Renal Effects of Incretin

Diabetic nephropathy (DN) is one of the major diabetic microvascular complications, leading to chronic kidney disease (CKD) [52]. According to United States Renal Data System (USRDS), up to 44% of patients with type 2 diabetes in the United States develop overt DN (USRDS 2007 Annual Data Report. Bethesda, MD: National Institute of Diabetes and Digestive and Kidney Diseases, National Institutes of Health, U.S. Department of Health and Human Services; 2007).

GLP-1 has been reported to elicit renal protective effects against DN [11, 54]. Specifically, GLP-1 decreases inflammatory and oxidative stress markers in glomerular endothelial cells [11, 55].

In kidney, GLP-1R were mainly detected in renal glomeruli but not in tubules. Recent studies highlighted the lack of specificity of multiple anti-GLP-1R antibody [51, 63]. However, Fujita et al. clearly showed the presence of GLP-1R in renal glomeruli using in situ hybridization, supporting previous reports [64]. We have shown that exendin-4, a GLP-1R agonist, activates the cAMP/PKA signaling pathway, resulting in increased phospho-c-Raf (Ser259) levels which could inhibit phospho-c-Raf (Ser338)/phospho-Erk1/2/PAI-1 signaling activated by angiotensin II or PKCβ [11]. Interestingly, PKCβ increases the levels of ubiquitinated GLP-1R, decreasing GLP-1R protein levels in the glomeruli (Figure 1).

In contrast, PKCα, another PKC isoform, decreases RNA levels of GLP-1R in the pancreas [65]. Additionally, we showed that exendin-4 decreased the mRNA levels of inflammatory markers CD68, PAI-1, and CXCL2 in the renal cortex of diabetic rodents [11] (in diabetic WT mice, decreased by 52 ± 7, 24 ± 9, and 36 ± 11%, resp.; Figure 2). Other researchers have demonstrated the presence of the same mechanism in mesangial cells, showing GLP-1-induced increases in cAMP to suppress the inflammatory response against AGEs by decreasing the expression of receptor for AGEs (RAGE) [66]. GLP-1 decreases albuminuria and ameliorates mesangial expansion, which is a typical pathological feature of DN [11, 54]. 8-OHdG and malondialdehyde (MDA), markers of oxidative stress, are significantly increased in diabetic and insulin-resistant conditions [55]. Administration of GLP-1R agonist liraglutide was shown to decrease the levels of these oxidative stress markers and ameliorate renal function in diabetic rats [56]. GLP-1 directly suppresses transforming growth factor- (TGF-) β signal, which is related to glomerular injury, mesangial matrix expansion, and increasing extracellular matrix in DN [55]. Furthermore, the results from the Akita $Glp1r^{-/-}$ mice showed severe mesangial expansion and increases in glomerular ROS, upregulated renal NADPH oxidase, and decreased renal cAMP/PKA activity [64]. Taking these reports together, GLP-1 may have renoprotective effects at least in rodent DN models.

While a relatively small number of studies have demonstrated the effectiveness of GLP-1 therapy on human DN, intravenous infusion of GLP-1 in insulin-resistant states was shown to increase sodium excretion, reduce H$^+$ secretion, and reduce glomerular hyperfiltration, leading to renoprotective effects [67]. Interestingly, our recent findings show that GLP-1R protein levels were decreased in the renal cortex of patients with type 1 diabetes of extreme duration (Mima A, King GL, unpublished observation).

6. Renal Effects of DPP-4 Inhibitors

Several DPP-4 inhibitors were reported to ameliorate renal function and pathology in DN. Linagliptin has been reported to decrease renal fibrosis following diabetes-induced endothelial-to-mesenchymal transition through an effect mediated by microRNA 29s [57]. Vildagliptin was reported to elicit renoprotective effects, such as a reduction in albuminuria [68] and decreased ECM deposition in the diabetic glomeruli by reducing the levels of DPP-4 and increasing levels of GLP-1 [69]. Furthermore, as we have previously shown using GLP-1R agonist exendin-4 [11], vildagliptin decreased the oxidative stress in the kidney of rat model of type 2 diabetes [70]. Additionally, sitagliptin ameliorated diabetes-induced renal pathological changes accompanied by decreased lipid peroxidation [71]. In patients with type 2 diabetes, sitagliptin and alogliptin reduced albuminuria and 8-OHdG, markers of oxidative stress, and increased urinary cAMP levels, leading to renoprotective effects [49]. Recent subanalysis study of SAVOR-TIMI 53 shows that saxagliptin significantly decreases albuminuria in both microalbuminuria and overt proteinuria state of type 2 DN patients (Frederich B et al.

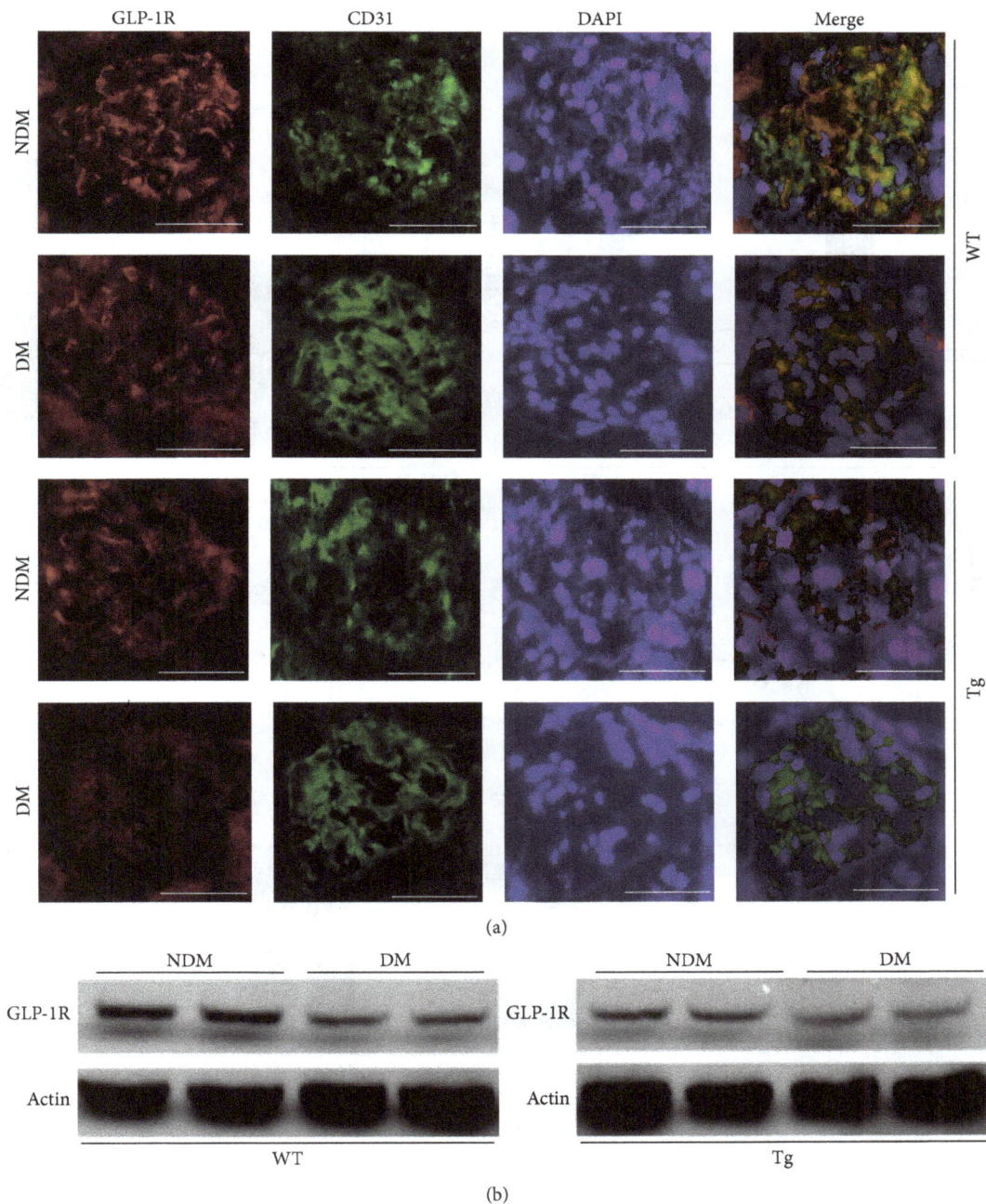

FIGURE 1: Overexpression of PKCβ2 in mouse glomerular endothelial cells (EC-PKCβ2Tg) and decreased glucagon-like peptide-1 receptors in diabetes. (a) Immunostaining of GLP-1R and CD31, showing merged images of the glomeruli. (b) Immunoblots of GLP-1R from renal cortex of mice. Images are reproduced from Mima et al. [11], with permission from Diabetes ©2012.

presentation abstract; American Diabetes Association 74th Scientific Sessions, 2014). Furthermore, the MARLINA-T2D trial will examine the effect of linagliptin on albuminuria in people with type 2 diabetes [53] (Table 1). However, it seems that the renoprotective effects of DPP-4 inhibitors found in most studies depend on the amelioration of glycemic control or increased GLP-1 levels. Therefore, further studies are needed to clarify the effects of DPP-4 inhibitors on DN.

7. Cardiovascular Effects of Incretin-Based Therapeutic Agents

A number of studies have demonstrated the effects of incretins on macrovascular complications, including coronary artery disease (CAD), atherosclerosis, and cerebrovascular disease [72]. Intravenous administration of GLP-1 reduced infarct size after the occlusion of left anterior descending

(a)

(b)

(c)

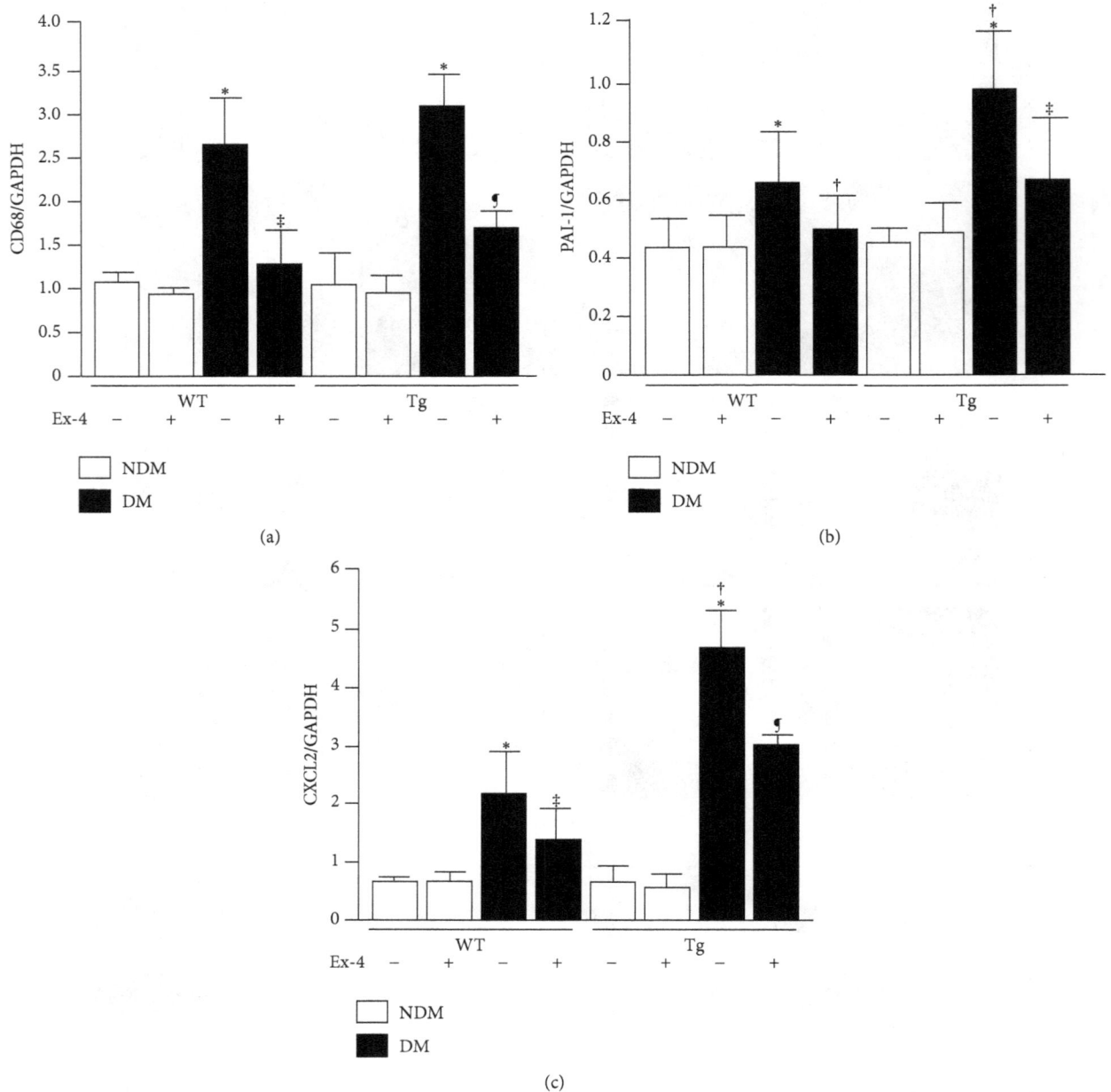

FIGURE 2: Effect of exendin-4 treatment on inflammatory markers in EC-PKCβ2Tg mice. (a) CD68 mRNA expression in the renal cortex of each group. $^*P < 0.05$ versus WT/NDM/exendin-4($-$), $^\dagger P < 0.05$ versus WT/DM/exendin-4($-$), and $^\ddagger P < 0.05$ versus EC-PKCβ2Tg/DM/exendin-4($-$). $N = 6$ in nondiabetic WT + vehicle, nondiabetic WT + Ex-4, diabetic WT + vehicle, diabetic WT + Ex-4, nondiabetic EC-PKCβ2Tg + Ex-4, and diabetic EC-PKCβ2Tg + Ex-4 groups; $n = 7$ in nondiabetic EC-PKCβ2Tg + vehicle and diabetic EC-PKCβ2Tg + vehicle groups. (b) PAI-1 mRNA expression in the renal cortex of each group. $^*P < 0.05$ versus WT/NDM/exendin-4($-$), $^\dagger P < 0.05$ versus WT/DM/exendin-4($-$), and $^\ddagger P < 0.05$ versus EC-PKCβ2Tg/DM/exendin-4($-$). $N = 6$ in nondiabetic WT + vehicle, nondiabetic WT + Ex-4, diabetic WT + vehicle, diabetic WT + Ex-4, nondiabetic EC-PKCβ2Tg + Ex-4, and diabetic EC-PKCβ2Tg + Ex-4 groups; $n = 7$ in nondiabetic EC-PKCβ2Tg + vehicle and diabetic EC-PKCβ2Tg + vehicle groups. (c) CXCL2 mRNA expression in the renal cortex of each group. $^*P < 0.05$ versus WT/NDM/exendin-4($-$), $^\dagger P < 0.05$ versus WT/DM/exendin-4($-$), and $^\ddagger P < 0.05$ versus EC-PKCβ2Tg/DM/exendin-4($-$). $n = 6$ in nondiabetic WT + vehicle, nondiabetic WT + Ex-4, diabetic WT + vehicle, diabetic WT + Ex-4, nondiabetic EC-PKCβ2Tg + Ex-4, and diabetic EC-PKCβ2Tg + Ex-4 groups; $n = 7$ in nondiabetic EC-PKCβ2Tg + vehicle and diabetic EC-PKCβ2Tg + vehicle groups. Reproduction from Mima et al. [11] with permission from Diabetes ©2012.

TABLE 1: Clinical trials and animal studies of selected incretin-based agents for kidney disease.

Study (drug)	Numbers	Treatment plan	Outcome
Hattori [48] (sitagliptin and alogliptin; 2014)	Sitagliptin and alogliptin; 12	Sitagliptin 50 mg/day for 4 weeks (first period; baseline), alogliptin 25 mg/day for 4 weeks (second period), and sitagliptin 50 mg/day for 4 weeks (third period)	Significant decreases in albuminuria after the change from sitagliptin to alogliptin (81.0 ± 52.4 to 33.9 ± 23.9 mg/g Cr; $P < 0.05$)
Frederich et al. (presentation abstract; American Diabetes Association 74th Scientific Sessions, 2014) Subanalysis study of SAVOR-TIMS53 (saxagliptin; 2013)	Saxagliptin, 2043; placebo, 799	Saxagliptin 2.5, 5, or 10 mg/day (24 weeks)	Significant increases in negative rate of albuminuria (4.6% versus 13.4%)
Groop et al. [53] (linagliptin (MARLINA-T2D); ongoing)	A total of 350 eligible individuals are randomized in a 1:1 ratio to receive linagliptin or placebo	Linagliptin 5 mg/day for 24 weeks	
Mima et al. [11] (exendin-4)	STZ-induced diabetic mice + exendin-4; 6 STZ-induced diabetic mice + vehicle; 6	Exendin-4 (1.0 nmol/kg/day) was administered intraperitoneally for 6 months	Significant decreases in albuminuria (by 27 ± 10%; $P < 0.05$) and mesangial expansion (by 38 ± 10%; $P < 0.05$) compared to DM + vehicle
Park et al. [54] (exendin-4)	*db/db* mice + exendin-4; 8 *db/db* mice + vehicle; 8	Exendin-4 (1.0 nmol/kg/day) was administered intraperitoneally for 8 weeks	Significant decreases in albuminuria ($P < 0.01$), mesangial matrix fraction ($P < 0.05$), and macrophages infiltration in glomeruli ($P < 0.01$)
Kodera et al. [55] (exendin-4)	STZ-induced diabetic rats + exendin-4; 6 STZ-induced diabetic rats + vehicle; 6	Exendin-4 (10 μg/kg/BW) was administered intraperitoneally for 8 weeks	Significant decreases in albuminuria ($P < 0.05$), mesangial matrix expansion ($P < 0.001$), and ICAM-1 expression in glomeruli ($P < 0.01$)
Hendarto et al. [56] (liraglutide)	STZ-induced diabetic rats + liraglutide; STZ-induced diabetic rats + vehicle	Liraglutide (0.3 mg/kg/12 h) was administered with subcutaneous injection for 4 weeks	Significant decreases in albuminuria ($P < 0.01$), NOX4 in glomeruli ($P < 0.05$), and TGF-β expression in glomeruli ($P < 0.01$)
Kanasaki et al. [57] (linagliptin)	STZ-induced diabetic mice + linagliptin; 5-6 STZ-induced diabetic mice + vehicle; 7-8	Linagliptin (5 mg/kg BW/day) in drinking water for 4 weeks	Significant decreases in albuminuria ($P < 0.05$) and mesangial matrix expansion ($P < 0.01$)

STZ, streptozotocin; BW, body weight; ICAM-1, intercellular adhesion molecule-1; TGF-β, transforming growth factor-β.

coronary artery in rats [73]. Administration of liraglutide could increase the expression of cardioprotective genes, leading to beneficial effects on cardiac tissues [12]. Additionally, GLP-1 treatment has been reported to significantly reduce infarct size and improve cardiac function in pigs [74]. We have shown that GLP-1 incubation increases cAMP and PKA levels in glomerular endothelial cells [11]. Similarly, GLP-1 was found to increase cAMP levels in cardiomyocytes, leading to cardioprotective effects [73]. Like GLP-1, GIP also may have vascular protective effects. Recently, elegant work by Nogi et al. shows that GIP inhibits infiltration of macrophages, resulting in decreases in atherosclerotic lesions in both diabetic and nondiabetic mice lacking apolipoprotein E [75]. In Liraglutide Effect and Action in Diabetes: Evaluation of Cardiovascular Outcome Results (LEADER) clinical trial, the effects of GLP-1R agonist liraglutide will be examined for much longer periods [76]. However, even among patients with normal renal function, increases in serum levels of lipase and amylase (reported to be nearly 25% higher than in controls) without symptoms of acute pancreatitis were recognized in this trial [77].

Several studies have shown that DPP-4 inhibitors exhibit cardioprotective effects. Sitagliptin was reported to improve the recovery of left ventricular end-diastolic pressure (LVEDP) in rodents [60, 61]. Furthermore, sitagliptin reduced the size of myocardial infarct area in animal studies [60]. Similar to the effects we reported in the glomerulus [11], the cardioprotective effects are derived from the activation of the GLP-1/cAMP/PKA signaling pathway [60]. Reduced exacerbation of left ventricular function and myocardial dysfunction was reported in DPP-4-null rodents, as compared to wild-type animals, in an induced model of heart failure [58]. Treatment with vildagliptin reduced cardiomyocyte apoptosis and fibrosis in mice, improving the survival rate [62]. In agreement with the outcomes of animal studies, oral administration of DPP-4 inhibitor sitagliptin ameliorated myocardial stunning in response to catecholamine overload in patients with type 2 diabetes and coronary artery disease with normal resting LV function [78]. In contrast to this favorable result, the combination therapy using sitagliptin and granulocyte colony-stimulating factor did not alter the left ventricle ejection fraction (LVEF) at 6-month follow-up (Franz WM et al. presentation abstract; American Heart Association, 2011). Another study using a DPP-4 inhibitor, Saxagliptin Assessment of Vascular Outcomes Recorded in Patients with Diabetes Mellitus-Thrombolysis in Myocardial Infarction 53 (SAVOR-TIMI 53), demonstrated somewhat disappointing results, with more patients hospitalized for heart failure in the saxagliptin group than in the placebo group [79]. The study of the effects of vildagliptin administration demonstrated increased LV end-diastolic and end-systolic volumes (McMurray J. presentation abstract; European Society of Cardiology Annual Meeting, 2013). Similarly, the Examination of Cardiovascular Outcomes with Alogliptin versus Standard of Care (EXAMINE) cardiovascular outcome trial did not observe a reduction in cardiovascular events [80]. In contrast to the relatively short examination period in these studies, Trial Evaluating Cardiovascular Outcomes with Sitagliptin (TECOS) study [59] examined clinical outcomes over much longer periods. Regarding this clinical trial, a recent study reported no increase in admission to hospital for heart failure in the sitagliptin comparing to placebo group [81]. The results were different between SAVOR-TIMI 53 and TECOS; increases in cardiovascular events were recognized in patients with elevated levels of natriuretic peptides, previous heart failure, or chronic kidney disease in SAVOR-TIMI 53, while in TECOS, renal insufficiency patients were excluded. We cannot find any effects of incretin-based therapeutics on macrovascular diseases, but observational period is relatively short in these studies, when compared to UKPDS that showed favorable macrovascular outcomes [1, 2]. Furthermore, the Evaluation of Lixisenatide in Acute coronary syndrome (ELIXA) also showed no increase in admission to hospital for heart failure (Pfeffer MA et al. presentation abstract; American Diabetes Association, 2015). Indeed, it is possible that inhibition of DPP-4 decreases LV function indicated by previous studies, but we have to evaluate these update results described above to clarify the safety of incretin-based therapeutic agents (Table 2).

8. Cerebrovascular Effects of Incretin-Based Therapeutic Agents

Previous animal studies showed GLP-1's neuroprotective effects on cerebral ischemia in diabetes. Administration of exendin-4 after cerebral ischemia reduced cerebral infarction area and neurological disorders. As in the case with our results, exendin-4 increased the cAMP/PKA in nerve cells [11], leading to neuroprotective effects. Unlike GLP-1, no study has been carried out about the neuroprotective effects using GIP, though $GIPr^{-/-}$ mice showed impaired learning and neurogenesis [82]. Consistent with GLP-1's neuroprotective effects on cerebral ischemia, the DPP-4 inhibitor, linagliptin, also could reduce ischemic brain damage in diabetic rodents [83]. Further, it seems that the neuroprotective effects are independent from glycemic control and probably mediated by GLP-1, because sulfonylurea glimepiride did not show the same favorable effects though it decreased blood glucose level [83].

9. The Effects of Incretin-Based Therapeutic Agents on Diabetic Retinopathy

Diabetic retinopathy (DR) is recognized in a majority of diabetic patients and is one of the major causes of blindness [84, 85]. Chronic hyperglycemic state is a major cause of DR, as supported by the findings of DCCT and UKPDS studies [86, 87]. Also, inflammation and oxidative stress play a significant role in the development of DR [17]. Recent studies suggest that the effects of GLP-1 on the retinal functions could be of significance in the treatment of DR [88]. GLP-1R is expressed in the cells of the retinal ganglion, Müller cells, and pigment epithelial cells [88]. Subcutaneous injection of exendin-4 prevented the decreases in retinal cells and retinal thickness in a rat model of diabetes [88]. Exendin-4 was demonstrated to regulate the Bax/Bcl-2 ratio, leading to neuroprotective effects and prevention of hyperglycemia-induced injury to retinal ganglion cells [89]. Furthermore, intravitreal injection of exendin-4 protected the retina by upregulating the excitatory amino acid transporter expression in the retina [88]. Larger studies, including clinical trials in human patients, are needed to clearly show the potential effectiveness of GLP-1 for DR.

Like incretins, DPP-4 inhibitors also elicit beneficial effects against DR, with oral administration of sitagliptin preventing the pathological changes in the blood-retinal barrier in a rat model of type 2 diabetes [90]. Our recent study showed retinal inflammation to be significantly increased in both diabetes and insulin resistance [17]. Sitagliptin reduced the levels of IL-1β, a marker of diabetes-induced retinal inflammation. Furthermore, sitagliptin elicited beneficial effects against the diabetes-induced decrease in circulating CD34$^+$ cells, which are enriched in endothelial progenitor cells, compromising the repair process in the damaged vasculature [90]. However, the possibility that the activation of retinal GLP-1R leads to antiapoptotic effects in the retinal endothelial cells could not be excluded, and the actual mechanism and effect remain to be elucidated in further studies in rodents.

TABLE 2: Clinical trials and animal studies of selected incretin-based agents for cardiovascular disease.

Study (drug)	Patient numbers	Treatment plan	Outcome
Ku and Su [58] (sitagliptin; 2014)	Sitagliptin, 19; placebo 31	Sitagliptin (100 mg/day) was administered for 4 weeks	Significant improvement in myocardial function and reduction in postischemic stunning (ejection fraction, 70.5 ± 7.0 versus 65.7 ± 8.0%; $P < 0.0001$; strain rate in ischemic segments, -2.27 ± 0.65 versus $-1.988 \pm 0.58\,s^{-1}$; $P = 0.001$)
Green et al. [59] (sitagliptin (TECOS); 2015)	Sitagliptin, 839; placebo, 851 (primary outcome)	Sitagliptin 100 mg/day (or 50 mg/day if the baseline GFR was ≥30 and <50 mL per minute per 1.73 m²) Median follow-up was 3.0 years	Sitagliptin was noninferior to placebo for the primary compositive cardiovascular outcome (hazard ratio, 0.98; 95% CI, 0.88 to 1.09; $P < 0.001$). Rates of hospitalization for heart failure did not differ between the two groups (hazard ratio, 1.00; 95% CI, 0.83 to 1.20; $P = 0.98$)
Pfeffer et al. (presentation abstract; American Diabetes Association 75th Scientific Sessions, 2015 Lixisenatide (ELIXA); 2015)	Lixisenatide, 3034; placebo, 3034	Lixisenatide 10–20 μg/day Median follow-up was 2.1 years	Lixisenatide was noninferior to placebo for the primary compositive cardiovascular outcome (hazard ratio, 0.97; 95% CI, 0.85 to 1.10). Rates of hospitalization for heart failure did not differ between the two groups (hazard ratio, 0.94; 95% CI, 0.78 to 1.13). Rates of mortality (hazard ratio, 0.94; 95% CI, 0.78 to 1.13)
Ye et al. [60] (Sitagliptin)	Mice underwent coronary ligation + sitagliptin 10; mice underwent coronary ligation + vehicle 10	Sitagliptin (300 mg/kg/day) was administered by oral gavage for 3 or 14 days	Significant decreases in infarct size (24.3 ± 0.7% in 3 days; $P < 0.05$ and 16.9 ± 0.6%; $P < 0.001$ in 14 days)
Gomez et al. [61]	Hybrid (landrace and large white) pigs with BNP infusion + sitagliptin; 6 Placebo; 6	Sitagliptin (30 mg/kg/BW) was orally administered for 3 weeks	An increase in stroke volume was observed in the sitagliptin group compared with placebo (+24 + 6% versus −17 + 7%, $P < 0.01$). Glomerular filtration rate declined at week 4 compared with baseline in the placebo group (1.3 + 0.4 versus 2.3 + 0.3 mL/kg/min, $P < 0.01$)
Takahashi et al. [62]	Mice underwent transverse aortic constriction + sitagliptin; 40 Mice underwent transverse aortic constriction + vehicle; 41	Vildagliptin (10 mg/kg/BW day) was administered by drinking water	Improvement of both LV dilatation and dysfunction in the transverse aortic constriction group ameliorated ($P < 0.05$)

GFR, glomerular filtration rate; BW, body weight; BNP, brain natriuretic peptide.

10. The Effects of Incretin-Based Therapeutic Agents on Diabetic Neuropathy

Chronic hyperglycemic state and impaired insulin signaling induce neurological disorders including peripheral nerve system [91, 92]. It has been reported that the effects of GLP-1 and GIP on the peripheral nervous system could be of significance in diabetic neuropathy. GLP-1 or exendin-4 significantly increased the neurite outgrowth of dorsal root ganglion neurons of rodents [93]. Furthermore, exendin-4 ameliorated the delayed motor and sensory nerve conduction [94]. In diabetic rats, the size of myelinated fibers and the ratio of axon/fiber area were decreased, while administration of exendin-4 significantly ameliorated these disorders [94]. Considering these results, GLP-1 could be a useful treatment for diabetic neuropathy.

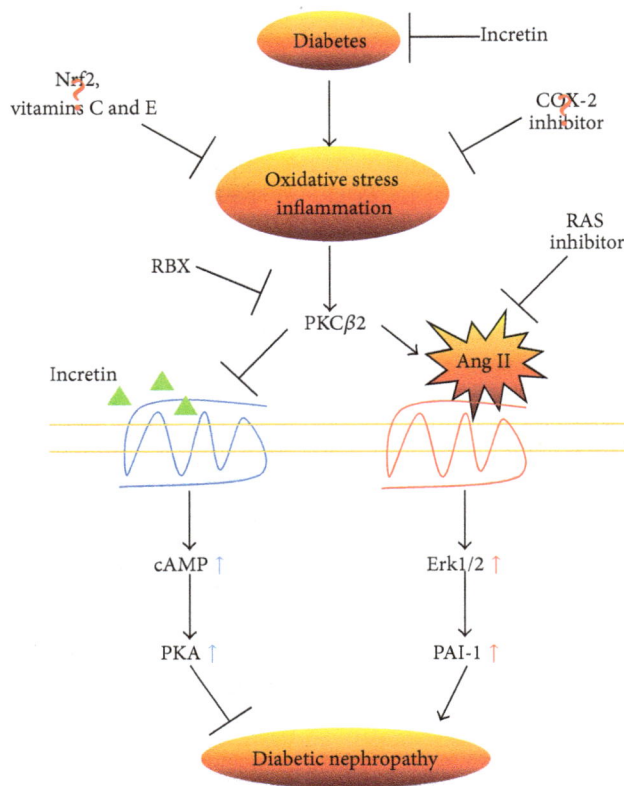

FIGURE 3: Schematic representation of potential protective factors, including incretin and biological targets of PKC activation that could prevent the progression to diabetic nephropathy. Nrf2, nuclear factor erythroid 2-related factor 2; COX-2, cyclooxygenase-2; RAS, renin angiotensin system; RBX, ruboxistaurin; PKC, protein kinase C; Ang II, angiotensin II; cAMP, cyclic adenosine monophosphate; Erk, extracellular signal-regulated kinase; PKA, protein kinase A; PAI-1, plasminogen activator inhibitor-1.

11. Summary

Both diabetes and insulin resistance induce macro- and microvascular complications. Recent novel therapies for diabetes using incretin or DPP-4 inhibitors elicit biological vasoprotective effects that surpass glycemic control. Incretin-based therapies for diabetic vascular complications show potential as promising for the prevention of diabetic vascular complications, though the activation of PKCβ2 and angiotensin II could inhibit this therapeutic effect. Different from proposed therapies, such as antioxidant or anti-inflammatory drugs, incretin-based therapies could be beneficial (Figure 3). However, most favorable results appear to be realized in animal disease models. Thus, large-scale clinical trials should be performed to assess the effects of incretin-based treatments on diabetic vascular complications.

Conflict of Interests

No potential conflict of interests relevant to this paper was reported.

Acknowledgments

Preparation of this publication was supported by grants to Akira Mima from Grant-in-Aid for Scientific Research (26461230) from Japan Society for the Promotion of Science and Japan Health Foundation. Akira Mima reports receiving speaker fees from MSD, Novartis, Takeda, Otsuka, Kyowa Kirin, Eli Lilly, Chugai, Mitsubishi Tanabe, Kissei, Torii, Astellus, Bayer, and Boehringer Ingelheim.

References

[1] The Diabetes Control and Complications Trial Research Group, "The effect of intensive treatment of diabetes on the development and progression of long-term complications in insulin-dependent diabetes mellitus," *The New England Journal of Medicine*, vol. 329, pp. 977–986, 1993.

[2] UK Prospective Diabetes Study (UKPDS) Group, "Intensive blood-glucose control with sulphonylureas or insulin compared with conventional treatment and risk of complications in patients with type 2 diabetes (UKPDS 33)," *The Lancet*, vol. 352, no. 9131, pp. 837–853, 1998.

[3] D. M. Nathan, P. A. Cleary, J.-Y. C. Backlund et al., "Intensive diabetes treatment and cardiovascular disease in patients with type 1 diabetes," *The New England Journal of Medicine*, vol. 353, no. 25, pp. 2643–2653, 2005.

[4] R. R. Holman, S. K. Paul, M. A. Bethel, D. R. Matthews, and H. A. W. Neil, "10-Year follow-up of intensive glucose control in type 2 diabetes," *The New England Journal of Medicine*, vol. 359, no. 15, pp. 1577–1589, 2008.

[5] D. Koya and G. L. King, "Protein kinase C activation and the development of diabetic complications," *Diabetes*, vol. 47, no. 6, pp. 859–866, 1998.

[6] K. Naruse, C. Rask-Madsen, N. Takahara et al., "Activation of vascular protein kinase C-beta; inhibits Akt-dependent endothelial nitric oxide synthase function in obesity-associated insulin resistance," *Diabetes*, vol. 55, no. 3, pp. 691–698, 2006.

[7] M. Kitada, Z. Zhang, A. Mima, and G. L. King, "Molecular mechanisms of diabetic vascular complications," *Journal of Diabetes Investigation*, vol. 1, no. 3, pp. 77–89, 2010.

[8] S. G. Coca, F. Ismail-Beigi, N. Haq, H. M. Krumholz, and C. R. Parikh, "Role of intensive glucose control in development of renal end points in type 2 diabetes mellitus: systematic review and meta-analysis," *Archives of Internal Medicine*, vol. 172, no. 10, pp. 761–769, 2012.

[9] S. Zoungas, A. Patel, J. Chalmers et al., "Severe hypoglycemia and risks of vascular events and death," *The New England Journal of Medicine*, vol. 363, no. 15, pp. 1410–1418, 2010.

[10] D. J. Drucker, "The biology of incretin hormones," *Cell Metabolism*, vol. 3, no. 3, pp. 153–165, 2006.

[11] A. Mima, J. Hiraoka-Yamomoto, Q. Li et al., "Protective effects of GLP-1 on glomerular endothelium and its inhibition by PKCβ activation in diabetes," *Diabetes*, vol. 61, no. 11, pp. 2967–2979, 2012.

[12] M. H. Noyan-Ashraf, M. Abdul Momen, K. Ban et al., "GLP-1R agonist liraglutide activates cytoprotective pathways and improves outcomes after experimental myocardial infarction in mice," *Diabetes*, vol. 58, no. 4, pp. 975–983, 2009.

[13] R. E. Amori, J. Lau, and A. G. Pittas, "Efficacy and safety of incretin therapy in type 2 diabetes: systematic review and meta-analysis," *Journal of the American Medical Association*, vol. 298, no. 2, pp. 194–206, 2007.

[14] S. Devaraj, A. T. Cheung, I. Jialal et al., "Evidence of increased inflammation and microcirculatory abnormalities in patients with type 1 diabetes and their role in microvascular complications," *Diabetes*, vol. 56, no. 11, pp. 2790–2796, 2007.

[15] A. Treszl, L. Szereday, A. Doria, G. L. King, and T. Orban, "Elevated C-reactive protein levels do not correspond to autoimmunity in type 1 diabetes," *Diabetes Care*, vol. 27, no. 11, pp. 2769–2770, 2004.

[16] H. Ha, M. R. Yu, Y. J. Choi, M. Kitamura, and H. B. Lee, "Role of high glucose-induced nuclear factor-κB activation in monocyte chemoattractant protein-1 expression by mesangial cells," *Journal of the American Society of Nephrology*, vol. 13, no. 4, pp. 894–902, 2002.

[17] A. Mima, W. Qi, J. Hiraoka-Yamomoto et al., "Retinal not systemic oxidative and inflammatory stress correlated with VEGF expression in rodent models of insulin resistance and diabetes," *Investigative Ophthalmology and Visual Science*, vol. 53, no. 13, pp. 8424–8432, 2012.

[18] C.-C. Wu, J.-S. Chen, K.-C. Lu et al., "Aberrant cytokines/chemokines production correlate with proteinuria in patients with overt diabetic nephropathy," *Clinica Chimica Acta*, vol. 411, no. 9-10, pp. 700–704, 2010.

[19] A. Mima, W. Qi, and G. L. King, "Implications of treatment that target protective mechanisms against diabetic nephropathy," *Seminars in Nephrology*, vol. 32, no. 5, pp. 471–478, 2012.

[20] P. Xia, T. Inoguchi, T. S. Kern, R. L. Engerman, P. J. Oates, and G. L. King, "Characterization of the mechanism for the chronic activation of diacylglycerol-protein kinase C pathway in diabetes and hypergalactosemia," *Diabetes*, vol. 43, no. 9, pp. 1122–1129, 1994.

[21] G. L. King, M. Kunisaki, Y. Nishio, T. Inoguchi, T. Shiba, and P. Xia, "Biochemical and molecular mechanisms in the development of diabetic vascular complications," *Diabetes*, vol. 45, supplement 3, pp. S105–S108, 1996.

[22] M. Kitada, D. Koya, T. Sugimoto et al., "Translocation of glomerular p47phox and p67phox by protein kinase C-β activation is required for oxidative stress in diabetic nephropathy," *Diabetes*, vol. 52, no. 10, pp. 2603–2614, 2003.

[23] A. D. Hodgkinson, T. Bartlett, P. J. Oates, B. A. Millward, and A. G. Demaine, "The response of antioxidant genes to hyperglycemia is abnormal in patients with type 1 diabetes and diabetic nephropathy," *Diabetes*, vol. 52, no. 3, pp. 846–851, 2003.

[24] Z. Zhang, K. Apse, J. Pang, and R. C. Stanton, "High glucose inhibits glucose-6-phosphate dehydrogenase via cAMP in aortic endothelial cells," *The Journal of Biological Chemistry*, vol. 275, no. 51, pp. 40042–40047, 2000.

[25] L. A. Brondani, B. M. de Souza, G. C. K. Duarte et al., "The UCP1 -3826A/G polymorphism is associated with diabetic retinopathy and increased UCP1 and MnSOD2 gene expression in human retina," *Investigative Ophthalmology & Visual Science*, vol. 53, no. 12, pp. 7449–7457, 2012.

[26] A. Mezzetti, F. Cipollone, and F. Cuccurullo, "Oxidative stress and cardiovascular complications in diabetes: isoprostanes as new markers on an old paradigm," *Cardiovascular Research*, vol. 47, no. 3, pp. 475–488, 2000.

[27] M. Kakimoto, T. Inoguchi, T. Sonta et al., "Accumulation of 8-hydroxy-2′-deoxyguanosine and mitochondrial DNA deletion in kidney of diabetic rats," *Diabetes*, vol. 51, no. 5, pp. 1588–1595, 2002.

[28] J. Leinonen, T. Lehtimäki, S. Toyokuni et al., "New biomarker evidence of oxidative DNA damage in patients with non-insulin-dependent diabetes mellitus," *FEBS Letters*, vol. 417, no. 1, pp. 150–152, 1997.

[29] R. E. Gilbert, S. A. Kim, K. R. Tuttle et al., "Effect of ruboxistaurin on urinary transforming growth factor-β in patients with diabetic nephropathy and type 2 diabetes," *Diabetes Care*, vol. 30, no. 4, pp. 995–996, 2007.

[30] D. Koya, I.-K. Lee, H. Ishii, H. Kanoh, and G. L. King, "Prevention of glomerular dysfunction in diabetic rats by treatment with d-alpha-tocopherol," *Journal of the American Society of Nephrology*, vol. 8, no. 3, pp. 426–435, 1997.

[31] J.-R. Koo and N. D. Vaziri, "Effects of diabetes, insulin and antioxidants on NO synthase abundance and NO interaction with reactive oxygen species," *Kidney International*, vol. 63, no. 1, pp. 195–201, 2003.

[32] G. T. Mustata, M. Rosca, K. M. Biemel et al., "Paradoxical effects of green tea (*Camellia sinensis*) and antioxidant vitamins in diabetic rats: improved retinopathy and renal mitochondrial defects but deterioration of collagen matrix glycoxidation and cross-linking," *Diabetes*, vol. 54, no. 2, pp. 517–526, 2005.

[33] H. Zheng, S. A. Whitman, W. Wu et al., "Therapeutic potential of Nrf2 activators in streptozotocin-induced diabetic nephropathy," *Diabetes*, vol. 60, no. 11, pp. 3055–3066, 2011.

[34] H. Li, L. Zhang, F. Wang et al., "Attenuation of glomerular injury in diabetic mice with tert-butylhydroquinone through nuclear factor erythroid 2-related factor 2-dependent antioxidant gene activation," *American Journal of Nephrology*, vol. 33, no. 4, pp. 289–297, 2011.

[35] P. Palsamy and S. Subramanian, "Resveratrol protects diabetic kidney by attenuating hyperglycemia-mediated oxidative stress and renal inflammatory cytokines via Nrf2-Keap1 signaling," *Biochimica et Biophysica Acta—Molecular Basis of Disease*, vol. 1812, no. 7, pp. 719–731, 2011.

[36] P. E. Pergola, M. Krauth, J. W. Huff et al., "Effect of bardoxolone methyl on kidney function in patients with T2D and stage 3b-4 CKD," *American Journal of Nephrology*, vol. 33, no. 5, pp. 469–476, 2011.

[37] P. E. Pergola, P. Raskin, R. D. Toto et al., "Bardoxolone methyl and kidney function in CKD with type 2 diabetes," *The New England Journal of Medicine*, vol. 365, no. 4, pp. 327–336, 2011.

[38] A. Psichas, F. Reimann, and F. M. Gribble, "Gut chemosensing mechanisms," *The Journal of Clinical Investigation*, vol. 125, no. 3, pp. 908–917, 2015.

[39] B. P. Bullock, R. S. Heller, and J. F. Habener, "Tissue distribution of messenger ribonucleic acid encoding the rat glucagon-like peptide-1 receptor," *Endocrinology*, vol. 137, no. 7, pp. 2968–2978, 1996.

[40] Ö. Erdogdu, D. Nathanson, Å. Sjöholm, T. Nyström, and Q. Zhang, "Exendin-4 stimulates proliferation of human coronary artery endothelial cells through eNOS-, PKA- and PI3K/Akt-dependent pathways and requires GLP-1 receptor," *Molecular and Cellular Endocrinology*, vol. 325, no. 1-2, pp. 26–35, 2010.

[41] T. Nyström, M. K. Gutniak, Q. Zhang et al., "Effects of glucagon-like peptide-1 on endothelial function in type 2 diabetes patients with stable coronary artery disease," *The American Journal of Physiology—Endocrinology and Metabolism*, vol. 287, no. 6, pp. E1209–E1215, 2004.

[42] T. P. Vahl, M. Tauchi, T. S. Durler et al., "Glucagon-Like Peptide-1 (GLP-1) receptors expressed on nerve terminals in the portal vein mediate the effects of endogenous GLP-1 on glucose

tolerance in rats," *Endocrinology*, vol. 148, no. 10, pp. 4965–4973, 2007.

[43] A. Ojima, T. Matsui, S. Maeda, M. Takeuchi, and S. Yamagishi, "Glucose-dependent insulinotropic polypeptide (GIP) inhibits signaling pathways of advanced glycation end products (AGEs) in endothelial cells via its antioxidative properties," *Hormone and Metabolic Research*, vol. 44, no. 7, pp. 501–505, 2012.

[44] L. A. Nikolaidis, D. Elahi, T. Hentosz et al., "Recombinant glucagon-like peptide-1 increases myocardial glucose uptake and improves left ventricular performance in conscious dogs with pacing-induced dilated cardiomyopathy," *Circulation*, vol. 110, no. 8, pp. 955–961, 2004.

[45] M. Monami, N. Marchionni, and E. Mannucci, "Glucagon-like peptide-1 receptor agonists in type 2 diabetes: a meta-analysis of randomized clinical trials," *European Journal of Endocrinology*, vol. 160, no. 6, pp. 909–917, 2009.

[46] M. Monami, I. Iacomelli, N. Marchionni, and E. Mannucci, "Dipeptydil peptidase-4 inhibitors in type 2 diabetes: a meta-analysis of randomized clinical trials," *Nutrition, Metabolism and Cardiovascular Diseases*, vol. 20, no. 4, pp. 224–235, 2010.

[47] J. Matsubara, S. Sugiyama, K. Sugamura et al., "A dipeptidyl peptidase-4 inhibitor, des-fluoro-sitagliptin, improves endothelial function and reduces atherosclerotic lesion formation in apolipoprotein edeficient mice," *Journal of the American College of Cardiology*, vol. 59, no. 3, pp. 265–276, 2012.

[48] S. Hattori, "Sitagliptin reduces albuminuria in patients with type 2 diabetes," *Endocrine Journal*, vol. 58, no. 1, pp. 69–73, 2011.

[49] H. Fujita, H. Taniai, H. Murayama et al., "DPP-4 inhibition with alogliptin on top of angiotensin II type 1 receptor blockade ameliorates albuminuria via up-regulation of SDF-1α in type 2 diabetic patients with incipient nephropathy," *Endocrine Journal*, vol. 61, no. 2, pp. 159–166, 2014.

[50] M. Arakawa, T. Mita, K. Azuma et al., "Inhibition of monocyte adhesion to endothelial cells and attenuation of atherosclerotic lesion by a glucagon-like peptide-1 receptor agonist, exendin-4," *Diabetes*, vol. 59, no. 4, pp. 1030–1037, 2010.

[51] N. Panjwani, E. E. Mulvihill, C. Longuet et al., "GLP-1 receptor activation indirectly reduces hepatic lipid accumulation but does not attenuate development of atherosclerosis in diabetic male *ApoE$^{-/-}$* mice," *Endocrinology*, vol. 154, no. 1, pp. 127–139, 2013.

[52] A. Mima, "Diabetic nephropathy: protective factors and a new therapeutic paradigm," *Journal of Diabetes and Its Complications*, vol. 27, no. 5, pp. 526–530, 2013.

[53] P. H. Groop, M. E. Cooper, V. Perkovic et al., "Dipeptidyl peptidase-4 inhibition with linagliptin and effects on hyperglycaemia and albuminuria in patients with type 2 diabetes and renal dysfunction: rationale and design of the MARLINA-T2D trial," *Diabetes & Vascular Disease Research*, vol. 12, no. 6, pp. 455–462, 2015.

[54] C. W. Park, H. W. Kim, S. H. Ko et al., "Long-term treatment of glucagon-like peptide-1 analog exendin-4 ameliorates diabetic nephropathy through improving metabolic anomalies in db/db mice," *Journal of the American Society of Nephrology*, vol. 18, no. 4, pp. 1227–1238, 2007.

[55] R. Kodera, K. Shikata, H. U. Kataoka et al., "Glucagon-like peptide-1 receptor agonist ameliorates renal injury through its anti-inflammatory action without lowering blood glucose level in a rat model of type 1 diabetes," *Diabetologia*, vol. 54, no. 4, pp. 965–978, 2011.

[56] H. Hendarto, T. Inoguchi, Y. Maeda et al., "GLP-1 analog liraglutide protects against oxidative stress and albuminuria

in streptozotocin-induced diabetic rats via protein kinase A-mediated inhibition of renal NAD(P)H oxidases," *Metabolism: Clinical and Experimental*, vol. 61, no. 10, pp. 1422–1434, 2012.

[57] K. Kanasaki, S. Shi, M. Kanasaki et al., "Linagliptin-mediated DPP-4 inhibition ameliorates kidney fibrosis in streptozotocin-induced diabetic mice by inhibiting endothelial-to-mesenchymal transition in a therapeutic regimen," *Diabetes*, vol. 63, no. 6, pp. 2120–2131, 2014.

[58] H.-C. Ku and M.-J. Su, "DPP4 deficiency preserved cardiac function in abdominal aortic banding rats," *PLoS ONE*, vol. 9, no. 1, Article ID e85634, 2014.

[59] J. B. Green, M. A. Bethel, S. K. Paul et al., "Rationale, design, and organization of a randomized, controlled Trial Evaluating Cardiovascular Outcomes with Sitagliptin (TECOS) in patients with type 2 diabetes and established cardiovascular disease," *American Heart Journal*, vol. 166, no. 6, pp. 983–989.e7, 2013.

[60] Y. Ye, K. T. Keyes, C. Zhang, J. R. Perez-Polo, Y. Lin, and Y. Birnbaum, "The myocardial infarct size-limiting effect of sitagliptin is PKA-dependent, whereas the protective effect of pioglitazone is partially dependent on PKA," *American Journal of Physiology: Heart and Circulatory Physiology*, vol. 298, no. 5, pp. H1454–H1465, 2010.

[61] N. Gomez, K. Touihri, V. Matheeussen et al., "Dipeptidyl peptidase IV inhibition improves cardiorenal function in overpacing-induced heart failure," *European Journal of Heart Failure*, vol. 14, no. 1, pp. 14–21, 2012.

[62] A. Takahashi, M. Asakura, S. Ito et al., "Dipeptidy -peptidase IV inhibition improves pathophysiology of heart failure and increases survival rate in pressure-overloaded mice," *The American Journal of Physiology—Heart and Circulatory Physiology*, vol. 304, no. 10, pp. H1361–H1369, 2013.

[63] C. Pyke and L. B. Knudsen, "The glucagon-like peptide-1 receptor—or not?" *Endocrinology*, vol. 154, no. 1, pp. 4–8, 2013.

[64] H. Fujita, T. Morii, H. Fujishima et al., "The protective roles of GLP-1R signaling in diabetic nephropathy: possible mechanism and therapeutic potential," *Kidney International*, vol. 85, no. 3, pp. 579–589, 2014.

[65] G. Xu, H. Kaneto, D. R. Laybutt et al., "Downregulation of GLP-1 and GIP receptor expression by hyperglycemia: possible contribution to impaired incretin effects in diabetes," *Diabetes*, vol. 56, no. 6, pp. 1551–1558, 2007.

[66] Y. Ishibashi, Y. Nishino, T. Matsui, M. Takeuchi, and S.-I. Yamagishi, "Glucagon-like peptide-1 suppresses advanced glycation end product-induced monocyte chemoattractant protein-1 expression in mesangial cells by reducing advanced glycation end product receptor level," *Metabolism: Clinical and Experimental*, vol. 60, no. 9, pp. 1271–1277, 2011.

[67] J.-P. Gutzwiller, S. Tschopp, A. Bock et al., "Glucagon-like peptide 1 induces natriuresis in healthy subjects and in insulin-resistant obese men," *The Journal of Clinical Endocrinology & Metabolism*, vol. 89, no. 6, pp. 3055–3061, 2004.

[68] W. J. Liu, S. H. Xie, Y. N. Liu et al., "Dipeptidyl peptidase IV inhibitor attenuates kidney injury in streptozotocin-induced diabetic rats," *The Journal of Pharmacology and Experimental Therapeutics*, vol. 340, no. 2, pp. 248–255, 2012.

[69] L. L. F. Glorie, A. Verhulst, V. Matheeussen et al., "DPP4 inhibition improves functional outcome after renal ischemia-reperfusion injury," *The American Journal of Physiology—Renal Physiology*, vol. 303, no. 5, pp. F681–F688, 2012.

[70] P. Vavrinec, R. H. Henning, S. W. Landheer et al., "Vildagliptin restores renal myogenic function and attenuates renal sclerosis

independently of effects on blood glucose or proteinuria in Zucker Diabetic Fatty rat," *Current Vascular Pharmacology*, vol. 12, no. 6, pp. 836–844, 2014.

[71] C. Mega, E. T. de Lemos, H. Vala et al., "Diabetic nephropathy amelioration by a low-dose sitagliptin in an animal model of type 2 diabetes (Zucker diabetic fatty rat)," *Experimental Diabetes Research*, vol. 2011, Article ID 162092, 12 pages, 2011.

[72] B. B. Dokken, L. R. La Bonte, G. Davis-Gorman, M. K. Teachey, N. Seaver, and P. F. McDonagh, "Glucagon-like peptide-1 (GLP-1), immediately prior to reperfusion, decreases neutrophil activation and reduces myocardial infarct size in rodents," *Hormone and Metabolic Research*, vol. 43, no. 5, pp. 300–305, 2011.

[73] M. Matsubara, S. Kanemoto, B. G. Leshnower et al., "Single dose GLP-1-tf ameliorates myocardial ischemia/reperfusion injury," *The Journal of Surgical Research*, vol. 165, no. 1, pp. 38–45, 2011.

[74] L. Timmers, J. P. S. Henriques, D. P. V. de Kleijn et al., "Exenatide reduces infarct size and improves cardiac function in a porcine model of ischemia and reperfusion injury," *Journal of the American College of Cardiology*, vol. 53, no. 6, pp. 501–510, 2009.

[75] Y. Nogi, M. Nagashima, M. Terasaki, K. Nohtomi, T. Watanabe, and T. Hirano, "Glucose-dependent insulinotropic polypeptide prevents the progression of macrophage-driven atherosclerosis in diabetic apolipoprotein E-null mice," *PLoS ONE*, vol. 7, no. 4, Article ID e35683, 2012.

[76] S. P. Marso, N. R. Poulter, S. E. Nissen et al., "Design of the liraglutide effect and action in diabetes: evaluation of cardiovascular outcome results (LEADER) trial," *American Heart Journal*, vol. 166, no. 5, pp. 823.e5–830.e5, 2013.

[77] W. M. Steinberg, M. A. Nauck, B. Zinman et al., "LEADER 3-lipase and amylase activity in subjects with type 2 diabetes baseline data from over 9000 subjects in the LEADER trial," *Pancreas*, vol. 43, no. 8, pp. 1223–1231, 2014.

[78] L. M. McCormick, A. C. Kydd, P. A. Read et al., "Chronic dipeptidyl peptidase-4 inhibition with sitagliptin is associated with sustained protection against ischemic left ventricular dysfunction in a pilot study of patients with type 2 diabetes mellitus and coronary artery disease," *Circulation: Cardiovascular Imaging*, vol. 7, no. 2, pp. 274–281, 2014.

[79] B. M. Scirica, D. L. Bhatt, E. Braunwald et al., "Saxagliptin and cardiovascular outcomes in patients with type 2 diabetes mellitus," *The New England Journal of Medicine*, vol. 369, no. 14, pp. 1317–1326, 2013.

[80] W. B. White, C. P. Cannon, S. R. Heller et al., "Alogliptin after acute coronary syndrome in patients with type 2 diabetes," *The New England Journal of Medicine*, vol. 369, no. 14, pp. 1327–1335, 2013.

[81] J. B. Green, M. A. Bethel, P. W. Armstrong et al., "Effect of sitagliptin on cardiovascular outcomes in type 2 diabetes," *The New England Journal of Medicine*, vol. 373, pp. 232–242, 2015.

[82] E. Faivre, V. A. Gault, B. Thorens, and C. Hölscher, "Glucose-dependent insulinotropic polypeptide receptor knockout mice are impaired in learning, synaptic plasticity, and neurogenesis," *Journal of Neurophysiology*, vol. 105, no. 4, pp. 1574–1580, 2011.

[83] V. Darsalia, H. Ortsäter, A. Olverling et al., "The DPP-4 inhibitor linagliptin counteracts stroke in the normal and diabetic mouse brain: a comparison with glimepiride," *Diabetes*, vol. 62, no. 4, pp. 1289–1296, 2013.

[84] R. Klein, B. E. K. Klein, and S. E. Moss, "Epidemiology of proliferative diabetic retinopathy," *Diabetes Care*, vol. 15, no. 12, pp. 1875–1891, 1992.

[85] J. W. Miller, A. P. Adamis, and L. P. Aiello, "Vascular endothelial growth factor in ocular neovascularization and proliferative diabetic retinopathy," *Diabetes/Metabolism Reviews*, vol. 13, no. 1, pp. 37–50, 1997.

[86] E. M. Kohner, I. M. Stratton, S. J. Aldington, R. R. Holman, and D. R. Matthews, "Relationship between the severity of retinopathy and progression to photocoagulation in patients with Type 2 diabetes mellitus in the UKPDS (UKPDS 52)," *Diabetic Medicine*, vol. 18, no. 3, pp. 178–184, 2001.

[87] The Diabetes Control and Complications Trial/Epidemiology of Diabetes Interventions and Complications Research Group, "Retinopathy and nephropathy in patients with type 1 diabetes four years after a trial of intensive therapy," *The New England Journal of Medicine*, vol. 342, pp. 381–389, 2000.

[88] Y. Zhang, J. Zhang, Q. Wang et al., "Intravitreal injection of exendin-4 analogue protects retinal cells in early diabetic rats," *Investigative Ophthalmology & Visual Science*, vol. 52, no. 1, pp. 278–285, 2011.

[89] Z. Fu, H.-Y. Kuang, M. Hao, X.-Y. Gao, Y. Liu, and N. Shao, "Protection of exenatide for retinal ganglion cells with different glucose concentrations," *Peptides*, vol. 37, no. 1, pp. 25–31, 2012.

[90] A. Gonçalves, E. Leal, A. Paiva et al., "Protective effects of the dipeptidyl peptidase IV inhibitor sitagliptin in the blood-retinal barrier in a type 2 diabetes animal model," *Diabetes, Obesity and Metabolism*, vol. 14, no. 5, pp. 454–463, 2012.

[91] A. O. Colby, "Neurologic disorders of diabetes mellitus. I," *Diabetes*, vol. 14, pp. 424–429, 1965.

[92] A. O. Colby, "Neurologic disorders of diabetes mellitus. Ii," *Diabetes*, vol. 14, no. 8, pp. 516–525, 1965.

[93] T. Himeno, H. Kamiya, K. Naruse et al., "Beneficial effects of exendin-4 on experimental polyneuropathy in diabetic mice," *Diabetes*, vol. 60, no. 9, pp. 2397–2406, 2011.

[94] W. J. Liu, H. Y. Jin, K. A. Lee, S. H. Xie, H. S. Baek, and T. S. Park, "Neuroprotective effect of the glucagon-like peptide-1 receptor agonist, synthetic exendin-4, in streptozotocin-induced diabetic rats," *British Journal of Pharmacology*, vol. 164, no. 5, pp. 1410–1420, 2011.

18

Free Fatty Acids Activate Renin-Angiotensin System in 3T3-L1 Adipocytes through Nuclear Factor-kappa B Pathway

Jia Sun,[1] Jinhua Luo,[2] Yuting Ruan,[1] Liangchang Xiu,[3] Bimei Fang,[4] Hua Zhang,[1] Ming Wang,[5] and Hong Chen[1]

[1]Department of Endocrinology, Zhujiang Hospital, Southern Medical University, Guangzhou, China
[2]Department of Geratology, The Affiliated Hospital of Guangdong Medical College, Guangdong Medical College, Zhanjiang, Guangdong, China
[3]Department of Epidemiology and Medical Statistics, School of Public Health, Guangdong Medical College, Dongguan, Guangdong, China
[4]Second Clinical School of Medicine, Southern Medical University, Guangzhou, China
[5]Nephrology Center of Integrated Traditional Chinese and Western Medicine, Zhujiang Hospital, Southern Medical University, Guangzhou, China

Correspondence should be addressed to Ming Wang; wming1999@163.com and Hong Chen; rubychq@163.com

Academic Editor: Xingxing Kong

The activity of a local renin-angiotensin system (RAS) in the adipose tissue is closely associated with obesity-related diseases. However, the mechanism of RAS activation in adipose tissue is still unknown. In the current study, we found that palmitic acid (PA), one kind of free fatty acid, induced the activity of RAS in 3T3-L1 adipocytes. In the presence of fetuin A (Fet A), PA upregulated the expression of angiotensinogen (AGT) and angiotensin type 1 receptor (AT_1R) and stimulated the secretion of angiotensin II (ANG II) in 3T3-L1 adipocytes. Moreover, the activation of RAS in 3T3-L1 adipocytes was blocked when we blocked Toll-like receptor 4 (TLR4) signaling pathway using TAK242 or NF-κB signaling pathway using BAY117082. Together, our results have identified critical molecular mechanisms linking PA/TLR4/NF-κB signaling pathway to the activity of the local renin-angiotensin system in adipose tissue.

1. Introduction

Activation of the renin-angiotensin system (RAS) is instrumental in regulating blood pressure and fluid balance. RAS activation is also associated with impaired differentiation of preadipocytes [1] and increased lipolysis and enhanced oxidative stress and inflammatory response [2–8]. Defects in the system are associated with obesity, type 2 diabetes, and cardiovascular diseases. RAS are found in a number of tissues, including kidneys, heart, and nervous and immune systems. Components of RAS, including renin, angiotensinogen (AGT), angiotensin-converting enzyme (ACE), and angiotensins I, II, and III (ANG I, ANG II, and ANG III), have also been found in adipose tissue [9, 10]. It is well established that free fatty acids (FFAs) are activators of RAS in leukocytes [11, 12]. However, whether FFAs play a role in the activation

of RAS in adipocytes is unclear. It has been shown that the levels of FFAs originating from lipolysis in adipocytes are significantly increased in peripheral circulation as well as local tissues in obese humans and animals [13, 14]. It has been hypothesized that RAS could regulate adipocyte differentiation through Ang II and the adipocyte AT_1R in mice [15]. Therefore, FFAs may directly regulate RAS activation in adipose tissue which might be a trigging mechanism of glucose and lipid metabolism disorder and obesity-related diseases. FFA components such as palmitic acid (PA) and lauric acid can bind to Toll-like receptor 4 (TLR4) with the assistance of the endogenous ligand, fetuin A (Fet A), thus mediating the activation of TLR4 and NF-κB pathways and leading to the inflammatory cascade [14]. TLR4 is a member of the family of Toll-like receptors (TLRs), which can activate mitogen-activated protein kinase and nuclear factor

κB (NF-κB) to regulate inflammatory and immune responses after binding to ligands [16]. Moreover, a recent study has demonstrated that active TLR4 can induce the activation of RAS in hepatocytes [17] and cardiac muscle cells [18]. Therefore, we hypothesize that palmitic acid (PA) triggers the TLR4 signaling pathway, leading to RAS activation in adipocytes.

2. Material and Methods

2.1. Reagents. We purchased 3T3-L1 preadipocyte line from ATCC (CL-173); Dulbecco's Modified Eagle Medium (DMEM) with 25 mM D-glucose from HyClone (USA); Dexamethasone (DXM), Isobutylmethylxanthine (IBMX), 4% paraformaldehyde, Oil Red O, Irbesartan, and Captopril from Sigma (Sigma-Aldrich, St. Louis, USA); dimethyl sulfoxide (DMSO) from Invitrogen (USA); Ang II Enzyme-linked immunosorbent assay kit from Cusabio (Wuhan, China); Anti-TLR4 antibody from Abnova (Taiwan, China); anti-AGT antibody from Merck (Merck Millipore, Darmstadt, Germany); anti-AT$_1$R antibody and anti-GAPDH antibody from Santa Cruz (CA, USA); Anti-α-tubulin antibody from Cell Signaling Technology (Beverly, MA, USA); and horseradish peroxidase-linked goat-anti-rabbit antibody from KPL (Gaithersburg, MD, USA).

2.2. Cell Culture, Differentiation, and Identification. 3T3-L1 preadipocytes were subcultured with 25 mM D-glucose DMEM. Two days after confluence, the cells were differentiated to adipocytes using the same medium containing 10% fetal bovine serum (FBS, HyClone), supplemented with 10 μg/mL insulin, 1 μM DXM, and 0.5 mM IBMX. This medium was replaced with a fresh medium containing insulin 48 hours later, after which the medium was replaced every other day. Approximately 90%–95% of cells differentiated into mature adipocytes on days 8–10 of culture, which were used in the experiments. After the 3T3-L1 preadipocytes were completely differentiated, 4% paraformaldehyde was added to the culture dish and maintained for 10 min, stained with Oil Red O staining for 30 min, followed by stain extraction and observation using a microscope.

2.3. Preparation of Palmitic Acid. Palmitic acid (PA) and bovine serum albumin (BSA) were purchased from Sigma (Sigma-Aldrich, St. Louis, USA). PA were dissolved completely in 0.1 M NaOH at 70°C and then complexed with 9.5 mL 10% BSA at 55°C for 10 min such that a final PA concentration of 5 mM was achieved. Stock solutions were stored at 4°C after filtration or diluted with DMEM to one-tenth (500 μM PA) or one-twentieth (250 μM PA) that were prepared fresh before experiments.

2.4. Enzyme-Linked Immunosorbent Assay. 3T3-L1 adipocytes were treated, respectively, with DMEM, DMEM + 0.1% BSA, DMEM + 0.1% BSA + 10 μg/mL Fet A, or DMEM + 0.1% BSA + 500 μM PA for 3 hours or treated in 500 μM PA + Fet A condition for 1, 3, or 5 hours. In other experiments, 3T3-L1 adipocytes were treated with 250 μM PA + 10 μg/mL Fet A or 500 μM PA + 10 μg/mL Fet A in the same vehicle, containing DMEM and 0.1% BSA, for 3 hours. The supernatants were collected and the concentrations of ANG II were determined by double antibody sandwich method, using Ang II *Enzyme-linked immunosorbent assay* kit. The OD values were measured by a microplate reader, and then ANG II concentration was calculated.

2.5. Quantitative RT-PCR. Amplification and detection of RNA were performed in an ABI Prism 7300 Sequence Detection System using SYBR Green (Applied Biosystems, Foster City, CA, USA), according to the manufacturer's instructions. Primers for quantitative RT-PCR were designed based on sequences from the GenBank, as follows. The relative mRNA expression level was calculated using the comparative expression level $2^{-\Delta\Delta CT}$ method:

TLR4: F: 5$'$-GCATCATCTTCATTGTCCTTGA-3$'$,
R: 5$'$-CTTGTTCTTCCTCTGCTGTTTG-3$'$;
AGT: F: 5$'$-CCTTCCATCTCCTTTACCACAA-3$'$,
R: 5$'$-GCAGGGTCTTCTCATTCACAG-3$'$;
AT$_1$R: F: 5$'$-TGCCATGCCCATAACCATCTG-3$'$,
R: 5$'$-CGTGCTCATTTTCGTAGACAGG-3$'$;
GAPDH: F: 5$'$-GGAAGCCCATCACCATCTT-3$'$,
R: 5$'$-GGTTCACACCCATCACAAACAT-3$'$.

2.6. Western Blotting Analysis. Protein extract was separated on a 15% SDS-polyacrylamide gel and electrophoretically transferred onto a PDVF membrane (Millipore, Etten-Leur, The Netherlands). Membranes were blocked overnight with 5% nonfat dried milk and incubated for 2 h after washing with TBST (10 mM Tris, pH 8.0, 150 mM NaCl, and 0.1% Tween 20), and the membranes were incubated for 1 h with horseradish peroxidase-linked goat-anti-rabbit antibody. The membranes were washed again with TBST, and the proteins were visualized using ECL chemiluminescence.

2.7. Immunofluorescence Double Staining. 3T3-L1 adipocytes were treated with 500 μM PA after pretreatment with two kinds of RAS blocking agents, respectively; one is an angiotensin receptor blocking agent (ARB), Irbesartan, with 10 μM concentration; the other is an inhibitor of ACE (ACEI), Captopril, with 10 μM concentration. Cells were then fixed by paraformaldehyde after the supernatant was removed. FITC + DAPI double staining method was used to detect nuclear translocation of the p65 subunit of NF-κB.

2.8. Statistical Analysis. All statistical analyses were performed using SPSS version 16.0 software. Results were presented as means ± SD. Student's *t*-test was used to compare the means between two samples and statistical comparisons of more than two groups were performed using one-way analysis of variance (ANOVA); post hoc tests were performed using LSD test or Tamhane's T2 test. P values < 0.05 were considered statistically significant.

3. Results

3.1. Combined Fet A and PA Upregulated the Expressions of AGT, AT$_1$R, and TLR4 and Stimulated the Secretion of ANG II in 3T3-L1 Adipocytes. To investigate whether the involvement of Fet A has an effect on the components of RAS

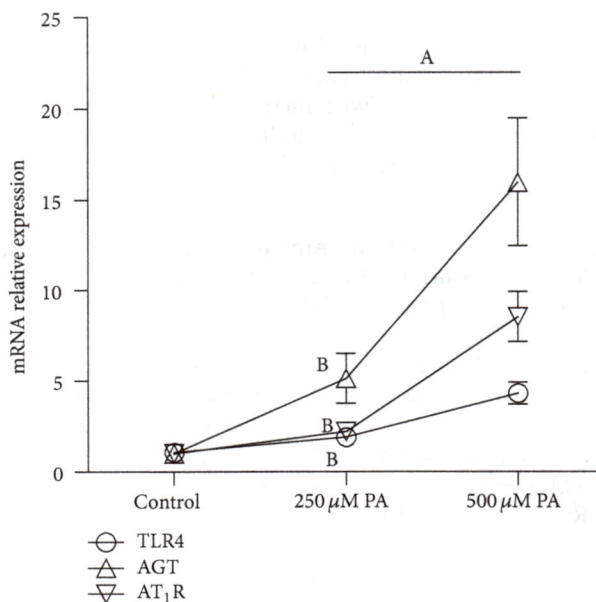

FIGURE 1: mRNA expression of TLR4, AGT, and AT_1R in 3T3-L1 adipocytes induced by PA. Data are presented as mean ± SD. (A) $P < 0.05$ versus control, (B) $P < 0.05$ versus 500 μM PA ($\overline{x} \pm s$, $n = 9$).

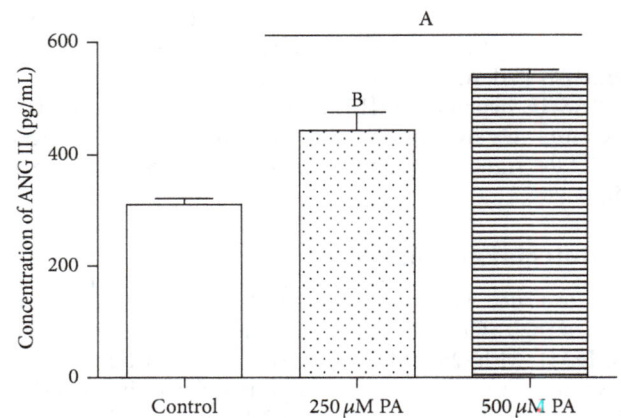

FIGURE 2: Concentrations of ANG II secreted by 3T3-L1 adipocytes after being treated by different concentrations of PA. Data are presented as mean ± SD. (A) $P < 0.05$ versus control, (B) $P < 0.05$ versus 500 μM PA ($\overline{x} \pm s$, $n = 6$).

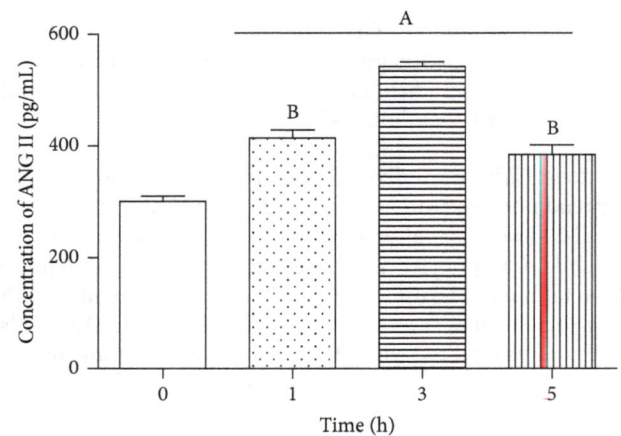

FIGURE 3: Concentrations of ANG II secreted by 3T3-L1 adipocytes after being treated with PA + Fet A at different time. Data are presented as mean ± SD. (A) $P < 0.05$ versus control, (B) $P < 0.05$ versus 3 h ($\overline{x} \pm s$, $n = 6$).

induced by PA in adipocytes, we conducted the following experiments. 3T3-L1 adipocytes were treated with DMEM, DMEM + 0.1% BSA, DMEM + 0.1% BSA + 10 μg/mL Fet A, or DMEM + 0.1% BSA + 500 μM PA for 3 hours, respectively. We found that there were no significant differences in mRNA expressions of AGT, AT_1R and secretion of ANG II between groups. In particular, treatment group of PA or Fet A alone has no significant effect in mRNA expressions of RAS components ($P > 0.05$) (data not shown). In contrast, when 3T3-L1 adipocytes were treated with DMEM + 0.1% BSA + 250 μM PA + 10 μg/mL Fet A or DMEM + 0.1% BSA + 500 μM PA + 10 μg/mL Fet A for 3 hours, PA increased the mRNA expressions of TLR4, AGT, and AT_1R (Figure 1) and the secretion of ANG II (Figure 2). We also test the optimal Fet A and PA treatment time for the secretion of ANG II. We found that the optimal time was 3 hours and time longer than 3 hours caused unspecific effect (Figure 3).

3.2. Combination of Fet A + PA Totally Lost the Effect on the Expressions of AGT and AT_1R in the 3T3-L1 Adipocytes When Blocking TLR4 Beforehand.

To investigate whether TLR4 is the medium of PA affecting RAS component expression, we pretreated 3T3-L1 adipocytes with 5 μM TLR4 inhibitor-TAK242 for 1 hour and then treated with DMEM + 0.1% BSA or DMEM + 0.1% BSA + 500 μM PA + 10 μg/mL Fet for 3 hours, respectively. Compared with the Fet A + PA alone group, TLR4 inhibitor-TAK242 completely blocked the expressions of AGT and AT_1R in the mRNA level (Figure 4) and protein level (Figure 6).

3.3. Combination of Fet A + PA Only Partly Lost the Effect on Expressions of AGT and AT_1R in the 3T3-L1 Adipocytes When Blocking NF-κB Beforehand.

To investigate whether NF-κB is the medium of PA affecting the expression of RAS components, we pretreated 3T3-L1 adipocytes with 1 μM NF-κB inhibitor-BAY117082 for 1 hour and then treated with DMEM + 0.1% BSA or DMEM + 0.1% BSA + 500 μM PA + 10 μg/mL Fet for 3 hours, respectively. Compared with the Fet A + PA alone group, NF-κB inhibitor-BAY117082 only partly blocked the expressions of AGT and AT_1R in the mRNA level (Figure 5) and protein level (Figure 6).

3.4. Combination of Fet A + PA Enabled the Translocation of p65 Subunit of NF-κB to the Nucleus in the 3T3-L1 Adipocytes, and the Effect Was Blocked by RAS Inhibitors.

3T3-L1 adipocytes were treated with DMEM + 0.1% BSA (group 1) or DMEM + 0.1% BSA + 500 μM PA + 10 μg/mL Fet A (group 2) for 3 hours or pretreated with DMEM + 10 μM Irbesartan for 1 hour followed by DMEM + 0.1% BSA + 500 μM PA + 10 μg/mL Fet A for 3 hours (group 3) or pretreated with DMEM + 10 μM Captopril for 1 hour followed

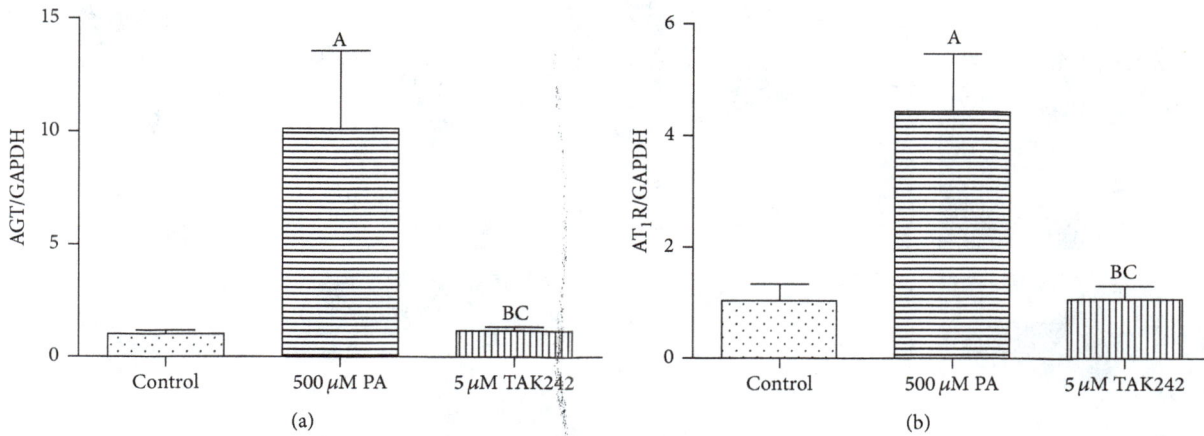

(a)

(b)

FIGURE 4: TAK242 pretreatment prevented upregulation of AGT and AT_1R mRNA expressions. Data are presented as mean ± SD. (A) $P < 0.05$ versus control, (B) $P < 0.05$ versus PA group, and (C) $P > 0.05$ versus control ($\overline{x} \pm s$, $n = 9$).

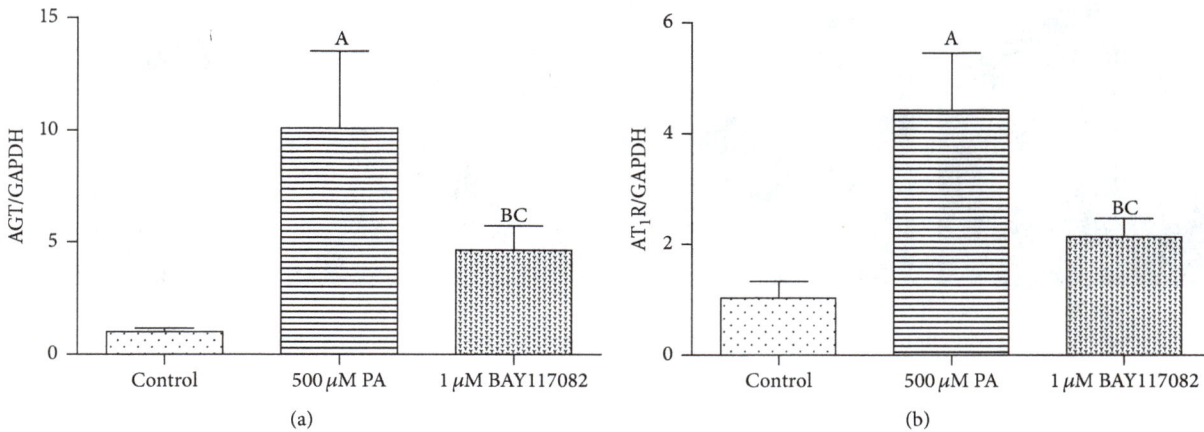

(a)

(b)

FIGURE 5: BAY117082 pretreatment partly prevented upregulation of AGT and AT_1R mRNA expressions. Data are presented as mean ± SD. (A) $P < 0.05$ versus control, (B) $P < 0.05$ versus PA group, and (C) $P > 0.05$ versus control ($\overline{x} \pm s$, $n = 9$).

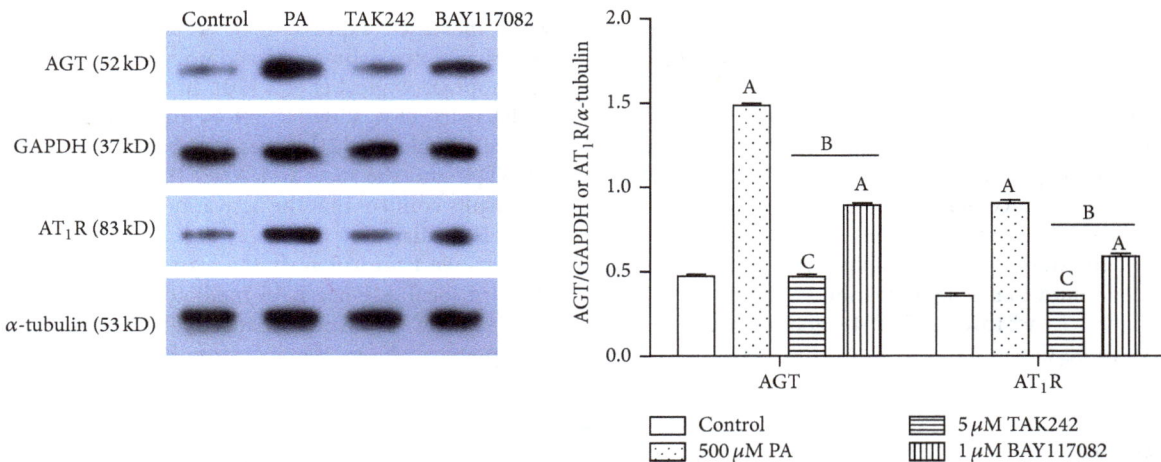

FIGURE 6: Effects of PA with or without TLR4/NF-κB inhibitors on AGT and AT_1R protein expression in the 3T3-L1 adipocytes. Data are presented as mean ± SD. (A) $P < 0.05$ versus control, (B) $P < 0.05$ versus 500 μM PA, and (C) $P > 0.05$ versus control ($\overline{x} \pm s$, $n = 3$).

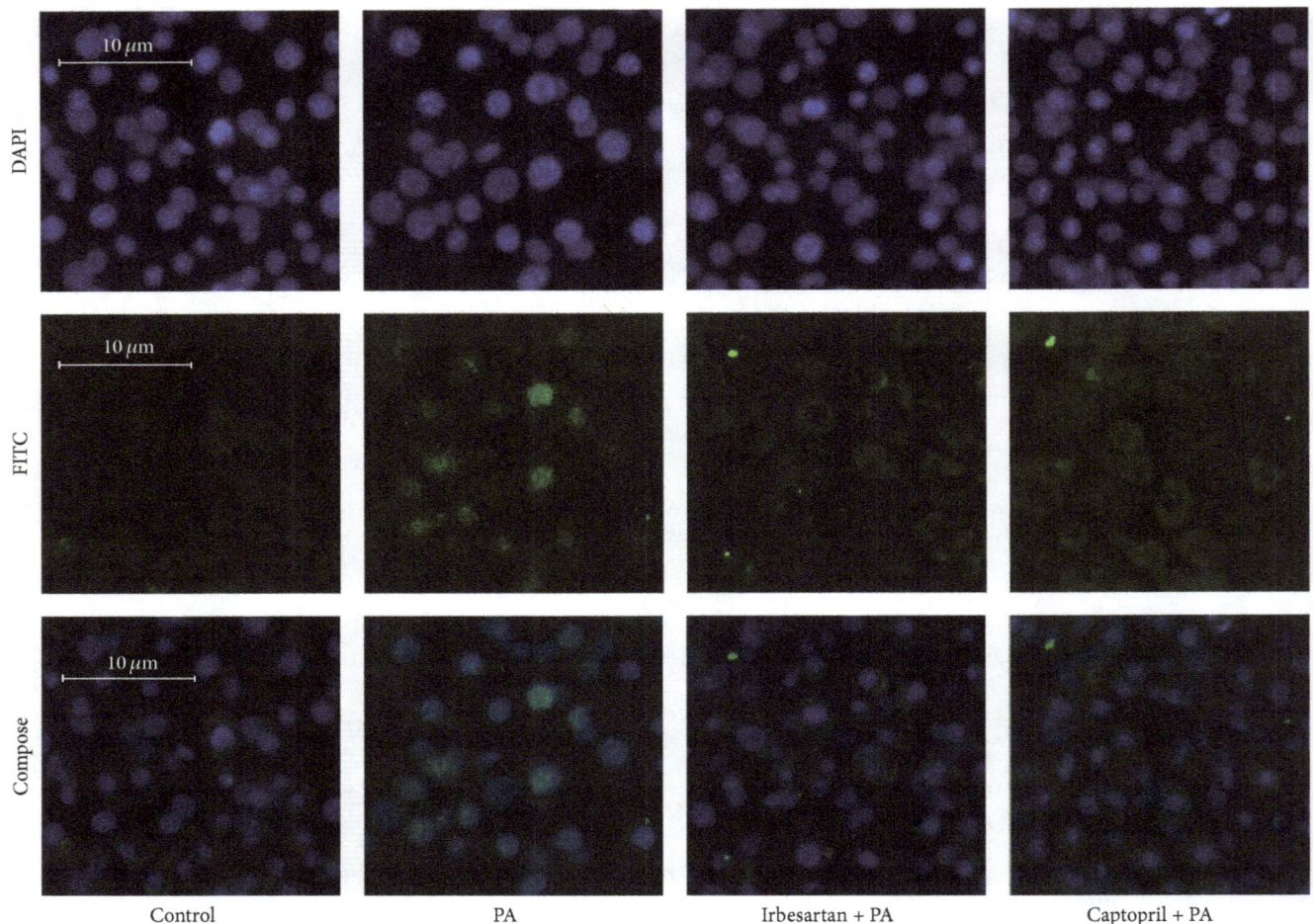

FIGURE 7: Effect of PA with or without Irbesartan or Captopril pretreatment on NF-κB p65 subunit translocation in 3T3-L1 adipocytes. DAPI: DAPI staining of nucleus; FITC: FITC staining of NF-κB p65 subunit; Compose: composite images of DAPI and FITC.

by DMEM + 0.1% BSA + 500 μM PA + 10 μg/mL Fet A (group 4) for 3 hours. The intensity of green fluorescence of FITC in the nucleus of group 2 was stronger, and the cytoplasm of group 2 was weaker than the other 3 groups. The intensity of green fluorescence of FITC in the nucleus and cytoplasm was almost similar in the control (group 1), Irbesartan pretreatment (group 3), and Captopril pretreatment (group 4) groups (Figure 7).

In summary, we found that PA upregulated the expressions of AGT and AT$_1$R in both gene and protein level, as well as the gene expression of TLR4 in 3T3-L1 adipocytes. The PA-induced enhancement of AGT resulted in increasing secretion of ANG II, which is believed to be a crucial early step in the development of adipocytes inflammation. Moreover, we found that RAS activation mediated by PA in adipocytes needs to act through TLR4 signaling pathway but not entirely to be dependent on TLR4 downstream NF-κB pathway.

4. Discussion

AGT, the precursor of ANG II, is mainly expressed in adipocytes [19], which is an important component of RAS in adipose tissue. AGT gets converted to ANG II after being catalyzed by the components of RAS-renin and ACE and the increased generation of ANG II responses to upregulation of AGT expression [4]. Therefore, AGT expression is the symbol of local RAS activation [2, 8, 10]. In addition to the elevation of AGT expression, local RAS activation is often accompanied by the increased expression of AT$_1$R, which is the major ANG II receptor expressed in adipocytes, mediating a series of pathophysiological effects [20]. In current study, we show that PA with Fet A, a liver secretory glycoprotein which exists in blood circulation [21], upregulated the expression of AGT and AT$_1$R and the secretion ANG II in 3T3-L1 adipocytes. Our results confirm that the activation of RAS in the adipose tissues is mediated by PA.

Next, we try to identify the signaling pathways of activation of local adipose RAS mediated by PA infusion. We found that PA with Fet A induced TLR4 activation in 3T3-L1 adipocytes. To further confirm PA-mediated activation of the adipose RAS through TLR4 signaling pathways, TLR4 blocker TAK242 was used to block TLR4 signal pathway before addition of PA and Fet A. We found that the TLR4 blocker completely prevented elevating expressions of AGT, ANG II, and AT$_1$R, confirming that activation of adipose RAS depends on the TLR4 signaling pathway.

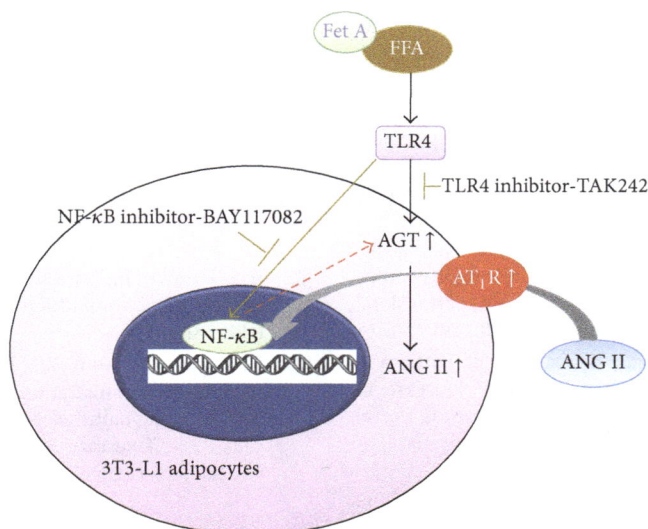

FIGURE 8: Mechanism of RAS activation induced by FFA (PA) in 3T3-L1 adipocytes.

NF-κB, a nuclear transcription factor [22], also upregulated AGT and AT$_1$R, the RAS components, in rat vascular smooth muscle cells [23] and preglomerular vascular smooth muscle cells [23]. Previous studies also found that Ang II could activate NF-κB and its downstream inflammatory pathways [20]. To examine whether NF-κB is involved in the activation of adipocyte RAS, we tested the expressions of AGT, ANGII, and AT$_1$R in PA with Fet A induced RAS activation after using NF-κB inhibitors. We found that PA with Fet A still caused a marginal increase in the expressions of AGT, ANGII, and AT$_1$R with the pretreatment of NF-κB inhibitors. Together, our results suggest that the activation of adipose RAS completely depends on the TLR4 signaling pathway but only partly depends on NF-κB although NF-κB can be activated by TLR4 signaling pathways.

To further vindicate the PA/TLR4/NF-κB signaling pathway, we examined the effect of PA with Fet A on the nuclear translocation of NF-κB. We found that PA with Fet A stimulated the nuclear translocation of NF-κB P65, resulting in eventually increasing NF-κB activity in 3T3-L1 adipocytes. However, this effect is diminished or partly prevented by ACEI or ARB pretreatment, further indicating that PA-induced activation of adipose RAS is correlated with NF-κB activation.

We present a schematic diagram to explain the pathways of activation of adipose RAS induced by PA/Fed A through TLR4/NF-κB signaling pathway in 3T3-L1 adipocytes (Figure 8). When combining act with Fed A, PA enhances TLR4/NF-κB activity, subsequently upregulating the gene and protein expression of AGT and AT$_1$R in adipocytes. PA-induced enhancement of AGT results in increasing secretion of ANG II, which is a crucial early step in the development of adipocytes inflammation. Moreover, the adipose RAS activation mediated by PA/TLR4 is not entirely dependent on NF-κB.

Our findings identify a potential mechanism involved in the pathogenesis of obesity-related diseases.

Conflict of Interests

The authors declare that there is no conflict of interests regarding the publication of this paper.

Authors' Contribution

Jia Sun and Jinhua Luo contributed equally to this work and they are co-first authors.

Acknowledgments

This work was supported by grants to Jia Sun (National Natural Science Foundation of China no. 81300689; the Seedling Projects of Science Foundation of Guangdong Province of China, 2013LYM_0008; the Ministry of Education Foundation of China, 2013443312005) and Ming Wang (National Natural Science Foundation of China, 81403215).

References

[1] Y. Tomono, M. Iwai, S. Inaba, M. Mogi, and M. Horiuchi, "Blockade of AT1 receptor improves adipocyte differentiation in atherosclerotic and diabetic models," *American Journal of Hypertension*, vol. 21, no. 2, pp. 206–212, 2008.

[2] F. Jing, M. Mogi, and M. Horiuchi, "Role of renin-angiotensin-aldosterone system in adipose tissue dysfunction," *Molecular and Cellular Endocrinology*, vol. 378, no. 1-2, pp. 23–28, 2013.

[3] W. A. Banks, L. M. Willoughby, D. R. Thomas, and J. E. Morley, "Insulin resistance syndrome in the elderly: assessment of functional, biochemical, metabolic, and inflammatory status," *Diabetes Care*, vol. 30, no. 9, pp. 2369–2373, 2007.

[4] K. Putnam, R. Shoemaker, F. Yiannikouris, and L. A. Cassis, "The renin-angiotensin system: a target of and contributor to dyslipidemias, altered glucose homeostasis, and hypertension of the metabolic syndrome," *American Journal of Physiology—Heart and Circulatory Physiology*, vol. 302, no. 6, pp. H1219–H1230, 2012.

[5] T. Suganami, M. Tanaka, and Y. Ogawa, "Adipose tissue inflammation and ectopic lipid accumulation," *Endocrine Journal*, vol. 59, no. 10, pp. 849–857, 2012.

[6] G. Giacchetti, L. A. Sechi, C. A. Griffin, B. R. Don, F. Mantero, and M. Schambelan, "The tissue renin-angiotensin system in rats with fructose-induced hypertension: overexpression of type 1 angiotensin II receptor in adipose tissue," *Journal of Hypertension*, vol. 18, no. 6, pp. 695–702, 2000.

[7] K. Gorzelniak, S. Engeli, J. Janke, F. C. Luft, and A. M. Sharma, "Hormonal regulation of the human adipose-tissue renin-angiotensin system: relationship to obesity and hypertension," *Journal of Hypertension*, vol. 20, no. 5, pp. 965–973, 2002.

[8] I. Hainault, G. Nebout, S. Turban, B. Ardouin, P. Ferré, and A. Quignard-Boulangé, "Adipose tissue-specific increase in angiotensinogen expression and secretion in the obese (fa/fa) Zucker rat," *The American Journal of Physiology—Endocrinology and Metabolism*, vol. 282, no. 1, pp. E59–E66, 2002.

[9] N. S. Kalupahana, F. Massiera, A. Quignard-Boulange et al., "Overproduction of angiotensinogen from adipose tissue induces adipose inflammation, glucose intolerance, and insulin resistance," *Obesity*, vol. 20, no. 1, pp. 48–56, 2012.

[10] N. S. Kalupahana and N. Moustaid-Moussa, "The adipose tissue renin-angiotensin system and metabolic disorders: a review of molecular mechanisms," *Critical Reviews in Biochemistry and Molecular Biology*, vol. 47, no. 4, pp. 379–390, 2012.

[11] Y. Azekoshi, T. Yasu, S. Watanabe et al., "Free fatty acid causes leukocyte activation and resultant endothelial dysfunction through enhanced angiotensin II production in mononuclear and polymorphonuclear cells," *Hypertension*, vol. 56, no. 1, pp. 136–142, 2010.

[12] S. Watanabe, T. Tagawa, K. Yamakawa, M. Shimabukuro, and S. Ueda, "Inhibition of the renin-angiotensin system prevents free fatty acid-induced acute endothelial dysfunction in humans," *Arteriosclerosis, Thrombosis, and Vascular Biology*, vol. 25, no. 11, pp. 2376–2380, 2005.

[13] G. Boden, "Free fatty acids (FFA), a link between obesity and insulin resistance," *Frontiers in Bioscience*, vol. 3, pp. d169–d175, 1998.

[14] D. Pal, S. Dasgupta, R. Kundu et al., "Fetuin-A acts as an endogenous ligand of TLR4 to promote lipid-induced insulin resistance," *Nature Medicine*, vol. 18, no. 8, pp. 1279–1285, 2012.

[15] K. Putnam, F. Batifoulier, K. G. Bharadwaj et al., "RAS regulate adipocyte differentiation through Ang II and the adipocyte AT1R in mice," *Endocrinology*, vol. 153, no. 10, pp. 4677–4686, 2012.

[16] H. Shi, M. V. Kokoeva, K. Inouye, I. Tzameli, H. Yin, and J. S. Flier, "TLR4 links innate immunity and fatty acid-induced insulin resistance," *The Journal of Clinical Investigation*, vol. 116, no. 11, pp. 3015–3025, 2006.

[17] Y. Shirai, H. Yoshiji, R. Noguchi et al., "Cross talk between toll-like receptor-4 signaling and angiotensin-II in liver fibrosis development in the rat model of non-alcoholic steatohepatitis," *Journal of Gastroenterology and Hepatology*, vol. 28, no. 4, pp. 723–730, 2013.

[18] J. Hua, Q. Peng, and H. Y. Wang, "Effect of activating toll like receptor 4 on AGT and AT1R in myocardiocytes," *Chinese Journal of Hypertension*, vol. 16, no. 4, pp. 336–339, 2008.

[19] V. Serazin, M.-N. Dieudonné, M. Morot, P. De Mazancourt, and Y. Giudicelli, "cAMP-positive regulation of angiotensinogen gene expression and protein secretion in rat adipose tissue," *The American Journal of Physiology—Endocrinology and Metabolism*, vol. 286, no. 3, pp. E434–E438, 2004.

[20] T. Skurk, V. van Harmelen, and H. Hauner, "Angiotensin II stimulates the release of interleukin-6 and interleukin-8 from cultured human adipocytes by activation of NF-κB," *Arteriosclerosis, Thrombosis, and Vascular Biology*, vol. 24, no. 7, pp. 1199–1203, 2004.

[21] L. Jinhua, S. Jia, and C. Dehong, "Effect of activating toll like receptor 4 on renin-angiotensin system in 3T3-L1 adipose cells," *Journal of Southern Medical University*, vol. 34, no. 6, pp. 787–791, 2014.

[22] A. S. Baldwin Jr., "The NF-κB and IκB proteins: new discoveries and insights," *Annual Review of Immunology*, vol. 14, no. 1, pp. 649–681, 1996.

[23] K. Miyata, R. Satou, W. Shao et al., "ROCK/NF-kappaB axis-dependent augmentation of angiotensinogen by angiotensin ii in primary-cultured preglomerular vascular smooth muscle cells," *The American Journal of Physiology—Renal Physiology*, vol. 306, no. 6, pp. F608–F618, 2014.

19

Lifestyle Interventions to Prevent Type 2 Diabetes: A Systematic Review of Economic Evaluation Studies

Koffi Alouki,[1] Hélène Delisle,[1] Clara Bermúdez-Tamayo,[2] and Mira Johri[3,4]

[1]*TRANSNUT, WHO Collaborating Centre on Nutrition Changes and Development, Department of Nutrition, Faculty of Medicine, University of Montreal, 2405 Chemin de la Côte Sainte-Catherine, Montreal, QC, Canada H3T 1A8*

[2]*Institut de Recherche en Santé Publique de l'Université de Montréal (IRSPUM), University of Montreal, 7101 Avenue du Parc, 3e Étage, Montréal, QC, Canada H3N 1X9*

[3]*Centre de Recherche du Centre Hospitalier de l'Université de Montréal (CRCHUM), Tour Saint-Antoine, 850 Rue Saint-Denis, Montréal, QC, Canada H2X 0A9*

[4]*Department of Health Administration, School of Public Health (ESPUM), Faculty of Medicine, University of Montreal, 7101 Avenue du Parc, 3e Étage, Montréal, QC, Canada H3N 1X9*

Correspondence should be addressed to Hélène Delisle; helene.delisle@umontreal.ca

Academic Editor: Mitsuhiko Noda

Objective. To summarize key findings of economic evaluations of lifestyle interventions for the primary prevention of type 2 diabetes (T2D) in high-risk subjects. *Methods.* We conducted a systematic review of peer-reviewed original studies published since January 2009 in English, French, and Spanish. Eligible studies were identified through relevant databases including PubMed, Medline, National Health Services Economic Evaluation, CINHAL, EconLit, Web of sciences, EMBASE, and the Latin American and Caribbean Health Sciences Literature. Studies targeting obesity were also included. Data were extracted using a standardized method. The BMJ checklist was used to assess study quality. The heterogeneity of lifestyle interventions precluded a meta-analysis. *Results.* Overall, 20 studies were retained, including six focusing on obesity control. Seven were conducted within trials and 13 using modeling techniques. T2D prevention by physical activity or diet or both proved cost-effective according to accepted thresholds, except for five inconclusive studies, three on diabetes prevention and two on obesity control. Most studies exhibited limitations in reporting results, primarily with regard to generalizability and justification of selected sensitivity parameters. *Conclusion.* This confirms that lifestyle interventions for the primary prevention of diabetes are cost-effective. Such interventions should be further promoted as sound investment in the fight against diabetes.

1. Background

Noncommunicable diseases (NCDs) are steadily rising, affecting both developing and developed countries. This is a consequence not only of population aging, but also of the nutrition transition towards westernized diets and sedentary lifestyles. The nutrition transition is fueled by socioeconomic and technological development as well as globalization and accelerated urbanization [1]. Among the nutrition-related NCDs, diabetes is a major concern because its prevalence is rapidly increasing worldwide and particularly so in developing countries. Nearly 387 million people were affected in 2013. This number is expected to reach 592 million by 2035, with the Middle East, South East Asia, and Africa showing the fastest increase in the number of cases [2]. According to the International Diabetes Federation, 80% of people suffering from diabetes live in low- and middle-income countries. Diabetes is associated with several complications, leading to morbidity, disability, and premature mortality [2, 3]. Type 2 diabetes (T2D) is by far the most common form of the disease. Diabetes also entails a heavy economic burden for patients, households, and healthcare systems [4, 5].

T2D is a lifestyle disease, which can and should be prevented by intensive lifestyle interventions, characterized by changes in dietary habits and increased physical activity. Indeed, lifestyle interventions at the prediabetes stage have proved successful at reducing the incidence of T2D by 28.5% to 58%, in China (Da Qing), India (Indian Diabetes Prevention Program: IDPP-1), Finland (Diabetes Prevention Program, DPP), and the United States (Diabetes Prevention Program and Outcomes Study, DPPOS) [6–8]. Weight control is key to the prevention and management of diabetes independent of dietary composition [9]. As obesity is a major risk factor for T2D, lifestyle interventions aimed at weight loss or control are also critical to prevent T2D. Except for India and China, few studies have been conducted to date on diabetes prevention programs in low- and middle-income countries. In developed nations and even more so in low-resource countries, healthcare spending is a critical economic and political issue [10]. A recent World Health Organization report recommended addressing common lifestyle risk factors for NCDs, considering their cost-effectiveness, and their relative ease, and speed of implementation [11]. In resource-limited settings in particular, decision makers require information on the economic burden of NCDs, particularly T2D, and of the potential added value of lifestyle interventions for health and development. The economic evaluation of various preventative interventions is important in view of the urgent need for developing countries to set these NCDs as a public health priority, of the rapid increase in diabetes prevalence and of substantial variations in lifestyle intervention components and delivery.

There are limited systematic reviews on this topic and the most recent ones covered the period of 1985–2008 [12, 13]. Most economic evaluations of T2D prevention programmes pertained to developed countries partly owing to lack of relevant data in developing countries, while cost-effectiveness tends to be context-specific [14]. Our objective was to review economic evaluation studies of lifestyle interventions for the primary prevention of T2D and also for the control of obesity as key risk factor, based on data published since 2009. This review was intended to update knowledge on the cost-effectiveness of T2D prevention.

2. Methods

2.1. Search Process. In order to identify all relevant studies performing an economic evaluation of lifestyle interventions to prevent T2D and for obesity control, we searched the following databases: PubMed, Medline, the British National Health Services Economic Evaluation (NHS EES), CINHAL, Econ Lit, Web of sciences, EMBASE, and Latin American and Caribbean Health Sciences Literature (LILACS). We restricted our search to studies published in French, English, or Spanish between January 2009 and December 2014 as previous systematic reviews included studies published between 1995 and 2008. We used medical subject headings (MeSH) and other relevant terms to the topic as major constructs to build our search strategy. The MeSH or other relevant terms are related to economic, diabetes, and intervention constructs. To combine these, we used boolean operators "AND" and "OR" as appropriate. In addition, the reference lists of all included studies were scanned to identify any additional potentially relevant reports. For example, the PubMed search combined (i) "Cost-benefit-analysis (MeSH)" OR "Costs and cost-analysis (MeSH)" OR "Cost-benefit (title)" OR "Cost-effectiveness (title)" OR "Cost-utility (title)" OR "Economic evaluation (title)" AND (ii) "Type 2 diabetes (MeSH)" OR "Non Insulin dependent diabetes (MeSH)" OR "Gestational diabetes (MeSH)" OR "Obesity (MeSH)" OR "Impaired glucose tolerance (title)" OR "Prediabetes (title)" AND (iii) "Diet (MeSH)" OR "Physical activity (MeSH)" OR "Diet therapy (MeSH)" OR "Lifestyle (MeSH)" OR "Risk reduction behaviour (MeSH)" OR "Prevention (title)" OR "Lifestyle modification (title)" OR "Lifestyle advice programme (title)" OR "Non pharmacological prevention (title)". Appendix shows the majors constructs used in our search strategy.

2.2. Study Selection. In order to select the relevant studies for this review, we screened titles and abstracts using a three-stage process. At the first stage, two authors (Koffi Alouki and Clara Bermúdez-Tamayo) independently selected studies based on abstracts and titles. They rejected clearly irrelevant titles, abstracts only, and duplicates. They cross-checked their results and retained candidate studies for full paper screening. Finally, studies were screened by reading the full papers. Through this process, the same coauthors resolved the disagreements. On the basis of full assessment and discussion of each study, they jointly selected the studies that were to be included in the review. This review was not blinded.

The study selection was guided by the following inclusion criteria:

(i) Original research articles published in peer-reviewed journals were candidates for inclusion.

(ii) Type of economic evaluation: the selected studies conducted a full economic evaluation as defined by Drummond et al. [47]. "Full economic evaluations" are studies in which a comparison of two or more treatments or care alternatives is undertaken and in which both the costs and outcomes of the alternatives are examined in terms of cost-effectiveness, cost-utility, or cost-benefit analyses.

(iii) The participants: the population groups targeted for the primary prevention of T2D were adult subjects (over 18 years old) who were at high risk of developing the disease because of obesity, impaired glucose tolerance, impaired fasting glycaemia, or gestational diabetes.

(iv) The interventions: we considered dietary modifications or physical activity or both to prevent T2D or control obesity.

(v) The comparison: any comparison arm or group used against the lifestyle intervention was accepted for this review.

(vi) Outcomes: these were cost per QALY (Quality Adjusted Life Years) gained, cost per life year gained, cost per DALY (Disability Adjusted Life Years) averted, cost per diabetes case averted, and other relevant outcomes.

(vii) Studies published between January 2009 and December 2014.

(viii) Studies that were published in English, French, or Spanish.

2.3. Data Extraction and Synthesis. The first reviewer (Koffi Alouki) extracted data using a standardized data extraction form built according to the Consolidated Health Economic Evaluation Statement (CHEERS) [15]. The second reviewer (Clara Bermúdez-Tamayo) checked that the extracts and discrepancies were resolved through discussion. A third reviewer was not necessary as all queries were resolved by consensus. Data extracted included the type of economic evaluation, subjects' characteristics (e.g., age, biological and anthropometric characteristics), intervention details (e.g., duration, location, intensity, and mode of delivery of the intervention), comparator, analytical model used, effectiveness data, sensitivity analysis, and reported outcomes relevant to the review. Fields extracted are summarised in Table 1. There are some trial-based type studies while others relied on model-based studies or previous trial results to extrapolate by using modeling techniques, something which was previously highlighted in the literature [10]. The interventions compared, the population groups targeted, and the outcomes reported also varied across studies. For these reasons we chose a narrative approach for this systematic review, as is usually done for systematic reviews of economic evaluations.

2.4. Assessment of Study Quality. We used the British Medical Journal (BMJ) quality assessment checklist, a 36-item scale, to assess the quality of the studies [36]. This checklist was developed with the aim of standardizing the presentation of study data, thereby contributing to the quality of economic evaluations. We also assessed any risk of bias due to conflicts of interest or sponsorship of studies. Each item was answered by "No" or "Yes" or "Not applicable." We gave a score of 0 if the answer was "Yes" and 1 if it was "No." Then we summed up the number of "No" responses to obtain a global score in which a higher score represented poorer quality. Two reviewers (Koffi Alouki, Clara Bermúdez-Tamayo) conducted this operation independently and disagreements were resolved through discussion. Quality rating was used to interpret the results but no study was excluded on this basis.

3. Results

3.1. Overview of Studies. The stages of the search process are illustrated in the flowchart of Figure 1. The search yielded 176 abstracts. After reviewing the abstracts, subsequent reference tracking, and excluding duplicate articles, we narrowed the focus to 56 candidate studies having performed an original economic evaluation. Further review of the full text resulted in 20 studies that met our inclusion criteria. Table 2 summarizes the retained study characteristics and the analytical approach used. The studies were conducted in the UK, USA, Canada, Australia, Germany, Finland, the Netherlands, Singapore, Sweden, and China. Three studies performed only a cost-effectiveness analysis while 13 studies assessed

only cost-utility. The four remaining studies combined cost-effectiveness and cost-utility analysis. There were 10 studies using a Markov-type model or a decision tree, or both, to make projections of the evolution of T2D [22–24, 26–29, 31, 33, 35]. Seven studies performed trial-based analyses [16–21, 30]. The period for which the potential benefit of the intervention was simulated ranged from three years to lifetime. The two studies targeting women with gestational diabetes were conducted throughout pregnancy [20, 31]. In eight studies [16, 17, 22, 23, 25, 27–29], data on efficacy and effectiveness used in simulations were drawn from the major randomized controlled trials on T2D prevention: DPPOS [37], DPP [38], and Da Qing [39]. In a further six studies, effectiveness data was based on synthesis of multiple studies [24, 31–35]. Six of the 20 studies used effectiveness data from a specific intervention conducted in the same country where the economic evaluation was carried out [18–21, 26, 30]. The items included in the cost calculations were obviously dependent on the study perspective. The cost to the healthcare system only or to the whole society was generally considered. Only two studies adopted a third payer perspective. The costs and the effectiveness were discounted using rates varying from 3% to 5% according to the countries. To test the robustness of the results, a sensitivity analysis was performed in most studies. It was not possible to identify the source of funding for only one study [27]. Among the other 19 studies, four had not reported any funding. Most studies (16/20) were funded by public agencies.

3.2. Description of Interventions. The interventions included in this review varied from the simple provision of information to active behaviour change schemes. The lifestyle changes described across studies pertained to diet, physical activity, or both. In some cases, the screening of subjects at high risk preceded the interventions without explicitly taking account of the screening in the cost calculations [17, 18, 24]. Of 10 model-based studies, seven simulated interventions based on the DPP [23–25, 28, 29] or the China Da Qing study [22, 27]. The DPP intervention goal was to achieve and maintain a weight reduction of at least 7% of initial body weight through diet and physical activity of moderate intensity, such as brisk walking for at least 150 minutes per week. The DPP program included a lifestyle curriculum, taught by case managers on a one-to-one basis during the first 24 weeks after enrollment. The teaching was flexible, culturally sensitive, and individualized. Subsequent individual sessions (usually monthly) and group sessions with the case managers were designed to reinforce the behavioral changes. The aim of nutritional counselling was to help the participants achieve a diet containing 10% of total energy intake as saturated fats, 5–10% as polyunsaturated fats, 25–30% as total fat (saturated, monounsaturated, polyunsaturated, and trans fatty acids), and 25 to 35 grams of fibre per day. One study described a commercial program consisting of a low-calorie diet and physical activity advice [31]. One study carried out the economic evaluation of the "DASH" diet (Dietary Approaches to Stop Hypertension) or a "low fat" diet [33] to reduce the disease burden related to excess body weight. The "DASH" diet emphasizes reduced consumption of fat, red meat,

TABLE 1: General features of selected studies.

Study	Country	Population	Intervention	Variables of interest	Comparison	Time horizon	Analytical approach	Study design
For diabetes prevention								
Herman et al. [16], 2012	USA	≥25 y.o. IGT/IFG, BMI ≥ 24 (≥22 for Asians)	DPP lifestyle modification	Diabetes cases prevented, QALYs	Metformin, placebo	10 years	Trial-based study	CU
Herman et al. [17], 2013	USA	≥25 y.o. IGT/IFG, BMI ≥ 24 (≥22 for Asian)	Lifestyle modification and metformin	Diabetes cases prevented, QALYs	Placebo	10 years	Trial-based study	CU
van Wier et al. [18], 2013	Netherlands	Adults aged 30–50 y at risk of T2D	Lifestyle intervention implemented in primary care	Risk of T2D, risk of CVD, and CVD mortality in the following 10 years	Provision of health brochures	10 years (duration 2 years)	Trial-based study	CU/CE
Sagarra et al. [19], 2014	Spain	Adults aged 45–75 y with IFG/IGT	Lifestyle intervention (individual or group intensive intervention)	Diabetes cases prevented, QALYs	Routine care	4 years	Trial-based study	CU/CE
Kolu et al. [20], 2013	Finland	≥40 years BMI ≥ 25 or IGT, history of macrosomia, and type 2 or type 1 diabetes in first- or second-degree relatives	Lifestyle modification	Health perception, birth weight, and quality of life	Routine care	37 weeks	Trial-based study	CU/CE
Oostdam et al. [21], 2012	Germany	Overweight pregnant women and at least one of the following: history of macrosomia, GDM, or first grade relative with diabetes or obese	Exercise program (FitFor2)	Maternal fasting blood glucose, QALYs, infant birth weight, and insulin sensitivity	Routine care	32 weeks	Trial-based study	CU
Liu et al. [22], 2013	China	Age ≥25 y, IGT	One-time screening for IGT/T2D with positive case receiving (i) lifestyle intervention/diet; (ii) lifestyle intervention/exercise; (iii) both diet and exercise; (iv) one-time screening alone.	Remaining survival years and QALYs	Control	40 years	Model-based study (decision tree and Markov)	CU
Png et al. [23], 2014	Singapore	Subjects with prediabetes (IFG/IGT)	Lifestyle modification	QALYs	Metformin/ placebo	3 years	Model-based study (decision tree)	CU
Bertram et al. [24], 2010	Australia	Age ≥45 y and high BMI, family history of T2D, or people from indigenous, and women with GDM	Diet and/or exercise,	Diabetes cases prevented, DALYs Averted	Acarbose, metformin, and orlistat	Lifetime	Model-based study (Markov)	CE
Mortaz et al. [25], 2012	Canada	Age ≥40 y and first-degree relative with T2D, high risk population groups (aboriginals, Hispanics, Asians, or Africans), and history of IGT/IFG, GDM, hypertension, dyslipidemia, overweight, abdominal obesity, and polycystic ovary	Screening followed by lifestyle intervention	QALYs	No screening	10 years/ lifetime	Model-based study (Markov)	CU

TABLE 1: Continued.

Study	Country	Population	Intervention	Variables of interest	Comparison	Time horizon	Analytical approach	Study design
Johansson et al. [26], 2009	Sweden	Age 30–56 y and at risk of chronic disease without known diabetes	Lifestyle intervention	QALYs	Routine care	10 years	Model-based study (Markov)	CU
Neumann et al. [27], 2011	Germany	Subjects at high risk of developing T2D	Lifestyle intervention	QALYs	Routine care	Lifetime	Model-based study (Markov)	CU
Palmer and Tucker [28], 2012	Australia	Mean age 50.6 y with IGT/IFG, BMI ≥ 34	Intensive lifestyle intervention, Metformin	QALYs	Control	Lifetime	Model-based study (Markov)	CU
Smith et al. [29], 2010	United States	BMI ≥ 25 and the 4 components of MetS as defined by NCEP/ATP III	Lifestyle intervention	QALYs	Routine care	3 years	Model-based study (Markov)	CU
For obesity control								
Tsai et al. [30], 2013	USA	BMI 30–50, plus abdominal obesity plus at least one of the 4 other MetS criteria	Brief lifestyle counselling	QALYs and kilograms lost per year	Routine care	2 years	Trial-based study	CU/CE
Cobiac et al. [31], 2010	Australia	Age ≥ 40 y and BMI ≥ 27	"Lighten up to Healthy Lifestyle" and "Weight Watchers"	Weight lost/DALYs averted	Routine care	12 months	Model-based study (Markov)	CE
Miners et al. [32], 2012	United Kingdom	Age ≥ 50 y and BMI ≥ 30	E- learning devices to promote healthy diet and physical activity	Weight lost/QALYs gained	Routine care	Lifetime	Model-based study (e-learning economic evaluation model)	CU
Forster et al. [33], 2011	Australia	Age ≥ 40 y and BMI ≥ 25	The Dietary Approach to Stop Hypertension (DASH) and low fat diet intervention	Weight lost/DALYs Averted	Routine care	100 years	Model-based study (Markov)	CE
Lewis et al. [34], 2014	UK	Adult subjects with BMI ≥ 30	Lighter Life total (a very low calorie diet total dietary replacement) weight reduction program and group support appropriate for obese people	Weight lost, QALYs gained	(A) With BMI ≥ 30 group: (1) no treatment, (2) lifestyle intervention, (3) weight watchers, (4) slimming world, and (5) lighter life total movement only (B) With BMI ≥ 40 group: (1) no treatment, (2) gastric banding, (3) gastric bypass, and (4) lighter life total movement only	10 years	Not specified	CU
Anokye et al. [35], 2011	United Kingdom	Age 40–60 y, sedentary lifestyle	Exercise Referral scheme in physical activity	QALYs	Routine care	Lifetime	Model-based study (decision tree)	CU

BMI: body mass index; CE: cost-effectiveness; CU: cost-utility; CVD: cardiovascular disease; DPP: diabetes prevention program; GDM: gestational diabetes mellitus; IGT/IFG: impaired glucose tolerance/impaired fasting glucose; T2D: type 2 diabetes.

TABLE 2: Economic evaluation details of studies.

Study	Currency, discount rate	Perspective	Costs	Effectiveness measure	Incremental cost-effectiveness ratio	Is intervention cost-effective? (benchmark)***
For diabetes preventions						
Herman et al. [16], 2012	US$, 2010, 3%	Health system and societal	Direct medical and nonmedical costs + intervention costs	QALYs	Lifestyle compared to placebo, health system perspective: 12,878$US/QALY; societal perspective: 23,597$US/QALY	Yes
Herman et al. [17], 2013	US$, 2010, 3%	Health system and societal	Direct medical and nonmedical costs + intervention costs	QALYs	(a) Health system perspective: cost saving (lifestyle versus placebo) cost saving (metformin versus placebo); (b) societal perspective: the ICER was 3,235$US/QALY (lifestyle versus placebo)	Yes
van Wier et al. [18], 2013	Euros, 2008	Societal	Intervention costs + productivity lost costs	QALYs, 9-year risk of developing T2D	−50,273€/QALY gained; the ICER of 9-year risk for developing T2D was −1416€ Lifestyle guidance offered by practice nurses was not more effective in reducing these risks than the provision of general health brochures	No
Sagarra et al. [19], 2014	Euros, 2007	Health system	Intervention costs	Diabetes cases prevented and QALYs	376.17€/case of T2D averted; 3243€/QALY gained	Yes
Kolu et al. [20], 2013	Euros, 2009	Societal	Direct medical costs + lost productivity costs + health care intervention costs	Health perceptions (visual analog scale), birth weight, 15D (quality of life)	Each gram of birth weight prevented requires an additional cost of €7; each perceived health gain requires additional cost of 1697€	No
Oostdam et al. [21], 2012	Euros, 2009	Societal	Direct and indirect costs	Maternal fasting blood glucose, QALYs gained, infant birth weight, and insulin sensitivity	Being not cost-effective versus control group for blood glucose, insulin sensitivity, infant birth weight, and QALYs gained	No
Liu et al. [22], 2013	US$, 2007, 3%	Societal	Direct and nonmedical costs, indirect costs	QALYs	Savings: US$ 2017 per subject	Yes
Png et al. [23], 2014	US$, 2012, 3%	Health system and societal	Direct medical costs, direct nonmedical costs, and indirect costs	QALYs	Health system perspective: US$ 17,184/QALY for lifestyle modification versus placebo; societal perspective: US$ 36,367/QALY	Yes (WHO benchmark)
Bertram et al. [24], 2010	AU$, 2010, 3%	Health system	Directs cost of each intervention	DALYs averted, diabetes cases averted	AU$ 23.000/DALY averted (diet and exercise); AU$ 22.000/DALY averted (metformin)	Yes

TABLE 2: Continued.

Study	Currency, discount rate	Perspective	Costs	Effectiveness measure	Incremental cost-effectiveness ratio	Is intervention cost-effective? (benchmark)***
Mortaz et al. [25], 2012	CAN$, 2010, 3%	Health system	Direct cost per person	QALYs	Conventional screening every 3 years was more effective over no screening	Yes
Johansson et al. [26], 2009	Krona, 2004, 3%	Societal	The societal costs	QALYs	For women QALY losses were lower and cost increases were lower; among men, the net costs were larger and QALYs lost were higher in all three treatments than in controls	Yes for women, No for men
Neumann et al. [27], 2011	Euros, 2007, 3%	Societal	Direct cost + interventions cost	QALYs	The ICERs were negative, for men and women who started the intervention when aged 30–50 years	Yes
Palmer and Tucker [28], 2012	AU$, 2009, 5%	Third-party payer and health system	Direct medical costs + intervention costs	QALYs	Intensive lifestyle change was cost-effective compared to controls	Yes
Smith et al. [29], 2010	US$, 2000, 3%	Societal	Direct costs + interventions costs	QALYs	$ 3,420/QALY due to decrease in diabetes incidence with intervention	Yes
For obesity control						
Tsai et al. [30], 2013	US$, 2010	Health system	Intervention costs + health care providers + medication	QALYs	$US 3134/QALY (BLC compared to usual care) $US 115397/QALY (EBLC compared to routine care)	Yes
Cobiac et al. [31], 2010	US$, 2003, 3%	Health system	Direct and intervention costs	DALYs averted	Both weight loss programmes produced small improvements in the exposed subjects compared to current practices	No
Miners et al. [32], 2012	£UK, 2009, 3,5%	Health system	Direct and intervention costs	QALYs	The lowest was 102,000£/QALY; however, scenario contains women associated with lower QALYs compared with men	No
Forster et al. [33], 2011	AUS$, 2003, 3%	Health system	The intervention + direct costs related to each state in the model	DALYs averted	AUS$ 12000/DALY averted (DASH diet) AUS$ 13000/DALY averted (low fat diet)	Yes
Lewis et al. [34], 2014	£UK, 2012, 3,5%	Health system	Intervention costs	QALYs	For subjects with BMI ≥30, lighter life is cost-effective; for subjects with BMI ≥40 eligible for bariatric surgery, gastric bypass is cost-effective	Yes
Anokye et al. [35], 2011	£UK, 2011, 3,5%	Third-party payer	Direct costs + intervention costs	QALYs	20,876£/QALY	Yes

BLC: brief lifestyle counselling; DALY: Disability Adjusted Life Year; DASH: dietary approach to stop hypertension; EBLC: enhanced brief lifestyle counselling; ICER: incremental cost-effectiveness ratio; MetS: metabolic syndrome; QALY: Quality Adjusted Life Year; VAS: visual analog scale; 15D: 15-Dimension.
*** According to authors conclusions about the value of one or more interventions to control obesity or prevent type 2 diabetes. One study used WHO benchmark to justify the conclusion as mentioned in bracket.

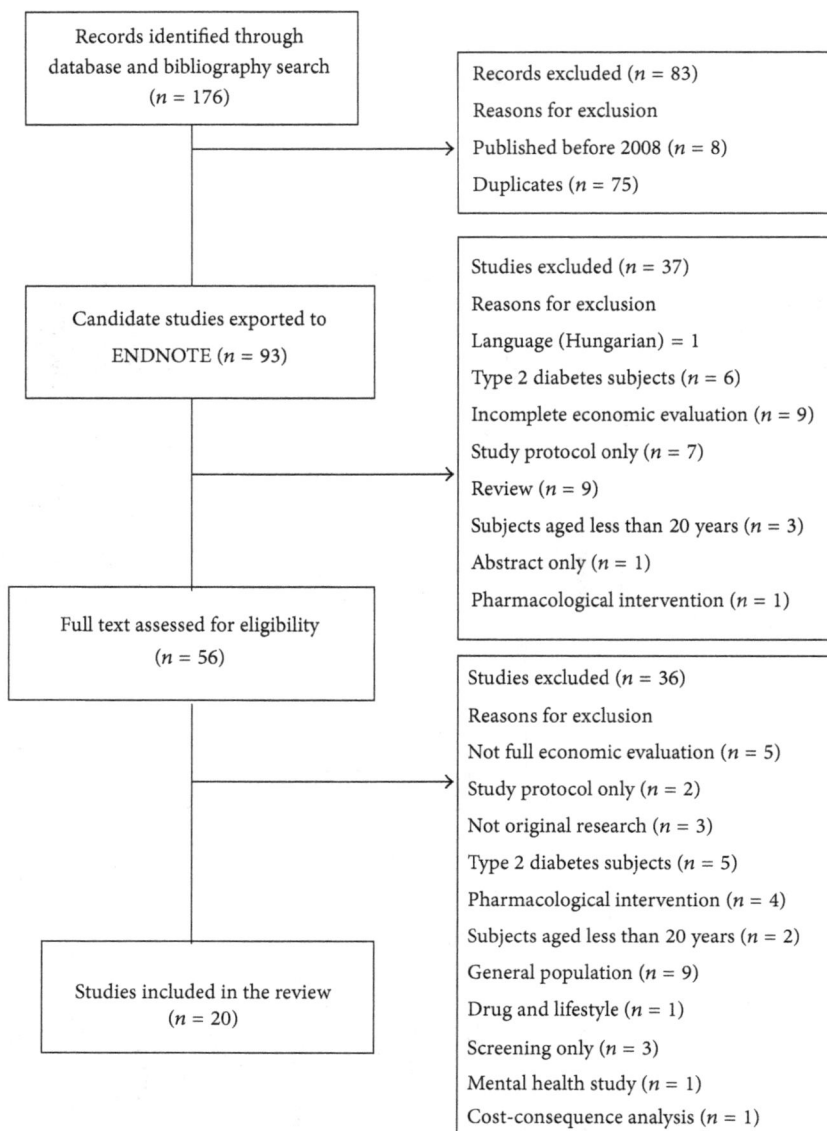

FIGURE 1: Flowchart of overall systematic search process.

sweets, and sugar-containing beverages, and the program recommends 180 minutes per week of moderate intensity physical activity. Individual or group sessions were held every 4 to 8 weeks. One study performed the economic analysis of lifestyle changes achieved through e-learning devices [32]. Another economic evaluation from the United Kingdom was conducted on a program focusing on very low-calorie diets [34]. Two studies reported on the economic evaluation of interventions consisting solely of physical activity [21, 35]. The first one was based on exercise referral schemes [40]. It took the form of a structured programme of exercise in a fitness centre and incorporating monitoring of individual performance. The second study pertained to sessions of physical activity that included 60 minutes of walking in addition to exercise. The exercise sessions consisted of aerobic and strength exercises. Depending on the studies,

the comparison (or control) interventions were common standard care, placebo, metformin (850 mg twice daily), or simple advice in writing for physical activity and nutrition.

3.3. Analysis of Costs. Reported costs depended on the chosen perspective, the nature of the intervention, the target population, and the time horizon. The various costs are shown in Table 2. There is no consistency across studies in the items included to estimate the costs of interventions. All studies considered direct costs including medical costs [16, 17, 20–23, 25, 30]. Medical records were the most common source for data on diabetes and complications. Generally, the direct medical costs were copayment fees for treatment, diagnostic testing, prescription drugs, and medical supplies. The direct costs also included the costs of visits to healthcare providers and exercise physiologist and metformin cost for controls. Direct nonmedical costs pertained to services such as transportation of subjects and family members to clinics, as well as special food in some instances. Lost income for the patients and their families and the costs of hiring nurses or care providers were recorded as indirect costs. Four studies [18, 20, 21, 23] reported on the estimated cost of productivity loss. In four of the 20 studies [22, 24, 25, 29], cost estimates were only presented as category totals, without breakdown into individual items and without a separate presentation of the resources needed for the interventions. Two studies described the unit costs of various resources, using the ingredient approach [27, 28]. Physical quantities of necessary inputs were counted and multiplied by unit prices to obtain total costs [41]. Pricing sources were reported in all studies. For most studies, price data came from healthcare facilities, from patient records, or else from estimates based on published data. Other costs such as transport were self-reported by the subjects. Seven studies recorded costs alongside the trials [17–19, 21]. Except for four studies [18–21], all studies discounted the costs by 3% to 5%.

3.4. Effectiveness Data. The effectiveness data were usually derived from major randomized controlled trials on T2D prevention [7, 17, 19, 38, 39]. Nearly one-third of studies estimated effectiveness based on meta-analyses or literature reviews [24, 31–35]. More than half the studies expressed intervention benefits in terms of QALYs gained. Three out of the 20 studies reported effectiveness as DALYs averted [24, 31, 33]. Diabetes cases averted by the interventions were reported in two studies [19, 24]. Another study estimated the delay in progression to T2D attributable to the lifestyle intervention [28]. One study reported change in utility as an outcome measure, based on the 15-dimension questionnaire tool (15D) to assess quality of life but without conversion to quality adjusted life years [20]. Several tools were used to assess the effects of interventions. Three studies used disability weights. Nine studies (9/20) used the EQ5D (EuroQoL 5-Dimension tool), three studies used the QWB-SA (Quality of Well Being-Self-Administered), two studies used the HRQoL (Health Related Quality of Life) system, one study used the VSA (Visual Scale Analog), and one study used the 15D or SF-36 (36-item short form survey instrument). Long-term assumptions about effectiveness were dissimilar. In some cases, the key assumption was that the expected effects of the intervention were for the short term with a linear decrease in effectiveness following the intervention [27]. Another study projected the same effectiveness during the whole duration of the time horizon projected. The probability of progressing from prediabetes to T2D in all studies using modeling techniques was always lower in the intervention arm consisting of lifestyle intervention than in the comparison arm, whether placebo, usual care, or metformin treatment. Assumptions regarding the effectiveness of screening were needed when screening was required before implementing interventions. The studies reported sensitivity and specificity of screening ranging from 75% to 100% [22, 25].

3.5. Cost-Effectiveness of Interventions. Cost-effectiveness results are presented in Table 2. Compared with usual care,

placebo, or metformin, interventions based on lifestyle modifications were reported as cost-effective in 15 of 20 studies [16, 17, 19, 22–30, 33–35]. The conclusions are usually based on the incremental cost-effectiveness ratio as applied in the study countries. One study considered the WHO threshold to decide on the cost-effectiveness [23], according to which intervention is considered highly cost-effective when the ICER is below the GDP (Gross Domestic Product) per capita and cost-effective when the ICER ranges from 1 to 3 times GDP per capita. When a strategy improves health outcomes at lower cost, it is considered to be dominant and it is obviously preferred as cost-effective. Those interventions that are less effective and more costly (considered as dominated interventions) or more costly and more effective but with a resulting more expensive ICER would unlikely be cost-effective; these studies were considered inconclusive. Three studies revealed that the interventions were dominant [17, 22, 27]. However, the results reported in four studies were less favourable. Oostdam et al. [21] reported that a lifestyle intervention implemented during 32 weeks and targeting at-risk pregnant women in Germany was not cost-effective. Similar results were also reported in another intensive lifestyle intervention targeting at-risk pregnant women [20]. One study reported that a lifestyle intervention offered by nurses was not more cost-effective in reducing T2D risk than the control intervention consisting in the provision of a general health brochure [18]. Johansson et al. [26] examined the cost-effectiveness of lifestyle by sex and concluded that intervention was only cost-effective among women.

Sensitivity analysis, which allows assessing the reliability and the generalizability of the results [42], was performed in all studies except one [34]. Over half the studies performed univariate sensitivity analysis and eight studies performed bivariate sensitivity analysis. Probabilistic sensitivity analysis was used in ten studies [18, 21, 24, 26–29, 31, 32, 35]. The input parameters that were analyzed through a range of assumed values were discounted cost and outcomes (QALYs gained), variations of intervention cost, variation of probability of transition between disease states considered, the duration of interventions, the size of the population at risk, and performance and frequency of screening test. Although the ICER was sensitive to changes in the above parameters, it remained acceptable for most studies, except for the three studies reporting that the intervention was not cost-effective [20, 27, 31].

3.6. Quality Assessment. Based on the BMJ checklist, the studies included in this review showed quality limitations in reporting as shown in Figure 2. The number of such limitations varied from 1 to 5. Only one study [19] had no methodological shortfall. Out of the remaining 20 studies, 15 presented at least two methodological limitations and five studies showed only one. More than half (12/20) of studies did not address the issue of generalizability. The justification of the parameters used for the sensitivity analysis was presented by only few studies. The models of five studies were not fully described or their choice was not justified. Three studies did not explicitly declare potential conflicts of

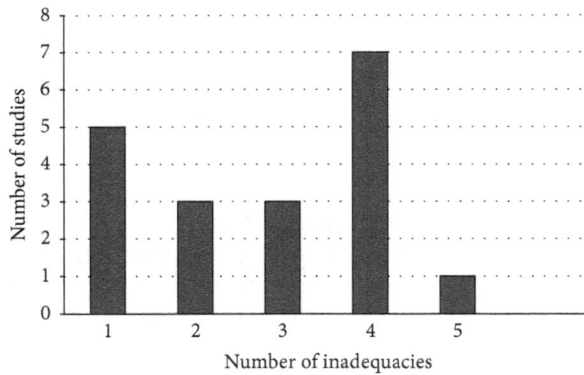

FIGURE 2: Limitations of studies as result of quality assessment.

interest. Eight studies did not report separately the resources for the interventions and their unit cost.

4. Discussion

The purpose of this systematic review was to describe economic evaluations of lifestyle interventions to prevent T2D or control obesity in high-risk population groups and which were carried out since 2009. Our review was focused exclusively on interventions targeting at-risk adult subjects. Lifestyle interventions in communities and schools for the primordial prevention of T2D were excluded as a recent review reported on their cost-effectiveness [13]. We identified 20 studies, mostly conducted in developed countries. Our results confirmed those of former reviews [12, 13], which concluded that lifestyle interventions through physical activity or diet or combining both were generally cost-effective, with a few exceptions. In our review, five out of the 20 studies were inconclusive. There was a trend for a higher proportion of interventions targeting the prevention of T2D compared to those focusing on obesity to be cost-effective (11/14 versus 4/6, resp.). The inconclusive studies [18, 20, 21, 31, 32] included one on the prevention of T2D, two on the prevention of gestational diabetes among pregnant women, and two on obesity control. These studies were more costly with less effectiveness or more costly with higher effectiveness but resulting in a more expensive incremental cost-effectiveness ratio compared with standard care (or control treatment). Three of the seven studies conducted within trial were nonconclusive compared with three of the 13 studies based on models. This would suggest that model-based studies tend to overestimate cost-effectiveness. The short duration of some studies may also explain the absence of significant changes in the outcomes. Another inconclusive study pertained to an e-based intervention, which may not induce enough motivation for change. Overall, there was considerable heterogeneity in the nature of lifestyle interventions across studies, which hampered comparisons and possibly contributed to the inconsistencies in outcome findings. Study results could be influenced by intervention components, selection of participants, and methodological

and modeling choices [43]. Additionally, thresholds of cost-effectiveness varied across countries and studies.

4.1. Which Outcomes, Which Costs, and Which Time Horizon? Few studies evaluated effectiveness in terms of QALY although it is known that diabetes is associated with deterioration of the quality of life. QALY is a relevant parameter that allows comparisons of the burden of disease in terms of quality and quantity [44]. Most studies of this review used EQ-5D and few used HRQoL and SF-36. Preference-based health state classification systems were preferred in most studies to objective methods of evaluation of health states. McDonough and Tosteson [45] showed that, among studies that compared alternative preference-based systems, the EQ-5D tended to provide larger change scores and therefore more favourable results than the Health Utility Index (HUI), while the SF-6D provided smaller change scores and therefore less favourable ratios than the other systems. Hence, the choice of outcome as a measure of effectiveness has an impact on reported results. All studies reported costs in local currency and prices. Cost variations were due primarily to the chosen perspective (societal/health system or third party), to the various inputs for the interventions, and to differences of care unit costs across countries. The lifestyle interventions involved several health professionals, which explains the higher costs of these interventions compared to controls. In some but not all simulation studies, the costs of health infrastructure and training of personnel were also provided. Such inclusive costs would be particularly useful for low-resource countries where health systems are ill-prepared to tackle a chronic disease like T2D [46]. Few studies complied with the recommendation to present quantity and unit cost of inputs separately from total cost as advocated in the guidelines [36], resulting in lack of the information required for the replication of the intervention in other settings. Additionally, the reported costs were often incomplete. For instance, if a societal perspective is adopted, the costs related to lost productivity, premature mortality, and permanent and temporary disability should be computed which is not always the case. As stated in the guidelines [47, 48], the future costs beyond one-year time should be discounted, which was done in most studies and using different discount rates. Some interventions did not use discounting due to their short duration. Although the selected rates were not justified in most studies, they probably reflect the fact that there are no universally accepted discount rates for economic evaluations studies [47]. The time horizon should be long enough to capture any significant difference between the intervention and the comparison groups in terms of costs and outcomes [48]. Yet, it appeared too short in some studies to appraise and capture long-term impact of interventions. Particularly, in the management of obesity or gestational diabetes, the inconclusive results may be partly ascribed to too short interventions to capture the long-term benefits. The costs for treating T2D complications are onerous, and the temporal horizon of some studies based on model assumptions cannot guarantee that the complications will not appear later on. The conclusions regarding cost-effectiveness should therefore be taken with caution. Weight loss is also an objective of T2D prevention interventions.

However, without sustained compliance of subjects with advocated lifestyle changes, weight regain over the long-term can alter the quality of life and impinge on the estimated cost-effectiveness of interventions. Considering exclusively the short-term effects of obesity control interventions can indeed be misleading [49]. For this reason, it is not impossible that the cost-effectiveness of some interventions reviewed here and focusing on obesity was overestimated.

Trial-based studies limited the results of interventions to health gains over the course of the intervention. In contrast, studies supported by models were based on assumptions on a longer temporal horizon. This approach, however, would omit taking into account other relevant events that may occur later on that will have an impact on the costs and on the quality of life or other outcomes [10]. Additionally, the nature of the model inevitably has a bearing on the estimated cost-effectiveness of the interventions.

4.2. What about T2D Modeling? The analytical models varied across studies. Modeling diabetes evolution showed variations among studies with regard to the shift from normal glycaemia to prediabetes and then to diabetes and finally to the complications. With the exception of one study, the models however seemed to be consistent with the natural evolution of the disease as described in the literature [50]. The accuracy of the models is one of the criteria for sound economic evaluations, and it reflects the ability to capture the evolution of the pathology in a real situation [51, 52]. Yet, in some studies, the models showed complication states without disclosing the nature of the complications. Another limitation of most models is that complications are taken separately into account while subjects living with T2D can have several complications. Some studies [23, 25] did not consider the likelihood of glycaemia returning to normal in subjects with prediabetes. The simplification of analytical models may not help to consider these subtleties during the course of evolution of the disease in a real situation.

Most simulated interventions were based on epidemiological studies of T2D prevention that provide the reference evidence for lifestyle interventions as relevant strategy to prevent diabetes. The randomized controlled trials that measured the long-term effects in real life situations after cessation of the active intervention [37, 39] therefore provide important new data for the simulation studies to better estimate the long-term effectiveness of interventions to prevent diabetes. However, the efficacy observed in controlled experimental conditions is different from the expected effectiveness in the real world because of subject selection, recruitment, and follow-up and other factors that have a bearing on economic outcomes [10, 53]. Moreover, in some model-based studies, the at-risk subjects may not accurately match the at-risk subjects of the original studies, so that the assumed effectiveness in these studies is uncertain. The effectiveness of interventions in the real world often falls a long way short of the maximum efficacy shown in trials [54]. For instance, a retrospective observational analysis of overweight and obese subjects demonstrated that, compared with the 58% reduction in risk of progression to diabetes seen in the DPP trial, risk reduction for incident diabetes

in subjects who participated in the study in an intense and sustained way was lower [55]. The effectiveness was also shown to vary according to the setting of the intervention [56].

4.3. Quality of Studies. Assessment of quality of studies revealed methodological shortcomings. Most articles lacked one or several reporting items of the BMJ checklist for quality of economic evaluation studies although this checklist was issued before these studies were conducted. Another limitation observed is the lack of a clear description of the models [34], while the guidelines recommend transparency in their description [47]. In some cases, the models did not adequately capture the natural history of the disease, leading to questionable conclusions. Conversely, in another study [27], the model did not include the complication state, which would have been relevant in the natural history of diabetes. However, although we performed an evaluation of the quality of studies, we deliberately chose not to exclude any study on that basis. In any case, excluding the poorer quality studies would not have altered the conclusions.

4.4. Strengths and Weaknesses of the Review. We used a comprehensive electronic search strategy using preestablished criteria in common medical literature databases. As all studies are not referenced in electronic databases, we revisited the bibliography of each selected study to ensure that our search was exhaustive. Two reviewers cross-checked the database to identify the relevant studies. At variance with previous reviews on the economic evaluation of T2D prevention studies, ours also included intervention studies targeting obesity as main risk factor for T2D and not only the interventions aiming directly at T2D prevention. Our review also updates the results of these former reviews. Ours also encompassed the assessment of study quality based on the BMJ guidelines designed for the critical appraisal of economic evaluation studies. We adopted a dichotomous scale for each item, however, which does not reflect the level of completeness of the information reported for each item considered. It is also recognized that limiting the candidate studies to those published in French, English, and Spanish is a potential source of publication bias. Due to the heterogeneity in the methods and results of the different studies, we were not able to perform a meta-analysis, which is usually considered the "gold standard" but which is not often feasible with economic evaluation studies.

5. Conclusion

The present review on the cost-effectiveness of lifestyle modification interventions showed, with only a few exceptions, that these interventions targeting adult subjects at high risk for diabetes were cost-effective despite different assumptions regarding disease progression and variations in the delivery of these interventions. The results are consistent with conclusions of former reviews, confirming the importance of lifestyle interventions combining diet and physical activity to prevent diabetes in at-risk population groups. This review

Table 3: List of combinations of terms used for research studies in the database.

Economic concepts	Type 2 diabetes concepts	Intervention concepts
	MeSH terms	
Cost-benefit analysis Cost and cost analysis	Type 2 diabetes mellitus Noninsulin dependent diabetes mellitus Gestational diabetes	Diet Physical activity Diet therapy Lifestyle Risk reduction behaviour
	Title terms	
Cost-effectiveness Cost-utility Economic outcomes Cost outcomes Economic evaluation Cost	Impaired glucose tolerance Prediabetes	Prevention Lifestyle modification Nonpharmacological prevention Primary prevention Nutritional intervention Dietary intervention Nutrition counselling Prevention programme Lifestyle advice programme

also broke new ground by assessing the methodological limitations of the economic evaluations and the quality of reporting, to aid in interpretation of results. Lifestyle interventions should be further stressed as an effective strategy to prevent or delay diabetes. Unfortunately, few studies have been conducted in resource-poor countries in spite of a dire need for such data, and the findings from developed countries are not entirely relevant. Future research should address the effectiveness and cost-effectiveness of such interventions in low-income country settings, where the prevalence of T2D is soaring. Meanwhile, the data of the present review provide compelling arguments for policy makers to implement measures to prevent T2D.

Appendix

See Table 3.

Conflict of Interests

The authors declare that no conflict of interests is present in this paper.

Acknowledgments

This study was undertaken within the framework of the project "Pôle Francophone Africain sur le Double Fardeau Nutritionnel," funded by the Canadian International Development Agency (CIDA), Canada (Project DFN S064359). The first author received scholarships from the Islamic Development Bank and from the Faculty of Medicine of University of Montreal for his Ph.D. program in international nutrition.

References

[1] B. M. Popkin, "Global nutrition dynamics: the world is shifting rapidly toward a diet linked with noncommunicable diseases," *American Journal of Clinical Nutrition*, vol. 84, no. 2, pp. 289–298, 2006.

[2] IDF, *International Diabetes Federation Diabetes Atlas*, International Diabetes Federation (IDF), 6th edition, 2014.

[3] J. C. N. Mbanya, A. A. Motala, E. Sobngwi, F. K. Assah, and S. T. Enoru, "Diabetes in sub-Saharan Africa," *The Lancet*, vol. 375, no. 9733, pp. 2254–2266, 2010.

[4] J. M. Kirigia, H. B. Sambo, L. G. Sambo, and S. P. Barry, "Economic burden of diabetes mellitus in the WHO African region," *BMC International Health and Human Rights*, vol. 9, article 6, 2009.

[5] A. Ankotche, Y. Binan, A. Leye et al., "Graves conséquences du coût financier du diabète sur sa prise en charge, en dehors des complications, en Afrique sub-saharienne: l'exemple de la Côte-d'Ivoire," *Médecine des Maladies Métaboliques*, vol. 3, no. 1, pp. 100–105, 2009.

[6] Q. Gong, E. W. Gregg, J. Wang et al., "Long-term effects of a randomised trial of a 6-year lifestyle intervention in impaired glucose tolerance on diabetes-related microvascular complications: the China da Qing Diabetes Prevention Outcome Study," *Diabetologia*, vol. 54, no. 2, pp. 300–307, 2011.

[7] A. Ramachandran, C. Snehalatha, S. Mary, B. Mukesh, A. D. Bhaskar, and V. Vijay, "The Indian Diabetes Prevention Programme shows that lifestyle modification and metformin prevent type 2 diabetes in Asian Indian subjects with impaired glucose tolerance (IDPP-1)," *Diabetologia*, vol. 49, no. 2, pp. 289–297, 2006.

[8] T. J. Orchard, M. Temprosa, E. Barrett-Connor et al., "Long-term effects of the diabetes prevention program interventions on cardiovascular risk factors: a report from the DPP Outcomes Study," *Diabetic Medicine*, vol. 30, no. 1, pp. 46–55, 2013.

[9] S. M. Islam, T. D. Purnat, N. T. Phuong, U. Mwingira, K. Schacht, and G. Fröschl, "Non–Communicable Diseases (NCDs) in developing countries: a symposium report," *Globalization and Health*, vol. 10, article 81, 2014.

[10] D. J. Cohen and M. R. Reynolds, "Interpreting the results of cost-effectiveness studies," *Journal of the American College of Cardiology*, vol. 52, no. 25, pp. 2119–2126, 2008.

[11] WHO, "Package of Essential Noncommunicable (PEN) Disease Interventions for Primary Health Care in Low-Resource Settings," 2010.

[12] R. Li, P. Zhang, L. E. Barker, F. M. Chowdhury, and X. Zhang, "Cost-effectiveness of interventions to prevent and control

diabetes mellitus: a systematic review," *Diabetes Care*, vol. 33, no. 8, pp. 1872–1894, 2010.

[13] S. Saha, U.-G. Gerdtham, and P. Johansson, "Economic evaluation of lifestyle interventions for preventing diabetes and cardiovascular diseases," *International Journal of Environmental Research and Public Health*, vol. 7, no. 8, pp. 3150–3195, 2010.

[14] T. A. Gaziano, G. Galea, and K. S. Reddy, "Scaling up interventions for chronic disease prevention: the evidence," *The Lancet*, vol. 370, no. 9603, pp. 1939–1946, 2007.

[15] D. Husereau, M. Drummond, S. Petrou et al., "Consolidated Health Economic Evaluation Reporting Standards (CHEERS) statement," *The BMJ*, vol. 346, article f1049, 2013.

[16] W. H. Herman, S. L. Edelstein, R. E. Ratner et al., "The 10-year cost-effectiveness of lifestyle intervention or metformin for diabetes prevention: an intent-to-treat analysis of the DPP/DPPOS," *Diabetes Care*, vol. 35, no. 4, pp. 723–730, 2012.

[17] W. H. Herman, S. L. Edelstein, R. E. Ratner et al., "Effectiveness and cost-effectiveness of diabetes prevention among adherent participants," *American Journal of Managed Care*, vol. 19, no. 3, pp. 194–202, 2013.

[18] M. F. van Wier, J. Lakerveld, S. D. M. Bot, M. J. M. Chinapaw, G. Nijpels, and M. W. van Tulder, "Economic evaluation of a lifestyle intervention in primary care to prevent type 2 diabetes mellitus and cardiovascular diseases: a randomized controlled trial," *BMC Family Practice*, vol. 14, no. 1, article 45, 2013.

[19] R. Sagarra, B. Costa, J. J. Cabré, O. Solà-Morales, and F. Barrio, "Lifestyle interventions for diabetes mellitus type 2 prevention," *Revista Clínica Española*, vol. 214, no. 2, pp. 59–68, 2014.

[20] P. Kolu, J. Raitanen, P. Rissanen, and R. Luoto, "Cost-effectiveness of lifestyle counselling as primary prevention of gestational diabetes mellitus: findings from a cluster-randomised trial," *PLoS ONE*, vol. 8, no. 2, Article ID e56392, 2013.

[21] N. Oostdam, J. Bosmans, M. G. A. J. Wouters, E. M. W. Eekhoff, W. van Mechelen, and M. N. M. van Poppel, "Cost-effectiveness of an exercise program during pregnancy to prevent gestational diabetes: results of an economic evaluation alongside a randomised controlled trial," *BMC Pregnancy and Childbirth*, vol. 12, article 64, 2012.

[22] X. Liu, C. Li, H. Gong et al., "An economic evaluation for prevention of diabetes mellitus in a developing country: a modelling study," *BMC Public Health*, vol. 13, article 729, 2013.

[23] M. E. Png, J. S. Yoong, and S. Petta, "Evaluating the cost-effectiveness of lifestyle modification versus metformin therapy for the prevention of diabetes," *PLoS ONE*, vol. 9, no. 9, Article ID e107225, 2014.

[24] M. Y. Bertram, S. S. Lim, J. J. Barendregt, and T. Vos, "Assessing the cost-effectiveness of drug and lifestyle intervention following opportunistic screening for pre-diabetes in primary care," *Diabetologia*, vol. 53, no. 5, pp. 875–881, 2010.

[25] S. Mortaz, C. Wessman, R. Duncan, R. Gray, and A. Badawi, "Impact of screening and early detection of impaired fasting glucose tolerance and type 2 diabetes in Canada: a Markov model simulation," *Clinicoecon and Outcomes Research*, vol. 4, pp. 91–97, 2012.

[26] P. Johansson, C.-G. Östenson, A. M. Hilding, C. Andersson, C. Rehnberg, and P. Tillgren, "A cost-effectiveness analysis of a community-based diabetes prevention program in Sweden," *International Journal of Technology Assessment in Health Care*, vol. 25, no. 3, pp. 350–358, 2009.

[27] A. Neumann, P. Schwarz, and L. Lindholm, "Estimating the cost-effectiveness of lifestyle intervention programmes to prevent diabetes based on an example from Germany: Markov modelling," *Cost Effectiveness and Resource Allocation*, vol. 9, no. 1, article 17, 2011.

[28] A. J. Palmer and D. M. D. Tucker, "Cost and clinical implications of diabetes prevention in an Australian setting: a long-term modeling analysis," *Primary Care Diabetes*, vol. 6, no. 2, pp. 109–121, 2012.

[29] K. J. Smith, H. E. Hsu, M. S. Roberts et al., "Cost-effectiveness analysis of efforts to reduce risk of type 2 diabetes and cardiovascular disease in southwestern Pennsylvania, 2005–2007," *Preventing Chronic Disease*, vol. 7, no. 5, article A109, 2010.

[30] A. G. Tsai, T. A. Wadden, S. Volger et al., "Cost-effectiveness of a primary care intervention to treat obesity," *International Journal of Obesity*, vol. 37, supplement 1, pp. S31–S37, 2013.

[31] L. Cobiac, T. Vos, and L. Veerman, "Cost-effectiveness of weight watchers and the lighten up to a healthy lifestyle program," *Australian and New Zealand Journal of Public Health*, vol. 34, no. 3, pp. 240–247, 2010.

[32] A. Miners, J. Harris, L. Felix, E. Murray, S. Michie, and P. Edwards, "An economic evaluation of adaptive e-learning devices to promote weight loss via dietary change for people with obesity," *BMC Health Services Research*, vol. 12, article 190, 2012.

[33] M. Forster, J. L. Veerman, J. J. Barendregt, and T. Vos, "Cost-effectiveness of diet and exercise interventions to reduce overweight and obesity," *International Journal of Obesity*, vol. 35, no. 8, pp. 1071–1078, 2011.

[34] L. Lewis, M. Taylor, J. Broom, and K. L. Johnston, "The cost-effectiveness of the Lighter Life weight management programme as an intervention for obesity in England," *Clinical Obesity*, vol. 4, no. 3, pp. 180–188, 2014.

[35] N. K. Anokye, P. Trueman, C. Green, T. G. Pavey, M. Hillsdon, and R. S. Taylor, "The cost-effectiveness of exercise referral schemes," *BMC Public Health*, vol. 11, article 954, 2011.

[36] M. F. Drummond and T. O. Jefferson, "Guidelines for authors and peer reviewers of economic submissions to the BMJ. The BMJ Economic Evaluation Working Party," *British Medical Journal*, vol. 313, no. 7052, pp. 275–283, 1996.

[37] W. C. Knowler, S. E. Fowler, R. F. Hamman et al., "10-Year follow-up of diabetes incidence and weight loss in the Diabetes Prevention Program Outcomes study," *The Lancet*, vol. 374, no. 9702, pp. 1677–1686, 2009.

[38] J. Tuomilehto, J. Lindström, J. G. Eriksson et al., "Prevention of type 2 diabetes mellitus by changes in lifestyle among subjects with impaired glucose tolerance," *The New England Journal of Medicine*, vol. 344, no. 18, pp. 1343–1350, 2001.

[39] G. Li, P. Zhang, J. Wang et al., "The long-term effect of lifestyle interventions to prevent diabetes in the China Da Qing Diabetes Prevention Study: a 20-year follow-up study," *The Lancet*, vol. 371, no. 9626, pp. 1783–1789, 2008.

[40] NICE, *Modelling the Cost Effectiveness of Physical Activity Interventions*, National Institute for Health and Clinical Excellence (NICE), London, UK, 2006.

[41] B. Johns, T. Adam, and D. B. Evans, "Enhancing the comparability of costing methods: cross-country variability in the prices of non-traded inputs to health programmes," *Cost Effectiveness and Resource Allocation*, vol. 4, article 8, 2006.

[42] D. Walker and J. A. Fox-Rushby, "Allowing for uncertainty in economic evaluations: qualitative sensitivity analysis," *Health Policy and Planning*, vol. 16, no. 4, pp. 435–443, 2001.

[43] M. Brisson and W. J. Edmunds, "Impact of model, methodological, and parameter uncertainty in the economic analysis of vaccination programs," *Medical Decision Making*, vol. 26, no. 5, pp. 434–446, 2006.

[44] R. D. Goldney, P. J. Phillips, L. J. Fisher, and D. H. Wilson, "Diabetes, depression, and quality of life: a population study," *Diabetes Care*, vol. 27, no. 5, pp. 1066–1070, 2004.

[45] C. M. McDonough and A. N. A. Tosteson, "Measuring preferences for cost-utility analysis: how choice of method may influence decision-making," *PharmacoEconomics*, vol. 25, no. 2, pp. 93–106, 2007.

[46] J.-B. Echouffo-Tcheugui and A.-P. Kengne, "A United Nation high level meeting on chronic non-communicable diseases: utility for Africa?" *Pan African Medical Journal*, vol. 11, article 71, 2012.

[47] M. F. Drummond, M. J. Sculpher, G. W. Torrance, J. B. O'Brien, and L. G. Stoddart, *Methods for the Economic Evaluation of Health Care Programmes*, Oxford University Press, New York, NY, USA, 3rd edition, 2005.

[48] ACMTS, *Lignes Directrices de l'Évaluations Economique des Techonologies de Santé au Canada*, Agence Canadienne des Médicaments et des Technologies de la Santé (ACMTS), Ottawa, Canada, 3rd edition, 2006.

[49] L. Sutton, A. Karan, and A. Mahal, "Evidence for cost-effectiveness of lifestyle primary preventions for cardiovascular disease in the Asia-Pacific Region: a systematic review," *Globalization and Health*, vol. 10, no. 1, article 79, 2014.

[50] J. B. Echouffo-Tcheugui, M. K. Ali, S. J. Griffin, and K. M. V. Narayan, "Screening for type 2 diabetes and dysglycemia," *Epidemiologic Reviews*, vol. 33, no. 1, pp. 63–87, 2011.

[51] D. M. Eddy, "Accuracy versus transparency in pharmacoeconomic modelling: finding the right balance," *PharmacoEconomics*, vol. 24, no. 9, pp. 837–844, 2006.

[52] Z. Philips, L. Ginnelly, M. Sculpher et al., "Review of guidelines for good practice in decision-analytic modelling in health technology assessment," *Health Technology Assessment*, vol. 8, no. 36, pp. 1–158, 2004.

[53] R. Kahn and M. B. Davidson, "The reality of type 2 diabetes prevention," *Diabetes Care*, vol. 37, no. 4, pp. 943–949, 2014.

[54] N. J. Wareham, "Mind the gap: efficacy versus effectiveness of lifestyle interventions to prevent diabetes," *The Lancet Diabetes & Endocrinology*, vol. 3, no. 3, pp. 160–161, 2015.

[55] S. L. Jackson, Q. Long, M. K. Rhee et al., "Weight loss and incidence of diabetes with the Veterans Health Administration MOVE! lifestyle change programme: an observational study," *The Lancet Diabetes & Endocrinology*, vol. 3, no. 3, pp. 173–180, 2015.

[56] R. Whittemore, "A systematic review of the translational research on the Diabetes Prevention Program," *Translational Behavioral Medicine*, vol. 1, no. 3, pp. 480–491, 2011.

20

Treatment with Tacrolimus and Sirolimus Reveals No Additional Adverse Effects on Human Islets *In Vitro* Compared to Each Drug Alone but They Are Reduced by Adding Glucocorticoids

Kristine Kloster-Jensen,[1,2,3] **Afaf Sahraoui,**[1,2,3] **Nils Tore Vethe,**[4] **Olle Korsgren,**[5,6] **Stein Bergan,**[4,7] **Aksel Foss,**[1,2,3] **and Hanne Scholz**[1,2,3]

[1]*Department of Transplant Medicine, Oslo University Hospital, P.O. Box 4950, 0424 Oslo, Norway*
[2]*Institute for Surgical Research, Oslo University Hospital, P.O. Box 4950, 0424 Oslo, Norway*
[3]*Institute of Clinical Medicine, University of Oslo, P.O. Box 1171, Blindern, 0318 Oslo, Norway*
[4]*Department of Pharmacology, Oslo University Hospital, P.O. Box 4950, 0424 Oslo, Norway*
[5]*Science for Life Laboratory, Department of Immunology, Genetics and Pathology, Uppsala University, Box 815, 75108 Uppsala, Sweden*
[6]*Department of Clinical Immunology, Genetics and Pathology, Rudbeck Laboratory, Uppsala University Hospital, 75185 Uppsala, Sweden*
[7]*School of Pharmacy, University of Oslo, P.O. Box 1171, Blindern, 0318 Oslo, Norway*

Correspondence should be addressed to Kristine Kloster-Jensen; kkjensen@rr-research.no

Academic Editor: Laurent Crenier

Tacrolimus and sirolimus are important immunosuppressive drugs used in human islet transplantation; however, they are linked to detrimental effects on islets and reduction of long-term graft function. Few studies investigate the direct effects of these drugs combined in parallel with single drug exposure. Human islets were treated with or without tacrolimus (30 μg/L), sirolimus (30 μg/L), or a combination thereof for 24 hrs. Islet function as well as apoptosis was assessed by glucose-stimulated insulin secretion (GSIS) and Cell Death ELISA. Proinflammatory cytokines were analysed by qRT-PCR and Bio-Plex. Islets exposed to the combination of sirolimus and tacrolimus were treated with or without methylprednisolone (1000 μg/L) and the expression of the proinflammatory cytokines was investigated. We found the following: (i) No additive reduction in function and viability in islets existed when tacrolimus and sirolimus were combined compared to the single drug. (ii) Increased expression of proinflammatory cytokines mRNA and protein levels in islets took place. (iii) Methylprednisolone significantly decreased the proinflammatory response in islets induced by the drug combination. Although human islets are prone to direct toxic effect of tacrolimus and sirolimus, we found no additive effects of the drug combination. Short-term exposure of glucocorticoids could effectively reduce the proinflammatory response in human islets induced by the combination of tacrolimus and sirolimus.

1. Introduction

Despite promising results in islet transplantation, glycaemic control is gradually impaired due to progressive graft dysfunction [1, 2]. The initial loss of islets immediately after islet transplantation is a result of inflammatory events and an alloantigen-nonspecific inflammatory process where inflammatory cytokines play a part in cellular injury to islets.

Another major reason for graft dysfunction is toxicity caused by the use of immunosuppressive drug therapy. The common immunosuppressive protocols used in clinical islet transplantation include induction therapy with either ATG or IL-2 receptor monoclonal antibody, followed by maintenance treatment including that of tacrolimus and sirolimus [1]. Tacrolimus, a CNI (calcineurin inhibitor), is the pillar of immunosuppressive therapy in both solid organ and islet transplantation because of its efficacy in preventing acute rejection and improving short-term graft survival [1, 3]. Tacrolimus inhibits insulin secretion and reduces islets viability [4–6]. Sirolimus is an mTOR (mammalian target of rapamycin) inhibitor, which inhibits cell proliferation and reduces allograft rejection resulting in improved long-term graft survival [7, 8]. Sirolimus decreases insulin secretion in islets, impairs revascularization, and reduces angiogenesis [9–11]; however the impact of these effects on transplanted islets is not fully characterized [12]. To what extent the combination treatment of sirolimus and tacrolimus shows additive toxicity to islets is not fully elucidated and few studies compare the direct effects on human islets of this drug combination *in vitro* [13, 14].

The instant inflammatory reaction observed in the peritransplant period after human islet transplantation leads to loss of more than 50% of the injected islets within the first hour [2, 15, 16]. Several approaches such as inhibition of specific cytokines such as TNF alpha and IL-1beta have been studied to evaluate potency in helping reduce this effect [17, 18]. Glucocorticoids are well-known immunosuppressive agents in transplantation, with strong anti-inflammatory properties by inhibiting production of several cytokine and chemokine. But because glucocorticoids have diabetogenic effects *in vivo* and directly impair insulin secretion, they have mostly been excluded from the immunosuppressive regimens in clinical islet transplantation after presentation of the Edmonton protocol. We have previously shown that short-term use of methylprednisolone during islet culturing prior to transplantation is effective for maintaining islet viability by reducing the proinflammatory cytokines production even though insulin secretion was temporarily suppressed [19].

This study was undertaken to elaborate on the direct effects of the combination treatment with tacrolimus and sirolimus on the function and viability in human islets compared to the effect of each drug alone. Finally we also investigated the effect of methylprednisolone, a glucocorticoid, on human islets after treatment with the combination of tacrolimus and sirolimus.

2. Materials and Methods

2.1. Islet Isolation and Culture. Human islets were isolated from 5 human pancreata obtained from multiorgan donors (one female and four males) after appropriate consent in the islet isolation laboratory facility at The Nordic Network for Clinical Islet Transplantation, Uppsala University Hospital, Sweden, according to the automated method refined by the Nordic Network for Islet Transplantation [20]. Approval of the experimental use of the islets was granted by the local Institutional Ethical Committee and performed in accordance with the principles of the Declaration of Helsinki 2000. The average donor age was 53 years (range 39–60 years), the body mass index (BMI) 26.6 kg/m^2 (range 22–32 kg/m^2). All donors met the criteria with glycosylated haemoglobin A1c below 6.5% (48 mmol/mol) [21]. Islet preparations were maintained in culture medium CMRL1066 (Mediatech), supplemented with 10% ABO-compatible serum, 10 mM Hepes, and 1% penicillin/streptomycin/L-glutamine (Invitrogen), at

37°C (5% CO_2) for the first 24 hours after isolation. After a medium change, the islets were maintained at 22°C (5% CO_2) until being used in experiments.

2.2. Immunosuppressive Drugs and Culturing. Between 2 and 5 days after isolation, equal aliquots of clinical grade islet preparations (purities from 75 ± 20% and viability of 85 ± 5%) were placed into 90 mm Petri dishes and cultured with tacrolimus 30 μg/L (37 nM), sirolimus 30 μg/L (33 nM) (Sigma-Aldrich, St. Louis, MO), or the combination thereof for 24 hours at 37°C (5% CO_2). Each experiment comprised control and stimulated islets from the same donor. In parallel experiments methylprednisolone (1000 μg/L) was added or not to the combined treatment of tacrolimus and sirolimus for 24 hours at 37°C (5% CO_2). We used our previous investigation into the blood through concentrations of methylprednisolone after a bolus dose of 500 mg intravenously in liver transplant recipients, to select the dose to use in *in vitro* exposure [22, 23]. We have also shown that 48 hours use of different doses of methylprednisolone to human islets *in vitro* reduced the viability and insulin secretion, without representing a durable detrimental effect [19]. Many transplant centers include a single dose of methylprednisolone as premedication prior to islet transplant [24]. Based on these findings, we selected 100 mg as the dose for the present study in order to investigate the anti-inflammatory effects of methylprednisolone on immunosuppressive exposed human islets.

Following treatment, cultured supernatants were collected and human islets were hand-picked into columns, washed two times with ice-cold phosphate buffered saline (PBS) before being used for either RNA extraction or lysed in 200 μL MiliQ water before homogenization by sonication, and then stored at −70°C until analyses with RT-PCR or multiplex bioassay (Bio-Plex human cytokine assay), respectively. The drug concentrations were selected to simulate toxic blood drug concentrations observed in portal vein immediately after transplantation [25]. Generally the therapeutic level of both FK506 (Tacrolimus) and rapamycin (Sirolimus) is assumed to be between 5 and 15 μg/L, although it may reach toxic levels of 20–25 μg/L [26]. Animal studies have shown that portal vein peak concentrations after 2 hours of tacrolimus and sirolimus are 5–7 times higher than the mean 24 hours through systemic level [25]. To represent a high level of drug concentration we therefor chose to use 30 μg/L. All drugs were solved in methanol and diluted in cell culture medium to reach their final concentrations.

2.3. Glucose-Stimulated Insulin Secretion Assay. Following treatment, twenty islets were hand-picked, transferred into 12 Transwell trays (Costar, Cambridge, MA, USA), and preincubated in Krebs-Ringer bicarbonate buffer (11.5 mM NaCl, 0.5 mM KCl, 2.4 mM NaHCO$_3$, 2.2 mM CaCl$_2$, 1 mM MgCl$_2$, 20 mM HEPES, and 2 mg/L albumin: all Sigma-Aldrich) containing 1.67 mmol/L glucose (Fresenius Kabi, Halden, Norway) at 37°C (5% CO_2) for 30 min before the islets were incubated for 40 min in fresh Krebs-Ringer bicarbonate buffer containing 1.67 mmol/L glucose (basal insulin secretion). Finally, the islets were incubated for 40 min in fresh

Krebs-Ringer bicarbonate buffer containing 20.0 mmol/L glucose (for stimulated insulin secretion). The supernatants were subsequently collected, and insulin concentration was measured using a human insulin enzyme immunoassay (EIA) (Mercodia AB, Uppsala, Sweden). Stimulation index (SI) expresses the islets capacity for insulin secretion and is calculated as the ratio of insulin secretion at 20.0 mmol/L to 1.67 mmol/L glucose/40 min.

2.4. Detection of Cell Apoptosis and Cell Death.
Assessment of apoptosis in islets was measured by the detection of DNA-histone complexes present in the cytoplasmic fraction of the cells using Cell Death Detection ELISA^{PLUS} (Roche, Basel, Switzerland) according to the instructions of the manufacturer.

2.5. Real-Time Quantitative PCR.
Total RNA was isolated from frozen islet pellets using the RNeasy Mini Kit (Qiagen, Hilden, Germany) according to manufacturer's guidelines. The concentration of all RNA samples was quantified using a NanoDrop ND-1000 UV/Vis spectrophotometer (Saveen Werner AB, Sweden), and 1 μg total RNA was reverse-transcribed using the High-Capacity cDNA Archive Kit according to the instructions of the manufacturer (Applied Biosystems, Forster City, CA, USA). Quantification of mRNA expression was performed using the following TaqMan assays: human IL-1β: Hs00174097m1 and IL-8: Hs00174103m1 with an ABI 7900HT Fast Real-Time PCR System (Applied Biosystems). Results were normalised to the housekeeping gene beta-actin and data were analysed using the $2^{-\Delta\Delta Ct}$ method.

2.6. Measurement of Proinflammatory Cytokines.
Concentrations of IL-8 and IL-6 were measured in islet lysate utilizing multiplex technology on a Multiplex Analyser (BioRad, Hercules, CA) following the instructions of the manufacturer. Each sample was correlated to the protein content of the islet lysate measured by protein assay kit (BCA; Pierce, Rockford, IL, USA).

2.7. Statistical Analyses.
Results are presented as mean ± SEM. Statistical analyses were performed with Kruskal-Wallis one-way analysis of variance (ANOVA) followed by unpaired t-test. Differences were considered significant at levels of $p < 0.05$. Statistical analyses were performed using GraphPad Prism 5.0 (GraphPad Software, CA, USA).

3. Results

3.1. No Additive Adverse Effect on Human Islet Function by the Combination Treatment with Tacrolimus and Sirolimus Compared to Tacrolimus Alone.
To investigate the effect of tacrolimus and sirolimus on human islets function compared to either drug alone, we performed a glucose challenge test after 24 hours of exposure to either tacrolimus or sirolimus or the combination thereof. The insulin release from control islets was significantly increased in response to stimulation with high glucose (20 mM) solution compared to low glucose

(1.67 mM) solution (Figure 1(a)). The combination treatment of tacrolimus and sirolimus resulted in a slight increase of basal insulin secretion and a reduced glucose-stimulated insulin secretion after stimulation with high glucose solution (Figure 1(a)). These results lead to a significant reduction of the stimulation index (SI) compared to untreated islets ($p = 0.0193$; Figure 1(b)). When methylprednisolone was added to the combination treatment we found no altered basal insulin secretion level in human islets after incubation in low glucose solution, whereas we found reduced insulin secretion after 1 hour in high glucose solution (Figure 1(a)), which led to a reduced SI ($p = 0.0057$; Figure 1(b)). As previously reported, tacrolimus treated islets show a significant reduction in capacity for stimulated insulin secretion (Figure 1(a)) [4] with no effects on the insulin content [5]. This suppression of high glucose-induced insulin release is also expressed by the reduced stimulation index compared to untreated control ($p = 0.0400$; Figure 1(b)). Following the incubation with sirolimus alone, the islets presented an almost normal insulin secretion both at basal and at stimulated level ($p = 0.273$), in accordance with previous findings [12]. Importantly when we compared the effects of the combination to each drug alone, we did not find additional deleterious effects of the combined treatment compared to tacrolimus alone on the GSIS in human islets (Figures 1(a) and 1(b)).

3.2. The Combination Treatment of Tacrolimus and Sirolimus Induced Apoptosis in Human Islets.
In order to investigate its potential role in the reduction of islets function, we characterized apoptosis by measurements of the double-stranded DNA breaks using Cell Death ELISA^{PLUS}. Human islets treated with the combination of tacrolimus and sirolimus or sirolimus alone showed a significantly increased apoptosis ($p < 0.05$; Figure 1(c)) whereas tacrolimus exposure alone did not affect the apoptosis. In addition, the combination of tacrolimus and sirolimus with methylprednisolone showed no significant difference compared to untreated controls suggesting that methylprednisolone helps reduce apoptosis in islets exposed to the drug combination.

3.3. Treatment with Tacrolimus and Sirolimus Induces Expression of Proinflammatory Cytokines.
To further characterize the molecular mechanisms associated with the detrimental effect of tacrolimus and sirolimus, we studied the expression (mRNA and protein) of the proinflammatory cytokines, IL-8, IL-6, and IL-1beta, known mediators causing pancreatic islet dysfunction and apoptosis [27, 28]. We found increased mRNA expression levels of IL-1beta (Figure 2(a)) and IL-8 (Figure 2(b)) in human islets after exposure to the combined treatment with tacrolimus and sirolimus as well as each of the drugs alone, compared to untreated controls. However, no additive elevation of the mRNA expression of neither IL-1beta (Figure 2(a)) nor IL-8 (Figure 2(b)) in the combination treatment compared to either drug alone was observed. Correspondingly, we found a significant increased protein expression of IL-8 (Figure 3(a)) and IL-6 (Figure 3(b)) in human islets.

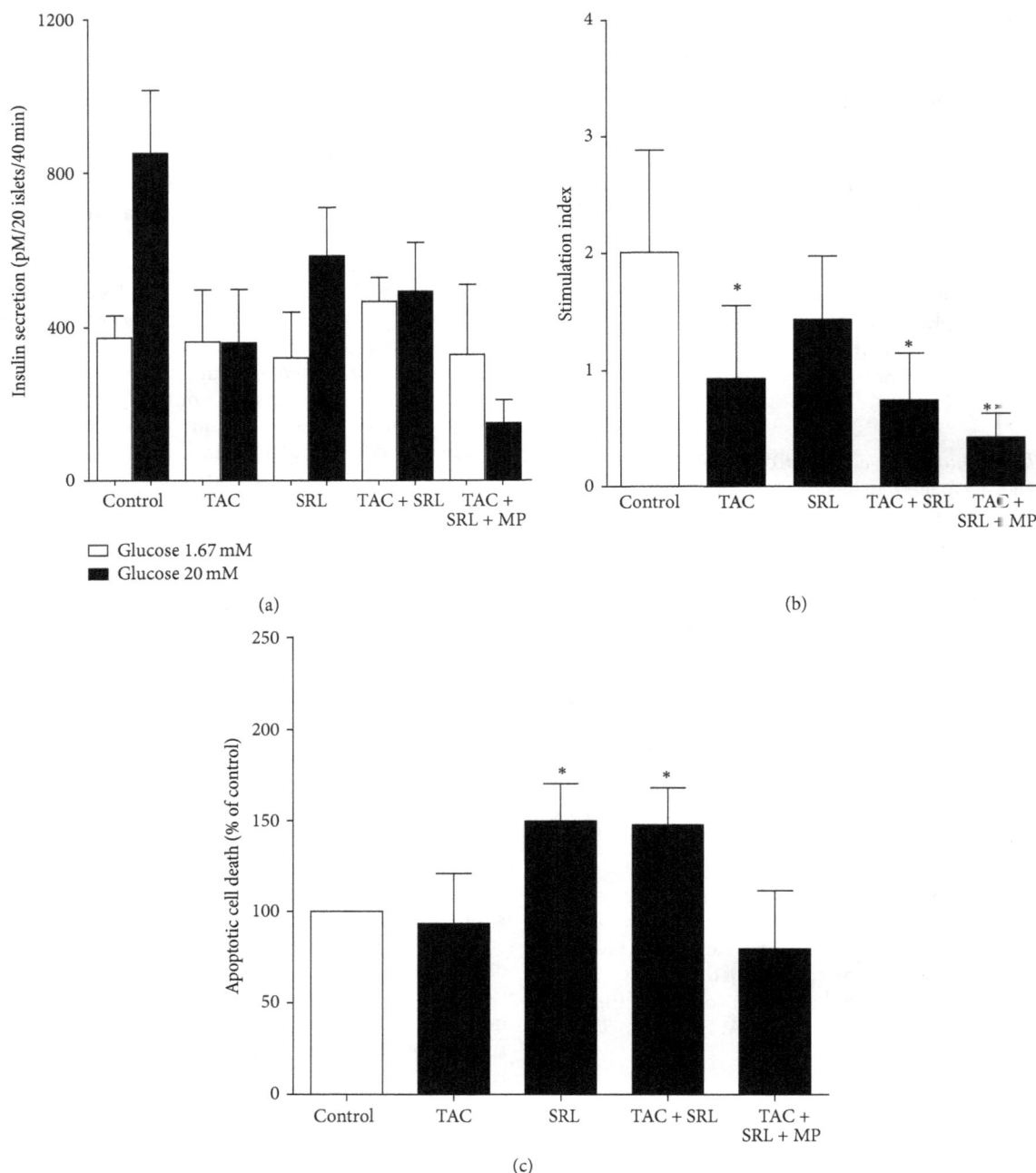

FIGURE 1: The effect of immunosuppressant drugs on human islets function and survival. Human islets treated without or with tacrolimus (TAC 30 μg/L), sirolimus (SRL 30 μg/L), or a combination thereof with or without methylprednisolone (MP 100 ng/L) for 24 h. (a) Glucose-stimulated insulin secretion (GSIS) and (b) corresponding stimulation index (SI) (ratio stimulated to basal glucose-stimulated insulin secretion) in human islets as described in Section 2. (c) Apoptotic cell death measured by the Cell Death Detection ELISA[PLUS] in human islet following the same culture conditions. Data are presented as means ± SEM of five separate experiments from five different donors. $^*p < 0.05$, $^{**}p < 0.006$ versus control.

3.4. Methylprednisolone Reduce the Proinflammatory Response Induced by the Combined Treatment with Tacrolimus and Sirolimus. Adding methylprednisolone to the combination treatment caused a significant reduction in gene expression of IL-8 ($p = 0.0023$) and IL-1beta ($p = 0.0027$) (Figure 4(a)) in the human islets. This reduction was followed by significantly reduced protein levels of IL-8 ($p = 0.0115$) and IL-6

($p = 0.0001$) in human islets compared to the combination alone (Figure 4(b)).

4. Discussion

Many studies compare the direct effects of immunosuppressive drug regimens on islets in vitro, but few are on human

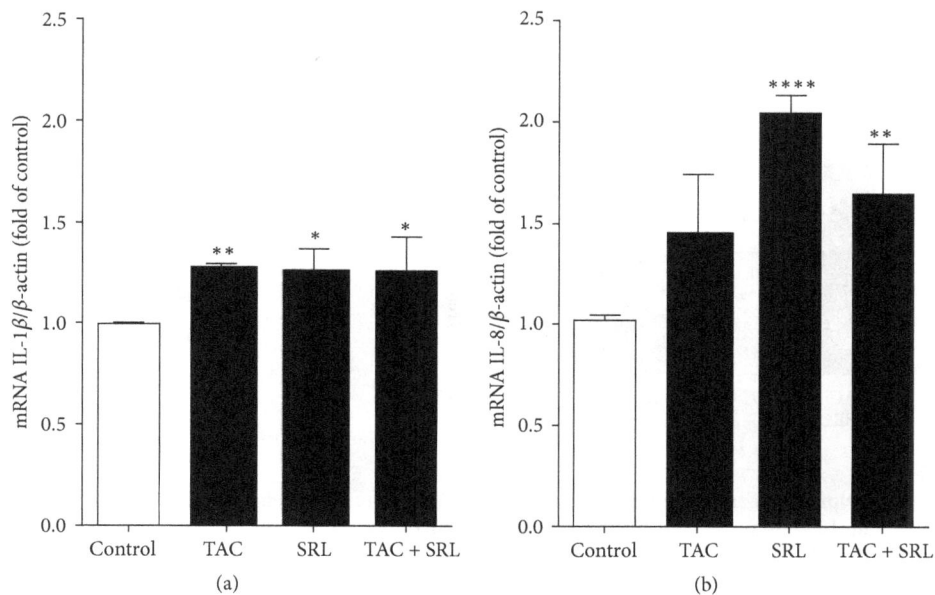

FIGURE 2: The effect of immunosuppressant drugs on gene expression of IL-1beta and IL-8 in human islets. Human islets cultured without or with tacrolimus (TAC 30 μg/L), sirolimus (SRL 30 μg/L), or a combination thereof for 24 hours were tested for gene expression of (a) IL-1beta and (b) IL-8 by qPCR in relation to the control gene β-actin. Data are presented as mean ± SEM of four separate experiments from four different donors. $^*p < 0.05$, $^{**}p < 0.005$, and $^{****}p < 0.0001$ versus control.

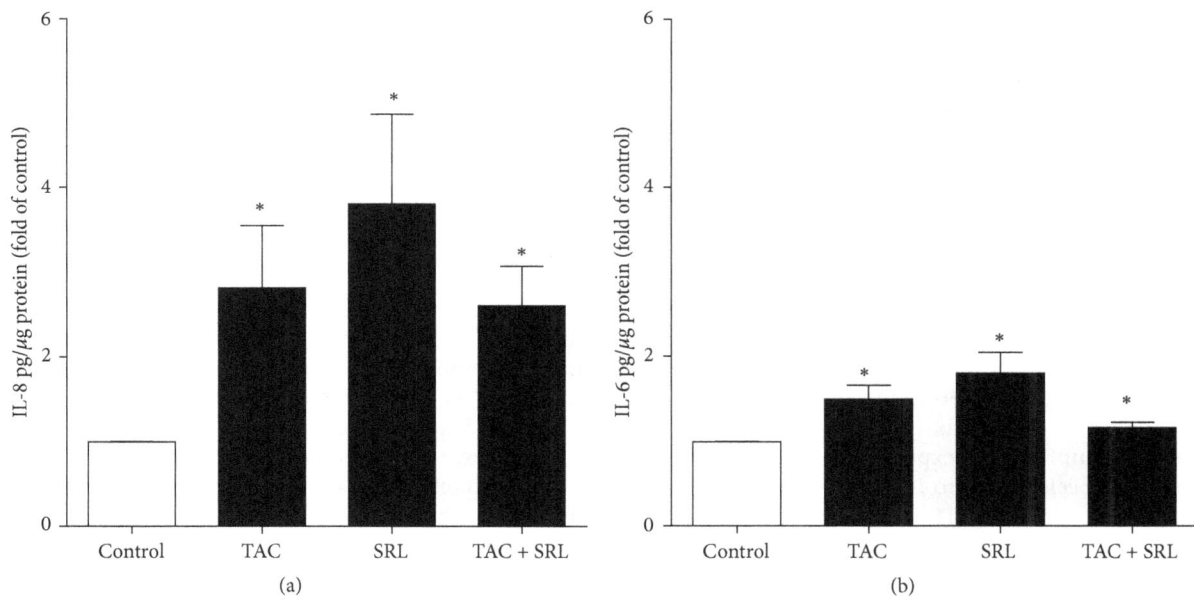

FIGURE 3: The effect of immunosuppressant drugs on protein release of IL-8 and IL-6 in human islets. Human islets cultured without or with tacrolimus (TAC 30 μg/L), sirolimus (SRL 30 μg/L), or a combination thereof for 24 hours. Protein levels of (a) IL-8 and (b) IL-6 in human islets were investigated in cell lysate using multiplex bead-based cytokine assay (Bio-Plex Human Cytokine Group 1). Data is presented as mean ± SEM of four separate experiments from four different donors. $^*p < 0.05$ versus control.

islets. And although a wide range of clinical observations involve drug regimens few studies compare the effects of regimens to the effects of the drugs alone [1, 29, 30].

In this study we investigate the impact of the combined drug therapy of tacrolimus and sirolimus on islets compared to the exposure to each drug alone. Also, we explore how this drug combination is influenced by methylprednisolone. In summary, we found that the combination of tacrolimus and sirolimus does not reduce human islet function and survival more than each of the drugs alone, nor does it further increase

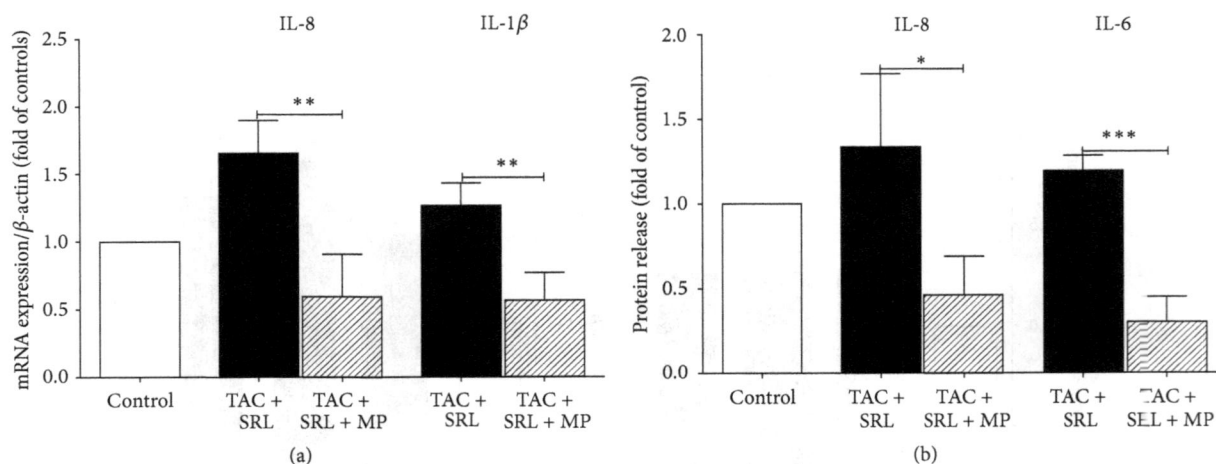

FIGURE 4: The effect of methylprednisolone on the inflammatory potential in human islets. Human islets cultured with tacrolimus (TAC 30 µg/L), sirolimus (SRL 30 µg/L), with or without methylprednisolone (MP 1000 ng/L), for 24 hours were tested for (a) gene expression of IL-1beta and IL-8 and (b) protein release of IL-8 and IL-6. The fold change represents the expression of target genes in isolated islets relative to the β-actin mRNA level. Data is presented as mean ± SEM of four separate experiments from four different donors. $^{*}p < 0.05$, $^{**}p < 0.005$, and $^{***}p < 0.0005$ versus control.

proinflammatory cytokine expression. Methylprednisolone reduced the proinflammatory cytokine expression induced by the combination of tacrolimus and sirolimus.

In our data islets function was reduced when exposed to tacrolimus whereas sirolimus exposure did not significantly influence islet function. This is consistent with clinical observations where islets cultured with the combination tacrolimus and sirolimus decrease GSIS [31, 32]. Despite different mechanisms of action, tacrolimus [4, 6] and sirolimus [12, 31, 33, 34] ultimately reduced islet function. Sirolimus is known to influence glucose homeostasis through reduction in mitochondrial ATP production, decrease in beta cell proliferation, and impairing of insulin secretion and resistance as a consequence of chronicle exposure [11, 35]. Since our study was an acute in vitro study it is likely that deteriorating effects of sirolimus would be masked by the short exposure time.

Apoptosis is a major cause of islet cell loss in the early posttransplantation period [36] and it is triggered by the isolation process, islet hypoxia [37], and proinflammatory cytokines [38]. Human islets exposed to either sirolimus or tacrolimus have been shown to induce apoptosis in human islets regardless of added dose [4, 9, 29]. But tacrolimus is also shown not to cause significant apoptosis in beta-cells [6, 39], which correlates well with our findings of no increase in cell death following tacrolimus exposure. Short time exposure of tacrolimus has recently been shown to highly suppress insulin secretion in human islets without changing intracellular insulin content or viability [40]. This is consistent with our study (Figure 1(c)) and others [6, 39]. Sirolimus reduced the survival of islets, supporting the findings from previous studies showing that sirolimus conclusively causes detrimental effects on beta-cells survival and cell apoptosis both in murine and in human beta-cells [9, 41] and increased apoptosis [9, 29].

Following islet transplantation proinflammatory cytokines such as IL-1beta and IL-8 are activated [42] suggesting an alloantigen nonspecific, inflammatory process [42, 43]. We observed a significantly increased expression of IL-1beta, IL-8, and IL-6 on mRNA and protein levels in islets exposed to tacrolimus and sirolimus equally in the combination and single drugs. Our observation could therefore illustrate a reciprocal inhibition of the two drugs [13] or that maximum intervention has been reached. Others have shown that sirolimus and tacrolimus have anti-inflammatory properties [44–47]. Compared to our data they use longer exposure time and lower drug dose, which are reasonable explanations for these differences.

Tacrolimus and sirolimus are structurally similar and both bind to FK506 binding proteins to form immunosuppressive complexes; however they are not considered antagonistic to one another [48]. We found no significant difference in impact on islets exposed to the drug combinations compared to each drug alone. One explanation for this could be that tacrolimus and sirolimus exert opposite effects and inhibit the actions of each other [13, 14, 49]. Another explanation could be that both drugs act by means of a common immunosuppressant binding protein or yet unidentified intracellular proteins. We recently published a paper where we found a difference in intracellular uptake of drugs when tacrolimus and sirolimus are given in combination compared to separately [50]. Even though it has been debatable we cannot exclude an antagonism between tacrolimus and sirolimus [48, 51] or that there is a distinction between high and low dose being essential for the drug-drug interaction [52].

It is well known that corticosteroid induces hyperglycemia mainly by reducing insulin-mediated glucose uptake. But the direct beta-cells toxicity through inhibition of insulin production and secretion is still controversial; most likely it depends on dose and exposure time [19, 53]. Improvement in the outcome of islet transplantation after the Edmonton protocol is partially due to steroid-free immunosuppressive protocol [1]. To enhance therapeutic efficacy while minimizing the toxicity of each drug multiple immunosuppressive drugs are being used in transplantation. Due to proinflammatory cytokines impact on islet survival, induction therapy has shifted from interleukin-2 receptor antagonist alone to a variety of new T-cell depleting antibodies, TNF alpha inhibitors, CXCR1/2 blocker, and several others [1, 54]. Our findings support that induction treatment may be needed to reduce inflammatory reactions during transplantation. We found that methylprednisolone reduced cytokine and chemokine production from islet preparations; this accords well with previous findings [55, 56]. On the other hand steroids are also known to reduce insulin secretion from beta-cells [57]; fortunately this is not permanent state [19] and a brief exposure to steroids in the preculturing phase even improves survival in an experimental mouse model. The proinflammatory cytokine production caused by sirolimus and tacrolimus was suppressed by methylprednisolone. Because of their diabetogenic properties it is still controversial whether glucocorticoids are deleterious to islets in the acute phase of transplantation. Indeed, a new trend according to the latest CITR report demonstrates that glucocorticoids are used after first infusion in approximately 17% of islet transplant patients as part of the immunosuppressive treatment, while at 6 months only 6% use these drugs [1]. Our results support short-term use of methylprednisolone as an inhibitor of the cytokine release following tacrolimus and sirolimus.

In conclusion, the *ex vivo* exposure of human islets to tacrolimus, sirolimus, and the combination of the two reduces islet function and survival and increases proinflammatory cytokines in the islets. The proinflammatory response of the tacrolimus-sirolimus combination was reduced by short-term exposure to methylprednisolone. These findings provide a basis for further investigations into the drug interactions between tacrolimus and sirolimus that can help tailor immunosuppressive regimens for islet transplant recipients.

Abbreviations

CNI: Calcineurin inhibitor
GSIS: Glucose-stimulated insulin secretion.

Conflict of Interests

All authors state that they have no conflict of interests.

Authors' Contribution

Kristine Kloster-Jensen, Afaf Sahraoui, Aksel Foss, Olle Korsgren, and Hanne Scholz participated in the research design and reviewed/edited the paper, Nils Tore Vethe, Stein Bergan contributed to the scientific discussion and reviewed/edited the paper, and Kristine Kloster-Jensen, Hanne Scholz performed the experiments and wrote the paper.

Acknowledgments

Human islets were provided through the JDRF Award 31-2008-413 (ECIT Islet for Basic Research Programs). The authors are grateful to the Nordic Network for Clinical Islet Transplantation and thank Odd Fellow Medical Research foundation, The Norwegian Diabetes Association, and a grant from South-Eastern Norway Regional Health Authority.

References

[1] F. B. Barton, M. R. Rickels, R. Alejandro et al., "Improvement in outcomes of clinical islet transplantation: 1999-2010," *Diabetes Care*, vol. 35, no. 7, pp. 1436–1445, 2012.

[2] O. Korsgren, T. Lundgren, M. Felldin et al., "Optimising islet engraftment is critical for successful clinical islet transplantation," *Diabetologia*, vol. 51, no. 2, pp. 227–232, 2008.

[3] T. R. Srinivas and H.-U. Meier-Kriesche, "Minimizing immunosuppression, an alternative approach to reducing side effects: objectives and interim result," *Clinical Journal of the American Society of Nephrology*, vol. 3, supplement 2, pp. S101–S116, 2008.

[4] M. Bugliani, M. Masini, R. Liechti et al., "The direct effects of tacrolimus and cyclosporin A on isolated human islets: a functional, survival and gene expression study," *Islets*, vol. 1, no. 2, pp. 106–110, 2009.

[5] R. G. Radu, S. Fujimoto, E. Mukai et al., "Tacrolimus suppresses glucose-induced insulin release from pancreatic islets by reducing glucokinase activity," *American Journal of Physiology—Endocrinology and Metabolism*, vol. 288, no. 2, pp. E365–E371, 2005.

[6] N. Rostambeigi, I. R. Lanza, P. P. Dzeja et al., "Unique cellular and mitochondrial defects mediate FK506-induced islet beta-cell dysfunction," *Transplantation*, vol. 91, no. 6, pp. 615–623, 2011.

[7] B. Kaplan, Y. Qazi, and J. R. Wellen, "Strategies for the management of adverse events associated with mTOR inhibitors," *Transplantation Reviews*, vol. 28, no. 3, pp. 126–133, 2014.

[8] L. Rostaing and N. Kamar, "mTOR inhibitor/proliferation signal inhibitors: entering or leaving the field?" *Journal of Nephrology*, vol. 23, no. 2, pp. 133–142, 2010.

[9] A. D. Barlow, J. Xie, C. E. Moore et al., "Rapamycin toxicity in MIN6 cells and rat and human islets is mediated by the inhibition of mTOR complex 2 (mTORC2)," *Diabetologia*, vol. 55, no. 5, pp. 1355–1365, 2012.

[10] C. T. Bussiere, J. R. T. Lakey, A. M. J. Shapiro, and G. S. Korbutt, "The impact of the mTOR inhibitor sirolimus on the proliferation and function of pancreatic islets and ductal cells," *Diabetologia*, vol. 49, no. 10, pp. 2341–2349, 2006.

[11] S.-B. Yang, H. Y. Lee, D. M. Young et al., "Rapamycin induces glucose intolerance in mice by reducing islet mass, insulin content, and insulin sensitivity," *Journal of Molecular Medicine*, vol. 90, no. 5, pp. 575–585, 2012.

[12] S. Marcelli-Tourvieille, T. Hubert, E. Moerman et al., "In vivo and in vitro effect of sirolimus on insulin secretion," *Transplantation*, vol. 83, no. 5, pp. 532–538, 2007.

[13] B. E. Bierer, P. S. Mattila, R. F. Standaert et al., "Two distinct signal transmission pathways in T lymphocytes are inhibited by complexes formed between an immunophilin and either FK506 or rapamycin," *Proceedings of the National Academy of Sciences of the United States of America*, vol. 87, no. 23, pp. 9231–9235, 1990.

[14] R. E. Morris, B. M. Meiser, J. Wu, R. Shorthouse, and J. Wang, "Use of rapamycin for the suppression of alloimmune reactions in vivo: schedule dependence, tolerance induction, synergy with cyclosporine and FK 506, and effect on host-versus-graft

and graft-versus-host reactions," *Transplantation Proceedings*, vol. 23, no. 1, pp. 521–524, 1991.

[15] A. Citro, E. Cantarelli, and L. Piemonti, "Anti-inflammatory strategies to enhance islet engraftment and survival," *Current Diabetes Reports*, vol. 13, no. 5, pp. 733–744, 2013.

[16] H. Johansson, A. Lukinius, L. Moberg et al., "Tissue factor produced by the endocrine cells of the islets of langerhans is associated with a negative outcome of clinical islet transplantation," *Diabetes*, vol. 54, no. 6, pp. 1755–1762, 2005.

[17] B. J. Hering, R. Kandaswamy, J. D. Ansite et al., "Single-donor, marginal-dose islet transplantation in patients with type 1 diabetes," *The Journal of the American Medical Association*, vol. 293, no. 7, pp. 830–835, 2005.

[18] M. McCall, R. Pawlick, T. Kin, and A. M. J. Shapiro, "Anakinra potentiates the protective effects of etanercept in transplantation of marginal mass human islets in immunodeficient mice," *American Journal of Transplantation*, vol. 12, no. 2, pp. 322–329, 2012.

[19] T. Lund, B. Fosby, O. Korsgren, H. Scholz, and A. Foss, "Glucocorticoids reduce pro-inflammatory cytokines and tissue factor in vitro and improve function of transplanted human islets in vivo," *Transplant International*, vol. 21, no. 7, pp. 669–678, 2008.

[20] M. Goto, T. M. Eich, M. Felldin et al., "Refinement of the automated method for human islet isolation and presentation of a closed system for in vitro islet culture," *Transplantation*, vol. 78, no. 9, pp. 1367–1375, 2004.

[21] M. Stahle, A. Foss, B. Gustafsson et al., "Clostripain, the missing link in the enzyme blend for efficient human islet isolation," *Transplantation Direct*, vol. 1, no. 5, pp. 1–6, 2015.

[22] I. Sæves, P.-D. Line, and S. Bergan, "The pharmacokinetics of prednisolone and prednisone in adult liver transplant recipients early after transplantation," *Therapeutic Drug Monitoring*, vol. 34, no. 4, pp. 452–459, 2012.

[23] I. Sæves, N. T. Vethe, and S. Bergan, "Quantification of 6 glucocorticoids in human plasma by liquid chromatography tandem mass spectrometry: method development, validation, and assessment of matrix effects," *Therapeutic Drug Monitoring*, vol. 33, no. 4, pp. 402–410, 2011.

[24] A. M. Posselt, M. D. Bellin, M. Tavakol et al., "Islet transplantation in type 1 diabetics using an immunosuppressive protocol based on the anti-LFA-1 antibody efalizumab," *American Journal of Transplantation*, vol. 10, no. 8, pp. 1870–1880, 2010.

[25] A. M. J. Shapiro, H. L. Gallant, G. H. Er et al., "The portal immunosuppressive storm: relevance to islet transplantation?" *Therapeutic Drug Monitoring*, vol. 27, no. 1, pp. 35–37, 2005.

[26] S. M. Tsunoda and F. T. Aweeka, "Drug concentration monitoring of immunosuppressive agents: focus on tacrolimus, mycophenolate mofetil and sirolimus," *BioDrugs*, vol. 14, no. 6, pp. 355–369, 2000.

[27] N. R. Barshes, S. Wyllie, and J. A. Goss, "Inflammation-mediated dysfunction and apoptosis in pancreatic islet transplantation: implications for intrahepatic grafts," *Journal of Leukocyte Biology*, vol. 77, no. 5, pp. 587–597, 2005.

[28] S. Negi, A. Jetha, R. Aikin, C. Hasilo, R. Sladek, and S. Paraskevas, "Analysis of beta-cell gene expression reveals inflammatory signaling and evidence of dedifferentiation following human islet isolation and culture," *PLoS ONE*, vol. 7, no. 1, Article ID e30415, 2012.

[29] J. D. Johnson, Z. Ao, P. Ao et al., "Different effects of FK506, rapamycin, and mycophenolate mofetil on glucose-stimulated insulin release and apoptosis in human islets," *Cell Transplantation*, vol. 18, no. 8, pp. 833–845, 2009.

[30] B. W. Paty, J. S. Harmon, C. L. Marsh, and R. P. Robertson, "Inhibitory effects of immunosuppressive drugs on insulin secretion from HIT-T15 cells and Wistar rat islets," *Transplantation*, vol. 73, no. 3, pp. 353–357, 2002.

[31] P. Gillard, Z. Ling, C. Mathieu et al., "Comparison of sirolimus alone with sirolimus plus tacrolimus in type 1 diabetic recipients of cultured islet cell grafts," *Transplantation*, vol. 85, no. 2, pp. 256–263, 2008.

[32] D. L. Roelen, V. A. L. Huurman, R. Hilbrands et al., "Relevance of cytotoxic alloreactivity under different immunosuppressive regimens in clinical islet cell transplantation," *Clinical and Experimental Immunology*, vol. 156, no. 1, pp. 141–148, 2009.

[33] N. Niclauss, D. Bosco, P. Morel, L. Giovannoni, T. Berney, and G. Parnaud, "Rapamycin impairs proliferation of transplanted islet β cells," *Transplantation*, vol. 91, no. 7, pp. 714–722, 2011.

[34] N. Zhang, D. Su, S. Qu et al., "Sirolimus is associated with reduced islet engraftment and impaired β-cell function," *Diabetes*, vol. 55, no. 9, pp. 2429–2436, 2006.

[35] M. Shimodahira, S. Fujimoto, E. Mukai et al., "Rapamycin impairs metabolism-secretion coupling in rat pancreatic islets by suppressing carbohydrate metabolism," *The Journal of Endocrinology*, vol. 204, no. 1, pp. 37–46, 2010.

[36] L. Moberg, H. Johansson, A. Lukinius et al., "Production of tissue factor by pancreatic islet cells as a trigger of detrimental thrombotic reactions in clinical islet transplantation," *The Lancet*, vol. 360, no. 9350, pp. 2039–2045, 2002.

[37] Z. Ma, N. Moruzzi, S.-B. Catrina, V. Grill, and A. Björklund, "Hyperoxia inhibits glucose-induced insulin secretion and mitochondrial metabolism in rat pancreatic islets," *Biochemical and Biophysical Research Communications*, vol. 443, no. 1, pp. 223–228, 2014.

[38] S. Paraskevas, W. P. Duguid, D. Maysinger, L. Feldman, D. Agapitos, and L. Rosenberg, "Apoptosis occurs in freshly isolated human islets under standard culture conditions," *Transplantation Proceedings*, vol. 29, no. 1-2, pp. 750–752, 1997.

[39] I. Hernández-Fisac, J. Pizarro-Delgado, C. Calle et al., "Tacrolimus-induced diabetes in rats courses with suppressed insulin gene expression in pancreatic islets," *American Journal of Transplantation*, vol. 7, no. 11, pp. 2455–2462, 2007.

[40] B. L. Gala-Lopez, A. R. Pepper, R. L. Pawlick et al., "Anti-aging glycopeptide protects human islets against tacrolimus-related injury and facilitates engraftment in mice," *Diabetes*, 2015.

[41] E. Bell, X. Cao, J. A. Moibi et al., "Rapamycin has a deleterious effect on MIN-6 cells and rat and human islets," *Diabetes*, vol. 52, no. 11, pp. 2731–2739, 2003.

[42] U. Johansson, A. Olsson, S. Gabrielsson, B. Nilsson, and O. Korsgren, "Inflammatory mediators expressed in human islets of Langerhans: implications for islet transplantation," *Biochemical and Biophysical Research Communications*, vol. 308, no. 3, pp. 474–479, 2003.

[43] M. J. Cowley, A. Weinberg, N. W. Zammit et al., "Human islets express a marked proinflammatory molecular signature prior to transplantation," *Cell Transplantation*, vol. 21, no. 9, pp. 2063–2078, 2012.

[44] J. M. B. Del Castillo, M. C. García-Martín, J. Arias-Díaz, E. Giné, E. Vara, and J. L. B. Cantero, "Antiapoptotic effect of tacrolimus on cytokine-challenged human islets," *Cell Transplantation*, vol. 18, no. 10-11, pp. 1237–1246, 2009.

[45] A. Mita, C. Ricordi, A. Miki et al., "Anti-proinflammatory effects of sirolimus on human islet preparations," *Transplantation*, vol. 86, no. 1, pp. 46–53, 2008.

[46] B. M. Rau, C. M. Krüger, C. Hasel et al., "Effects of immuno-suppressive and immunostimulative treatment on pancreatic injury and mortality in severe acute experimental pancreatitis," *Pancreas*, vol. 33, no. 2, pp. 174–183, 2006.

[47] A. M. J. Shapiro, W. L. Suarez-Pinzon, R. Power, and A. Rabinovitch, "Combination therapy with low dose sirolimus and tacrolimus is synergistic in preventing spontaneous and recurrent autoimmune diabetes in non-obese diabetic mice," *Diabetologia*, vol. 45, no. 2, pp. 224–230, 2002.

[48] M. D. Vu, S. Qi, D. Xu et al., "Tacrolimus (FK506) and sirolimus (rapamycin) in combination are not antagonistic but produce extended graft survival in cardiac transplantation in the rat," *Transplantation*, vol. 64, no. 12, pp. 1853–1856, 1997.

[49] F. J. Dumont, M. R. Melino, M. J. Staruch, S. L. Koprak, P. A. Fischer, and N. H. Sigal, "The immunosuppressive macrolides FK-506 and rapamycin act as reciprocal antagonists in murine T cells," *The Journal of Immunology*, vol. 144, no. 4, pp. 1418–1424, 1990.

[50] K. Kloster-Jensen, N. T. Vethe, S. Bremer et al., "Intracellular sirolimus concentration is reduced by tacrolimus in human pancreatic islets in vitro," *Transplant International*, vol. 28, no. 10, pp. 1152–1161, 2015.

[51] H. Chen, S. Qi, D. Xu et al., "Combined effect of rapamycin and FK 506 in prolongation of small bowel graft survival in the mouse," *Transplantation Proceedings*, vol. 30, no. 6, pp. 2579–2581, 1998.

[52] M. J. Barten, F. Streit, M. Boeger et al., "Synergistic effects of sirolimus with cyclosporine and tacrolimus: analysis of immunosuppression on lymphocyte proliferation and activation in rat whole blood," *Transplantation*, vol. 77, no. 8, pp. 1154–1162, 2004.

[53] C. Lambillotte, P. Gilon, and J.-C. Henquin, "Direct gluco-corticoid inhibition of insulin secretion. An in vitro study of dexamethasone effects in mouse islets," *The Journal of Clinical Investigation*, vol. 99, no. 3, pp. 414–423, 1997.

[54] M. D. Bellin, F. B. Barton, A. Heitman et al., "Potent induction immunotherapy promotes long-term insulin independence after islet transplantation in type 1 diabetes," *American Journal of Transplantation*, vol. 12, no. 6, pp. 1576–1583, 2012.

[55] A. C. Liberman, J. Druker, M. J. Perone, and E. Arzt, "Gluco-corticoids in the regulation of transcription factors that control cytokine synthesis," *Cytokine & Growth Factor Reviews*, vol. 18, no. 1-2, pp. 45–56, 2007.

[56] R. I. Scheinman, A. Gualberto, C. M. Jewell, J. A. Cidlowski, and A. S. Baldwin Jr., "Characterization of mechanisms involved in transrepression of NF-κB by activated glucocorticoid receptors," *Molecular and Cellular Biology*, vol. 15, no. 2, pp. 943–953, 1995.

[57] F. Delaunay, A. Khan, A. Cintra et al., "Pancreatic β cells are important targets for the diabetogenic effects of glucocorticoids," *The Journal of Clinical Investigation*, vol. 100, no. 8, pp. 2094–2098, 1997.

21

Influence of Acute High Glucose on Protein Abundance Changes in Murine Glomerular Mesangial Cells

**Michelle T. Barati,[1] James C. Gould,[1,2] Sarah A. Salyer,[1,3] Susan Isaacs,[1]
Daniel W. Wilkey,[1] and Michael L. Merchant[1]**

[1]*Kidney Disease Program, Department of Medicine, University of Louisville, Louisville, KY 40202, USA*
[2]*Harvard Medical School, Boston, MA 02115, USA*
[3]*Tuskegee University School of Veterinary Medicine, Tuskegee, AL 36088, USA*

Correspondence should be addressed to Michael L. Merchant; mlmerc02@louisville.edu

Academic Editor: Feng Zheng

The effects of acute exposure to high glucose levels as experienced by glomerular mesangial cells in postprandial conditions and states such as in prediabetes were investigated using proteomic methods. Two-dimensional gel electrophoresis and matrix assisted laser desorption ionization time of flight mass spectrometry methods were used to identify protein expression patterns in immortalized rat mesangial cells altered by 2 h high glucose (HG) growth conditions as compared to isoosmotic/normal glucose control (NG*) conditions. Unique protein expression changes at 2 h HG treatment were measured for 51 protein spots. These proteins could be broadly grouped into two categories: (1) proteins involved in cell survival/cell signaling and (2) proteins involved in stress response. Immunoblot experiments for a protein belonging to both categories, prohibitin (PHB), supported a trend for increased total expression as well as significant increases in an acidic PHB isoform. Additional studies confirmed the regulation of proteasomal subunit alpha-type 2 and the endoplasmic reticulum chaperone and oxidoreductase PDI (protein disulfide isomerase), suggesting altered ER protein folding capacity and proteasomal function in response to acute HG. We conclude that short term high glucose induces subtle changes in protein abundances suggesting posttranslational modifications and regulation of pathways involved in proteostasis.

1. Introduction

Renal glomerular mesangial cells (GMCs) functions are altered in diabetic nephropathy by chronic exposure to high glucose (HG) or exposure to glycated albumin [1–4]. The early effects of hyperglycemia are thought to be dominated by hemodynamic factors including glomerular hyperfiltration and shear stress leading to damage by microalbuminuria or proteinuria [5–10]. The early histopathology of diabetic nephropathy is characterized by a thickening of the glomerular basement membrane (GBM) and an accumulation of extracellular matrix (ECM) in the glomerular mesangium. The damaging effects of chronic hyperglycemia on various kidney glomerular cell types such as mesangial cells, podocytes, and endothelial cells have been intensely studied.

The theories that have been addressed include increased substrate channeling into the polyol pathway and the hexosamine pathways and increased production of reactive oxygen species (ROS) and activation of protein kinase C (via advanced glycation end-products (AGE), diacylglycerols (DAG), and/or reactive oxygen species (ROS)) [11–13]. These advances in our understanding of the effects of chronic hyperglycemia on renal physiology have not been matched by understanding of the effects of acute (2 h) hyperglycemic conditions episodically experienced by cells like the GMC in states such as prediabetes. We hypothesize that understanding these acute changes induced by hyperglycemia might yield insight into the mechanisms through which chronic hyperglycemia disrupts mechanisms used to maintain normal glomerular function.

2. Material and Methods

2.1. Cell Culture.

The rat GMC line CRL-2573 (ATCC) maintained normal growth media (DMEM: 5 mM D-glucose, 15% FBS) under 5% CO_2 at 37°C. The cells (passages 10–15) were plated in Corning T25 flasks and cultured until 70–80% confluence was reached. Normal media were removed from cells and replaced with DMEM supplemented with 0.5% FBS/5 mM D-glucose. After 24 h, media were removed and replaced with isoosmotic-normal glucose (NG*) media (DMEM-5 mM D-glucose, 20 mM mannitol, and 0.5% FBS) or high glucose (HG) media (DMEM: 25 mM D-glucose, 0 mM mannitol, and 0.5% FBS), for 2 h. For 2DE analysis, after 2 h treatment, the total protein was collected as previously described [14] using IPG rehydration buffer supplemented with protease inhibitors.

2.2. Cell Viability.

Cell viability was determined after 2 h HG and NG* treatment using the MTT assay [15] as described by the manufacturer (Sigma, St. Louis, MO, USA).

2.3. Two-Dimensional Electrophoresis (2DE) and Image Acquisition.

2DE experiments were conducted as reported previously [14]. Murine GMC protein (75 µg) was rehydrated overnight into IPG (pH 3–10; 7 cm; Invitrogen) strips. The strip was focused for a total of 1200–1300 Vh with a final 30 min focusing period at 2000 V constant. Proteins were separated in the second dimension on 4–12% Bis-Tris mini gels (8 cm × 8 cm). The gel slabs were fixed in 10% methanol and 7% acetic acid and then transferred to SYPRO-Ruby protein gel stain (Molecular Probes, Oregon, USA) for 18 hours. Gels were scanned using a PerkinElmer ProXpress CCD-based digital imager at 50 µm resolution. The gel/stain exposure and emission acquisition times were varied to maximize the detector response while avoiding detector saturation. The image files were matched, reference gels were created, and spot volumes were determined using Progenesis Discovery software (Nonlinear Dynamics, Newcastle upon Tyne, UK). A student's t-test is used to evaluate all matched spot pairs. Protein spots that were found to have variable spot volumes between samples were statistically compared by spot mean and SEM.

2.4. Proteomic Analyses.

Protein gel spots were digested as previously described [14]. MALDI-TOF and TOF/TOF MS data were acquired on the tryptic digests using an AB4700 Proteomics Analyzer (Applied Biosystems, Foster City, CA) and analyzed using Matrix Science Mascot (ver. 2.0) as described previously [16]. Data was analyzed assuming (a) monoisotopic peptides masses, (b) cysteine carbamidomethylation, (c) variable oxidation of methionine, (d) maximum of one missed trypsin cleavage, and (e) a mass accuracy of greater than 150 ppm for MS data and 0.3 Da for MS-MS data against the SwissProt (release 52.0, 20070307) protein database (261513 sequences; 95638062 residues) constrained to the mammalian (50870 sequences) taxa. Limitation of the original protein mass was not employed within the Mascot search. Protein identifications were accepted for protein identifications that include using MASCOT MS + MS/MS analysis with significant MOWSE scores ($p < 0.05$; for MS MOWSE score of 60 which equals significance and for MS/MS MOWSE peptide ion score alone of 40 which equals significance).

2.5. Confocal Microscopy.

Confocal microscopy images were obtained as previously described [17]. Briefly, multichambered cover glass wells (Nunc, Naperville, CT) were seeded with GMC cells. Cells were serum starved with 0.5% FBS-NG medium 24 h before 2 h glucose treatment. Cells were rinsed three times with PBS that contained calcium and magnesium and fixed in 3.7% paraformaldehyde in PBS for 10 min, followed by permeabilization with 0.025% NP-40 in PBS for 15 min. Cells were incubated with primary antibody (1:250 anti-PHB in PBS/0.025% NP-40) at 20°C, rinsed five times with PBS/0.025% NP-40, and incubated with the Alexa Fluor 488 conjugated secondary antibody (1:1000) at 20°C. The cells were rinsed five times with PBS/0.025% NP-40, incubated with 300 nM DAPI for 5 min, and rinsed three times with PBS. Images were acquired using a Zeiss confocal microscope and analyzed using LSM510 software. Z scan analysis was performed by scanning at 1 µm intervals and three-dimensional reconstruction of the fluorescence images. The images for PHB and for DAPI were merged in a single image to elucidate PHB cellular distribution. Fluorescence intensity measurements (mean fluorescence intensity per $µm^2$) were computed per cell (n = 4-5 cells per treatment replicate per treatment condition) and used to estimate differences in PHB nuclear and cytoplasmic distribution.

2.6. Protein Immunoblotting (IB).

1DE and 2DE protein immunoblots (IB) were conducted as previously described [14]. Total cell lysate samples were separated by 2DE (n = 3 HG, n = 3 NG*). For 2DE IB analysis, following IEF of mesangial proteins, the plastic backing of the IPG strips was trimmed off. The acidic most point of the strip was aligned in the IPG well of the Bis-Tris mini gels adjacent to the MW standard lane of the minigel. This procedure insured uniform alignment of IPG strips to the MW standards, in order to compare PHB migration pattern between experimental conditions. Following 1DE or 2DE electrophoresis and transfer, membranes were immunoblotted for PHB (Santa Cruz Biotechnologies, Santa Cruz, CA) at a 1:1000 dilution in 5% albumin in Tris-Tween-20 buffered saline (TTBS). PHB spots were imaged on film with luminol images aligned and quantified by densitometry analysis comparing the means of the acidic third and basic third of the PHB charge trains to the total train densitometry. Additional antibodies used for 1DE immunoblots were anti PDI (Stressgen; San Diego, CA) at a concentration of 1:10,000 and PSMA2 (Cell Signaling; Danvers, MA) at a concentration of 1:1000.

2.7. Analysis of Protein Expressional Networks.

Ingenuity Pathways Analysis bioinformatic tool (Ingenuity Systems, Mountain View, CA) uses a curated database (Ingenuity Systems Knowledge Base) of previously published findings on mammalian biology from the public literature to evaluate proteins lists inclusive of expression ratios for protein

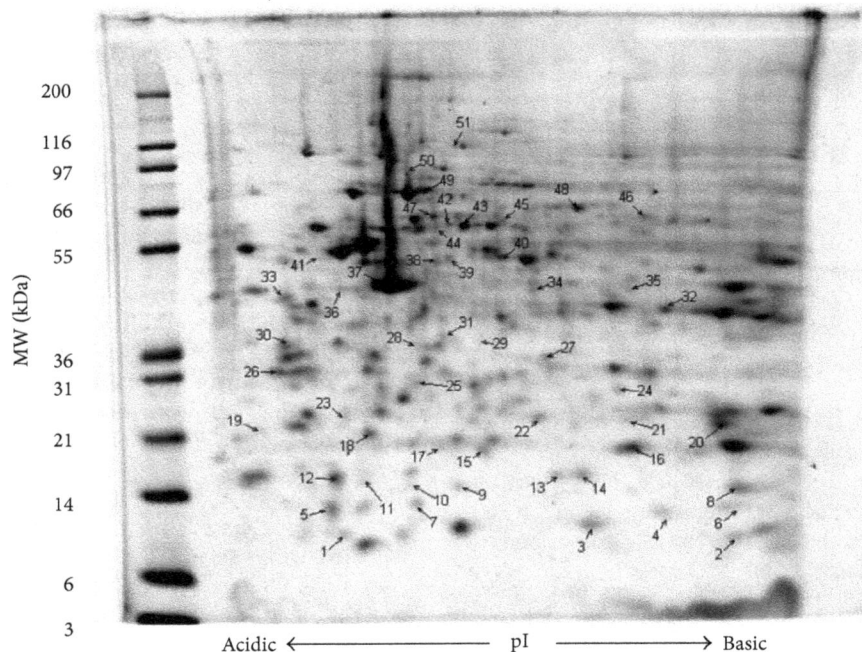

FIGURE 1: Murine GMC proteome altered by acute (2 h) exposure to HG culture conditions. GMC cells were grown to 80% confluence and were serum-starved (0.5% FBS) overnight, and were treated for 2 h with 25 mM glucose (HG) or 5 mM glucose + 20 mM mannitol (NG*) as an isoosmotic control. Cells were lysed using 2DE buffer and 75 μg protein used for 2DE analysis. Proteins whose expression is altered by 2 h HG are annotated on the gel with identifications provided in Table 1. Data are representative of five individual gels for HG and for NG* conditions.

expressional patterns. The purpose of the evaluation is to establish within the lists of provided expressional data relational networks of protein interactions (e.g., direct protein-protein interaction and transcriptional control). Analysis of submitted protein lists with expressional ratios using the Ingenuity knowledge base was used to identify direct interactions between mammalian orthologs.

Murine GMC proteins demonstrating statistically significant expression between 2 h HG and 2 h NG* as well were analyzed by the Ingenuity Knowledge Base and Pathways Analysis tool. The data output identifies nodes characterizing individual proteins and edges characterizing biological relationships. Putative protein networks are rank ordered according to p value ($-\log_{10}{}^{P}$), where the p value is a measure of random association of the listed proteins.

2.8. Statistical Analysis. Statistical analysis of relative spot pixel intensity from 2D gels (n = 5, 2 h each group) and analysis of PHB, PDI, or PSMA2 for HG versus NG* expression by IB was performed using two-tailed, unpaired t-test. p values < 0.05 were considered significant.

3. Results

3.1. Alteration of Protein Expression by Acute High Glucose. Based on the MTT assay results (data not shown), GMC viability did not statistically vary between 2 h HG and NG* treatments. To determine proteins regulated by 2 h HG treatment, protein spot volume lists were curated by

first estimating intergel variability in matched protein spot volumes (averaged CV for 20 matched spots = 0.17). Next, all intraglucose treatment matched gel spot volumes having a CV greater than 0.35 (2 × CV) were discarded. Fifty-one (51) protein spots had a spot volume CV of less than 0.35 and uncorrected t-test values of ≤0.05. Thirty-five protein spots had increased expression and 16 protein spots had decreased expression with 2 h HG treatment and all were analyzed using proteomic methods based on MASCOT MOWSE scoring including MALDI TOF/TOF peptide fragmentation (sequence tagging) data with a significance p value ≤ 0.05 for all the reported protein identities. A representative 2DE gel image (with annotations) and tabulated information for 51 regulated protein spots are provided (Figure 1; Table 1). In general, all proteins identified were observed migrating in the gels at the correct molecular weight plus or minus 10% except for gel spot 5. Cofilin-1 was identified migrating at a molecular weight of approximately 9000 Da and a pI of 5.3. Cofilin-1 nominally has a translated molecular weight of 18,749 Da and a pI of 8.2. Two additional cofilin-1 containing gel spots as well as one HSP10 containing gel spot were observed to focus on isoelectric points less than 0.5 pH units, more acidic than expected. Twenty-three proteins were observed to focus on isoelectric points greater than 0.5 pH units, more basic than expected. The remaining gel spots identified proteins within 0.5 pH units of the expected pI.

3.2. Analysis of Protein Expressional Networks. Bioinformatic analysis of protein expression in 2 h NG* versus 2 h HG

TABLE 1

Spot	Protein name	Gene product	(HG/NG*)	Theoretical M_r	Theoretical pI	Observed M_r	Observed pI	IPA network	Percent coverage
1	Not identified		1.23						
2	10 kDa heat-shock protein, mitochondrial	CH10_RAT	2.37	10895	8.9	8000	8.3	n/a	77
3	Calpactin I light chain	S10AA_RAT	1.37	11182	6.3	8000	7.4	1	45
4	Macrophage migration inhibitory factor	MIF_RAT	1.34	12640	6.8	9000	7.8	3	26
5	Cofilin-1	COF1_RAT	1.5	18749	8.2	9000	5.3	n/a	34
6	Not identified		1.70						
7	Not identified		1.24						
8	Profilin-1	PROF1_RAT	1.34	15119	8.5	15000	8.4	1	45
9	Cystatin B	CYTB_RAT	0.82	11303	5.9	10000	6.5	2	80
10	Not identified		0.66						
11	Coactosin-like protein	COTL1_MOUSE	1.74	16048	5.3	16000	5.5	1, 2	37
12	Galectin-1	LEG1_RAT	1.23	15189	5.1	15000	5.3	3	61
13	Histidine triad nucleotide-binding protein 1	HINT1_MOUSE	1.39	13882	6.4	11000	7.3	3	49
14	40S ribosomal protein S12	RS12_RAT	1.34	14858	6.8	15000	7.2	2	44
15	Nucleoside diphosphate kinase A (NDK A)	NDKA_RAT	1.68	17296	6.0	16000	6.6	3	39
16	Nucleoside diphosphate kinase B	NDKB_RAT	1.26	17386	6.9	18000	7.6	1	66
17	Not identified		1.89						
18	Eukaryotic translation initiation factor 5A	IF5A1_RAT	1.23	17049	5.1	20000	5.6	2	43
	MIR-interacting saposin-like protein	MSAP_MOUSE		21096	5.0	20000	5.6	n/a	29
19	Not identified		1.64						
20	Cofilin-1	COF1_RAT	1.63	18749	8.2	21000	8	1	65
21	Cofilin-1	COF1_RAT	1.59	18749	8.2	21000	7.6	1	60
22	Cofilin-1	COF1_RAT	1.57	18749	8.2	21000	7	1	54
23	Not identified		1.61						
24	Proteasome subunit alpha type 1	PSA2_RAT	1.54	26024	6.9	23000	7.5	1	47
25	Heat-shock protein beta-1	HSPB1_RAT	2.31	22936	6.1	23000	6.1	1	39
	Phosphoserine phosphatase	SERB_RAT		25180	5.5	23000	6.1	n/a	33
26	14-3-3 protein epsilon	1433E_RAT	1.37	29326	4.6	30000	4.8	1	29
27	Proteasome subunit alpha type 2	PSA1_RAT	1.78	29784	6.2	31000	7.2	1	36
28	Prohibitin	PHB_RAT	2.24	29859	5.6	32000	6.1	2	62
29	Not identified		2.33						
30	Proliferating cell nuclear antigen	PCNA_RAT	1.46	29072	4.6	34000	4.9	1	31
31	Heat-shock protein beta-1	HSPB1_MOUSE	0.70	23057	6.1	35000	6.3	n/a	25
32	Annexin A2	ANXA2_RAT	0.83	38939	7.6	40000	7.8	1	56
33	Reticulocalbin 3 precursor	RCN3_HUMAN	1.80	37470	4.7	41000	4.9	2	20
34	Macrophage capping protein	CAPG_RAT	1.53	39060	6.1	41000	6.9	3	20
35	Acetyl-CoA acetyltransferase, cytosolic	THIC_RAT	2.15	41538	6.9	41000	7.7	3	28
36	SUMO-activating enzyme subunit 1	SAE1_RAT	2.15	38945	5.0	41000	5.4	2	54
37	Actin, cytoplasmic-1 (beta-actin)	ACTB_RAT	0.58	42052	5.3	42000	5.7	1	30
	Actin, cytoplasmic-2 (gamma-actin)	ACTG_RAT		42108	5.3	42000	5.7	1	30
38	Not identified		0.6						
39	Actin-like protein 3	ARP3_MOUSE	0.53	47783	5.6	50000	6.5	1	38
40	Enolase 1	ENOA_RAT	0.60	47440	6.2	52000	6.7	1	38
	RAB GDP dissociation inhibitor beta	GDIB_RAT		51018	5.9	52000	6.7	n/a	34
41	Not identified		0.37						
42	Not identified		0.71						
43	Protein disulfide-isomerase A3 (ERp57)	PDIA3_RAT	0.78	57044	5.9	58000	6.4	3	50
44	GRP58	HNRPK_RAT	0.68	51230	5.4	57000	6.3	1	31
45	Not identified		2.21						
46	Heterogeneous nuclear ribonucleoprotein L	HNRPL_MOUSE	1.40	60712	6.7	58000	7.8	2	25
47	T-complex protein 1, epsilon subunit	TCPE_RAT	0.78	59955	5.5	58000	6.3	1	34

TABLE 1: Continued.

| Spot | Protein name | Gene product | (HG/NG*) | Theoretical | | Observed | | IPA network | Percent coverage |
				M_r	pI	M_r	pI		
48	Hsc70/Hsp90-organizing protein	STIP1_RAT	1.16	63158	6.4	65000	7.2	1	38
49	GRP 75	GRP75_RAT	0.82	74097	6.0	75000	6.1	1	31
50	Not identified		1.35						
51	RAB 6 interacting protein 2 (ERC protein 1)	GANAB_MOUSE	0.68	107300	5.7	116000	6.4	2	21

Murine GMC protein expression at 2 h culture HG versus 2 h culture NG*.

was achieved using the Ingenuity Knowledge Base and Pathways Analysis tools. The top three canonical pathways determined to be activated from 2 h acute high glucose exposure were actin-based motility by Rho, RhoA signaling, and the protein ubiquitination pathway. Analysis of protein expressional networks from murine GMC 2 h NG* and 2 h HG protein expressional data suggested three primary expression networks. Network 1 (score 49) addressed cancer, reproductive system disease, and hematological disease and included 25 identified proteins out of 35 total network components (Figure 2(a)). Network 2 (score 19) addressed cell death and survival, drug metabolism, and lipid metabolism and included 9 identified proteins out of 35 protein nodes (Figure 2(b)). Network 3 (score 14) addressed cellular movement, cellular compromise, cellular function, and maintenance and was composed of 7 identified proteins out of 29 possible network proteins. Prominent nodes within Network 1 were centered on signaling proteins including proteins involved with ubiquitination, cyclin D, ERK1/ERK2 MAP-Kinase, HSP90, ROCK, and histones h3 and h4. Prominent nodes in network 2 were centered on the VEGF, TNF, TGFβ1, tumor protein 53 (TP53), and ubiquitination.

3.3. Immunochemical Analysis for the Effect of High Glucose on the Expression of Proteins. Immunoblot (IB) analyses of the selected proteins were used to confirm the 2DE findings. Prohibitin (PHB) was selected for confirmation as it was one of the most strongly regulated protein spots and was also a component of IPA Network 2 with direct interaction with a prominent network node of TNF. The expression by 1DE (Figures 3(a) and 3(b)) supported a trend in increased total PHB abundance, but 2DE IB analysis of 2 h GMC cells cultured in HG and NG* showed a HG responsive and statistically significant ($p < 0.02$) increase in the acidic end of the PHB charge train (Figure 4). Confocal microscopy (Figures 5(a) and 5(b)) suggested that high glucose resulted in a statistically significant (p value < 0.0001) increased fractional abundance of PHB in the nucleus of the GMC.

Based on bioinformatics analysis defining regulation of protein ubiquitination pathways in one of the top three canonical pathways regulated, as well as a prominent node in protein expression Networks 1 and 2, we next analyzed the expression of proteins involved in protein homeostasis and found them to be regulated by 2DE analysis. Proteasome subunit alpha-type 2 (PSMA2) was confirmed to be increased in mesangial cells exposed to high glucose concentrations for 2 h (Figure 6). Comparative 2DE analysis also defined decreased expression of ER chaperone proteins such as PDI

and GRP58, which may lead to increased unfolded protein load in mesangial cells and induction of proteasomal degradation processes. Immunoblot analysis of mesangial proteins for PDI confirmed 2DE findings of decreased expression of PDI (Figure 6).

4. Discussion

GMCs participate in glomerular growth and differentiation as well as in regulation of glomerular blood flow [3, 4]. It is well established that chronic hyperglycemia such as in an uncontrolled diabetic state detrimentally affects the renal glomerulus and produces a pathologic GMC phenotype [18–22]. On the other hand, a gap in knowledge exists for changes in GMC function and protein expression patterns which occur in individuals who experience longer postprandial elevated plasma glucose levels [23]. Therefore to ascertain the effects of short term high glucose conditions encountered by GMC in subpathologic/prediabetic states, we conducted proteomic studies comparing mesangial protein expression after 2 h HG conditions against mesangial protein expression after 2 h NG* growth conditions. The analysis of cell viability at 2 h in the treatment conditions determined that mesangial cell viability was not decreased by the treatment conditions and time. The protein expression differences observed between the growth conditions were not therefore attributed to variable degrees of cell proliferation. Expressional regulation of 51 identified protein spots were observed under the conditions of 2 h HG. These proteins can be grouped as follows: cytoskeletal proteins, calcium/phospholipid binding proteins, chaperones, and proliferation and signaling-related proteins.

Increased glucose levels are known to stimulate a variety of responses within GMC including remodeling of cytoskeletal elements like actin and actin binding proteins [24]. Two upregulated spots were identified as cofilin-1 and cofilin-2 and demonstrated a 55–60% increased expression. Cofilins are actin binding proteins that affect the mobility of actin monomers at the ends of actively growing actin filaments and increase actin filament turnover. Cofilins bind and sever the pointed actin ends and increase the actin monomer pool. During conditions of stress, cofilins participate in the nuclear import of actin [24]. Two protein spots demonstrating reduced expression by HG, identified as the actin capping proteins, F-actin capping protein β-subunit, and actin-like protein 3. Each of these proteins migrated at the expected M_r and pI. These proteins, respectively, demonstrated a 30% and 50% decreased presence in the 2DE gels.

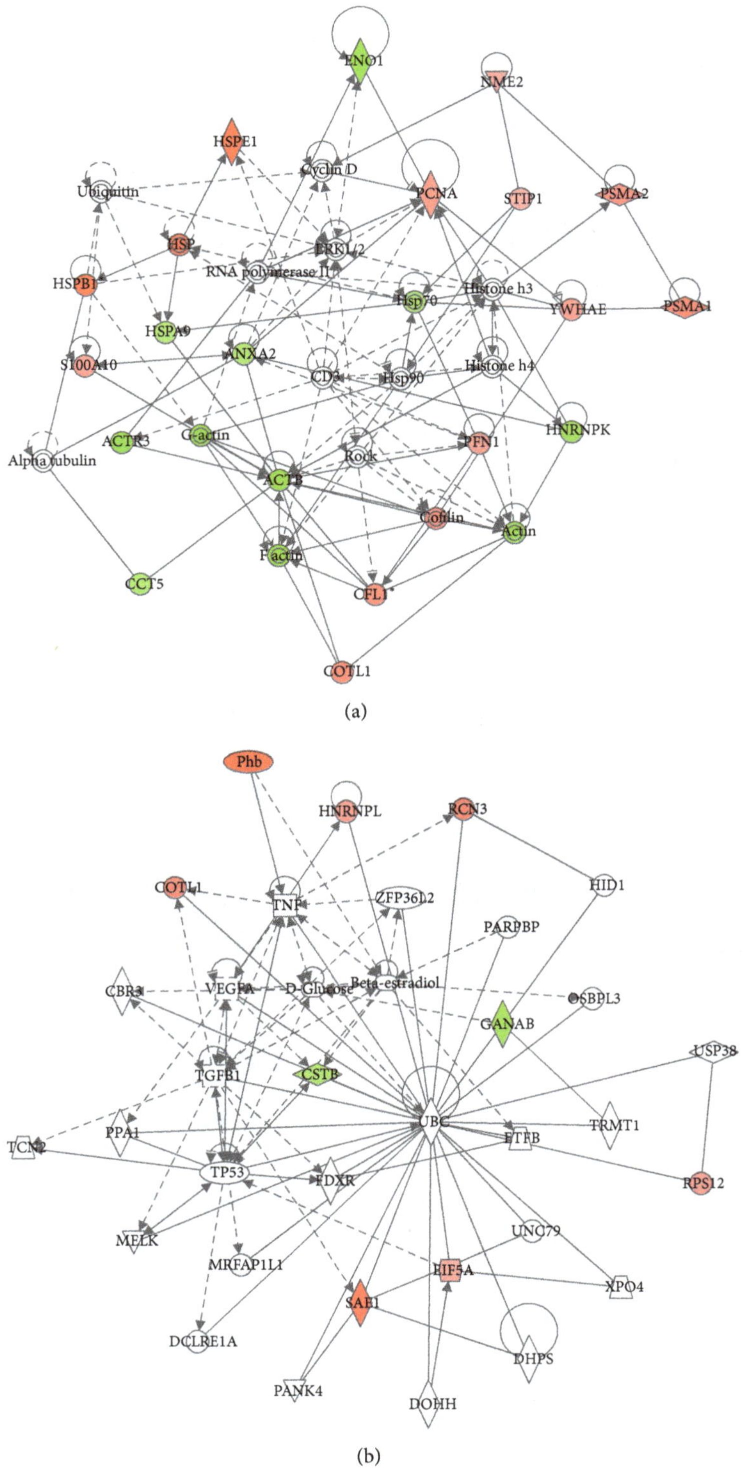

(a)

(b)

FIGURE 2: Network analysis of protein expression patterns using Ingenuity Pathways Analysis. (a) The top scoring network (Network 1) addressed cancer, reproductive system disease, and hematological disease and included 25 identified proteins out of 35 total network components. The score 49 suggests the odds of 1 out of 10^{49} for assembling randomly these protein identifications out of the existing murine protein database. (b) Network 2, defined by IPA, includes PHB. For (a) and (b), red indicates protein spots whose spot volume increased with 2 h high glucose. Green indicates proteins spots whose spot volume decreased with 2 h high glucose.

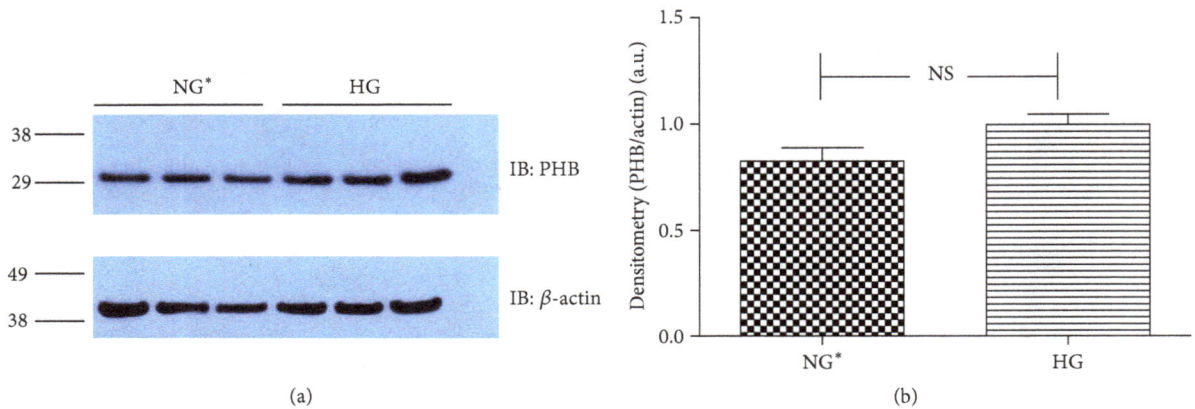

(a)   (b)

FIGURE 3: Validation of 2DE results for the enhanced PHB expression. Murine GMCs were cultured and treated for 2 h with HG and NG* as described. Cells were lysed in 2DE buffer, diluted into Laemmli buffer, and used for immunoblot experiments (a) and quantification of 1DE IB experiments for PHB expression normalized to total actin expression (b). Data is presented as a mean of three experiments. Statistical analysis of differences between the means of HG and NG* was achieved by t-test.

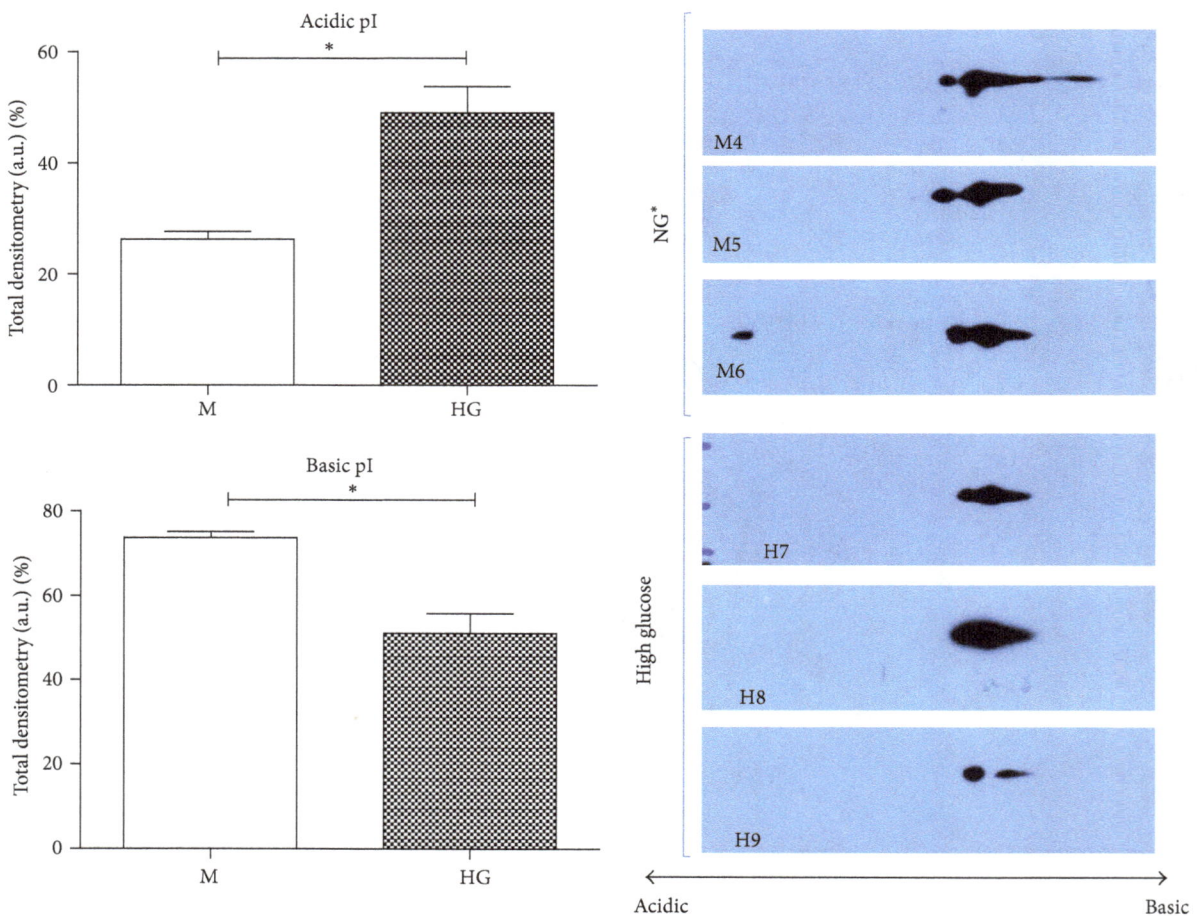

FIGURE 4: 2DE immunoblot experiments were used to determine the effects of HG and NG* on PHB isoforms. Following the transfer and development of PHB IB, images were aligned and densitometric measurements were estimated using ImageJ for the acidic one-third of the PHB charge train and for the basic two-thirds of the PHB charge train (IB images on right). Fractional values for PHB charge train components (acid and basic ends) were used to determine statistical significance differences (left bar graphs). M is the same as NG* (5 mM D-glucose + mannitol); HG is 25 mM D-glucose. *p value < 0.01.

(a)

(b)

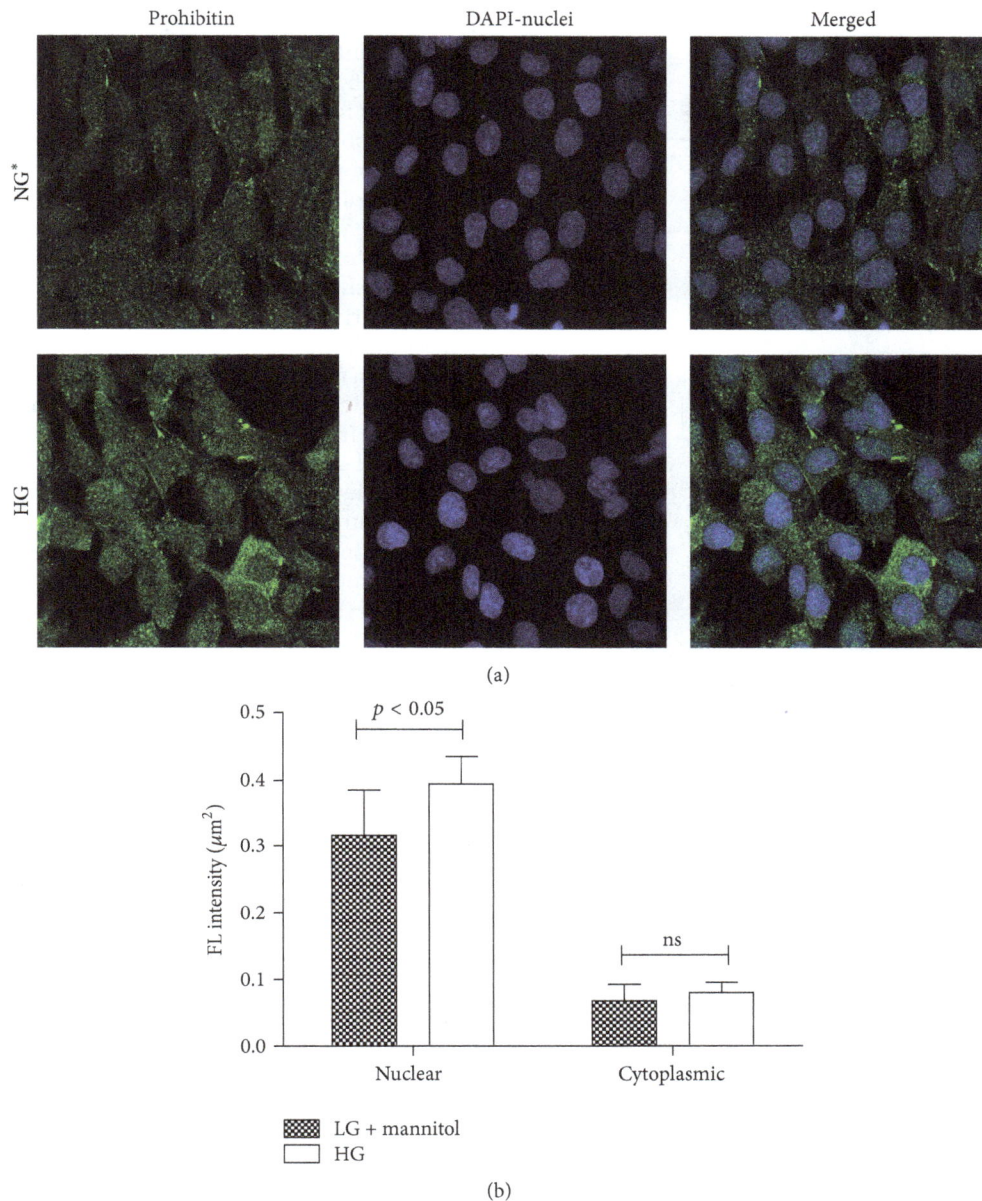

FIGURE 5: (a) Murine GMCs were seeded into 8-well chambered cover glass, grown, and treated as described in the methods. PHB detection was with the same primary antibody as used for IB. PHB detection with an Alexa Fluor 488 conjugated secondary antibody (green). Nuclei were stained with DAPI (blue). Confocal software was used to estimate pixel density in GMC and in nuclei (as defined by DAPI). Nuclei pixel density was subtracted from total density and plotted (b). Differences were estimated by t-test with significance at p value < 0.05.

Additionally, an acidic isoform of the intermediate filament protein vimentin was downregulated.

Calpactin light chain (also referred to as S100A10 or p11) functions as a ligand of annexin II (annexin $II_2 : p11_2$) [25–27]. Calpactin and annexin II were shown here to be upregulated by approximately 37% and 23%, respectively by acute hyperglycemic conditions. Calpactin complexed to annexin II is known to interact with the C-terminus of cytosolic phospholipase A2 and inhibits cPLA2 activity thus reducing inflammatory responses from the release of arachidonic acid [28]. Upregulation of reticulocalbindin 3 is necessary for increased sequestration of Ca^{2+}. The increased Ca^{2+} is in turn needed by other proteins found in the reticuloplasm like GRP78 or PDIA3 [29]. These observations of regulated changes in actin cytoskeletal protein and calcium binding protein expression, when taken together, are consistent with the known responses of mesangial cells to HG under more chronic conditions [30, 31].

Molecular chaperones have been well described in the literature as protein quality control managers that assist with the maintenance of cellular function in the face of stress conditions like heat stress, osmotic stress, or oxidant

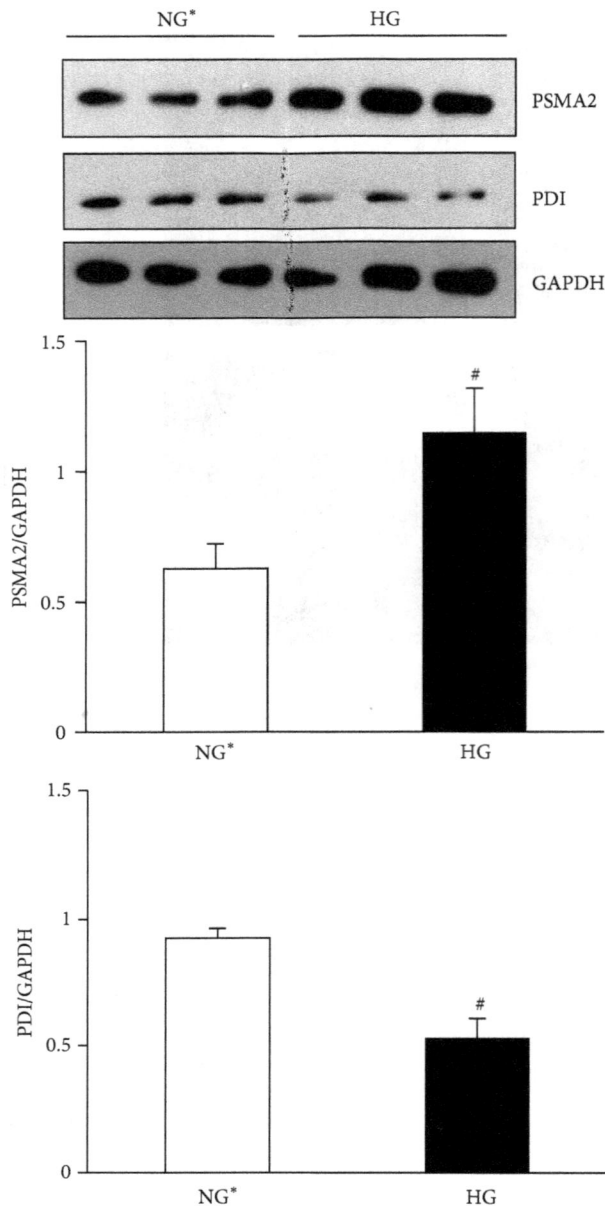

FIGURE 6: Correlative validation of 2DE results for the regulation of pathways involved in proteostasis. Immunoblot analysis of PSMA2 and PDI from mesangial cells cultured for 2 h in HG or NG* medium. Expression of PSMA2 increased whereas PDI decreased following 2 h HG. Bar graphs, densitometric quantitation of PSMA2 or PDI normalized to GAPDH for each lane. Data are average ± SEM #$p < 0.05$ versus NG*.

stress. Specific chaperones are spatially organized throughout the cell via organellar localization [32, 33]. The bulk of all mitochondrial proteins are synthesized under the direction of cell nuclear transcripts in the cytoplasm [34]. High molecular weight proteins are trafficked through and between the mitochondrial membranes and into mitochondrial matrix and require protein folding chaperone such as PHB and HSP10 for efficient protein folding [35]. A protein spot containing

PHB, possibly a posttranslationally modified form causing an acidic shift in PHB pI, was found to exhibit expressional regulation by 2DE, 2DE IB and increased nuclear localization by confocal microscopy analysis, following acute (2 h) glucose exposure in GMCs. PHB has been reported to exist as a membrane resident chaperone that participates in the protein folding pathway of mitochondrial-derived integral membrane proteins like COX2p and COX3p. Moreover, movement of PHB between the mitochondria and nucleus has been shown to play an important role in signaling mitochondrial oxidant stress and regulating apoptosis and transcription during stress, highlighting the importance of this protein to mitochondrial-nuclear communication [36, 37]. In the current study, observations of increased acidic forms of PHB, increased PHB nuclear localization, increased HSP10, and decreased GRP75 at 2 h HG stimulation suggest that acute hyperglycemic conditions may promote protein-structural stress within the mitochondrial matrix promoting translocation of PHB to the nucleus for an as-of-yet determined reason in GMCs. In addition, bioinformatic analysis grouped PHB and additional proteins regulated by 2 h HG in a network including mediators known to be involved in the pathogenesis of diabetic nephropathy and fibrosis, such as TGFβ, VEGF, and TNF [1, 38], highlighting a potentially novel role for PHB in GMC responses to HG.

One aspect of cell cycle control is polyubiquitination of cytoplasmic or nuclear proteins [39]. Polyubiquitination is a trigger for the trafficking of the modified protein to the proteasome for degradation. A second aspect of cell cycle control is exercised through monoubiquitination of nuclear proteins like histones [40–42]. Our observations with increased expression of PSMA2 are specific to acute exposure of cells to medium containing high glucose as compared to isoosmotic low glucose medium and suggest the likelihood of increased proteasomal activity. These findings are in part supported by the observations of decreased ubiquitinated cytosolic proteins in mesangial cells with 2 h high glucose concentrations (data not shown). Together, increased expression of PSMA2 and decreased expression of PDI with acute exposure to high glucose concentrations suggest regulation of pathways involved in proteostasis and/or cell stress response. In the ER, PDI serves an oxidoreductase chaperone regulating disulfide bonds [43] and its activity is decreased in liver cells of diabetic mice [44]. Furthermore, kidneys and liver of diabetic mice also have decreased expression of PDI [45, 46] Decreased expression of PDI in response to high glucose may alter protein maturation in the ER, triggering a stress response which includes increased protein degradation by the proteasome. The mechanism of decreased PDI expression in mesangial cells by acute exposure to high glucose remains to be defined.

In conclusion, the proteomics data and bioinformatic data analysis suggests that murine GMCs respond to acute HG via expression of proteins related by pathways regulating protein posttranslational modification and protein stability. These acute differences may also be important for cellular function as reported for GMCs treated with longer more chronic hyperglycemic time points of differences in specific protein abundance such as enolase, actin, and annexin proteins [30].

Conflict of Interests

The authors have no conflict of interests to disclose.

Acknowledgment

The authors would like to acknowledge the support of the funding from the National Institutes of Health K01-DK080951 to Michelle T. Barati.

References

[1] S. Chen, M. P. Cohen, G. T. Lautenslager, C. W. Shearman, and F. N. Ziyadeh, "Glycated albumin stimulates TGF-beta 1 production and protein kinase C activity in glomerular endothelial cells," *Kidney International*, vol. 59, no. 2, pp. 673–681, 2001.

[2] D. W. Powell, R. C. Mifflin, J. D. Valentich, S. E. Crowe, J. I. Saada, and A. B. West, "Myofibroblasts. I. Paracrine cells important in health and disease," *American Journal of Physiology—Cell Physiology*, vol. 277, no. 1, pp. C1–C9, 1999.

[3] J. E. B. Reusch, "Diabetes, microvascular complications, and cardiovascular complications: what is it about glucose?" *Journal of Clinical Investigation*, vol. 112, no. 7, pp. 986–988, 2003.

[4] J. D. Stockand and S. C. Sansom, "Glomerular mesangial cells: electrophysiology and regulation of contraction," *Physiological Reviews*, vol. 78, no. 3, pp. 723–744, 1998.

[5] S. L. Carney, N. L. M. Wong, and J. H. Dirks, "Acute effects of streptozotocin diabetes on rat renal function," *Journal of Laboratory and Clinical Medicine*, vol. 93, no. 6, pp. 950–961, 1979.

[6] J. S. Christiansen, J. Gammelgaard, M. Frandsen, and H.-H. Parving, "Increased kidney size, glomerular filtration rate and renal plasma flow in short-term insulin-dependent diabetics," *Diabetologia*, vol. 20, no. 4, pp. 451–456, 1981.

[7] T. H. Hostetter, H. G. Rennke, and B. M. Brenner, "The case for intrarenal hypertension in the initiation and progression of diabetic and other glomerulopathies," *The American Journal of Medicine*, vol. 72, no. 3, pp. 375–380, 1982.

[8] S. Stackhouse, P. L. Miller, S. K. Park, and T. W. Meyer, "Reversal of glomerular hyperfiltration and renal hypertrophy by blood glucose normalization in diabetic rats," *Diabetes*, vol. 39, no. 8, pp. 989–995, 1990.

[9] G. Stalder and R. Schmid, "Severe functional disorders of glomerular capillaries and renal hemodynamics in treated diabetes mellitus during childhood," *Annales Paediatrici*, vol. 193, pp. 129–138, 1959.

[10] R. Zatz, T. W. Meyer, H. G. Rennke, and B. M. Brenner, "Predominance of hemodynamic rather than metabolic factors in the pathogenesis of diabetic glomerulopathy," *Proceedings of the National Academy of Sciences of the United States of America*, vol. 82, no. 17, pp. 5963–5967, 1985.

[11] M. Brownlee, "Biochemistry and molecular cell biology of diabetic complications," *Nature*, vol. 414, no. 6865, pp. 813–820, 2001.

[12] M. Brownlee, "The pathobiology of diabetic complications: a unifying mechanism," *Diabetes*, vol. 54, no. 6, pp. 1615–1625, 2005.

[13] F. P. Schena and L. Gesualdo, "Pathogenetic mechanisms of diabetic nephropathy," *Journal of the American Society of Nephrology*, vol. 16, supplement 1, pp. S30–S33, 2005.

[14] M. T. Barati, M. L. Merchant, A. B. Kain, A. W. Jevans, K. R. McLeish, and J. B. Klein, "Proteomic analysis defines altered cellular redox pathways and advanced glycation end-product metabolism in glomeruli of db/db diabetic mice," *American Journal of Physiology—Renal Physiology*, vol. 293, no. 4, pp. F1157–F1165, 2007.

[15] T. Mosmann, "Rapid colorimetric assay for cellular growth and survival: application to proliferation and cytotoxicity assays," *Journal of Immunological Methods*, vol. 65, no. 1-2, pp. 55–63, 1983.

[16] C. Smith, M. Merchant, A. Fekete et al., "Splice variants of neuronal nitric oxide synthase are present in the rat kidney," *Nephrology Dialysis Transplantation*, vol. 24, no. 5, pp. 1422–1428, 2009.

[17] M. L. Merchant, B. A. Perkins, G. M. Boratyn et al., "Urinary peptidome may predict renal function decline in type 1 diabetes and microalbuminuria," *Journal of the American Society of Nephrology*, vol. 20, no. 9, pp. 2065–2074, 2009.

[18] M. E. Cooper, "Interaction of metabolic and haemodynamic factors in mediating experimental diabetic nephropathy," *Diabetologia*, vol. 44, no. 11, pp. 1957–1972, 2001.

[19] R. M. Mason and N. A. Wahab, "Extracellular matrix metabolism in diabetic nephropathy," *Journal of the American Society of Nephrology*, vol. 14, no. 5, pp. 1358–1373, 2003.

[20] T. Nishikawa, D. Edelstein, and M. Brownlee, "The missing link: a single unifying mechanism for diabetic complications," *Kidney International, Supplement*, vol. 58, pp. S26–S30, 2000.

[21] N. A. Wahab, K. Harper, and R. M. Mason, "Expression of extracellular matrix molecules in human mesangial cells in response to prolonged hyperglycaemia," *Biochemical Journal*, vol. 316, no. 3, pp. 985–992, 1996.

[22] G. Wolf, "New insights into the pathophysiology of diabetic nephropathy: from haemodynamics to molecular pathology," *European Journal of Clinical Investigation*, vol. 34, no. 12, pp. 785–796, 2004.

[23] J. Fan, S. J. May, Y. Zhou, and E. Barrett-Connor, "Bimodality of 2-h plasma glucose distributions in whites: the Rancho Bernardo study," *Diabetes Care*, vol. 28, no. 6, pp. 1451–1456, 2005.

[24] M. R. Clarkson, M. Murphy, S. Gupta et al., "High glucose-altered gene expression in mesangial cells. Actin-regulatory protein gene expression is triggered by oxidative stress and cytoskeletal disassembly," *The Journal of Biological Chemistry*, vol. 277, pp. 9707–9712, 2002.

[25] R. Bianchi, G. Pula, P. Ceccarelli, I. Giambanco, and R. Donato, "S-100 protein binds to annexin II and p11, the heavy and light chains of calpactin I," *Biochimica et Biophysica Acta (BBA)— Protein Structure and Molecular Enzymology*, vol. 1160, no. 1, pp. 67–75, 1992.

[26] Y. Miura, M. Kano, K. Abe, S. Urano, S. Suzuki, and T. Toda, "Age-dependent variations of cell response to oxidative stress: proteomic approach to protein expression and phosphorylation," *Electrophoresis*, vol. 26, no. 14, pp. 2786–2796, 2005.

[27] S. Réty, J. Sopkova, M. Renouard et al., "The crystal structure of a complex of p11 with the annexin II N-terminal peptide," *Nature Structural Biology*, vol. 6, no. 1, pp. 89–95, 1999.

[28] L. Parente and E. Solito, "Annexin 1: more than an anti-phospholipase protein," *Inflammation Research*, vol. 53, no. 4, pp. 125–132, 2004.

[29] D. Burdakov, O. H. Petersen, and A. Verkhratsky, "Intraluminal calcium as a primary regulator of endoplasmic reticulum function," *Cell Calcium*, vol. 38, no. 3-4, pp. 303–310, 2005.

[30] S. P. Ramachandra Rao, R. Wassel, M. A. Shaw, and K. Sharma, "Profiling of human mesangial cell subproteomes reveals a role for calmodulin in glucose uptake," *American Journal of Physiology—Renal Physiology*, vol. 292, no. 4, pp. F1182–F1189, 2007.

[31] C. Whiteside, S. Munk, E. Ispanovic et al., "Regulation of mesangial cell alpha-smooth muscle actin expression in 3-dimensional matrix by high glucose and growth factors," *Nephron Experimental Nephrology*, vol. 109, no. 2, pp. e46–e56, 2008.

[32] F.-X. Beck, R. Grünbein, K. Lugmayr, and W. Neuhofer, "Heat shock proteins and the cellular response to osmotic stress," *Cellular Physiology and Biochemistry*, vol. 10, no. 5-6, pp. 303–306, 2000.

[33] F.-X. Beck, W. Neuhofer, and E. Müller, "Molecular chaperones in the kidney: distribution, putative roles, and regulation," *The American Journal of Physiology—Renal Physiology*, vol. 279, no. 2, pp. F203–F215, 2000.

[34] J. M. Herrmann and K. Hell, "Chopped, trapped or tacked—protein translocation into the IMS of mitochondria," *Trends in Biochemical Sciences*, vol. 30, no. 4, pp. 205–212, 2005.

[35] L. G. J. Nijtmans, L. De Jong, M. A. Sanz et al., "Prohibitins act as a membrane-bound chaperone for the stabilization of mitochondrial proteins," *The EMBO Journal*, vol. 19, no. 11, pp. 2444–2451, 2000.

[36] A. S. Kathiria, M. A. Butcher, J. M. Hansen, and A. L. Theiss, "Nrf2 is not required for epithelial prohibitin-dependent attenuation of experimental colitis," *American Journal of Physiology—Gastrointestinal and Liver Physiology*, vol. 304, no. 10, pp. G885–G896, 2013.

[37] S. R. Sripathi, W. He, C. L. Atkinson et al., "Mitochondrial-nuclear communication by prohibitin shuttling under oxidative stress," *Biochemistry*, vol. 50, no. 39, pp. 8342–8351, 2011.

[38] Y.-J. Liang, J.-H. Jian, Y.-C. Liu et al., "Advanced glycation end products-induced apoptosis attenuated by PPARdelta activation and epigallocatechin gallate through NF-kappaB pathway in human embryonic kidney cells and human mesangial cells," *Diabetes/Metabolism Research and Reviews*, vol. 26, no. 5, pp. 406–416, 2010.

[39] O. Kerscher, R. Felberbaum, and M. Hochstrasser, "Modification of proteins by ubiquitin and ubiquitin-like proteins," *Annual Review of Cell and Developmental Biology*, vol. 22, pp. 159–180, 2006.

[40] C.-F. Kao, C. Hillyer, T. Tsukuda, K. Henry, S. Berger, and M. A. Osley, "Rad6 plays a role in transcriptional activation through ubiquitylation of histone H2B," *Genes & Development*, vol. 18, no. 2, pp. 184–195, 2004.

[41] J. C. Tanny, H. Erdjument-Bromage, P. Tempst, and C. D. Allis, "Ubiquitylation of histone H2B controls RNA polymerase II transcription elongation independently of histone H3 methylation," *Genes & Development*, vol. 21, no. 7, pp. 835–847, 2007.

[42] P. Zhu, W. Zhou, J. Wang et al., "A histone H2A deubiquitinase complex coordinating histone acetylation and H1 dissociation in transcriptional regulation," *Molecular Cell*, vol. 27, no. 4, pp. 609–621, 2007.

[43] F. R. M. Laurindo, L. A. Pescatore, and D. de Castro Fernandes, "Protein disulfide isomerase in redox cell signaling and homeostasis," *Free Radical Biology and Medicine*, vol. 52, no. 9, pp. 1954–1969, 2012.

[44] G. Nardai, K. Stadler, E. Papp, T. Korcsmáros, J. Jakus, and P. Csermely, "Diabetic changes in the redox status of the microsomal protein folding machinery," *Biochemical and Biophysical Research Communications*, vol. 334, no. 3, pp. 787–795, 2005.

[45] M. T. Barati, D. W. Powell, B. D. Kechavarzi et al., "Differential expression of endoplasmic reticulum stress-response proteins in different renal tubule subtypes of OVE26 diabetic mice," *Cell Stress and Chaperones*, 2015.

[46] N. Yamagishi, T. Ueda, A. Mori, Y. Saito, and T. Hatayama, "Decreased expression of endoplasmic reticulum chaperone GRP78 in liver of diabetic mice," *Biochemical and Biophysical Research Communications*, vol. 417, no. 1, pp. 364–370, 2012.

22

Effectiveness of a Peer Support Programme versus Usual Care in Disease Management of Diabetes Mellitus Type 2 regarding Improvement of Metabolic Control: A Cluster-Randomised Controlled Trial

Tim Johansson,[1] Sophie Keller,[1] Henrike Winkler,[2] Thomas Ostermann,[3] Raimund Weitgasser,[4,5] and Andreas C. Sönnichsen[6]

[1] *Institute of General Practice, Family Medicine, and Preventive Medicine, Paracelsus Medical University, 5020 Salzburg, Austria*
[2] *Paris Lodron University, 5020 Salzburg, Austria*
[3] *Centre for Integrative Medicine, University of Witten/Herdecke, 58448 Witten, Germany*
[4] *Department of Internal Medicine, Wehrle-Diakonissen Hospital, 5026 Salzburg, Austria*
[5] *Paracelsus Medical University, 5020 Salzburg, Austria*
[6] *Institute of General Practice and Family Medicine, University of Witten/Herdecke, 58448 Witten, Germany*

Correspondence should be addressed to Raimund Weitgasser; raimund.weitgasser@pkwd.at

Academic Editor: Rodica Pop-Busui

Aim. Testing the effectiveness of peer support additionally to a disease management programme (DMP) for type 2 diabetes patients. *Methods.* Unblinded cluster-randomised controlled trial (RCT) involving 49 general practices, province of Salzburg, Austria. All patients enrolled in the DMP were eligible, $n = 337$ participated (intervention: 148 in 19 clusters; control: 189 in 20 clusters). The peer support intervention ran over 24 months and consisted of peer supporter recruitment and training, and group meetings weekly for physical exercise and monthly for discussion of diabetes related topics. *Results.* At two-year follow-up, adjusted analysis revealed a nonsignificant difference in HbA_{1c} change of 0.14% (21.97 mmol/mol) in favour of the intervention (95% CI −0.08 to 0.36%, $p = 0.22$). Baseline values were 7.02 ± 1.25% in the intervention and 7.08 ± 1.25 in the control group. None of the secondary outcome measures showed significant differences except for improved quality of life (EQ-5D-VAS) in controls (4.3 points on a scale of 100; 95% CI 0.08 to 8.53, $p = 0.046$) compared to the intervention group. *Conclusion.* Our peer support intervention as an additional DMP component showed no significant effect on HbA_{1c} and secondary outcome measures. Further RTCs with a longer follow-up are needed to reveal whether peer support will have clinically relevant effects. *Trial Registration.* This trial has been registered with Current Controlled Trials Ltd. (ISRCTN10291077).

1. Introduction

The prevalence of type 2 diabetes is estimated to be 6% (42.08 mmol/mol) for the adult population of Austria [1], thus posing a relevant threat to population health. Guideline adherent, structured treatment and management of the disease as proposed by disease management programmes (DMPs) are seen as the best strategy in the prevention of diabetic complications, but evidence from RCTs and systematic reviews on DMPs reveal only modest effects on patient

care [2, 3], especially regarding the frequency of clinically relevant endpoints [4]. The Austrian DMP "Therapie Aktiv," implemented by statutory health insurance in 2007, had no significant effects on metabolic control in a cluster-randomised trial [5] and an open follow-up study [6].

While DMPs have been shown to improve process quality of care [5], they insufficiently address lifestyle changes like physical activity. A logical next step in the improvement of DMPs is therefore the design and implementation of additional components addressing these deficits. Most promising components are interventions to increase physical activity, to decrease caloric intake, and to improve patient education. A Cochrane review on exercise in patients with type 2 diabetes showed that physical activity significantly reduced HbA_{1c} by 0.62% (−16.72 mmol/mol) [7]. Reduced caloric intake and increased physical activity led to weight loss and to a significant improvement of metabolic control and risk factor profile in the Look-AHEAD trial [8, 9]. Patient education has been shown to improve metabolic control in several systematic reviews [10–12]. On the other hand, in all the studies cited above, success and improvement have been moderate and were achieved by quite intensive interventions involving professional support which can hardly be implemented on a population-wide level due to economic and structural reasons.

An alternative might be to emphasize self-management and peer-to-peer motivation instead of professionally dominated educational interventions. Thus a combination of traditional disease management with ongoing peer support may be a promising approach in diabetes care that deserves further evaluation. The idea of peer support goes back as far as the late 1980s, when the impact of diabetes education and peer support were first evaluated [13]. A systematic review of controlled intervention studies on the effect of social and peer support in diabetes identified six randomised trials that all showed some beneficial effects [14] but further studies questioned these early positive results. Although some evidence for the effectiveness of ongoing peer support on metabolic control has been presented [15, 16], a systematic review found this evidence to be too limited to support firm recommendations and calls for further well-designed studies [17]. No such studies have been done on the implementation of long-term peer support programmes added to a traditional DMP. We therefore designed the peer support programme "Aktivtreff Diabetes" as an additional component of the Austrian DMP "Therapie Aktiv" for type 2 diabetes and evaluated the effectiveness of the programme in a cluster-randomised controlled trial.

2. Methods

2.1. Design.
We designed our evaluation study as a pragmatic cluster-randomised controlled trial set in general practices in the province of Salzburg in Austria.

2.2. Participants.
We invited all 77 surgeries actively administering the DMP "Therapie Aktiv" in Salzburg to recruit participants for the study. All 1327 patients enrolled in the DMP were eligible to participate. We encouraged general practitioners to continuously recruit patients within a recruitment period of eight months (September 2010–April 2011). In addition, Salzburg public health insurance sent an invitation letter to all patients enrolled in the DMP. All patients willing to participate were included in the study after obtaining written informed consent according to the declaration of Helsinki. Exclusion criteria were the following: type 1 diabetes, dementia or major psychiatric illness, advanced neoplastic disease, or other diseases with drastically reduced life expectancy by physician judgement.

2.3. Intervention.
The intervention was carried out over a period of two years from May 2011 to May 2013 and consisted of four elements which were implemented in addition to the ongoing DMP.

2.3.1. Recruitment of Peer Supporters.
General practitioners suggested two peer supporters per intervention group who were made familiar with the details of the study and invited to the peer supporter training. Peer supporters are nonprofessionals who have type 2 diabetes. The peer supporters' main tasks were the following: organization of group meetings and exercise units as well as log of attendance, facilitation of group discussions on diabetes related topics, support of physically weak group members, and motivation of unmotivated participants. Throughout all responsibilities, peer supporters were encouraged to rather give support than advice. They played a crucial role as contact persons for the participants and for the research team. Peer supporters were reimbursed with 10€ per group meeting.

2.3.2. Peer Supporter Training.
During the first year of intervention peer supporters received six sessions of training (four hours each). We compiled a standardised curriculum for the training in order to assure reproducibility within the trial and for any application afterwards. Professionals trained peer supporters addressing the following topics: the concept of peer support, organisation of group meetings, physical activity, recommendations for the treatment and management of type 2 diabetes, motivation, medical aspects of diabetes, nutrition, experience, and feedback.

2.3.3. Physical Exercise Meetings.
Peer groups consisting of 8–12 participants met once every week for at least one hour of physical outdoor activity such as (Nordic) walking combined with other exercises. The first meetings were facilitated by a physical education trainer to get the groups started and familiarise them with the intervention and exercises. Thereafter, groups met largely autonomously and trainers supported the groups only when needed. The peer groups were regularly provided with instruction sheets (nine in total) showing and explaining exercises for mobilisation, coordination, and strength training.

2.3.4. Peer Group Meetings (Table 1).
Once a month groups held conversational and educational meetings focusing on personal, social, and emotional topics in the context of diabetes. The meetings were moderated alternately by peer supporters and health professionals and offered the opportunity to ask particular questions and expand and consolidate knowledge about diabetes. To assure standardisation and coverage of the most important topics, we developed a curriculum. It guided participants through subject areas that changed every other month and provided matched topics for every single session. Prior to each meeting, all participants received a newsletter addressing the corresponding topic including the latest scientific findings.

Patients in the control groups received standard care according to the DMP "Therapie Aktiv" which enforces care

TABLE 1: Topics for the group meetings and newsletters.

Year	Month	Topic/newsletter	Professional
2011	10–12	Healthy diet: dietary change step by step	Nutritionist
2012	01	Self-motivation and group motivation	—
	02	Lifestyle changes	Psychologist
	03	Daily self-management, medical checks	—
	04	Diabetes: therapy, blood glucose measurement	General practitioner
	05	Sweeteners	—
	06	Weight loss, weight control	Nutritionist
	07	Physical activity in daily routine	—
	08	Physical activity and motivational problems	Sports scientist
	09	Cardiovascular risk management	General practitioner
	10	Prevention of diabetic complications	—
	11	Glycaemic index and glycaemic load	Nutritionist
	12	Prevention of weight gain at Christmas	—
2013	01	Diabetes and depression	Psychologist
	02	Diabetes and alcohol; smoking cessation	—

according to international guidelines regarding monitoring, diagnostics, and treatment of type 2 diabetes.

2.4. Outcomes. The primary outcome measure was the difference in change of HbA_{1c} (%, resp., mmol/mol, determined by HPLC using a Menarini HA-8180 HPLC Analyser) from baseline to 24 months between the intervention and control groups. Prespecified secondary outcome measures comprised quality of life EQ-5D-3L index and EQ-5D visual analogue scale (VAS) [18], improved control of cardiovascular risk factors (systolic and diastolic blood pressure measured in the general practices according to standard WHO criteria using locally available gauged blood pressure monitors, total cholesterol, HDL cholesterol, and triglycerides, determined at local laboratories with automated clinical chemistry analysers, and LDL cholesterol, determined using the Friedewald equation), lowering of global cardiovascular risk (UKPDS-Risk Engine 2.0) [19], change in body weight (body mass index (BMI)), and smoking cessation (self-reported).

All primary and secondary outcomes were measured between October 2010 and April 2011 for baseline and between October 2012 and April 2013 for follow-up.

Baseline and follow-up data were recorded pseudonymised by the general practitioners using the structured documentation sheet of the disease management programme "Therapie Aktiv" and case report forms which were then sent to the study centre. We checked all forms for completeness and plausibility. In case of missing or implausible data, we contacted the responsible general practitioner.

2.5. Sample Size. We calculated sample size for $\alpha = 0.05$ and $\beta = 0.20$, proposing 0.5% (−18.03 mmol/mol) difference between intervention and control groups in change of HbA_{1c} from baseline to final examination at 24 months. Using an estimated standard deviation of 1.2% (−10.38 mmol/mol) for HbA_{1c} change, a sample size of 181 patients (91 per arm) was required. Assuming an intracluster correlation coefficient of 0.05 (derived from our previous study [5]) and an average cluster size of 12 patients per peer group, we estimated a design effect of $D = 1 + (12 - 1) \times 0.05 = 1.55$. Thus, the sample size increased to 280 patients (140 per arm). Allowing for up to 20% loss to follow-up, the sample size was adjusted to 175 patients per arm or a total of 350 patients.

2.6. Randomisation. To assure concealment of allocation, all patients were cluster-randomised by electronic sequence generation using Research Randomizer [20] after completion of recruitment and allocation of patients to prospective peer groups as clusters. Clustering was performed by the study management grouping 8–12 patients living close to each other into a cluster to facilitate face-to-face meetings. If there were a sufficient number of patients in a region, we aimed to group younger patients (<65 years) and older patients (≥65 years) in separate clusters. This resulted in three categories of clusters: category 1: mostly patients <65 years; category 2: mostly patients ≥65 years; category 3: clusters with patients of all ages. Randomisation was stratified by cluster category. When participants signed up and were clustered, neither the study management nor physicians nor patients knew which group would participate in the peer support programme or serve as control, to assure concealment of allocation. Randomisation at the patient level would not have been feasible because the intervention addresses the group.

2.7. Blinding. Due to the nature of the intervention, blinding was not possible.

2.8. Statistical Analysis. All statistical analyses were performed with IBM SPSS Statistics 20.0. We evaluated our primary endpoint in an intention-to-treat analysis according to the CONSORT guidelines for the reporting of cluster-randomised controlled trials [21]. For missing data regarding HbA_{1c} we applied the method of last available data carried forward. For unadjusted, univariate analysis, we used an independent t-test (two-tailed) to detect significant differences between the intervention and the control group. Per-protocol analysis was performed for all secondary outcomes, using independent t-tests to detect differences between groups.

In addition to univariate analysis we used a mixed model approach to account for nesting of patients in peer groups and to adjust for covariates. We calculated intracluster correlation coefficients (ICC) and then adjusted for cluster effects, age, and baseline value.

2.9. Ethics Approval and Trial Registration. The study protocol was presented to the ethics committee of the province of Salzburg and received unconditional ethics approval on February 24, 2010. The study was registered with current controlled trials on November 17, 2010 (ISRCTN10291077).

3. Results

3.1. Participants, Recruitment. Forty-nine (63.6%) of the eligible general practices ($n = 77$) recruited patients for the study. A total of $n = 420$ (29.6%) of all eligible patients ($n = 1327$) initially signed up. Twenty-seven patients did not meet inclusion criteria. Fifty-six patients withdrew consent after randomisation (54 interventions, 2 controls), and 9 patients died (5 interventions, 4 controls), leaving 328 patients for intention-to-treat analysis (intervention group: $n = 143$; control group: $n = 185$). Figure 1 shows the CONSORT flow diagram of the study. For 23 patients (intervention group: $n = 4$; control group: $n = 19$) final HbA_{1c} had to be imputed using the last available data carried forward method due to loss to follow-up.

Recruitment took place from September 2010 to April 2011 and the intervention ran from May 2011 until May 2013. All practices and peer supporters continued to participate during the whole study period.

3.2. Process Evaluation. Peer supporters visited median 5 (0–6) of the six peer supporter training sessions. The median number of physical activity meetings per group was 86 (1–104) with an achievable maximum of 104 times (once per week for two years). The median number of physical activity meetings of individual patients was 23 (0–90). Physical education trainers supported the groups in 11% of all performed physical activity meetings (148 of 1344).

Peer groups met 12 (0–14) times for all educational and conversational meetings (67% of 15 possible meetings), and of these 8 (0–8) were supported by a professional. Individual patients participated in 4 (0–14) of these meetings (34% of all meetings). In total, 178 group meetings were performed by the peer groups, of which 126 (72.4%) were supported by a professional.

3.3. Baseline Data. The baseline characteristics of the participants were balanced between the study groups (Table 2).

3.4. Follow-Up Results. Using univariate analysis (independent t-test) or mixed models adjusting for baseline values and

TABLE 2: Baseline characteristics of participants.

	n (I/C)[a]	Intervention $n = 148$	Control $n = 189$
Age (years, SD)	148/189	62.2 (8.8)	63.6 (10.8)
Female (n, %)	148/189	76 (51.4)	97 (51.3)
Duration of diabetes (years, SD)	145/178	8.4 (7.1)	7.0 (5.6)
Smokers (n, %)	141/183	17 (12.1)	22 (12.0)
Married (n, %)	145/182	99 (68.3)	121 (66.5)
Low level of education[b] (n, %)	143/181	126 (88.1)	164 (90.6)
Retired (n, %)	145/183	95 (65.6)	126 (68.8)
Living alone (n, %)	144/178	30 (20.8)	37 (20.8)

[a]Variation of n due to missing values; I = intervention group, C = control group.
[b]Only grade school, apprenticeship.

cluster effects, we found no significant differences between the intervention group and the control group regarding our primary and most secondary outcomes (Tables 3 and 4). Quality of life decreased in the intervention group and slightly improved in the control group, with a significant difference between groups in favour of the controls (EQ-5D index and EQ-5D VAS, Table 3). Only the difference in EQ-5D-VAS remains significant after adjustment for baseline value and cluster effects (Table 4). There was no significant difference between the intervention and control groups regarding smoking cessation. Four of 124 patients (3.2%) in the intervention group stopped smoking compared to two of 146 (1.4%) patients in the control group ($p = 0.649$).

For safety reasons we calculated the relative risk of the intervention for death or cardiovascular events (per-protocol analysis). No significant differences between the two groups could be seen (Table 5).

4. Discussion

Our study showed that a group based peer support intervention as an additional component to a traditional disease management programme on type 2 diabetes in general practice is feasible. Although peer support appears to be a very promising approach, our intervention did not significantly improve clinical outcomes or risk profile. A slight negative effect could even be seen regarding health related quality of life.

As demonstrated by the UKPDS [22], HbA_{1c} levels gradually worsen over time with a rise of about 0.1% (−22.4 mmol/mol) per year. We therefore postulated an increase of HbA_{1c} of about 0.2% (−21.31 mmol/mol) in the control group and a small decrease of HbA_{1c} in the intervention group, basing our sample size calculation on a net difference of 0.5% (−18.03 mmol/mol) in HbA_{1c} change over the two years of follow-up. Our supposition was only partly fulfilled: While HbA_{1c} rose in controls it did not decrease in the intervention group but was only kept unchanged. We therefore missed

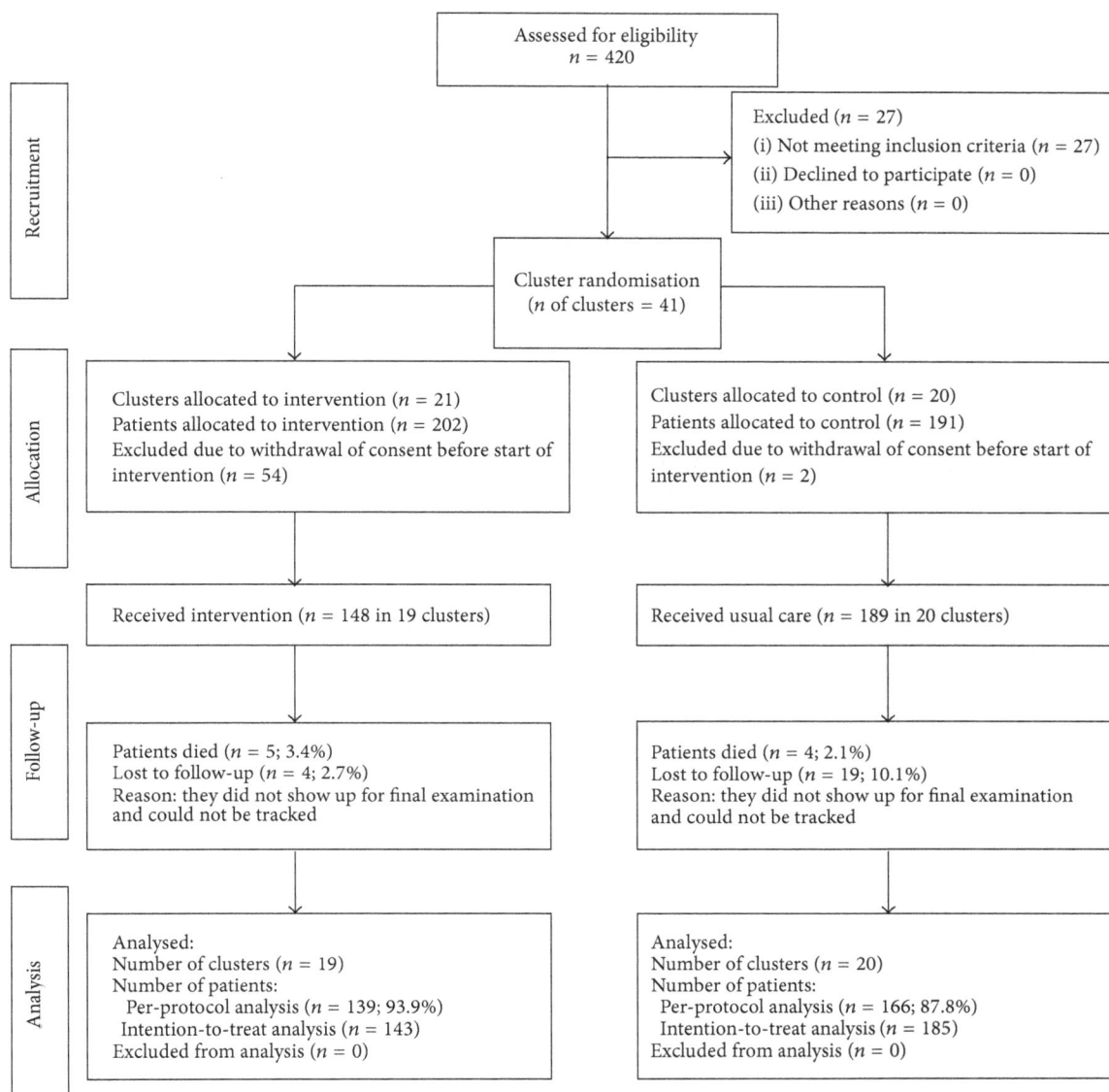

FIGURE 1: CONSORT diagram for recruitment and follow-up of clusters and participants.

to show a significant effect of our peer support intervention on our primary endpoint. A larger sample and a longer follow-up would be needed to show whether the peer support intervention can significantly prevent the rise in HbA_{1c} in the long run.

Our findings may at least partially be due to the well-controlled baseline values, leaving little room for improvement. Although general practitioners had been asked to recruit all patients with type 2 diabetes consecutively, we suspect that recruitment was performed differentially giving priority to well-controlled patients. Also, the intensity of the intervention may have been too low to demonstrate an effect on HbA_{1c}. Increased professional support would have intensified the intervention, but this would have been contradictory to our intention of implementing group based peer support with a main focus on patient self-management.

Due to withdrawal of consent, some groups were smaller than planned with a potentially negative impact on group dynamics.

Although quality of life was a predefined secondary outcome in our study we do not suggest to overestimate the marginally significant negative effect seen in our results. Firstly, a difference of 4 points on a VAS with 100 points does not seem clinically relevant. Secondly, this result could very well be due to chance in multiple testing. On the other hand, a decrease in quality of life as a consequence of our intervention cannot be ruled out and should be carefully considered as a possible detrimental effect of the programme. A reduction in well-being was also described in the study of Smith et al. who evaluated a peer support programme for type 2 diabetes mellitus in Ireland [23]. Smith postulates that peer support could cause peer supporters to focus on negative experiences

TABLE 3: Clinical outcomes at baseline and follow-up by study group.

	N^a	Intervention Mean (SD) baseline	Mean (SD) follow-up	N^a	Control Mean (SD) baseline	Mean (SD) follow-up	Mean difference between groups[b] (95% CI)	p-value[c]
				Primary endpoint				
HbA_{1c} (%)	143	7.02 (1.25)	7.05 (1.10)	185	7.08 (1.25)	7.21 (1.31)	0.10 (−0.14 to 0.35)	0.41
				Secondary endpoints				
				Laboratory results (mg/dL)				
Creatinine	139	0.86 (0.23)	0.90 (0.25)	162	0.96 (0.33)	1.00 (0.64)	0.01 (−0.07 to 0.10)	0.77
Triglycerides	139	150.8 (86.4)	147.9 (81.1)	164	151.7 (94.3)	147.2 (83.7)	−1.5 (−20.2 to 17.2)	0.88
Cholesterol	139	189.5 (40.1)	187.1 (40.3)	164	190.5 (44.8)	184.4 (40.6)	−3.6 (−12.8 to 5.5)	0.43
HDL	139	54.9 (14.4)	57.1 (18.7)	163	54.8 (16.4)	55.0 (15.0)	−2.0 (−4.9 to 0.9)	0.17
LDL	136	106.3 (35.9)	100.3 (37.0)	161	106.7 (38.9)	99.1 (35.7)	−1.1 (−9.3 to 7.1)	0.79
				Anthropometric measurements				
BMI (kg/m^2)	133	31.0 (5.3)	30.7 (5.3)	159	30.3 (4.8)	29.9 (4.9)	−0.1 (−0.6 to 0.3)	0.65
Systolic blood pressure (mmHg)	128	136.0 (15.7)	136.0 (15.7)	154	137.2 (17.9)	136.3 (15.8)	−1.0 (−5.2 to 3.2)	0.65
Diastolic blood pressure (mmHg)	128	80.8 (9.1)	80.4 (8.5)	154	80.4 (10.0)	80.8 (8.6)	0.8 (−1.7 to 3.2)	0.52
				UKPDS-Risk Engine: 10-year risk[f]				
CHD[d]	76	15.0 (9.3)	16.9 (11.0)	85	15.3 (9.9)	17.1 (9.6)	0.0 (−1.9 to 1.9)	0.99
Fatal CHD	76	10.2 (7.5)	12.2 (9.3)	85	10.2 (8.6)	12.1 (8.4)	−0.1 (−1.6 to 1.3)	0.85
Stroke	76	8.9 (7.3)	11.3 (9.4)	85	9.1 (8.4)	11.2 (9.2)	−0.4 (−1.2 to 0.3)	0.27
Fatal stroke	76	1.3 (1.3)	1.8 (1.8)	85	1.4 (1.5)	1.6 (1.4)	−0.2 (−0.5 to −0.0)	0.047
				Quality of life (EQ-5D)				
Index	128	0.90 (0.16)	0.87 (0.20)	149	0.88 (0.19)	0.88 (0.19)	0.04 (−0.0 to 0.1)	0.051
VAS[e]	117	75.1 (17.0)	72.8 (20.0)	130	70.9 (17.4)	73.7 (18.8)	5.2 (0.6 to 9.8)	0.03

[a]Variation of n due to missing values; BL = baseline; FU = follow-up.

[b]Mean difference between groups is calculated by subtracting mean pre-post-difference of the control group from mean pre-post-difference of the intervention group.

[d]Independent t-test, unadjusted.

[4]CHD = coronary heart disease.

[e]VAS = visual analogue scale.

[f]The reduced n is due to the fact that the UKPDS-risk engine can only be applied to patients in primary prevention.

which may have a negative effect on all participants. The increase of physical activity could also lead to discomfort in patients not used to exercising, thus compromising quality of life.

4.1. Comparison with Other Studies. Our results are in line with the majority of peer support trials that could not demonstrate a positive effect on HbA_{1c} [23–27]. Only very few controlled studies could show that peer support has a significant impact on glycaemic control in patients with type 2 diabetes [16, 28, 29]. All of the three positive studies were of short duration (≤6 months) and tested quite specific interventions like counselling via telephone or an online programme. According to the aforementioned systematic review, studies on peer support are in general heterogeneous in terms of setting, intervention, study design, length of follow-up, and outcome measures, and often the quality is low [17]. We could only identify one long-term randomised controlled trial exploring the effect of a peer group based intervention.

This Irish study, like our study, showed disappointing results regarding the effect of peer support on metabolic control and, as mentioned above, also detected a possible negative effect on quality of life [23]. Compared to our trial, the intervention examined in Smith's study was of very low intensity: Study participants had only nine meetings with peer supporters in two years, and peer supporters only had two evening training sessions. We hypothesized that our more intensive peer support intervention would have a more notable effect on HbA_{1c}. However, our results are consistent with the Irish peer support intervention. It remains unclear how to design and implement peer support as a structured intervention to effectively optimise metabolic control.

Some peer support studies for type 2 diabetes have shown benefits for participants using other outcome measures compared to HbA_{1c} such as healthier eating habits [27, 30, 31], health distress [16, 27, 28], blood pressure [32], BMI [30], or depression [31]. For all of these outcomes there exist other studies which did not find any effect [17], and in their

TABLE 4: Differences between groups regarding primary and secondary outcome measures, adjusted for baseline values, age, and ICC.

	n (I/C)	Mean difference between groups[b] (95%-CI)	ICC[a]	p value
Primary endpoint				
HbA_{1c} (%)	143/185	0.14 (−0.08 to 0.36)	−0.05	0.22
Secondary endpoints				
Laboratory results (mg/dL)				
Creatinine (mg/dL)	139/162	0.00 (−0.09 to 0.08)	−0.01	0.92
Triglycerides (mg/dL)	139/164	0.17 (−15.54 to 15.88)	0.00	0.98
Total cholesterol (mg/dL)	139/164	−2.28 (−10.05 to 5.48)	0.05	0.56
HDL cholesterol (mg/dL)	139/163	−1.94 (−4.69 to 0.81)	0.17	0.17
LDL cholesterol (mg/dL)	136/161	−0.37 (−7.48 to 6.74)	0.06	0.91
Anthropometric measurements				
BMI (kg/m^2)	133/159	−0.15 (−0.58 to 0.29)	−0.03	0.51
Systolic blood pressure (mmHg)	128/154	−0.56 (−3.96 to 2.84)	−0.05	0.75
Diastolic blood pressure (mmHg)	128/154	0.51 (−1.39 to 2.41)	−0.02	0.60
UKPDS-Risk Engine: 10-year risk[e]				
CHD[c]	76/85	0.10 (−1.75 to 1.95)	0.03	0.92
Fatal CHD	76/85	−0.09 (−1.53 to 1.36)	0.03	0.91
Stroke	76/85	−0.43 (−1.07 to 0.22)	−0.03	0.20
Fatal stroke	76/85	−0.22 (−0.44 to 0.00)	−0.07	0.053
Quality of life (EQ-5D)				
Index	128/149	0.04 (−0.00 to 0.08)	−0.01	0.08
VAS[d]	117/130	4.30 (0.08 to 8.53)	0.01	0.046

[a]ICC = intracluster correlation coefficient.
[b]Δ adjusted = adjusted mean difference, calculated using mixed models. Mean difference is calculated by subtracting mean pre-post-difference of the control group from mean pre-post-difference of the intervention group. Positive values indicate higher reductions in the intervention group compared to controls. Negative values indicate an increase in the intervention group compared to controls.
[c]CHD = coronary heart disease.
[d]VAS = visual analogue scale.
[e]The reduced n is due to the fact that the UKPDS-risk engine can only be applied to patients in primary prevention.

TABLE 5: Cardiovascular events and mortality.

Event	Intervention $n = 139$	Control $n = 166$	Relative risk	95% CI
Death	5	4	1.49	0.41 to 5.45
Myocardial infarction	2	4	0.60	0.11 to 3.21
Bypass or stenting	8	6	1.59	0.57 to 4.48
Stroke	2	1	2.39	0.22 to 26.06
Any cardiovascular event	9	8	1.34	0.53 to 3.39
Any cardiovascular event or death	13	12	1.29	0.61 to 2.74

systematic review Dale et al. draw the conclusion that no consistent evidence exists that supports a general benefit of peer support interventions [17].

4.2. Strengths and Limitations. This cluster-randomised controlled trial is one of the largest randomised trials on group peer support, and no existing controlled study provided longer follow-up than ours. Our peer support intervention was well designed, and process evaluation assured that the intervention was largely delivered as planned. Loss to follow-up (6.8%) was low, and the amount of missing data was

acceptable for a pragmatic trial. Diabetes care was well structured by the existing DMP in both the intervention and the control group, assuring that any differences in outcome could be attributed to the intervention and not to differences in standard health care delivery. All of these characteristics of our study assure a high degree of internal validity.

Nonetheless there are several sources of possible bias possibly compromising our study results. To avoid selection bias and to assure concealment of allocation, neither physicians nor patients knew at the time of signing up whether they would participate in the peer support programme or serve as controls. A number of patients dropped out after randomisation into the intervention group, presumably willing to participate in the study only as controls. Selection bias may have occurred here.

As mentioned above, differential recruitment of healthy patients by the general practitioners may have led to sampling bias or healthy user bias. There was little room for improvement of metabolic control in our study population which thwarted our power calculation. HbA_{1c} improvement by 0.5% is not a clinically realistic expectation when starting from a baseline HbA_{1c} of 7%. Our peer support intervention might therefore be more effective in patients with poor glycemic control. On the other hand, peer support is probably not suitable for all patients, and intentionally recruiting less well patients may lead to low participation rates in the group sessions, thus also compromising a possible effect.

Preselecting participants by restricting inclusion to patients enrolled in the DMP might be another source of sampling bias. In Salzburg, only about 10% of all patients with type 2 diabetes have been enrolled in the DMP at the beginning of our study. Thus external validity of our study is limited due to various reasons even though internal validity is high.

Attendance rates of the group sessions in our study were good but not excellent. Some patients only attended the discussion meetings and avoided the exercise meetings, thus compromising their chance to improve metabolic control by physical activity. Although patients and peer supporters were instructed and motivated to do additional exercising at home, most patients probably only participated in the physical activity group meetings once a week. This intervention may have been not sufficiently intense to exert an influence on our primary endpoint.

As the intervention made it necessary to preform groups of patients living close to each other, and due to the group based intervention, randomisation on the patient level was not possible. Bias due to cluster effects can be minimized by multilevel modelling but there remains a risk of cluster bias due to undetected confounders.

Our power calculation was based on a 0.5% (−18.03 mmol/mol) difference in HbA_{1c} reduction between intervention and control which was not achieved. Nonetheless HbA_{1c} increased by 0.1% (−22.4 mmol/mol) in controls, and this increase was apparently avoided by the peer support intervention. A much larger sample size and longer follow-up would be needed, though, to make this result significant.

As we know from the ACCORD study, low HbA_{1c} levels are not necessarily related to better outcome [33]. Therefore it might be postulated that HbA_{1c} is not a suitable outcome measurement in studies of type 2 diabetes. We agree to this postulate in intervention studies focused on drugs, but we believe that HbA_{1c} still is an acceptable outcome measure in studies focused on lifestyle changes. We evaluated clinically relevant outcomes like event rates and mortality as safety measures in our study, but follow-up certainly was not long enough to expect any significant effects of the intervention here.

4.3. Conclusions and Policy Implications. A group based peer support intervention as an additional component of a disease management programme on type 2 diabetes is feasible. It enables general practitioners to offer additional support to patients willing to be active and change their lifestyle, it requires minimal effort from the general practitioners, and it can be offered at low cost as the intervention is mainly carried out by the patients themselves. Our intervention tends to maintain HbA_{1c} while it gradually worsens in controls as has been shown in other studies like the UKPDS. Larger randomised controlled trials with a longer follow-up are needed to demonstrate the significance of this finding and to evaluate the effects of peer support on clinically relevant endpoints. To date, evidence is insufficient to give a general recommendation regarding the implementation of peer support programmes, but we believe that the concept provides an additional opportunity for chronically ill patients and therefore deserves further research.

Abbreviations

ACCORD:	Action to Control Cardiovascular Risk in Diabetes
BMI:	Body mass index
CHD:	Coronary heart disease
DMP:	Disease management programme
HbA_{1c}:	Haemoglobin A_{1c}
HDL:	High density lipoprotein
LDL:	Low density lipoprotein
UKPDS:	United Kingdom Prospective Diabetes Study
VAS:	Visual analogue scale.

Conflict of Interests

None of the authors have any additional conflict of interests.

Authors' Contribution

Tim Johansson and Sophie Keller contributed equally in writing the paper and carrying out the study. Andreas C. Sönnichsen designed the study and was principle investigator, supported by Raimund Weitgasser with diabetological expertise. Henrike Winkler and Raimund Weitgasser contributed substantially in designing and carrying out the study. Statistical analysis was performed by Thomas Ostermann, Sophie Keller, and Andreas C. Sönnichsen. All authors reviewed and approved the final paper.

Disclosure

Lilly Diabetes does not have privileged access to applications or to funded projects. Any results, including data and intellectual property rights, from funded projects will become the property of the International Diabetes Federation, which will put them in the public domain to the extent permitted by applicable data protection and privacy laws. Lilly Diabetes has one representative, as an observer with no voting rights, in the Executive Committee of BRIDGES and no representative in the Review Committee. Lilly Diabetes is not informed of the composition of the Review Committee. Lilly Diabetes does not have access to the data of this study and is not involved in the evaluation of these data.

Acknowledgments

The authors would like to thank all participating general practitioners of Salzburg and their teams, the peer support leaders, and patients for making this study possible. They also thank the scientific advisory board of the study, R. A. Gabbay, M.D., Ph.D., T. Tang, Ph.D., and P. Kowatsch, M.D., as well as the BRIDGES team, namely, R. L'Heveder, for their continuous support. This project was supported by a BRIDGES Grant (Bringing Research in Diabetes to Global Environments and Systems) from the International Diabetes Federation (Grant no. LT09-261). BRIDGES, an International Diabetes Federation Project, is supported by an educational grant from Lilly Diabetes.

References

[1] M. Stadler and R. Prager, "Type 2 diabetes mellitus-screening and prevention," *Wiener klinische Wochenschrift*, vol. 124, supplement 2, pp. 4–6, 2012.

[2] J. J. Ofman, E. Badamgarav, J. M. Henning et al., "Does disease management improve clinical and economic outcomes in patients with chronic diseases? A systematic review," *American Journal of Medicine*, vol. 117, no. 3, pp. 182–192, 2004.

[3] C. Pimouguet, M. Le Goff, R. Thiebaut, J. F. Dartigues, and C. Helmer, "Effectiveness of disease management programs for improving diabetes care: a meta-analysis," *Canadian Medical Association Journal*, vol. 183, pp. E115–E127, 2011.

[4] N. D. F. Olivarius, H. Beck-Nielsen, A. H. Andreasen, M. Hørder, and P. A. Pedersen, "Randomised controlled trial of structured personal care of type 2 diabetes mellitus," *British Medical Journal*, vol. 323, no. 7319, pp. 970–975, 2001.

[5] A. C. Sönnichsen, H. Winkler, M. Flamm et al., "The effectiveness of the Austrian disease management programme for type 2 diabetes: a cluster randomised controlled trial," *BMC family practice*, vol. 11, article 86, 2010.

[6] M. Flamm, S. Panisch, H. Winkler, T. Johansson, R. Weitgasser, and A. C. Sönnichsen, "Effectiveness of the Austrian disease management programme 'Therapie Aktiv' for type 2 diabetes regarding the improvement of metabolic control, risk profile and guideline adherence: 2 years of follow up," *Wiener Klinische Wochenschrift*, vol. 124, no. 17-18, pp. 639–646, 2012.

[7] D. E. Thomas, E. J. Elliott, and G. A. Naughton, "Exercise for type 2 diabetes mellitus," *Cochrane Database of Systematic Reviews*, vol. 3, Article ID CD002968, 2006.

[8] A. R. G. Look, X. Pi-Sunyer, G. Blackburn et al., "Reduction in weight and cardiovascular disease risk factors in individuals with type 2 diabetes: one-year results of the look AHEAD trial," *Diabetes Care*, vol. 30, pp. 1374–1383, 2007.

[9] R. R. Wing, J. L. Bahnson, G. A. Bray et al., "Long-term effects of a lifestyle intervention on weight and cardiovascular risk factors in individuals with type 2 diabetes mellitus: four-year results of the Look AHEAD trial," *Archives of Internal Medicine*, vol. 170, no. 17, pp. 1566–1575, 2010.

[10] S. E. Ellis, T. Speroff, R. S. Dittus, A. Brown, J. W. Pichert, and T. A. Elasy, "Diabetes patient education: a meta-analysis and meta-regression," *Patient Education and Counseling*, vol. 52, no. 1, pp. 97–105, 2004.

[11] T. Deakin, C. E. McShane, J. E. Cade, and R. D. Williams, "Group based training for self-management strategies in people with type 2 diabetes mellitus," *Cochrane Database of Systematic Reviews*, no. 2, Article ID CD003417, 2005.

[12] S. L. Norris, M. M. Engelgau, and K. M. V. Narayan, "Effectiveness of self-management training in type 2 diabetes: a systematic review of randomized controlled trials," *Diabetes Care*, vol. 24, no. 3, pp. 561–587, 2001.

[13] W. Wilson and C. Pratt, "The impact of diabetes education and peer support upon weight and glycemic control of elderly persons with noninsulin dependent diabetes mellitus (NIDDM)," *American Journal of Public Health*, vol. 77, no. 5, pp. 634–635, 1987.

[14] H. A. van Dam, F. G. van der Horst, L. Knoops, R. M. Ryckman, H. F. J. M. Crebolder, and B. H. W. van den Borne, "Social support in diabetes: a systematic review of controlled intervention studies," *Patient Education and Counseling*, vol. 59, no. 1, pp. 1–12, 2005.

[15] M. Heisler, S. Vijan, F. Makki, and J. D. Piette, "Diabetes control with reciprocal peer support versus nurse care management: a randomized trial," *Annals of Internal Medicine*, vol. 153, no. 8, pp. 507–515, 2010.

[16] K. Lorig, P. L. Ritter, D. D. Laurent et al., "Online diabetes self-management program: a randomized study," *Diabetes Care*, vol. 33, no. 6, pp. 1275–1281, 2010.

[17] J. R. Dale, S. M. Williams, and V. Bowyer, "What is the effect of peer support on diabetes outcomes in adults? A systematic review," *Diabetic Medicine*, vol. 29, no. 11, pp. 1361–1377, 2012.

[18] P. Clarke, A. Gray, and R. Holman, "Estimating utility values for health states of type 2 diabetic patients using the EQ-5D (UKPDS 62)," *Medical Decision Making*, vol. 22, no. 4, pp. 340–349, 2002.

[19] R. J. Stevens, V. Kothari, A. I. Adler, I. M. Stratton, and R. R. Holman, "The UKPDS risk engine: a model for the risk of coronary heart disease in type II diabetes (UKPDS 56)," *Clinical Science*, vol. 101, no. 6, pp. 671–679, 2001.

[20] G. C. Urbaniak and S. Plous, Research Randomizer, 2011, https://www.randomizer.org/.

[21] M. K. Campbell, G. Piaggio, D. R. Elbourne, and D. G. Altman, "Consort 2010 statement: extension to cluster randomised trials," *British Medical Journal*, vol. 345, no. 7881, Article ID e5661, 2012.

[22] UK Prospective Diabetes Study (UKPDS) Group, "Effect of intensive blood-glucose control with metformin on complications in overweight patients with type 2 diabetes (UKPDS 34)," *The Lancet*, vol. 352, no. 9131, pp. 854–865, 1998.

[23] S. M. Smith, G. Paul, A. Kelly, D. L. Whitford, E. O'Shea, and T. O'Dowd, "Peer support for patients with type 2 diabetes: cluster randomised controlled trial," *British Medical Journal*, vol. 342, Article ID d715, 2011.

[24] A. K. Baksi, M. Al-Mrayat, D. Hogan, E. Whittingstall, P. Wilson, and J. Wex, "Peer advisers compared with specialist health professionals in delivering a training programme on self-management to people with diabetes: a randomized controlled trial," *Diabetic Medicine*, vol. 25, no. 9, pp. 1076–1082, 2008.

[25] J. E. Cade, S. F. L. Kirk, P. Nelson et al., "Can peer educators influence healthy eating in people with diabetes? Results of

a randomized controlled trial," *Diabetic Medicine*, vol. 26, no. 10, pp. 1048–1054, 2009.

[26] T. C. Keyserling, C. D. Samuel-Hodge, A. S. Ammerman et al., "A randomized trial of an intervention to improve self-care behaviors of African-American women with type 2 diabetes: impact on physical activity," *Diabetes Care*, vol. 25, no. 9, pp. 1576–1583, 2002.

[27] K. Lorig, P. L. Ritter, F. J. Villa, and J. Armas, "Community-based peer-led diabetes self-management: a randomized trial," *Diabetes Educator*, vol. 35, no. 4, pp. 641–651, 2009.

[28] K. Lorig, P. L. Ritter, F. Villa, and J. D. Piette, "Spanish diabetes self-management with and without automated telephone reinforcement: two randomized trials," *Diabetes Care*, vol. 31, no. 3, pp. 408–414, 2008.

[29] F. T. Shaya, V. V. Chirikov, D. Howard et al., "Effect of social networks intervention in type 2 diabetes: a partial randomised study," *Journal of Epidemiology and Community Health*, vol. 68, no. 4, pp. 326–332, 2014.

[30] W. Anderson-Loftin, S. Barnett, P. Bunn, P. Sullivan, J. Hussey, and A. Tavakoli, "Soul food light: culturally competent diabetes education," *Diabetes Educator*, vol. 31, no. 4, pp. 555–563, 2005.

[31] R. E. Glasgow, S. M. Boles, H. G. McKay, E. G. Feil, and M. Barrera Jr., "The D-Net diabetes self-management program: long-term implementation, outcomes, and generalization results," *Preventive Medicine*, vol. 36, no. 4, pp. 410–419, 2003.

[32] C. J. Murrock, P. A. Higgins, and C. Killion, "Dance and peer support to improve diabetes outcomes in African American women," *Diabetes Educator*, vol. 35, no. 6, pp. 995–1003, 2009.

[33] H. C. Gerstein, M. E. Miller, R. P. Byington et al., "Effects of intensive glucose lowering in type 2 diabetes," *The New England Journal of Medicine*, vol. 358, pp. 2545–2559, 2008.

23

Community-Based Diabetes Screening and Risk Assessment in Rural West Virginia

Ranjita Misra,[1] Cindy Fitch,[2] David Roberts,[3] and Dana Wright[4]

[1] Department of Social & Behavioral Sciences, Robert C Byrd Health Science Center, School of Public Health, West Virginia University, 3313A, Morgantown, WV 26506-9190, USA

[2] Programs and Research, Extension Service, West Virginia University, P.O. Box 6031, 812 Knapp Hall, Morgantown, WV 26506-6031, USA

[3] WVU Extension Service, Lincoln and Boone Counties Extension Agent, Hamlin, WV, USA

[4] WVU Extension Services, 815 Alderson Street, Williamson, WV 25661, USA

Correspondence should be addressed to Ranjita Misra; ramisra@hsc.wvu.edu

Academic Editor: Ulrike Rothe

This project utilized a cross-sectional study design to assess diabetes risk among 540 individuals from 12 counties using trained extension agents and community organizations in West Virginia. Individuals were screened for diabetes using (1) the validated 7-item diabetes risk assessment survey and (2) hemoglobin A1c tests. Demographic and lifestyle behaviors were also collected. The average age, body mass index, and A1c were 51.2 ± 16.4, 31.1 ± 7.5, and 5.8 ± 0.74, respectively. The majority were females, Non-Hispanic Whites with no prior diagnosis of diabetes. Screenings showed that 61.8% of participants were at high risk for diabetes. Family history of diabetes (siblings or parents), overweight or obese status, sedentary lifestyle, and older age were commonly prevalent risk factors. Higher risk scores computed from the 7-item questions correlated positively with higher A1c ($r = 0.221$, $P < 0.001$). In multivariate logistic regression analyses, higher diabetes risk was predicted by obesity, older age, family history of hypertension, and gestational diabetes. Females were 4 times at higher risk than males. The findings indicated that community-based screenings were an effective way to assess diabetes risk in rural West Virginia. Linking diabetes screenings with referrals to lifestyle programs for high risk individuals can help reduce the burden of diabetes in the state.

1. Introduction

Diabetes affects 29.1 million Americans [1]. In adults, type 2 diabetes mellitus (T2DM) accounts for 90 to 95% of all cases. Despite emphasis on lifestyle modification and medications to treat T2DM, half of T2DM patients remain poorly controlled [2]. Consequently, it is the 7th leading cause of death due to complications such as heart disease and stroke, kidney failure, lower-limb amputations, and new cases of blindness. The economic burden of diabetes in 2012 was $245 billion for direct medical cost and $69 billion in indirect costs, such as disability, time lost from work, and premature death [3].

West Virginia Ranks 2nd in Prevalence of Diabetes among the 53 States and Territories. According to the 2012 Behavioral Risk Factor Surveillance System (BRFSS), diabetes prevalence in West Virginia was 13% (268,000 individuals), significantly higher than the national average of 10.2% [4]. Furthermore, another study estimated that 99,800 have undiagnosed diabetes [5] and possibly complications [6]. In addition, approximately 465,000 individuals have prediabetes. Factors that contribute to high rates of diabetes and prediabetes in West Virginia include aging population, physical inactivity, obesity, geography, lack of access to quality care, and the Appalachian culture of distrust of the healthcare system. It is estimated that the number of West Virginians living with diabetes (diagnosed and undiagnosed) will increase to 17% by 2025 from 268,000 to 314,000 [7]. The resulting medical and societal cost of diabetes will be $3.0 billion, a 25% increase from 2010 [7]. The average medical expenditures for patients with diabetes (nationally) were 2.3 times higher than those without diabetes [8]; glucose control was correlated with the medical cost, increasing significantly for every one percent increase in glycosylated hemoglobin (A1C) above 7%. Diagnosis and education to improve diabetes self-care management and health outcomes are limited due to lack of the patient's awareness of diabetes and its complications and convenient local screening and prevention programs. Patient care in the rural WV southern counties is limited, and interactions of individuals with diabetes with their providers are infrequent and ineffective for outpatient visits [9, 10].

Recent estimates claim that many individuals are not fully self-aware of their risk for diabetes. Misperceptions and lack of knowledge of their actual risk can put them on a fast track to developing diabetes if they do not reduce risk factors such as being overweight or obese, smoking, and physical inactivity. For example, in an international survey released by Health Dialog, 74% of American respondents said that obesity, unhealthy diet, and inadequate physical activity levels constitute the nation's biggest health issues [11]. Yet, 51% of the American respondents that were obese considered themselves to be healthy and 43% thought that their diets were good. This disconnect between what they know and how they apply that knowledge to themselves is quite concerning. Diabetes and its resulting comorbidities are of grave concern. Furthermore, evidence that behavioral lifestyle interventions can prevent or delay the development of type 2 diabetes and reduce risk factors for cardiovascular disease has been demonstrated in the US Diabetes Prevention Program [12, 13]. However, identification of individuals who are undiagnosed cases or at high risk is paramount before any intervention program can be launched to improve diabetes and CVD risk factors in community settings [14–16]. Several recent translations of the Diabetes Prevention Program and Finnish Diabetes Prevention Study have demonstrated encouraging effects across diverse settings, including churches [17, 18], community settings [16, 19], and YMCAs [18]. The personnel who implemented the intervention included health care professionals like nurses but also volunteer medical personnel, YMCA trainers, and community health workers.

Hence, the purpose if this study was to assess individual's diabetes risk in twelve rural counties of West Virginia using a noninvasive survey, followed up with glycosylated hemoglobin or A1c test to identify individuals with prediabetes and higher risk for diabetes. All high risk cases were referred to a self-management education and support program, the Dinning with Diabetes & Diabetes Prevention Program, and encouraged to visit a healthcare provider for follow-up care.

2. Methodology

The current project utilized a cross-sectional study design to assess diabetes risk using a partnership between the academic community, extension agents, and community organizations. The screenings were completed by extension agents who were part of our investigative team. Extension agents were trained to complete diabetes screenings (both surveys and A1c). They work with their local communities and provide

a range of community-based educational programs including the Dining with Diabetes program. Hence, using the WVUES network to test the effectiveness of diabetes screening in W.Va. counties was innovative and would allow for long-term sustainability of this model.

We used an established community-based approach, a network of community organizations, and the West Virginia University Extension Service (WVUES) Network for diabetes screenings and referral using extension agents. Prior to data collection, the extension agents were involved in the planning of the project, that is, finalization of sites and community events in all the twelve counties where data collection was completed, that is, McDowell, Logan, Boone, Lincoln, Cabell, Wirt, Braxton, Clay, Wood, Berkley, Jackson, and Greenbrier counties. Based on our initial discussion with the community coalitions and community leaders, several screenings were offered during week days and weekends to maximize participation.

The Community Health Care Centers in all the twelve counties surveyed for this project offered annual health fairs that allowed community agencies to set up informational booths to showcase services available in the area. County extension agents set up booths at these community health fairs to promote their services as well as diabetes screenings. Advertisement for screenings included free A1c testing during the event. While the health fair targets the general population, the majority of individuals who came to the booth were adults with some level of interest for assessing their diabetes risk. Interested participants completed a 2-page survey focused on family and personal health history and health behaviors, followed by A1c tests at the site (A1c tests were not mandatory but encouraged).

Diabetes screenings were also offered in conjunction with other scheduled community events such as parent/teacher nights at local high schools, information booths at basketball games, and scheduled library community events. These events were targeted to capture a diverse group of individuals. For example, the local library offers regular educational opportunities on topics that range from adult literacy to financial planning. Furthermore, in rural West Virginia communities, school and local sporting events are considered an important forum of civic engagement and provided our extension agents a greater access to individuals in the communities.

Participants included 540 individuals from 12 rural counties (521 zip codes) who were assessed for their risk for diabetes. Individuals aged 18 years and older were screened since younger participants are less likely to have diabetes. There were no exclusions by gender, but pregnant women were excluded due to their conditions. The majority of individuals who stopped by the booths and tables were interested and completed the health screening survey. While it is difficult to determine the number of uninterested participants in community events such as health fairs (as they could easily avoid the booth) or other events, it is likely that individuals who came to the extension booths for diabetes screenings are more likely to have greater health consciousness and/or worried about getting diabetes. Also, diabetes screenings scheduled at community events allowed for interested individuals to have fewer distractions of free give away materials that occurred during health fairs in other booths.

Approximately 50% of participants declined to complete the diabetes screenings at the health fairs and 20% at the library and community events. Why community events provided a greater response to the diabetes screenings remains an open empirical question for further investigation, and use of various community forums allowed for a greater representative sample in our study. However, the sample was biased towards a higher educated participant group as more than half of the participants were college graduates or had some college level education.

The survey and A1c testing were administered by the trained research team and information was collected during the 12 months of the study enrollment. The primary outcome was risk for diabetes.

2.1. Diabetes Risk Assessment. The main focus of this project was to identify individuals at high risk for diabetes without imposing tests that are difficult to perform or sustain in a community setting. Hence, we used an approach that combines a questionnaire and point-of-care capillary glycosylated hemoglobin tests to predict the risk for prediabetes or undiagnosed diabetes [20]. This approach involved three steps. (1) Completion of a validated and reliable 7-item diabetes risk assessment survey developed by the Centers for Disease Control and Prevention (CDC; http://www.cdc.gov/diabetes/prevention/pdf/prediabetestest.pdf): the questionnaire included age, weight for height, exercise, diabetes in the family, and delivery of a large baby. (2) Collection of a drop of whole blood by finger stick to assess the glycosylated hemoglobin (A1c) using point-of-care A1c Now monitoring kit by Bayer: the use of A1c was preferred over fasting or random glucose as it requires only a drop of capillary blood (finger prick), can be drawn by the extension agents, and can be completed at any time of the day. Hence, it was appropriate for community settings and reflects the average blood glucose levels in the past 3 months. The A1c Now is available for over-the-counter or professional use and is approved by the Food and Drug Administration for monitoring of A1c [21, 22]. Sicard and Taylor have shown that A1c Now has good accuracy and high correlation with standardized laboratory testing [23]. (3) A risk score of ≥9: medical history of the participants allowed us to identify those individuals with no prior diagnosis of diabetes by a health care provider; A1c levels of 5.7 and higher with no prior diagnosis allowed to identify individuals with prediabetes or possibly undiagnosed diabetes.

2.2. Healthy Lifestyle Habits. We assessed healthy lifestyle behaviors using one question on smoking status "do you smoke" with response options yes or no; food label reading behavior "do you read food labels" with response options yes or no; and two questions on physical activity "how often do you exercise for periods of at least 30 minutes" and "how do you rate your overall level of physical activity." Response options included less than once a week, 1-2 times per week, and 3-4 times per week and low, moderate, and high, respectively. Due to high correlation between the two

physical activity questions, the latter was used for analysis. In addition, information was collected on participants' demographic characteristics (age, gender, educational level, self-reported height and weight so that we can calculate the BMI, and educational level).

All analyses were done using the Statistical Program for Social Sciences (SPSS) system (version 21.0). Basic descriptive statistics were obtained for demographic, lifestyle, and diabetes risk factors. ANOVA with Post Hoc analysis was used to evaluate the difference in risk score by gender and educational status of respondents. The acceptance level for statistical significance was 0.05. Logistic regression analysis was used to estimate the factors that influence diabetes risk. The dependent variable was the low risk and higher risk group of participants. The following variables were included in the model: age, gender, education, body mass index, physical activity, tobacco use, current health status, family history of chronic diseases (diabetes and hypertension), and A1c. Individuals with prior diagnosis of diabetes ($n = 81$; 15%) were excluded from the multivariate analysis.

3. Results and Discussion

The sample comprised 538 individuals from 12 rural counties. The average age of the participants was 51.2 ± 16.4 years (range 18–89 years). The majority was female (78.8%), Non-Hispanic White (88.3%), with no prior diagnosis of diabetes (83.9%). Approximately half of the participants (43.3%) had a high school degree or less.

In terms of lifestyle behavior, 81.9% of participants indicated they do not smoke (4.3% did not provide the information); females had slightly higher smoking rates than males, but it did not significantly vary by gender. Approximately one-third or 37.5% reported sedentary lifestyle that is, at least 30 minutes of exercise less than once a week. While it is encouraging that two-thirds of the participants indicated they read food labels, 35.4% did not. Furthermore, females were significantly more likely to read food labels (68%) as compared to males (52%) ($P = 0.002$).

Mean body mass index (BMI) was 31, in the obese category; males (32.5 ± 7.7) were significantly more obese than females (30.7 ± 7.4; $P = 0.029$). Approximately one-third of the participants or 37.4% had high blood pressure and two-thirds (67.8%) indicated they had family history of high blood pressure.

Descriptive participant characteristics for low risk and high risk for prediabetes, and prior diagnosed diabetes are presented in Table 1. Significant differences were noted between the groups by age, body mass index, family history, and some of the lifestyle behaviors. Individuals with prior diagnosis of diabetes were more likely to be older, obese, and with a family history or medical history of hypertension. In addition, they also were less likely to be smokers, do vigorous activity, and be with no prior diagnosis of diabetes. Similarly, individuals at high risk for diabetes were older individuals (45 years of age and older), were obese, had a family/medical history of hypertension, and were female. Furthermore, they were more likely to read food labels and less likely to smoke than individuals with lower risk of diabetes (Table 1).

TABLE 1: Sample characteristics of participants by diagnosed diabetes and undiagnosed high risk and low risk ($N = 538$).

Variables	Diagnosed diabetes by a HCP ($n = 81$; 15.2%)		Undiagnosed; high risk ($n = 268$; 49.8%)		Low risk ($n = 184$; 34.2%)		P value
	Freq.	%	Freq.	%	Freq.	%	
Sex							**0.010**
Female	56	69.1	221	83.7	140	76.1	
Male	25	30.9	43	16.3	44	23.9	
Ethnicity							0.084
Non-Hispanic Whites	77	95.1	238	90.5	158	86.3	
Minorities	4	4.9	25	9.5	25	13.7	
Age			Mean = 51.2 ± 16.4 years				<0.001
18–44	13	16.0	40	15.2	134	72.8	
45–64	41	50.6	121	45.8	49	26.6	
≥65	27	33.3	103	39.0	1		
Education							0.382
≤High school grad	35	50.7	92	41.3	66	43.4	
College grad or some college	34	49.3	131	58.7	86	56.6	
Exercise at least 30 minutes							0.481
Less than once a week	35	43.8	107	40.7	63	34.8	
1-2 times per week	26	32.5	76	28.9	60	33.1	
3-4 or more times per week	19	23.8	80	30.4	58	32.0	
Body mass index			Mean = 31.1 ± 7.5				<0.001
Under/normal	5	6.5	38	15.6	55	31.6	
Overweight	22	28.6	85	34.8	53	30.5	
Obese	50	64.9	121	49.6	66	37.9	
Read food labels							0.008
Yes	53	66.3	182	70.5	101	56.1	
No	27		76		79		
Smoke							<0.001
Yes	11	13.8	21	8.1	42	24.3	
No	69	86.3	239	91.9	131	75.7	
History of hypertension							0.040
Yes	64	84.2	180	72.3	119	68.8	
No	12	15.8	69	27.2	54	31.2	
Family history of hypertension							<0.001
Yes	50	64.9	114	46.3	38	22.0	
No	27	35.1	132	53.7	135	78.0	

Note: HCP: healthcare provider.

3.1. Diabetes Risk. 81 individuals (15.1%) indicated they had a prior diagnosis of diabetes by a healthcare professional and hence were excluded from the diabetes risk assessment. The majority of participants (61.8%) were at high risk for prediabetes as they had a risk score of 9 points or higher. Mean risk score was 9.0 ± 4.83 for all participants without prior diagnosis of diabetes; mean score was 4.15 ± 2.46 for low risk and 12.35 ± 2.78 for high risk participants. According to the CDC's risk calculator, low risk for having diabetes is 3 to 8 points and high risk is 9 or more points; those with high risk are recommended to follow-up with their health care provider. The Diabetes Risk Calculator was developed and validated using data from NHANES III [20]. Analysis of the individual seven risk factors showed that the majority of participants had a family history of diabetes (siblings or parents; 65%), weighed more than their normal weight for

TABLE 2: Diabetes risk factors by low and high risk for prediabetes.

Diabetes risk factors	Low risk (n = 184)		High risk (n = 268)		P value
	Freq.	%	Freq.	%	
Baby weigh more than 9 pounds at birth*					**0.354**
No	156	88.1	249	86.5	
Yes	21	11.9	39	13.5	
Sister or brother with diabetes					**0.002**
No	153	79.3	210	66.9	
Yes	40	20.7	104	33.1	
Parent with diabetes					**0.106**
No	122	62.9	178	56.9	
Yes	72	37.1	135	43.1	
Weight is more than listed for height					**<0.001**
No	103	56.6	60	19.5	
Yes	79	43.4	247	80.5	
Less than 65 years and get little exercise/day					**<0.001**
No	177	94.7	188	60.1	
Yes	10	5.3	125	39.9	
45–64 years of age					**<0.001**
No	145	71.4	168	51.5	
Yes	58	28.6	158	48.5	
65 years or older					**<0.001**
No	203	100.0	194	59.1	
Yes	—	0.0	134	40.9	
	Mean	SD	Mean	SD	
Mean diabetes risk score	4.15	2.46	12.35	2.78	**<0.001**
Mean A1c	5.6	0.41	5.9	0.85	**<0.001**

Note: low risk for diabetes is defined by risk score < 9; high risk for prediabetes is defined by risk score ≥ 9.
*Only females were selected for this analysis.

height (66.7%), lead a sedentary lifestyle (37%), and were older in age (>45 years; 64%), all of which increased their risk for diabetes (Table 2).

Mean A1c was 5.6 ± 0.41 for the low risk group, 5.9 ± 0.85 for high risk group, and 7.2 ± 1.8 for participants with prior diagnosis of diabetes; A1c positively correlated with higher diabetes risk scores ($r = 0.221$, $P < 0.001$).

Results from the bivariate and multivariable logistic regression analyses are presented in Table 3. Logistic regression analysis estimated the factors that influenced diabetes risk for the two groups of participants: low risk and higher risk for diabetes. Important known risk factors were controlled in the model: age, gender, education, body mass index, physical activity, tobacco use, current health status, family history of chronic diseases (diabetes and hypertension), and A1c. The results between the unadjusted and adjusted ORs were consistent, with the exception of gender; gender was statistically significant in the unadjusted models but approached significance in the adjusted models ($P = 0.07$). Association of diabetes risk score and family history of diabetes (sibling and parents), smoking status, and reading food labels were

significant in the unadjusted (bivariate) model but not in the adjusted model (Table 3). As shown in the adjusted model, overweight/obese and older respondents were significantly at higher risk. However, for females, having a history of gestational diabetes increased their risk twelvefold as compared to those with low risk (OR 12.2; 95% CI 2.6–56.9). Furthermore, participants with higher risk were approximately four times as likely to have a family history of hypertension as compared to those with low risk (OR 4.08; 95% CI 1.2–14.2). Individuals with increased risk were handed their risk score and available healthcare providers in the area; they were encouraged to make an appointment with their primary care provider or a health care provider.

The burden of diabetes appears to be particularly high in rural areas of the state, with more than 60% of participants without a previous diagnosis of diabetes being at high risk of developing type 2 diabetes. This concurs with the high burden of reported diabetes and its serious health and economic consequences for the individual and society and is a major public health problem, especially in a rural, medically underserved state such as West Virginia. Over the past several years,

TABLE 3: Logistic regression: predicting high risk for prediabetes[▽].

	Unadjusted		Adjusted[φ]	
	OR	95% CI	OR	95% CI
Sex				
Male			Reference	
Female	1.61**	1.01, 2.6	3.91+	0.89, 17.09
Education				
≤High school grad	0.92	0.60, 1.39	0.73	0.24, 2.19
College grad or some college			Reference	
Physical activity***				
Low	1.23	0.77, 1.95	0.96	0.28, 3.23
Moderate	0.92	0.56, 1.48	0.97	0.28, 3.29
High			Reference	
Siblings with diabetes				
Yes			Reference	
No	0.49**	0.30, 0.78	0.76	0.22, 2.65
Parents with diabetes				
Yes			Reference	
No	0.69+	0.46, 1.04	0.89	0.30, 2.60
Baby weigh more than 9 pounds at birth				
Yes			Reference	
No	1.10	0.59, 2.07	12.2**	2.6, 56.9
Family history of hypertension				
Yes			Reference	
No	0.85	0.55, 1.29	4.08*	1.18, 14.16
Medical history of hypertension				
Yes			Reference	
No	0.32	0.21, 0.50	0.58	0.20, 1.72
Read food labels				
Yes			Reference	
No	0.53**	0.36, 0.79	0.90	0.33, 2.45
Smoke				
Yes			Reference	
No	3.64**	2.07, 6.42	0.72	0.21, 2.39
A1c	2.87**	1.6, 5.2	1.14	0.60, 3.34
Age	1.10**	1.08, 1.12	1.15**	1.09, 1.20
BMI	1.05**	1.02, 1.08	1.23**	1.12, 1.36

[▽]Individuals with diagnosed diabetes cases by a healthcare professionals were deleted from the analysis.
P values: [+] <0.10, [*] <0.05, and [**] <0.01.
[***]Physical activity: low, exercise less than once a week of at least 30 minutes; moderate, exercise 1-2 times per week of at least 30 minutes; high, exercise 3-4 or more times per week of at least 30 minutes.
[φ]Adjusted ORs reflect the association between high risk prediabetes status and each variable, adjusting for all the other variables in the model.

WV has ranked among the highest in diabetes occurrence in the country [24] suggesting that West Virginians have a vulnerability that may have genetic and/or lifestyle causative links. Lack of access as well as having to travel far for care are reported as factors associated with lack of preventive healthcare, besides poor dietary habits, sedentary lifestyle, obesity, and overweight status and low health literacy which may play a role in the higher rates of diabetes in the state [25–28].

Use of community-based screenings may be critical for primary and secondary prevention, and to educate and identify those people who may be unaware of their high risk and to encourage them to seek medical care. Since most individuals with undiagnosed diabetes or at high risk are asymptomatic [29], use of simple, safe, and validated tests such as the one used in this project can inform rural West Virginians of their risk and consequences, available programs, and clinics for follow-up care and that the problem is amenable to prevention and control. Furthermore, our results showed that screening was successful for all ages, genders, and minorities and Non-Hispanic Whites (the majority in West Virginia). Yet in order for these community-based screenings to succeed, be sustained, and be effective in West Virginia, it is critical that barriers to care and disparities are also considered. Besides known barriers such as access to care and transportation, other factors that contribute to the diabetes disparities include lack of specialists skilled in diabetic care and a disconnect or distrust between patients and their providers [25, 30]. In prior studies participants perceived that providers did not have a strong understanding of their culture [30] and the need for culturally sensitive programs for West Virginians [31].

The cost of the diabetes screenings was reasonable ($10 per point-of-cost A1c kit) and allowed the project to be clinically, socially, and ethically acceptable for the extension agents. While it can be argued that A1c tests may not be cost-effective for all community-based diabetes screenings, the American Diabetes Association recommends testing to detect type 2 diabetes and prediabetes in asymptomatic adults who are overweight or obese and have one or more additional risk factors for diabetes and in all adults 45 years of age or older [32]. Stepwise screenings [33] can also be used for these community-based diabetes screenings with the first step of the screening to use the 7-item CDC survey followed by A1c tests for those with diabetes risk scores ≥9, however, in a rural state such as West Virginia which had disproportionally higher prevalence rates of obesity (1st) and diabetes (4th) nationally [34], and many people have limited or no access to routine medical care, universal screening using a method that does not require fasting is reasonable. Community-based diabetes screening inevitably involves some concern related to high risk individuals identified by screenings who may not get the care they need and/or follow-up with health care providers for care or additional diagnostic tests. These are valid concerns that bear further exploration and research but do not negate the benefit of this simple screening program that quantifies the risk of undiagnosed diabetes or prediabetes while there is still time to prevent progression and complications.

The low cost of A1c tests could be easily translated for any clinic and hospital and for health care professionals and the public. This the cost of the screening was very reasonable in relation to the expenditure on medical care as a whole and the benefits which far outweighed the time for program planning and implementation. Conducting diabetes screening and referrals also allowed the extension agents for community outreach in their counties to improve diabetes and health outcomes and possibly improve the quality of life. Since the extension agents are trusted members of the community, use of these agents can be a sustainable model for diabetes screenings in community settings.

Using the extension network as a future model for diabetes screenings, referrals and lifestyle programs in West Virginia are innovative for several reasons: (1) extension agents are embedded in the community; they know the leaders and the community resources very well; (2) no other state organization has the outreach or infrastructure; (3) offering community-based screenings falls in direct line with the mission and goals of the land grant university and allows for long-term sustainability of this model; and (4) lessons learned will be shared across state extension programs, providing additional capacity to translate this model widely. In addition, rural communities can also devote resources for these low-cost diabetes screenings to develop public/private and community partnership as the return on investment is high and the condition is amenable to prevention. However, there should be clear guidelines on the management of individuals with a positive test result in order to help to both prevent the disease through lifestyle and pharmacological intervention and reduce the morbidity and mortality associated with diabetes [20].

Results showed a wide gap in reported lifestyle behavior and their overweight and obesity status. For example, approximately two-thirds or 71% of the undiagnosed high risk individuals indicated that they read food labels when making food choices, yet, nearly half of the participants were obese according to their self-reported BMI rankings. This gap between perception and lifestyle behavior has been noted in the literature when individuals who are overweight or obese do not think they are so [11]. While no association existed between educational status and diabetes risk in the logistic regression analysis, more than half of the high risk participants had some college level education or a college degree suggesting that there exists a gap in educated participant's knowledge of risk factors (especially family history of diabetes and hypertension) and the ability to effectively apply that knowledge to lower risk. Furthermore, a lack of perceived personal risk among those with a family history of diabetes and hypertension in this study may be indicative of not applying the knowledge to themselves. This concurs with a national population-based diabetes survey [35] where participants with prediabetes and at risk did not perceive their risk to be high.

Females were at higher risk than males, possibility due to their higher BMI and gestational diabetes. The odds of having higher risk for diabetes was fourfold than males making it critical that public health education should highlight the gender disparity for primary and secondary prevention efforts. This discovery also makes a strong case for continued community-based educational efforts to improve awareness, even among educated individuals to improve preventive efforts such as the adoption of healthy lifestyle in order to reduce the risk of developing type 2 diabetes in rural West Virginia.

There are numerous positive results that were attained in this project. Conducting diabetes screening during health fairs and other public events allowed extension agents to provide greater access to community screening and referrals to health care providers and extension classes such as Dining with Diabetes and strengthened partnerships between community and clinical service agencies to reduce health disparities, improve diabetes and health outcomes, and improve quality of life. Since the extension agents are trusted members of the community, use of these agents can be a sustainable model for diabetes screenings in community settings. However, as future research and screening are conducted on community-based screenings and referrals for treatment, there should be clear guidelines on the management of individuals with a positive test result and consider how to support the autonomy of participants through the lifestyle intervention, diabetes management, and pharmacological intervention in order to help to both prevent the disease and reduce the morbidity and mortality associated with diabetes [20]. The results of the project will be used to develop additional, community-based, culturally competent diabetes prevention and management programs.

Results should be considered in context to the following limitations. One of the limitations of the present study is that a small number of minority adults participated in the screening. This discrepancy poses the threat that the results are only indicative of the non-Hispanic White population and not the population of rural West Virginia, as a whole. However, West Virginia is comprised of a predominantly non-Hispanic White population (97%) and our study represented more minorities than the general population of the state. Studies indicate that ethnicity and minority status are risk factor not only for having type 2 diabetes but also for increasing morbidity and mortality with the disease [36, 37]. Hence, efforts need to be made to improve screening in this group to improve inequalities and compliance as the A1c does not require a fasting blood test. Another potential weakness is that the information was self-reported. Individuals may have answered questions in a socially acceptable manner that would incorporate information bias. For example, reporting that they are physically active incorrectly lowers their risk score for early onset diabetes. Other potential samples include participants that may not be representative of the general West Virginia population as there was a bias towards a higher educated participant group in this study as well as those who may have been motivated to volunteer for the community diabetes screenings due to a greater awareness and/or worry about their health status. A higher risk of diabetes was also noted among females, despite having no gender differences observed in the prevalence of diagnosed diabetes cases in the West Virginia population, according to the Behavioral Risk Factor Surveillance System (BRFSS) data [38]. Hence, future studies may explore the replicability of the high risk among women in larger samples and population-based studies.

4. Conclusion

The findings clearly indicated that community based screening was an effective way to assess diabetes risk in rural West Virginia. The findings also indicated that there exists a gap between knowledge of diabetes risk factors and the need for screenings, referrals, and lifestyle programs to effectively lower those risks. Plans for future research include targeting minority groups within the state using similar community outlets and faith-based organizations and enhancing our data collection to include health literacy and more detailed diet and physical activity reports. While individual assessments

were beneficial, we feel association of their diabetes risk scores with clinical data (A1c) will be more informative for participants and motivate them to attend *Dining with Diabetes* classes and/or other diabetes education or lifestyle programs available in their communities.

Conflict of Interests

The authors declare that there is no conflict of interests regarding the publication of this paper.

Acknowledgments

The authors would like to thank Ami Cook, Gwen Crum, Kay Davis, Sue Flanagan, Patty Morrison, Brenda Porter, and Gina Taylor for their help in data collection. Project is funded by WVU Public Service Grant.

References

[1] CDC, *National Diabetes Fact Sheet: National Estimates and General Information on Diabetes and Prediabetes in the United States*, Edited by C.f.D.C.a.P. Department of Health and Human Services, Centers for Disease Control and Prevention, Atlanta, Ga, USA, 2011.

[2] H. E. Resnick, M. I. Harris, D. B. Brock, and T. B. Harris, "American Diabetes Association diabetes diagnostic criteria, advancing age, and cardiovascular disease risk profiles: results from the Third National Health and Nutrition Examination Survey," *Diabetes Care*, vol. 23, no. 2, pp. 176–180, 2000.

[3] CDC, *National Diabetes Fact Sheet*, Centers for Disease Control and Prevention, 2011.

[4] W. S. Data, *West Virginia Behavioral Risk Factor Surveillance System Report*, edited by: West Virginia Department of Health and Human Resources, Bureau for Public Health, Health Statistics Center, 2012, http://www.wvdhhr.org/bph/hsc/pubs/brfss/2012/BRFSS2012.pdf.

[5] Institute for Alternative Futures, *Diabetes 2025 Forecasting Model*, Institute for Alternative Futures, 2010.

[6] M. I. Harris and R. C. Eastman, "Early detection of undiagnosed diabetes mellitus: a US perspective," *Diabetes/Metabolism Research and Reviews*, vol. 16, no. 4, pp. 230–236, 2000.

[7] J. P. Boyle, T. J. Thompson, E. W. Gregg, L. E. Barker, and D. F. Williamson, "Projection of the year 2050 burden of diabetes in the US adult population: dynamic modeling of incidence, mortality, and prediabetes prevalence," *Population Health Metrics*, vol. 8, article 29, 2010.

[8] E. S. Huang, A. Basu, M. O'Grady, and J. C. Capretta, "Projecting the future diabetes population size and related costs for the U.S.," *Diabetes Care*, vol. 32, no. 12, pp. 2225–2229, 2009.

[9] Y. H. Tang, S. M. C. Pang, M. F. Chan, G. S. P. Yeung, and V. T. F. Yeung, "Health literacy, complication awareness, and diabetic control in patients with type 2 diabetes mellitus," *Journal of Advanced Nursing*, vol. 62, no. 1, pp. 74–83, 2008.

[10] K. G. Rowley, M. Daniel, K. Skinner, M. Skinner, G. A. White, and K. O'Dea, "Effectiveness of a community-directed 'healthy lifestyle' program in a remote Australian Aboriginal community," *Australian and New Zealand Journal of Public Health*, vol. 24, no. 2, pp. 136–144, 2000.

[11] Bupa Health Pulse, *Global Trends, Attitudes, and Influences*, International Healthcare survey, 2011.

[12] R. Ratner, R. Goldberg, S. Haffner et al., "Impact of intensive lifestyle and metformin therapy on cardiovascular disease risk factors in the diabetes prevention program," *Diabetes Care*, vol. 28, no. 4, pp. 888–894, 2005.

[13] W. C. Knowler, E. Barrett-Connor, S. E. Fowler et al., "Reduction in the incidence of type 2 diabetes with lifestyle intervention or metformin," *The New England Journal of Medicine*, vol. 346, no. 6, pp. 393–403, 2002.

[14] M. K. Kramer, A. M. Kriska, E. M. Venditti et al., "Translating the Diabetes Prevention Program: a comprehensive model for prevention training and program delivery," *American Journal of Preventive Medicine*, vol. 37, no. 6, pp. 505–511, 2009.

[15] L. Jackson, "Translating the diabetes prevention program into practice: a review of community interventions," *Diabetes Educator*, vol. 35, no. 2, pp. 309–320, 2009.

[16] P. Balagopal, N. Kamalamma, T. G. Patel, and R. Misra, "A community-based diabetes prevention and management education program in a rural village in India," *Diabetes Care*, vol. 31, no. 6, pp. 1097–1104, 2008.

[17] J. M. Boltri, Y. M. Davis-Smith, J. P. Seale, S. Shellenberger, I. S. Okosun, and M. E. Cornelius, "Diabetes prevention in a faith-based setting: results of translational research," *Journal of Public Health Management and Practice*, vol. 14, no. 1, pp. 29–32, 2008.

[18] R. T. Ackermann, E. A. Finch, E. Brizendine, H. Zhou, and D. G. Marrero, "Translating the diabetes prevention program into the community. The DEPLOY Pilot Study," *American Journal of Preventive Medicine*, vol. 35, no. 4, pp. 357–363, 2008.

[19] P. Balagopal, N. Kamalamma, T. G. Patel, and R. Misra, "A community-based participatory diabetes prevention and management intervention in rural India using community health workers," *Diabetes Educator*, vol. 38, no. 6, pp. 822–834, 2012.

[20] B. Balkau, "Screening for diabetes," *Diabetes Care*, vol. 31, no. 5, pp. 1084–1085, 2008.

[21] ADA, "Summary of revisions for the 2010 clinical practice recommendations," *Diabetes Care*, vol. 33, no. 1, supplement 1, p. s3, 2010.

[22] FDA, "OTC-Over the Counter Medical Devices," 2012, http://www.accessdata.fda.gov/scripts/cdrh/cfdocs/cfIVD/Search.cfm.

[23] D. A. Sicard and J. R. Taylor, "Comparison of point-of-care HbA$_{1c}$ test versus standardized laboratory testing," *Annals of Pharmacotherapy*, vol. 39, no. 6, pp. 1024–1028, 2005.

[24] J. Manchin, C. Curtis, N. M. Bazzle, C. Slemp, and J. L. Toth, *The Burden of Diabetes in West Virginia*, Edited by H. H. Resources, 2009.

[25] C. A. Coyne, C. Demian-Popescu, and D. Friend, "Social and cultural factors influencing health in southern West Virginia: a qualitative study," *Preventing Chronic Disease*, vol. 3, no. 4, article A124, 2006.

[26] S. A. Denham, L. E. Wood, and K. Remsberg, "Diabetes care: provider disparities in the US Appalachian region," *Rural and Remote Health*, vol. 10, no. 2, p. 1320, 2010.

[27] K. Huttlinger, J. Schaller-Ayers, and T. Lawson, "Health care in appalachia: a population-based approach," *Public Health Nursing*, vol. 21, no. 2, pp. 103–110, 2004.

[28] S. L. Smith and I. A. Tessaro, "Cultural perspectives on diabetes in an Appalachian population," *American Journal of Health Behavior*, vol. 29, no. 4, pp. 291–301, 2005.

[29] M. I. Harris, R. Klein, T. A. Welborn, and M. W. Knuiman, "Onset of NIDDM occurs at least 4–7 yr before clinical diagnosis," *Diabetes Care*, vol. 15, no. 7, pp. 815–819, 1992.

[30] E. L. McGarvey, M. Leon-Verdin, L. F. Killos, T. Guterbock, and W. F. Cohn, "Health disparities between appalachian and non-appalachian counties in Virginia USA," *Journal of Community Health*, vol. 36, no. 3, pp. 348–356, 2011.

[31] J. M. Boltri, Y. M. Davis-Smith, L. E. Zayas et al., "Developing a church-based diabetes prevention program with African Americans: focus group findings," *Diabetes Educator*, vol. 32, no. 6, pp. 901–909, 2006.

[32] American Diabetes Association, "Standards of medical care in diabetes—2013," *Diabetes Care*, vol. 36, supplement 1, pp. S11–S66, 2013.

[33] A. M. W. Spijkerman, M. C. Adriaanse, J. M. Dekker et al., "Diabetic patients detected by population-based stepwise screening already have a diabetic cardiovascular risk profile," *Diabetes Care*, vol. 25, no. 10, pp. 1784–1789, 2002.

[34] West Virginia Health Statistics Center, *West Virginia Behavioral Risk Factor Surveillance System Report, 2013*, West Virginia Health Statistics Center, 2015, http://www.wvdhhr.org/bph/hsc/pubs/brfss/2013/BRFSS2013.pdf.

[35] L. Piccinino, S. Griffey, J. Gallivan, L. D. Lotenberg, and D. Tuncer, "Recent trends in diabetes knowledge, perceptions, and behaviors: implications for national diabetes education," *Health Education & Behavior*, vol. 42, no. 5, pp. 687–696, 2015.

[36] A. Sheehy, N. Pandhi, D. B. Coursin et al., "Minority status and diabetes screening in an ambulatory population," *Diabetes Care*, vol. 34, no. 6, pp. 1289–1294, 2011.

[37] L. Meneghini, "Ethnic disparities in diabetes care: myth or reality?" *Current Opinion in Endocrinology, Diabetes and Obesity*, vol. 15, no. 2, pp. 128–134, 2008.

[38] West Virginia Health and Human Services, "HSC Statistical Brief No. 28. Diabetes and Health Equity in West Virginia: A Review," December 2015, http://www.wvdhhr.org/bph/hsc/pubs/briefs/028/brief28_20121220_health_eq_stat.pdf.

24

An Investigation into the Antiobesity Effects of *Morinda citrifolia* L. Leaf Extract in High Fat Diet Induced Obese Rats Using a ^{1}H NMR Metabolomics Approach

Najla Gooda Sahib Jambocus,[1] Nazamid Saari,[1] Amin Ismail,[2] Alfi Khatib,[3] Mohamad Fawzi Mahomoodally,[4] and Azizah Abdul Hamid[1,5]

[1]Faculty of Food Science and Technology, Universiti Putra Malaysia, 43400 Serdang, Selangor, Malaysia
[2]Faculty of Medicine and Health Sciences, Universiti Putra Malaysia, 43400 Serdang, Selangor, Malaysia
[3]Department of Pharmaceutical Chemistry, Kulliyyah of Pharmacy, International Islamic University Malaysia, 25200 Kuantan, Pahang, Malaysia
[4]Department of Health Sciences, Faculty of Science, University of Mauritius, 230 Réduit, Mauritius
[5]Halal Products Research Institute, Universiti Putra Malaysia, 43400 Serdang, Selangor, Malaysia

Correspondence should be addressed to Najla Gooda Sahib Jambocus; najla.goodasahib@gmail.com and Azizah Abdul Hamid; azizahah@upm.edu.my

Academic Editor: Michal Ciborowski

The prevalence of obesity is increasing worldwide, with high fat diet (HFD) as one of the main contributing factors. Obesity increases the predisposition to other diseases such as diabetes through various metabolic pathways. Limited availability of antiobesity drugs and the popularity of complementary medicine have encouraged research in finding phytochemical strategies to this multifaceted disease. HFD induced obese Sprague-Dawley rats were treated with an extract of *Morinda citrifolia* L. leaves (MLE 60). After 9 weeks of treatment, positive effects were observed on adiposity, fecal fat content, plasma lipids, and insulin and leptin levels. The inducement of obesity and treatment with MLE 60 on metabolic alterations were then further elucidated using a ^{1}H NMR based metabolomics approach. Discriminating metabolites involved were products of various metabolic pathways, including glucose metabolism and TCA cycle (lactate, 2-oxoglutarate, citrate, succinate, pyruvate, and acetate), amino acid metabolism (alanine, 2-hydroxybutyrate), choline metabolism (betaine), creatinine metabolism (creatinine), and gut microbiome metabolism (hippurate, phenylacetylglycine, dimethylamine, and trigonelline). Treatment with MLE 60 resulted in significant improvement in the metabolic perturbations caused obesity as demonstrated by the proximity of the treated group to the normal group in the OPLS-DA score plot and the change in trajectory movement of the diseased group towards the healthy group upon treatment.

1. Introduction

The new understanding of obesity and its related disorders has resulted in a renewed interest in finding antiobesity agents from nature, with partial success [1]. An established antiobesity agent, such as green tea polyphenols, is one of the few plants extracts reported to reduce weight in both animals and human subjects [2–4]. Others include extracts of Nomame Herba, cocoa, and chitin/chitosan [5–7]. While these studies yielded significant information on the effect of those plants on diet induced obesity and its biochemical changes, the overall effect on metabolic responses is relatively unknown.

Metabolomics as a new bioanalytical technique in obesity research is still largely unexplored. This "omics" technique is concerned with the high throughput identification and quantification of small molecules (<1500 Da) in the metabolome, the collection of small metabolites present in a cell, organ, or organism [8]. So far, the main application of the metabolomics approach has been in toxicological and pharmaceutical research, having the potential of "bridging Traditional Chinese Medicine (TCM) and molecular pharmacology" [9]. Metabolomics has been applied for extracts characterisation and quality control of herbal supplements [10]. In regard to disease biomarkers discovery, metabolomics, in combination with multivariate data analysis, has been used for the profiling of various biofluids [11, 12]. More specifically to obesity research, it has been used to discriminate between metabolites of the obese models and the healthy models [13–15]. Metabolites such as betaine, taurine, acetone/acetoacetate, phenylacetylglycine, pyruvate, lactate, and citrate were the main discriminating metabolites between the obese and lean groups [13]. There is also the emerging trend of using metabolomics as a platform to study the holistic efficacy of traditional medicine. ^{1}H NMR based metabolomics approach was used to assess the effect of Xue-Fu-Zhu-Yu decoction (XFZYD) on high fat diet induced hyperlipidemia in rats. Metabolomics analysis of the plasma, combined with multivariate data analysis, revealed that XFZYD improved hyperlipidemia by regulating major metabolic pathways such as decreasing the accumulation of ketone bodies, enhancing glutathione biosynthesis, and reversing disturbances in lipid and energy metabolism [16].

Morinda citrifolia L., commonly called noni or Indian Mulberry, was discovered by the Polynesians more than 2000 years ago and brought to southeast Asia during migration [17]. Different parts of the plant have a long history of safe use and were reported to have many health promoting properties [18] including antidyslipidemic effects in rats [19] and inhibition of digestive and metabolic lipases *in vitro* [20–22]. We recently showed (results under publication) that a rutin rich extract of *Morinda citrifolia* leaves (MLE60) prevented weight and fat mass gain in lean Sprague-Dawley rats fed with a high fat diet with an improvement in plasma lipids, leptin, and insulin profiles and increased fecal fat output.

In this study, we assessed the effects of the leaf extract in high fat diet induced obese male Sprague-Dawley rats, using a ^{1}H NMR metabolomics approach, analysing urine and serum for markers metabolites.

2. Methodology

2.1. Preparation of Morinda citrifolia Leaf Extract (MLE 60). Mature *M. citrifolia* leaves were obtained from 5 representative trees from Bukit Expo, Universiti Putra Malaysia, Serdang, Selangor, Malaysia. Voucher specimens were deposited at the herbarium, Institute of Bioscience, Universiti Putra Malaysia (SK2197/13), and species were confirmed as *M. citrifolia* L. The leaves were immediately quenched using liquid nitrogen and lyophilised under pressure (−50°C, 48–72 hours, LABONCO, Labonco Corporation, Kansas City, Missouri, USA) until constant weight. The dried plant sample was ground using a commercial grinder, sieved, and stored at −80°C until further use.

Dried plant materials were extracted with 60% ethanol at room temperature for 72 hours. Filtrate was collected every 24 hours and the pooled filtrate was rotary-evaporated under vacuum until being concentrated. The aqueous phase was

frozen at −80°C and lyophilised under pressure (−50°C, 48 hours) and stored at −80°C until future use. Extracts were prepared by dissolving weighed amount of extract in 0.03% carboxymethyl cellulose (CMC).

2.2. Animal Experiment. Male Sprague-Dawley rats (3 weeks old) were purchased from Sapphire Enterprise, Malaysia, and acclimatized for 10 days under standard laboratory conditions (12 h light/dark cycle, 55–60% relative humidity, 23–25°C). After acclimatization, rats were randomly divided into 2 groups based on assigned diets: standard rat chow (Gold Coin, Malaysia) and a high saturated fat diet for 12 weeks (MP Diets, USA). The body weight of each rat in both groups was recorded weekly to ensure development of obesity in the HFD group. After 12 weeks of the assigned diet, rats in the HFD group were then further divided into the following groups (*n* = 6), based on supplementation or nonsupplementation with MLE 60/Orlistat, and rats in both HFD and ND groups were continued on their respective diets:

(i) ND: normal diet only.

(ii) HFD: high fat diet only.

(iii) HFD + 250: high fat diet + 250 mg/kg body weight MLE 60.

(iv) HFD + 500: high fat diet + 500 mg/kg body weight MLE 60.

(v) HFD + OR: high fat diet + 30 mg/kg body weight Orlistat.

Orlistat, the currently available pancreatic lipase inhibitor, was used as positive control. An overview of the experiment is given in Figure 1.

2.3. Administration of MLE 60. Animals were allowed their respective diets *ad libitum* and required dosage of MLE 60 was given through gastric intubation. Volume of extracts given per day did not exceed 3 mL. Control groups (ND and HFD) received the vehicle (0.03% CMC) through gastric intubation. Body weight and food intake of each rat were recorded weekly.

2.4. Urine, Serum, and Feces Collection. Animals were placed in individual metabolic cages at the initial, middle, and final stages of the experiment. Urine was collected over 24 hours in tubes containing 1% sodium azide, transferred to urine specimen bottles, and stored at −80°C until being analysed. Blood samples were collected by cardiac puncture and serum and plasma samples were separated at 1500 ×g for 15 minutes and stored at −80°C for further analysis. Feces were collected and stored in airtight containers at −80°C for further analysis.

2.5. Sacrifice of Animals. After 12 weeks of obesity induction and 9 weeks of treatment, animals were weighed and sacrificed by cardiac puncture under an anaesthetic effect (xylazine + ketamine). Rats were deprived of food for 12 h prior to sacrifice. Serum and plasma samples were separated at 1500 ×g for 15 minutes and stored at −80°C

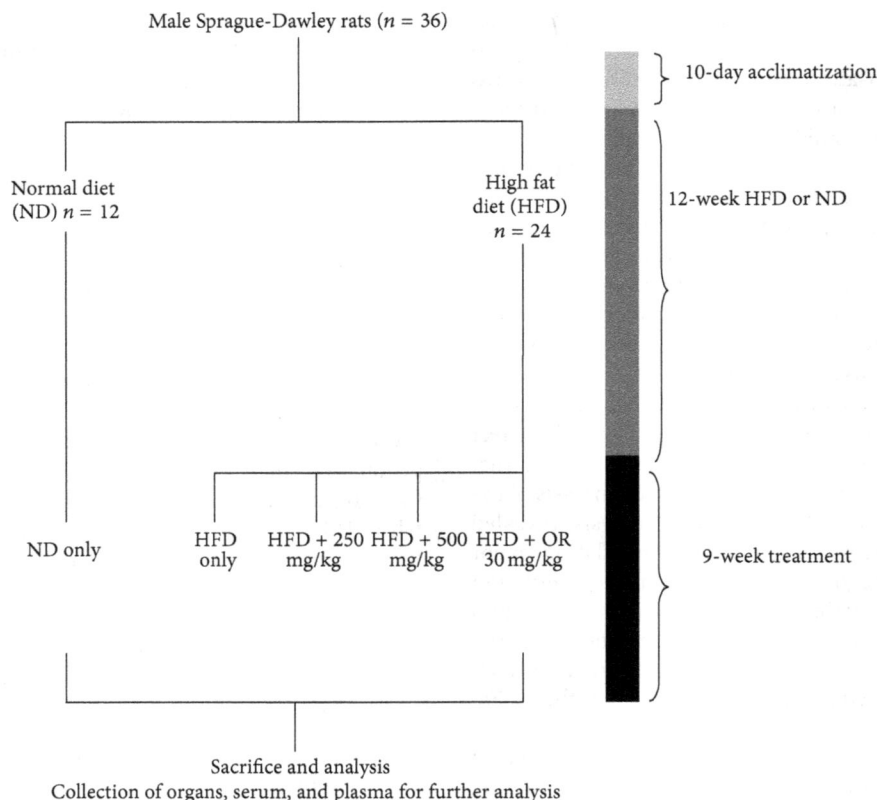

FIGURE 1: Schematic diagram of the experimental design to assess the antiobesity effect of MLE 60 in HFD induced obese male Sprague-Dawley rats.

for further analysis. All animals were handled according to the international principles of the Use and Handling of Experimental Animals (United States National Institute of Health, 1985) and all the protocols were approved by the Animal House and Use Committee of the Faculty of Medicine and Health Sciences, Universiti Putra Malaysia (Approval number UPM/FPSK/PADS/BR.UUH/00462).

2.6. Clinical Chemistry Measurements.
Various biochemical parameters were measured, including blood glucose (One Touch Basic glucose monitor, LifeScan), lipids profiles (Roche Diagnostics GmbH, Sandhofer Strasse, Mannheim), total cholesterol (TC), total triglycerides (TG), low density lipoprotein (LDL), high density lipoprotein (HDL), kidney function tests (creatinine and urea), liver function tests γ-glutamyltransferase (GGT), alanine aminotransferase (ALT), aspartate aminotransferase (AST), alkaline phosphatase (ALP), leptin (RayBio Rat Leptin ELISA kit, Cat# ELR-Leptin-001, Norcross, GA, USA), insulin (Mercodia Rat Insulin ELISA, Uppsala, Sweden), adiponectin (Assay-Max Rat Adiponectin ELISA kit, Cat# ERA2500-1), and ghrelin (RayBio Rat Ghrelin ELISA kit, Cat# EIA-GHR-1, Norcross, GS, USA). All procedures were carried out in accordance with the manufacturers' instruction.

2.7. Determination of Fecal Fat Content.
Fecal lipid content was determined according to a modified method of Tsujita

et al. [23]. Feces were collected at the initial and final stages of the experiment and stored at −80°C until further analysis. Feces (0.5 g) were soaked in 2 mL of deionized water for 24 hours at 4°C, followed by homogenisation by vortexing at high speed for 60 seconds. Lipids were extracted with 7.5 mL of methanol : chloroform (2 : 1, v : v) and shaken for 30 minutes, followed by addition of 2.5 mL of deionized water and 2.5 mL of chloroform and further shaking for 30 minutes. Mixture was then centrifuged at 2000 g for 15 min and the lipophilic layer from the extraction was collected and dried under vacuum. Total fat content was weighed using a laboratory balance.

2.8. ^1H NMR Analysis of Urine and Serum.
^{1}H NMR analysis of urine and serum was carried out following the method of Beckonert et al. [12]. Urine samples were thawed and centrifuged at 12 000 ×g for 10 minutes. 400 μL of the supernatant was mixed with 200 μL phosphate buffer solution consisting of 0.1% of 3-trimethylsilyl propionic-2,2,3,3-d4 acid sodium salt (TSP) as internal standard (adjusted to pH 7.4 using NaOD) and transferred into 5 mm NMR tubes. Spectra were acquired at 27°C on a Varian Unity INOVA 500 MHz spectrometer (Varian Inc., CA), with a frequency of 499.887 MHz. Standard one-dimensional (1D) NOESY-presat pulse sequence was used for suppression of the water peak. For each sample, 64 scans were recorded with an acquisition

time of 1.36 s, pulse width of 3.75 μs, and relaxation delay of 1.0 s.

For serum, thawed samples were centrifuged at 12 000 ×g for 10 minutes and 200 μL of the supernatant was mixed with 400 μL of phosphate buffer containing 0.2% TSP and transferred into 5 mm NMR tubes. In addition to the NOESY-preset experiments, water suppressed Carr-Purcell-Meiboom-Gull (CPMG) spin-echo pulse was performed to suppress broad signals from macromolecules. The CPMG spectra were acquired with 128 transients, with an acquisition time of 1.36 s, relaxation delay of 2.0 s, and number of loops of $n = 80$.

Additional two-dimensional ^{1}H-^{1}H J resolved and ^{1}H-^{13}C HMBC analysis was performed to confirm the identity of certain metabolites.

2.9. NMR Spectral Data Reduction and Multivariate Data Analysis.
Chenomx NMR Suite (Chenomx, Calgary, Canada) was used for metabolite identification and quantificaticn. Nonzero filled spectra were manually phased and baseline corrected, calibrated to TSP at 0.00 ppm. Processed spectra (δ 0–10 ppm) were segmented (0.04 ppm) using the profiler module. Residual signals of water (δ 4.75–δ 4.85) and urea (δ 5.50–δ 6.00 ppm) were excluded from analysis. Remaining bins were normalized to the sum of spectral integrals, extracted with Microsoft Excel, and imported into Simca-P software (Umetrics, Umeå, Sweden) for multivariate data analysis.

Multivariate data analysis was performed using the mean centering with Pareto scaling. Principal component analysis (PCA) was selected as the initial clustering method. Partial Least Squares Discriminant Analysis (PLS-DA) was further performed as a supervised pattern recognition analysis, which maximizes the variation between the different groups and identifies variables responsible for the separation. Orthogonal projections to latent structures-discriminant analysis (OPLS-DA) were also performed for biomarkers analysis between the obese and lean groups and any metabolite changes associated with MLE 60 treatment [24].

2.10. Statistical Analysis.
Data are expressed as mean ± standard deviation (SD). Difference between groups was determined by one-way analysis of variance (ANOVA, Minitab Version 14.0). Values were considered to be significantly different at the level of $p < 0.05$. For analysis of fecal fat content (week 6 and week 12) and body weight (before and after treatment), significance was further confirmed with one-sample t-test.

3. Results and Discussion

3.1. Induction of Obesity in Sprague-Dawley Rats Using a High Saturated Fat Diet.
After 12 weeks of either the HFD or the ND, rats on the HFD had significantly higher weight gain as compared to rats on the ND. Sprague-Dawley rats on the HFD put on 157.54 ± 39.54% of their original weight whereas rats on the ND gained 93.34 ± 13.82%. Other obesity related biomarkers such as total triglycerides (TG), total

TABLE 1: The plasma biochemistry of rats fed a normal diet (ND) or a high fat diet (HFD) for 12 weeks to induce obesity.

	ND	HFD
Total cholesterol (mmol/L)	1.28 ± 0.15[a]	1.16 ± 0.09[a]
HDL (mmol/L)	0.99 ± 0.16[a]	0.66 ± 0.08[b]
LDL (mmol/L)	0.28 ± 0.02[a]	0.23 ± 0.03[a]
Triglycerides (mmol/L)	0.43 ± 0.07[a]	0.91 ± 0.15[b]
Leptin (pg/mL)	719.30 ± 150.1[a]	1819.50 ± 150.1[b]
Insulin (μg/L)	0.20 ± 0.02[a]	1.30 ± 0.09[b]
Adiponectin (ng/mL)	7.40 ± 0.50[a]	6.11 ± 0.07[b]
Glucose (mmol/L)	5.68 ± 0.33[a]	6.26 ± 0.13[b]
Urea (μmol/L)	6.26 ± 0.81[a]	5.14 ± 0.80[a]
Creatinine (mmol/L)	55.20 ± 2.17[a]	51.60 ± 2.41[a]
GGT (U/L)	1.00 ± 0.00[a]	6.00 ± 0.84[b]
AST (U/L)	76.36 ± 3.16[a]	75.40 ± 1.29[a]
ALT (U/L)	37.64 ± 5.26[a]	30.82 ± 1.48[b]
ALP (U/L)	69.14 ± 9.98[a]	127.20 ± 5.07[b]

Different small letters indicate significant difference ($p < 0.05$) between ND and HFD groups as shown by analysis of variance (ANOVA) using Minitab Version 14.

cholesterol (TC), low density lipoprotein (LDL), and high density lipoprotein (HDL) levels in the plasma were also affected by the diet intervention (Table 1). Obese rats had lower HDL level (0.65 ± 0.08 mmol/L) as compared to lean rats (0.986 ± 0.16). There was no significant difference in the plasma TC and LDL content in both groups. The TG level was significantly ($p < 0.05$) elevated in the group fed the HFD (0.908±0.15 mmol/L) as compared to rats fed the ND (0.432± 0.07). Obese rats had higher fasting glucose levels than lean rats, though still in the normal range. Other obesity related adipocytic factors such as leptin and insulin were elevated in the obese models. Kidney function tests as measured by plasma urea and creatinine levels appeared normal, with no significant difference between the groups. In terms of liver function, GGT, ALT, and ALP levels were increased in obese rats fed the HFD. Hypercaloric diets ranging from 3.7 to 5.5 kcal/g result in models of obesity, which represent the aetiology of obesity at its best and reproduce its pathophysiological characteristics [25]. The increase in weight gain is gradual as the intervention progresses. Based on the changes in lipid profiles and other plasma biochemistries, our study, which uses HFD containing 36% of total calories from coconut oil, supports the theory that coconut/lard based high fat diets do model the metabolic disorders of human obesity in rodents [26, 27]. More specifically, a hydrogenated coconut oil (HCO) based HFD has previously caused weight gain, increased liver weight, and hyperlipidaemia in rats [28]. Based on the significant increase in body weight and other biochemical parameters measured, we can conclude that high fat diet induced obesity was successfully achieved in male Sprague-Dawley rats after a feeding period of 12 weeks.

3.2. ^{1}H NMR Spectra of Urine and Serum Metabolites of Sprague-Dawley Rats Fed HFD or ND for 12 Weeks.
Representatives of ^{1}H NMR spectra for the serum and urine samples

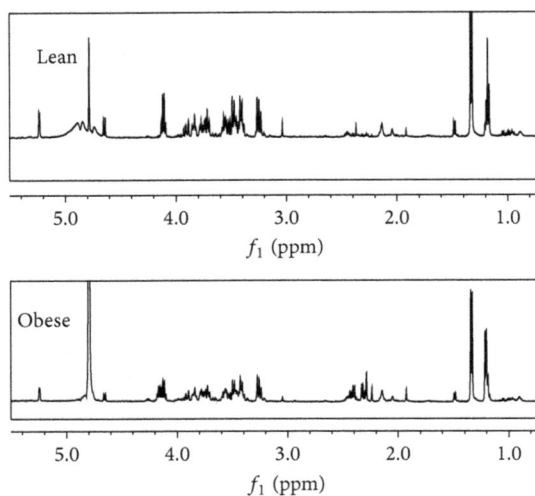

FIGURE 2: Typical 500 MHz ^{1}H NMR spectra of serum collected from a Sprague-Dawley rat fed a normal diet (lean) and a Sprague-Dawley rat fed a high fat diet (obese).

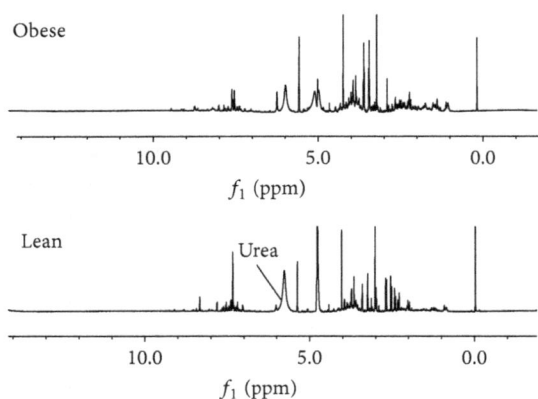

FIGURE 3: Typical 500 MHz ^{1}H NMR spectra of urine collected from a Sprague-Dawley rat fed a high fat diet (obese) and a Sprague-Dawley rat fed a normal diet (lean).

from an obese rat fed HFD and a lean rat fed ND for 12 weeks are shown in Figures 2 and 3, respectively. Expanded regions for better comparison are available in Supplementary Data sections in Supplementary Material available online at http://dx.doi.org/10.1155/2016/2391592. Metabolites were assigned based on previous studies [29, 30], the Chenomx NMR Suite, Version 7.7 (Chenomx Inc., Edmonton, AB, Canada), and the Human Urine and Serum Metabolome Databases [31, 32]. Additional two-dimensional ^{1}H-^{1}H J resolved and HMBC analysis was performed to aid in the identification of certain metabolites. A list of the identified metabolites, including their chemical shifts, is represented in Table 2.

CV ANOVA was used to test the significance of the models, whereby significance is achieved with a p value less than 0.05. Both PLS-DA and OPLS-DA models for urine and serum were validated accordingly (Table 3).

TABLE 2: ^{1}H NMR assignments of metabolites in rat's serum and urine.

Metabolites	Assignments	Chemical shifts	Samples
Urea	NH_2	5.78 (s)	U
Phenylacetylglycine	2,6-CH	7.42 (m)	U
	3,5-CH,	7.57 (m)	
	7-CH	7.65 (m)	
	10-CH	7.84 (m)	
Trigonelline	γCH_3	4.43 (s)	U
	C_2H	8.1 (m)	
	C_4H	8.8 (m)	
	C_5H,	9.1 (s)	
Hippurate	CH_2,	3.98 (d)	U
	CH	7.54 (d)	
	CH	7.65 (t)	
Acetate	CH_3	1.93 (s)	U, S
Dimethylamine	CH_3	2.71 (s)	U
Citrate	$1/2CH_2$	2.54 (d)	U
	$1/2CH_2$	2.66 (d)	
2-Oxoglutarate	CH_2	2.45 (t)	U
	CH_3	3.02 (t)	
Creatinine	CH_3,	3.06 (s)	U
	CH_2	4.06 (s)	
Lactate	CH_3,	1.34 (d)	U, S
	CH	4.11 (dd)	
B-Glucose	1-CH	4.66 (d)	U, S
α-Glucose	1-CH	5.22 (d)	U, S
Allantoin	CH	5.38 (s)	U
Glycine	CH_2	3.57 (s)	U
Taurine	CH_2S,	3.26 (t)	U, S
	CH_2-N	3.40 (t)	
TMAO	$N(CH_3)_3$	3.26 (s)	U
Alanine	βCH_3,	3.78 (dd)	S
	αCH	1.48 (d)	
Pyruvate	βCH_3	2.38 (s)	S
Succinate	CH	2.41 (s)	S
Acetoacetate	CH_3	2.27 (s)	S
3-Hydroxybutyrate	γCH_3	1.18 (d)	S
	βCH	4.23 (m)	
	αCH_2	2.31 (d)	
	αCH_2	2.38 (dd)	
2-Hydroxyisobutyrate	CH_3	1.34 (s)	S
Lipoprotein	$CH_3(CH_2)_n$	0.89 (m)	S
LDL/VLDL	$CH_3CH_2CH_2C=$	1.2–1.30 (m)	S

s: singlet; d: doublet; t: triplet; dd: doublet of doublets; m: multiplet.
S: serum; U: urine.

The variable importance in project (VIP) plots were generated to identify metabolites contributing significantly to the separation of the obese and the lean groups. A cut-off value of 0.7-0.8 for the VIP is generally acceptable. In this study, the cut-off value was set at 1.0 [24].

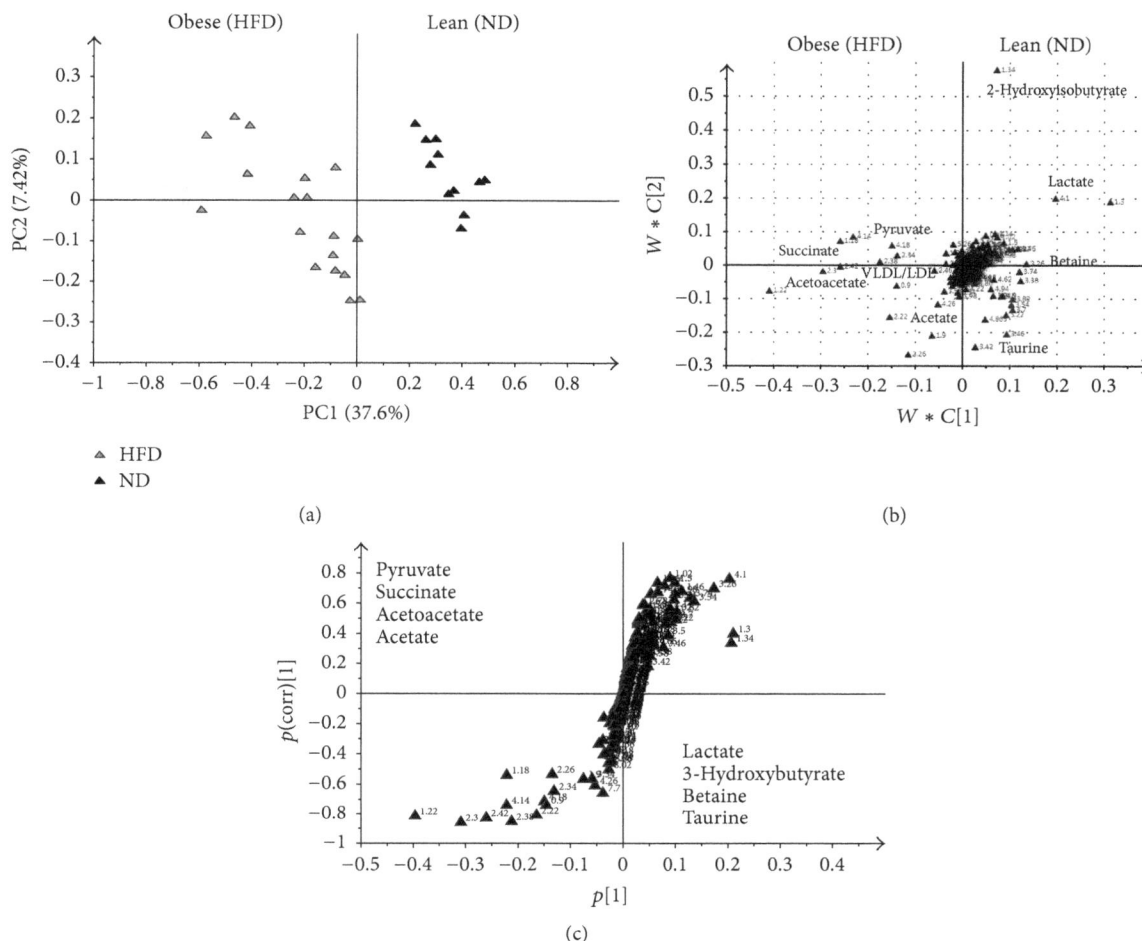

FIGURE 4: OPLS-DA derived score plot (a), loading plot (b), and S plot (c) obtained using ^{1}H NMR data for serum samples from Sprague-Dawley rats fed a high fat diet (HFD) or a normal diet (ND) for 12 weeks.

TABLE 3: PLSDA and OPLS-DA models validation for serum and urine of Sprague-Dawley rats fed a high fat diet (HFD) or a normal diet (ND) for 12 weeks.

Samples/models	R^2Y	Q^2Y	p CV ANOVA	Number of components
Serum				
PLS-DA	0.830	0.752	3.32×10^{-6}	2
OPLS-DA	0.987	0.936	4.26×10^{-7}	2
Urine				
PLS-DA	0.917	0.874	3.18×10^{-12}	3
OPLS-DA	0.959	0.923	1.89×10^{-12}	3

An OPLS-DA model was used to identify discriminating metabolites between the 2 groups fed the different diets. The OPLS-DA method is useful for biomarkers identification. The S plot was further used to visualise the influence of the variables in the model by considering both covariance $p(1)$ and correlation $p(corr)$ loadings profiles from the OPLS-DA model. This enables filtering interesting metabolites in

the projection. Ideal biomarkers have high magnitude and reliability values (Figures 4 and 5).

Induction of obesity was associated with increased serum levels of acetate, succinate, pyruvate, VLDL/LDL, and acetoacetate and decreased levels of lactate, 2-hydroxyisobutyrate, and betaine, among others (Figure 4). The same principle was applied to the analysis of urine and clear separation was obvious in the ^{1}H NMR profiles (Figure 5). Among the increased metabolites in the HFD group were the levels of creatinine, allantoin, taurine, and phenylacetylglycine, while the levels of 2-oxoglutarate, dimethylamine, citrate, and hippurate were decreased.

After 12 weeks of feeding on the HFD, male Sprague-Dawley rats had a significantly ($p < 0.05$) higher increase in body weight as compared to rats fed ND. Obese rats had higher plasma level of TG and lower level of HDL as compared to their lean counterparts. TC and LDL levels were not significantly changed in the 2 groups fed ND and HFD. ^{1}H NMR analysis of urine and serum revealed additional metabolic changes, beyond the measured small set of parameters. OPLS-DA analysis of serum ^{1}H NMR spectra revealed increased succinate, pyruvate, VLDL/LDL,

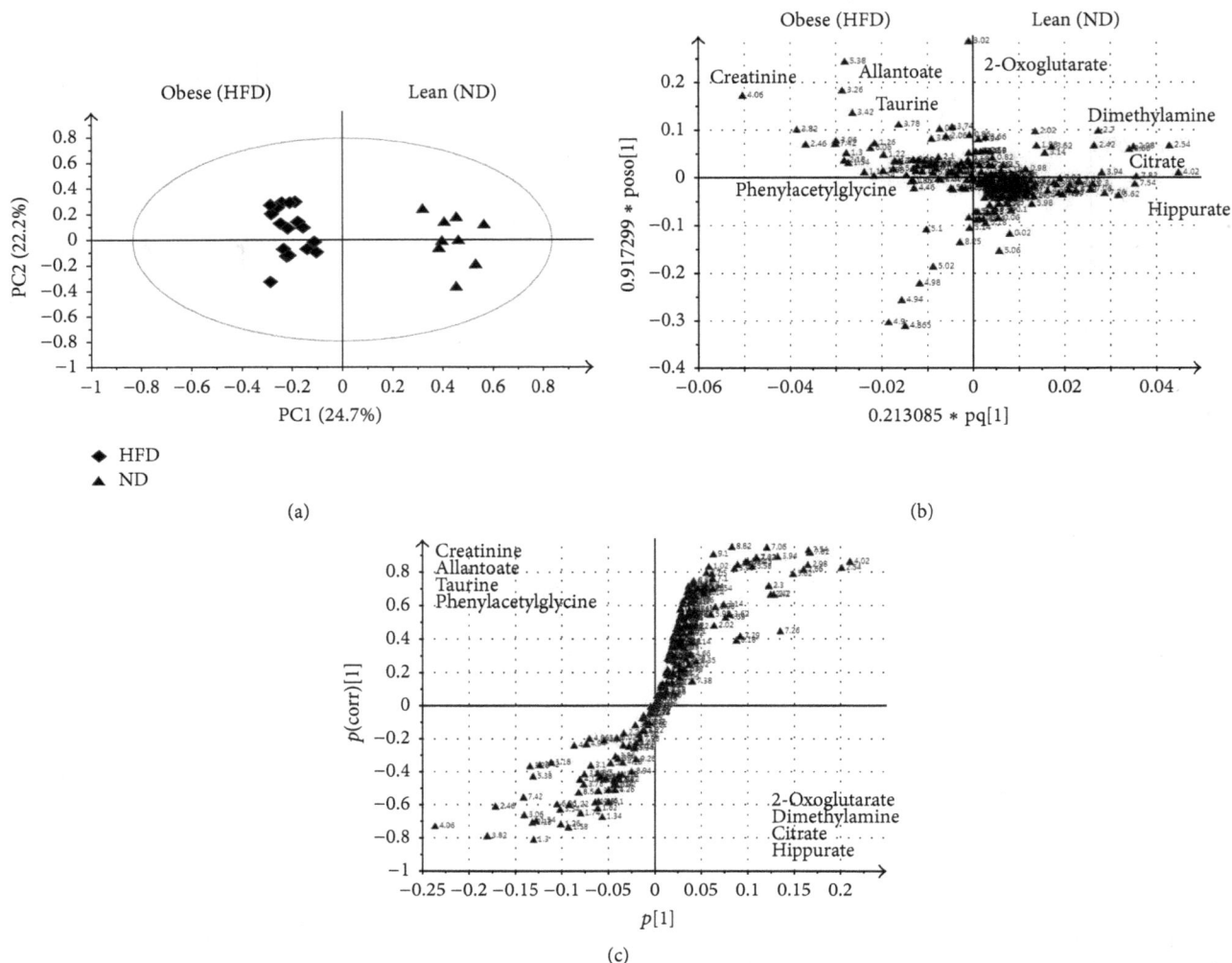

FIGURE 5: OPLS-DA derived score plot (a), loading plot (b), and S plot (c) obtained using ^{1}H NMR data for urine samples from Sprague-Dawley rats fed a high fat diet (HFD) or a normal diet (ND) for 12 weeks.

and acetoacetate and decreased lactate, betaine, and taurine levels in the HFD group. OPLS-DA analysis of urine samples showed that rats fed HFD had higher urinary content of creatinine, allantoin, taurine, and phenylacetylglycine and decreased levels of 2-oxoglutarate, dimethylamine, citrate, and hippurate.

All of these identified metabolites are related to various metabolic pathways, namely, the glucose metabolism and tricarboxylic acid (TCA) cycle, lipid metabolism, choline metabolism, amino acids metabolism, and creatinine metabolism.

Glucose Metabolism and TCA Cycle. Obese rats had higher succinate, pyruvate, acetoacetate, and acetate levels and decreased levels of lactate, 2-oxoglutarate, and citrate, all metabolites related to the glucose metabolism and the TCA cycle. These findings are consistent with other reports on the metabolomics studies of obesity [14, 33, 34]. This current study showed decreased serum lactate in obese rats fed HFD for 12 weeks, which is similar to the study of Song et al. [16]

where hyperlipidemic mice fed HFD had decreased level of lactate. The urine of Zucker rats and the serum of HFD mice also had lower lactate content than the normal weight rats and the serum [14, 35]. The reduced lactate levels can be explained by factors other than HFD induced obesity, including young age and activity [36].

HFD induced obese rats had lower urinary content of 2-oxoglutarate and citrate as compared to the lean rats. Previously, Schirra et al. [37] reported a decreased level of 2-oxoglutarate in 2 mutants groups studied for altered liver metabolism. The level of citrate in the plasma is regulated by insulin, glucose levels, fatty acid utilization, and cholesterol synthesis [38] and is usually increased in HFD obese models [39] and diabetic models [40]. However, consistent with our findings, HFD induced rodents have decreased urinary citrate levels [37] which is associated with insulin resistance in humans [41]. Independent measurement of plasma insulin in this study showed a 6-fold increase in the insulin level of HFD fed obese rats (1.29 μg/L) as opposed to the ND fed lean rats (0.21 μg/L), which indicates that the HFD not only induced obesity in the rodents, but also caused the model to be insulin resistant, most likely caused by decreased urinary citrate excretion due to an increase in metabolic acidosis [42].

With lactate being the precursor for gluconeogenesis, any fluctuation in lactate levels indicates perturbations in glucose production and lipid synthesis in the liver [43]. The downregulation of pyruvate dehydrogenase phosphatase in obese subjects has been reported to be a defect, which signals insulin resistance [44]. Elevated concentrations of pyruvate suggest increased glycogenolysis and glycolysis to meet exceeding energy demands, similarly to the observation of serum profile of obese growing pigs [45].

Lipid Metabolism. The levels of betaine and taurine were changed as a result of the HFD, revealing changes in lipid metabolic pathways. Serum profiles showed lower levels of taurine, while there was an increased level of urinary taurine content. Previous studies have reported reduced taurine content in the serum, urine, and liver of various rodent models [14]. However, also in accordance with our findings, Kim et al. [13] reported increased levels of taurine in the urine of HFD fed rats. Taurine plays various biological roles in the conjugation of cholesterol, antioxidation of bile acids, osmoregulation, and calcium signalling pathways [46, 47]. The supplementation of taurine showed amelioration in obesity most likely mediated by the ability of taurine to increase fatty acid oxidation [48]. This study shows decreased taurine in the obese group, suggesting decreased fatty acids oxidation and inhibition of taurine biosynthetic enzymes related to obesity, as observed by increased levels of LDL/VLDL shown in both serum spectra and actual measured values.

Choline Metabolism. Pertaining to choline metabolism, the level of betaine was decreased in the HFD group, similarly to most metabolomics based obesity studies reporting decreased hepatic and urinary betaine content in HFD fed rodents [33, 34] and decreased hippurate in the serum of HFD mice [38]. In humans, lowered betaine levels are associated with obesity related disorders such as metabolic disorders, lipid disorders, and type 2 diabetes [49]. Supplementation of betaine causes increase in metabolites in the carnitine biosynthesis pathway, reduced accumulation of triglycerides in the liver, with no effect on body weight gain and increase in adipose tissue mass [50].

Creatinine Metabolism. Feeding of HFD diet for 12 weeks resulted in increased creatinine levels in the urine samples, in line with other reports [37, 51, 52].

Amino Acids Metabolism. High level of serum acetoacetate might be the indication of depletion in leucine level, an amino acid involved in insulin signalling, protein synthesis of muscle mass, and production of alanine and glutamine [53]. Alanine peaks were more prominent in the serum spectra of the lean rats as compared to obese subjects.

Gut Microbiome Metabolism. Changes in specific metabolites support the idea that there is a link between obesity and the gut microbiome. HFD induced obese rats showed high urinary content of phenylacetylglycine and decreased levels of hippurate and dimethylamines, metabolites involved in the gut microbiome metabolism. Hippurate is produced in the gut by microorganisms using glycine and benzoic acid as building blocks [54]. Increased hippurate level in the urine has been associated with leanness [34] and this study confirms the findings from other studies [38] that HFD induced obesity is associated with decreased urinary level of hippurate in rodent models of obesity. Increased levels of phenylacetylglycine in Sprague-Dawley rats fed HFD have been previously reported [13]. High gainers fed HFD were associated with increased levels of phenylacetylglycine as compared to low gainers on ND, which indicates an increase in the precursors produced by gut microorganisms [55]. Moreover, reduced dimethylamine levels in the obese group reflect changes in the gut microbiome derived metabolism, similarly to what is observed in leptin-deficient ob/ob mice [56]. Trigonelline was also identified in the urine samples of lean rats. It is an indicator of niacin metabolism, an essential vitamin needed as coenzyme in carbohydrate and lipid metabolism. The body's requirements for niacin can be met by dietary intake or endogenous biosynthesis through tryptophan-mediated metabolism carried out by the liver and the gut microorganisms [57]. Obesity related stress causes depletion in the glutathione stores and the decrease of trigonelline is related to depletion of S-adenosylmethionine, used to make up the energy stores [58]. A strong link between human gut microbiome and obesity was established with decreased urinary excretion of hippurate, trigonelline, and xanthine and increased urinary excretion of 2-hydroxybutyrate and bariatric surgery induced weight loss resulted in the loss of typical obese metabotype [59].

3.3. Effect of 9-Week Treatment with 250/500 mg/kg of MLE in the Obese Rats Models. After 12 weeks of inducing obesity, rats on the HFD were further divided and received either MLE 60 (250 and 500 mg/kg), Orlistat (30 mg/kg), or the carrier vehicle (CMC). Obese rats were kept on the HFD while lean rats were continued on the ND. Body weight and food intake were recorded weekly and the plasma biochemistry was analysed at the end of the experiment (Table 4).

Although there was no significant weight loss in the obese group, receiving MLE 60 or Orlistat, further weight gain was prevented in the HFD + 500 and HFD + OR group. Treatment resulted in reduced visceral fat, with the HFD group having the highest amount (6.62 ± 1.54%). The treated groups had a reduced % of visceral fat ranging from 3.34 ± 0.99 for the HFD + OR group to 4.87 ± 0.96% for the HFD + 500 group. There was no significant difference in decrease of visceral fat between the obese rats receiving 500 mg/kg MLE 60 and rats receiving standard antiobesity drug, Orlistat. No significant difference was recorded in the daily food intake among all groups. At baseline (before treatment), there was no significant difference in the fecal fat excretion in the lean and obese rats. Treatment with 500 mg/kg MLE increased the fecal fat excretion (12.64 ± 1.73%), with a comparable effect to treatment with Orlistat (15.89 ± 1.62%). The fecal fat content

TABLE 4: The body weight, % visceral fat, food intake, % fecal fat excretion, and plasma biochemistry of HFD induced obese rats after 9 weeks of treatment with MLE 60 at 250 mg/kg and 500 mg/kg body and 30 mg Orlistat/kg body weight.

	HFD	HFD + 250	HFD + 500	HFD + OR	ND
Body weight (g)					
Initial (week 12)	559.20 ± 25.89^{Bb}	546.85 ± 83.20^{Bb}	544.29 ± 78.74^{Bb}	537.25 ± 93.83^{Bb}	379.33 ± 34.82^{Aa}
Final (week 21)	614.20 ± 131.58^{Bb}	605.57 ± 101.50^{Bb}	565.85 ± 87.47^{Bb}	553.13 ± 98.93^{Bb}	417.16 ± 32.99^{Aa}
Visceral fat (%)	6.62 ± 1.54^{c}	5.18 ± 0.40^{bc}	4.87 ± 0.963^{b}	3.34 ± 0.99^{b}	1.70 ± 0.28^{a}
Food intake (g/rat/day)	20.00 ± 3.09^{a}	19.08 ± 2.29^{a}	19.38 ± 2.01^{a}	19.08 ± 0.86^{a}	20.17 ± 1.35^{a}
Fecal fat content (%)					
Initial	6.18 ± 1.19^{aA}	7.35 ± 1.14^{aA}	6.31 ± 1.40^{aA}	6.12 ± 1.52^{aA}	7.64 ± 0.70^{aA}
Final	7.23 ± 1.01^{aC}	9.44 ± 1.07^{aC}	12.64 ± 1.73^{bB}	15.89 ± 1.62^{bA}	8.99 ± 0.61^{aC}
Total cholesterol (mmol/L)	1.43 ± 0.08^{b}	1.04 ± 0.01^{a}	0.94 ± 0.02^{a}	0.92 ± 0.07^{a}	1.29 ± 0.13^{b}
HDL (mmol/L)	0.82 ± 0.06^{b}	0.57 ± 0.12^{bc}	0.69 ± 0.07^{b}	0.56 ± 0.01^{c}	1.02 ± 0.09^{a}
LDL (mmol/L)	0.33 ± 0.07^{b}	0.22 ± 0.03^{ab}	0.17 ± 0.03^{a}	0.20 ± 0.04^{a}	0.21 ± 0.05^{a}
Triglycerides (mmol/L)	0.93 ± 0.16^{c}	0.72 ± 0.12^{bc}	0.50 ± 0.11^{ab}	0.58 ± 0.01^{ab}	0.42 ± 0.09^{a}
Leptin (pg/mL)	2119.50 ± 176.3^{b}	1563.30 ± 556.9^{ab}	1050.00 ± 229.3^{a}	1263.30 ± 30.10^{a}	1125.00 ± 117.60^{a}
Insulin (μg/L)	1.83 ± 0.10^{c}	0.71 ± 0.01^{b}	0.37 ± 0.13^{a}	0.47 ± 0.22^{ab}	0.31 ± 0.01^{a}
Ghrelin (ng/mL)	25.7 ± 3.71^{c}	54.57 ± 4.19^{a}	35.74 ± 1.68^{b}	37.63 ± 0.98^{b}	53.01 ± 1.95^{a}
Adiponectin (ng/mL)	8.61 ± 0.77^{b}	9.50 ± 0.23^{ab}	9.25 ± 0.50^{ab}	8.25 ± 0.44^{b}	9.87 ± 0.20^{a}
Glucose (mmol/L)	7.70 ± 0.78^{c}	6.85 ± 0.71^{bc}	5.83 ± 0.53^{ab}	4.98 ± 0.17^{a}	6.03 ± 0.17^{b}

Different small letters indicate significant difference ($p < 0.05$) between different groups and different capital letters indicate significant difference among the same group at different time points, as shown by analysis of variance (ANOVA) using Minitab Version 14.

in the control group (HFD only) remained unchanged after 9 weeks (7.23 ± 1.01%).

Few plasma parameters were measured after 9 weeks of treatment (Table 4). With regard to lipid profiles, treatment with both 500 mg MLE 60/kg and Orlistat improved the plasma LDL level, reducing its levels to the LDL profile of lean rats. The treatment, however, failed to improve HDL levels, with the HFD + OR group having the lowest plasma HDL content of 0.56 ± 0.01 mmol/L. Lean rats on the ND have the highest level of HDL, 1.02 ± 0.09 mmol/L. The most marked effect was in the TG content, whereby HFD + 500 (0.50±0.11) significantly improved the plasma TG level as compared to rats receiving the HFD only (0.93 ± 0.12).

The plasma insulin level was significantly improved in the HFD + 500 group (0.37 ± 0.13), which was similar to the ND group (0.31 ± 0.02). Similarly, plasma leptin levels were significantly improved in both HFD + 500 group (1050 ± 229 pg/mL) and HFD + OR group (1263 ± 30.10 pg/mL) as compared with the HFD group (2119 ± 176 pg/mL). Ghrelin levels were improved in all treated groups, with 250 mg/kg dosage being more potent, restoring the ghrelin levels to 54.57 ng/mL, not significantly different from the lean group (53.01 ng/mL). Adiponectin levels were not significantly different in the lean groups and the treated groups (9.25–9.87 ng/mL), except in the group treated with Orlistat (8.25 ng/mL), where the adiponectin level was not significantly different from the obese group (8.61 ng/mL). Treatment with 30 mg/kg Orlistat and 500 mg/kg MLE 60 had the most significant improvement.

In the previous section, rats fed HFD were associated with higher acetate and pyruvate and surprisingly lower lactate levels as opposed to lean rats fed ND. After an additional 9 weeks, rats fed HFD were still associated with higher acetate and pyruvate and also higher lactate level. Lactate is one of the key metabolites related to glucose metabolism and the TCA cycle, which has been reported to be higher in obese humans [60]. Increased lactate concentration has been attributed to the upregulation in anaerobic glycolysis in obese subjects and the balance between lactate production and lactate removal [14, 61]. The adipose tissue is one of the sites of lactate production, together with the skeletal muscles, erythrocytes, and brain [61, 62]. Increased lactate production can also reflect perturbations in glucose and lipid production in the liver due to the involvement of lactate as a precursor in gluconeogenesis [43] with increased serum lactate being associated with increased risk of mortality [63]. In this study, increased serum lactate in the HFD group can be attributed to the higher percentage of body fat as compared to the lean rats. Lactate levels in obese subjects are also highly dependent on insulin resistance [64]. In a study by Chen et al., normal weight subjects with normal blood glucose had the lowest plasma lactate levels, obese subjects with normal blood glucose had intermediate plasma lactate levels, and obese subjects with impaired blood glucose had the highest lactate levels. Consistent with these reports, this study shows that, after 21 weeks of feeding HFD, rats had higher insulin levels (1.83 μg/L) as compared to after 12 weeks of feeding (1.30 μg/L), which explains the elevated lactate levels in the obese groups. Treated groups had significant decrease in % of body fat and plasma insulin levels, which contributes to the decreased lactate plasma content [65].

Another metabolite, which was found to be strongly associated with obesity, is 2-hydroxyisobutyrate. It is involved in the gut microbiome metabolism and has been reported to

TABLE 5: Relative quantification of significant discriminating metabolites based on the concentration of 0.1% of 3-trimethylsilyl propionic-2,2,3,3-d4 acid sodium salt (TSP) as internal standard and quantified using Chenomx NMR Suite.

Metabolites	Chemical shifts	VIP value	HFD	ND	HFD + 250	HFD + OR	p value
Lactate	1.34 (d) 4.11 (dd)	2.46	1662.9 ± 51.9[c]	493.4 ± 73.1[a]	482.1 ± 55.9[a]	761.0 ± 33.6[b]	0.000
Alanine	3.78 (dd) 1.48 (d)	1.63	94.0 ± 3.03[b]	53.3 ± 13.48[a]	55.6 ± 3.52[a]	47.0 ± 2.50[a]	0.002
3-Hydroxybutyrate	1.18 (d) 4.23 (m) 2.31 (d) 2.38 (dd)	3.48	316.8 ± 23.17[b]	513.8 ± 74.20[a]	368.7 ± 24.00[ab]	396.9 ± 73.54[ab]	0.023
2-Hydroxyisobutyrate	1.34 (s)	5.60	232.5 ± 25.36[b]	153.8 ± 15.12[a]	143.9 ± 21.54[a]	182.1 ± 49.43[ab]	0.036
Pyruvate	2.38 (s)	2.19	55.6 ± 3.62[c]	18.7 ± 2.16[a]	31.1 ± 1.03[b]	28.3 ± 7.21[b]	0.000
Creatinine/creatine	3.06 (s) 4.06 (s)	1.28	45.1 ± 2.43[b]	25.6 ± 3.64[a]	23.3 ± 0.60[a]	39.5 ± 0.04[b]	0.000
α-Glucose	5.22 (d)	1.09	1116.4 ± 27.4[c]	458.1 ± 27.6[b]	511.7 ± 20.6[b]	206.4 ± 44.3[a]	0.000
Acetate	1.93 (s)	1.28	38.9 ± 2.80[b]	26.8 ± 4.42[a]	35.4 ± 1.50[b]	38.9 ± 2.61[b]	0.013

Different small letters indicate significant difference ($p < 0.05$) between different groups as shown by the analysis of variance (ANOVA) using Minitab Version 14.

be altered in leptin-deficient ob/ob mice [56] and increased in obese patients [66].

Regarding amino acid metabolism, serum alanine was increased in HFD group as compared to the lean group, in line with previous studies reporting increased alanine in the serum and liver of HFD induced mice and rats [39].

Obesity was characterised by decreased levels of 3-hydroxybutyrate, a metabolite of amino acid metabolism, which is associated with leanness and weight loss, where obese patients expressed the highest 3-hydroxybutyrate levels following bariatric surgery [66]. Early studies have also reported on the link between obesity and 3-hydroxybutyrate. Administration of the compound in obese subjects on low energy diets resulted in improved fat : lean ratio while not affecting weight loss [67]. The roles of acetoacetate and 3-hydroxybutyrate were further studied in obese and insulin dependent diabetic humans using a kinetic approach, to investigate ketone body metabolism. Obese subjects had lower ketone body de novo synthesis, with no significant clearance of 3-hydroxybutyrate from the normal healthy subjects, with 3-hydroxybutyrate being an important determinant in diabetic ketoacidosis [68]. Moreover, 3-hydroxybutyrate has also been associated with reduced food intake in obese subjects [69] and involved in the short-term and long-term effects of high fat diet in mice [14]. Won et al. also reported the downregulation of 2-hydroxybutyrate in both male and female leptin-deficient ob/ob mice [56].

In the metabolites identification, OPLS-DA model consisting of 2 groups at a time was employed, followed by the Shared and Unique Structure (SUS) plots, to compare biomarkers from 2 models.

Key discriminating metabolites as potential biomarkers in rat serum based on ^{1}H NMR loading plots in the HFD, HFD + 500, and ND groups were quantified, relative to the TSP in the serum samples. Statistical analysis (Minitab Version 14) was further employed to detect significance.

Focus was placed on metabolites with a VIP value of >1, as metabolites contributing more to the clustering of the different groups (Table 5).

There are limited studies, which have used a metabolomics approach to identify metabolic changes following intervention with drugs and therapeutics, including the phytochemical strategies for obesity, though the potential is vast [70]. However, there are few metabolomics based reports on weight loss as a result of weight loss intervention, including exercise and surgery. An energy-restricted diet for 8 weeks resulted in an improvement in glucose and lipid metabolism in overweight obese adults. Saturated fatty acids such as palmitic acid and stearic acid were significantly decreased as well as branched amino acid, isoleucine [71]. A lifestyle intervention in obese children, "Obeldicks," resulted in significant weight loss and abdominal obesity, modulated by the role of phosphatidylcholine metabolism. This particular study also highlights the large interindividual variation to lifestyle intervention and the possible need of a more individualised approach to lifestyle interventions [72]. ^{1}H NMR analysis also showed that while exercise can improve the metabolic disruptions associated with diet induced obesity, the effect cannot be cancelled out and diet predicts obesity better with a stronger influence on metabolites' profiles than exercise alone [14].

One of the few studies reporting the response of natural therapeutic agents in obese subjects assessed the effect of sea buckhorn and bilberry on serum metabolites in overweight women. No significant changes were observed in individual metabolites, though improvements in serum lipids and lipoproteins were observed [73]. The treatment of high fat diet induced hyperlipidemia with Xue-Fu-Zhu-Yu decoction was studied using a NMR based metabolomics approach. OPLS-DA analysis revealed the beneficial effects of the decoction, mainly through decrease in ketone bodies production, enhancement of biosynthesis, and modulation of lipid metabolism [16]. Dietary intervention of black soybean peptides in overweight human showed an increase in betaine, benzoic acid, pyroglutamic acid, and pipecolic acid, among others. VIP analysis showed L-proline, betaine, and lyso-PCs to be more correlated to the discrimination before and after treatment [74].

Treatment with MLE 60 at 250 mg/kg body weight improved serum levels of lactate, alanine, pyruvate, creatinine, and α-glucose, bringing their levels closer to the normal control whereas the level of 3-hydroxyisobutyrate, 3-hydroxybutyrate, and acetate remained unchanged. Similar improvements were achieved in the groups receiving 30 mg/kg body weight of Orlistat. The relative concentration of α-glucose was found to be most reduced, consistent with the actual biochemical measurement done previously where the Orlistat treated group had significantly lower plasma glucose (4.97 mmol/L) as compared to the lean group (6.02 mmol/L). This is consistent with the literature reporting that Orlistat in a weight loss regimen can significantly improve glucose tolerance and slows down the progression of type 2 diabetes and impaired glucose tolerance in clinical cases of obesity [75, 76].

Based on the relative quantification of certain metabolites (lactate, pyruvate, and glucose) in the treated groups, it is apparent that treatment with MLE 60 improved perturbations in various metabolic pathways, predominantly in the glucose and TCA cycle as reflected by positive modulations in lactate, pyruvate, and glucose levels. Disruptions in the creatinine and amino acid metabolic pathways were also improved as indicated by a reduction of creatinine and alanine accumulation in the obese groups treated with MLE 60. The levels of 3-hydroxyisobutyrate, a metabolite of the gut microbiome metabolism, were unchanged in the treated groups, suggesting that MLE 60 did not impact on the obesity-induced disruptions in the gut microbiome. Similarly, the levels of 2-hydroxybutyrate, a metabolite of amino acid metabolism, were also unchanged.

Obesity has been characterised by an elevated TCA function in diet induced hepatic insulin and fatty liver as well as decreased brain glucose metabolism, predominantly through the TCA cycle [77, 78]. Treatment with MLE 60 improved serum creatinine profiles as shown by ^{1}H NMR measurement as compared to nonsignificance observed when blood creatinine level was measured. Poor creatinine clearance is associated with weight gain and central obesity due to increased metabolic abnormalities as risk factors [79]. An increase in creatine kinase and adenylate kinase 1 activity was observed in obese subjects, attributed to a compensatory effect of the downregulation of muscle mitochondrial function, associated with obesity [80].

Hence, antiobesity agent which can positively influence these pathways as well as other parameters such as adipocytes factors and weight loss shows promise for weight management.

4. Conclusion

Based on the reported health properties of *M. citrifolia*, including the antiobesity activities, the aim of this study was to further explore the effect of a leaf extract, MLE 60, on obesity using a ^{1}H NMR metabolomic approach. ^{1}H NMR spectroscopy and multivariate data analysis revealed clear metabolic differences in the urine and serum samples of the HFD induced obese and lean rats. An OPLS-DA method was chosen to project maximum separation between the groups and to identify discriminating biomarkers. All multivariate models including PLS-DA and OPLS-DA were duly validated, using permutation tests, R^2Y, Q^2Y, and p CV ANOVA values. Several metabolites were identified in both the serum and urine samples, which were the basis of difference among the groups. These metabolites were involved in the glucose metabolism and TCA cycle (lactate, 2-oxoglutarate, citrate, succinate, pyruvate, and acetate), amino acid metabolism (alanine, 2-hydroxybutyrate), choline metabolism (betaine), creatinine metabolism (creatinine), and gut microbiome metabolism (hippurate, phenylacetylglycine, dimethylamine, and trigonelline). Some key metabolites were identified and quantified showing a statistically (p < 0.05) significant improvement in this treated group (500 mg/kg). This study, therefore, confirms the metabolic alteration caused by HFD induced obesity in a rat model and the improvement in certain metabolic pathways, upon treatment with MLE 60. It also provides additional information that ^{1}H NMR metabolomics can be a good approach to study the development of disease and response to treatment in obese subjects.

Conflict of Interests

The authors declare that there is no conflict of interests regarding the publication of this paper.

References

[1] J. W. Yun, "Possible anti-obesity therapeutics from nature—a review," *Phytochemistry*, vol. 71, no. 14-15, pp. 1625–1641, 2010.

[2] A. G. Dulloo, C. Duret, D. Rohrer et al., "Efficacy of a green tea extract rich in catechin polyphenols and caffeine in increasing 24-h energy expenditure and fat oxidation in humans," *The American Journal of Clinical Nutrition*, vol. 70, no. 6, pp. 1040–1045, 1999.

[3] P. Chantre and D. Lairon, "Recent findings of green tea extract AR25 (Exolise) and its activity for the treatment of obesity," *Phytomedicine*, vol. 9, no. 1, pp. 3–8, 2002.

[4] C. Lu, W. Zhu, C.-L. Shen, and W. Gao, "Green tea polyphenols reduce body weight in rats by modulating obesity-related genes," *PLoS ONE*, vol. 7, no. 6, Article ID e38332, 2012.

[5] L.-K. Han, Y. Kimura, and H. Okuda, "Reduction in fat storage during chitin-chitosan treatment in mice fed a high-fat diet," *International Journal of Obesity*, vol. 23, no. 2, pp. 174–179, 1999.

[6] M. Yamamoto, S. Shimura, Y. Itoh, T. Ohsaka, M. Egawa, and S. Inoue, "Anti-obesity effects of lipase inhibitor CT-II, an extract from edible herbs, Nomame Herba, on rats fed a high-fat diet," *International Journal of Obesity*, vol. 24, no. 6, pp. 758–764, 2000.

[7] A. M. M. Jalil, A. Ismail, P. P. Chong, M. Hamid, and S. H. S. Kamaruddin, "Effects of cocoa extract containing polyphenols and methylxanthines on biochemical parameters of obese-diabetic rats," *Journal of the Science of Food and Agriculture*, vol. 89, no. 1, pp. 130–137, 2009.

[8] J. B. German, B. D. Hammock, and S. M. Watkins, "Metabolomics: building on a century of biochemistry to guide human health," *Metabolomics*, vol. 1, no. 1, pp. 3–9, 2005.

[9] M. Wang, R.-J. A. N. Lamers, H. A. A. J. Korthout et al., "Metabolomics in the context of systems biology: bridging traditional Chinese medicine and molecular pharmacology," *Phytotherapy Research*, vol. 19, no. 3, pp. 173–182, 2005.

[10] B. Wu, S. Yan, Z. Lin et al., "Metabonomic study on ageing: NMR-based investigation into rat urinary metabolites and the effect of the total flavone of *Epimedium*," *Molecular BioSystems*, vol. 4, no. 8, pp. 855–861, 2008.

[11] K. S. Solanky, N. J. C. Bailey, B. M. Beckwith-Hall et al., "Application of biofluid ^{1}H nuclear magnetic resonance-based metabonomic techniques for the analysis of the biochemical effects of dietary isoflavones on human plasma profile," *Analytical Biochemistry*, vol. 323, no. 2, pp. 197–204, 2003.

[12] O. Beckonert, H. C. Keun, T. M. D. Ebbels et al., "Metabolic profiling, metabolomic and metabonomic procedures for NMR spectroscopy of urine, plasma, serum and tissue extracts," *Nature protocols*, vol. 2, no. 11, pp. 2692–2703, 2007.

[13] S.-H. Kim, S.-O. Yang, H.-S. Kim, Y. Kim, T. Park, and H.-K. Choi, "^{1}H-nuclear magnetic resonance spectroscopy-based metabolic assessment in a rat model of obesity induced by a high-fat diet," *Analytical and Bioanalytical Chemistry*, vol. 395, no. 4, pp. 1117–1124, 2009.

[14] G. E. Duggan, D. S. Hittel, C. C. Hughey, A. Weljie, H. J. Vogel, and J. Shearer, "Differentiating short- and long-term effects of diet in the obese mouse using ^{1}H-nuclear magnetic resonance metabolomics," *Diabetes, Obesity and Metabolism*, vol. 13, no. 9, pp. 859–862, 2011.

[15] E.-Y. Won, M.-K. Yoon, S.-W. Kim et al., "Gender specific metabolomic profiling of obesity in leptin deficient ob/ob mice by ^{1}H NMR spectroscopy," *PLoS ONE*, vol. 8, no. 10, Article ID e75998, 2013.

[16] X. Song, J. Wang, P. Wang, N. Tian, M. Yang, and L. Kong, "^{1}H NMR-based metabolomics approach to evaluate the effect of Xue-Fu-Zhu-Yu decoction on hyperlipidemia rats induced by high-fat diet," *Journal of Pharmaceutical and Biomedical Analysis*, vol. 78-79, pp. 202–210, 2013.

[17] J. Gerlach, "Native or introduced plant species," *Phelsuma*, vol. 4, pp. 70–74, 1996.

[18] A. R. Dixon, H. McMillen, and N. L. Etkin, "Ferment this: the transformation of Noni, a traditional Polynesian medicine (*Morinda citrifolia*, Rubiaceae)," *Economic Botany*, vol. 53, no. 1, pp. 51–68, 1999.

[19] S.-U. R. Mandukhail, N. Aziz, and A.-H. Gilani, "Studies on antidyslipidemic effects of *Morinda citrifolia* (Noni) fruit, leaves and root extracts," *Lipids in Health and Disease*, vol. 9, article 88, 2010.

[20] M. S. Pak-Dek, A. Abdul-Hamid, A. Osman, and C. S. Soh, "Inhibitory effect of *Morinda citrifolia* L. on lipoprotein lipase activity," *Journal of Food Science*, vol. 73, no. 8, pp. C595–C598, 2008.

[21] N. G. Sahib, A. A. Hamid, D. Kitts, M. Purnama, N. Saari, and F. Abas, "The effects of *Morinda citrifolia*, *Momordica charantia* and *Centella asiatica* extracts on lipoprotein lipase and 3T3-L1 preadipocytes," *Journal of Food Biochemistry*, vol. 35, no. 4, pp. 1186–1205, 2011.

[22] N. Gooda Sahib, A. Abdul Hamid, N. Saari, F. Abas, M. S. Pak Dek, and M. Rahim, "Anti-pancreatic lipase and antioxidant activity of selected tropical herbs," *International Journal of Food Properties*, vol. 15, no. 3, pp. 569–578, 2012.

[23] T. Tsujita, H. Takaichi, T. Takaku, S. Aoyama, and J. Hiraki, "Antiobesity action of epsilon-polylysine, a potent inhibitor of pancreatic lipase," *Journal of Lipid Research*, vol. 47, no. 8, pp. 1852–1858, 2006.

[24] L. Eriksson, E. Johansson, N. Kettanen-Wold, J. Trygg, C. Wikstrom, and S. Wold, *Multi- and Megavariate Data Analysis, Part 1. Basic Principles & Applications*, Umetrics Academy, Umea, Sweden, 2006.

[25] V. Von Diemen, E. N. Trindade, and M. R. M. Trindade, "Experimental model to induce obesity in rats," *Acta Cirurgica Brasileira*, vol. 21, no. 6, pp. 425–429, 2006.

[26] S. C. Woods, R. J. Seeley, P. A. Rushing, D. D'Alessio, and P. Tso, "A controlled high-fat diet induces an obese syndrome in rats," *Journal of Nutrition*, vol. 133, no. 4, pp. 1081–1087, 2003.

[27] R. Buettner, J. Schölmerich, and L. C. Bollheimer, "High-fat diets: modeling the metabolic disorders of human obesity in rodents," *Obesity*, vol. 15, no. 4, pp. 798–808, 2007.

[28] P. Yaqoob, E. J. Sherrington, N. M. Jeffery et al., "Comparison of the effects of a range of dietary lipids upon serum and tissue lipid composition in the rat," *The International Journal of Biochemistry and Cell Biology*, vol. 27, no. 3, pp. 297–310, 1995.

[29] J.-S. Tian, B.-Y. Shi, H. Xiang, S. Gao, X.-M. Qin, and G.-H. Du, "^{1}H-NMR-based metabonomic studies on the anti-depressant effect of genipin in the chronic unpredictable mild stress rat model," *PLoS ONE*, vol. 8, no. 9, Article ID e75721, 2013.

[30] N. Tian, J. Wang, P. Wang, X. Song, M. Yang, and L. Kong, "NMR-based metabonomic study of Chinese medicine Gegen Qinlian Decoction as an effective treatment for type 2 diabetes in rats," *Metabolomics*, vol. 9, no. 6, pp. 1228–1242, 2013.

[31] S. Bouatra, F. Aziat, R. Mandal et al., "The human urine metabolome," *PLoS ONE*, vol. 8, no. 9, Article ID e73076, 2013.

[32] N. Psychogios, D. D. Hau, J. Peng et al., "The human serum metabolome," *PLoS ONE*, vol. 6, no. 2, Article ID e16957, 2011.

[33] N. J. Serkova, M. Jackman, J. L. Brown et al., "Metabolic profiling of livers and blood from obese Zucker rats," *Journal of Hepatology*, vol. 44, no. 5, pp. 956–962, 2006.

[34] A. Waldram, E. Holmes, Y. Wang et al., "Top-down systems biology modeling of host metabotype-microbiome associations in obese rodents," *Journal of Proteome Research*, vol. 8, no. 5, pp. 2361–2375, 2009.

[35] L.-C. Zhao, X.-D. Zhang, S.-X. Liao, H.-Y. Wang, D.-H. Lin, and H.-C. Gao, "A metabonomic comparison of urinary changes in Zucker and GK rats," *Journal of Biomedicine and Biotechnology*, vol. 2010, Article ID 431894, 6 pages, 2010.

[36] A. A. Mahdi, S. Annarao, S. Tripathi et al., "Correlation of age related metabonomic changes in ^{1}H NMR serum and urine profiles of rats with cognitive function," *The Open Magnetic Resonance Journal*, vol. 1, no. 1, pp. 71–76, 2008.

[37] H. J. Schirra, C. G. Anderson, W. J. Wilson et al., "Altered metabolism of growth hormone receptor mutant mice: a combined NMR metabonomics and microarray study," *PLoS ONE*, vol. 3, no. 7, Article ID e2764, 2008.

[38] J. Shearer, G. Duggan, A. Weljie, D. S. Hittel, D. H. Wasserman, and H. J. Vogel, "Metabolomic profiling of dietary-induced insulin resistance in the high fat-fed C57BL/6J mouse," *Diabetes, Obesity and Metabolism*, vol. 10, no. 10, pp. 950–958, 2008.

[39] H. Li, Z. Xie, J. Lin et al., "Transcriptomic and metabonomic profiling of obesity-prone and obesity-resistant rats under high fat diet," *Journal of Proteome Research*, vol. 7, no. 11, pp. 4775–4783, 2008.

[40] D. C. DeVilliers, P. K. Dixit, and A. Lazarow, "Citrate metabolism in diabetes. I. Plasma citrate in alloxan-diabetic rats and in clinical diabetes," *Metabolism*, vol. 15, no. 5, pp. 458–465, 1966.

[41] A. Cupisti, M. Meola, C. D'Alessandro et al., "Insulin resistance and low urinary citrate excretion in calcium stone formers," *Biomedicine & Pharmacotherapy*, vol. 61, no. 1, pp. 86–90, 2007.

[42] G. Souto, C. Donapetry, J. Calviño, and M. M. Adeva, "Metabolic acidosis-induced insulin resistance and cardiovascular risk," *Metabolic Syndrome and Related Disorders*, vol. 9, no. 4, pp. 247–253, 2011.

[43] B. Xie, M. J. Waters, and H. J. Schirra, "Investigating potential mechanisms of obesity by metabolomics," *Journal of Biomedicine and Biotechnology*, vol. 2012, Article ID 805683, 10 pages, 2012.

[44] M. Piccinini, M. Mostert, G. Alberto et al., "Down-regulation of pyruvate dehydrogenase phosphatase in obese subjects is a defect that signals insulin resistance," *Obesity Research*, vol. 13, no. 4, pp. 678–686, 2005.

[45] Q. He, P. Ren, X. Kong et al., "Comparison of serum metabolite compositions between obese and lean growing pigs using an NMR-based metabonomic approach," *Journal of Nutritional Biochemistry*, vol. 23, no. 2, pp. 133–139, 2012.

[46] H. Satoh, "Cardioprotective actions of taurine against intracellular and extracellular calcium-induced effects," *Advances in Experimental Medicine and Biology*, vol. 359, pp. 181–196, 1994.

[47] Y. Nakaya, A. Minami, N. Harada, S. Sakamoto, Y. Niwa, and M. Ohnaka, "Taurine improves insulin sensitivity in the Otsuka Long-Evans Tokushima Fatty rat, a model of spontaneous type 2 diabetes," *American Journal of Clinical Nutrition*, vol. 71, no. 1, pp. 54–58, 2000.

[48] N. Tsuboyama-Kasaoka, C. Shozawa, K. Sano et al., "Taurine (2-aminoethanesulfonic acid) deficiency creates a vicious circle promoting obesity," *Endocrinology*, vol. 147, no. 7, pp. 3276–3284, 2006.

[49] M. Lever and S. Slow, "The clinical significance of betaine, an osmolyte with a key role in methyl group metabolism," *Clinical Biochemistry*, vol. 43, no. 9, pp. 732–744, 2010.

[50] J. Pekkinen, K. Olli, A. Huotari et al., "Betaine supplementation causes increase in carnitine metabolites in the muscle and liver of mice fed a high-fat diet as studied by nontargeted LC-MS metabolomics approach," *Molecular Nutrition & Food Research*, vol. 57, no. 11, pp. 1959–1968, 2013.

[51] M. S. Klein, C. Dorn, M. Saugspier, C. Hellerbrand, P. J. Oefner, and W. Gronwald, "Discrimination of steatosis and NASH in mice using nuclear magnetic resonance spectroscopy," *Metabolomics*, vol. 7, no. 2, pp. 237–246, 2011.

[52] J. B. Walker, "Metabolic control of creatine biosynthesis. II. Restoration of transamidinase activity following creatine repression," *The Journal of Biological Chemistry*, vol. 236, pp. 493–498, 1961.

[53] S. R. Kimball and L. S. Jefferson, "Regulation of protein synthesis by branched-chain amino acids," *Current Opinion in Clinical Nutrition and Metabolic Care*, vol. 4, no. 1, pp. 39–43, 2001.

[54] J. K. Nicholson, E. Holmes, and I. D. Wilson, "Gut microorganisms, mammalian metabolism and personalized health care," *Nature Reviews Microbiology*, vol. 3, no. 5, pp. 431–438, 2005.

[55] A. N. Phipps, J. Stewart, B. Wright, and I. D. Wilson, "Effect of diet on the urinary excretion of hippuric acid and other dietary-derived aromatics in rat. A complex interaction between diet, gut microflora and substrate specificity," *Xenobiotica*, vol. 28, no. 5, pp. 527–537, 1998.

[56] E.-Y. Won, M.-K. Yoon, S.-W. Kim et al., "Gender specific metabolomic profiling of obesity in leptin deficient ob/ob mice by 1H NMR spectroscopy," *PLoS ONE*, vol. 8, no. 10, Article ID e75998, 2013.

[57] S. Rezzi, Z. Ramadan, F.-P. J. Martin et al., "Human metabolic phenotypes link directly to specific dietary preferences in healthy individuals," *Journal of Proteome Research*, vol. 6, no. 11, pp. 4469–4477, 2007.

[58] J. Sun, L. K. Schnackenberg, R. D. Holland et al., "Metabonomics evaluation of urine from rats given acute and chronic doses of acetaminophen using NMR and UPLC/MS," *Journal of Chromatography B*, vol. 871, no. 2, pp. 328–340, 2008.

[59] R. Calvani, A. Miccheli, G. Capuani et al., "Gut microbiome-derived metabolites characterize a peculiar obese urinary metabotype," *International Journal of Obesity*, vol. 34, no. 6, pp. 1095–1098, 2010.

[60] C. B. Newgard, J. An, J. R. Bain et al., "A branched chain amino acid-related metabolic signature that differentiates obese and lean humans and contributes to insulin resistance," *Cell Metabolism*, vol. 9, no. 4, pp. 311–326, 2009.

[61] R. A. Kreisberg, "Glucose-lactate inter-relations in man," *The New England Journal of Medicine*, vol. 287, no. 3, pp. 132–137, 1972.

[62] P.-A. Jansson, A. Larsson, U. Smith, and P. Lönnroth, "Lactate release from the subcutaneous tissue in lean and obese men," *The Journal of Clinical Investigation*, vol. 93, no. 1, pp. 240–246, 1994.

[63] J. Aduen, W. K. Bernstein, T. Khastagir et al., "The use and clinical importance of a substrate-specific electrode for rapid determination of blood lactate concentrations," *The Journal of the American Medical Association*, vol. 272, no. 21, pp. 1678–1685, 2004.

[64] J. Lovejoy, F. D. Newby, S. S. P. Gebhart, and M. DiGirolamo, "Insulin resistance in obesity is associated with elevated basal lactate levels and diminished lactate appearance following intravenous glucose and insulin," *Metabolism*, vol. 41, no. 1, pp. 22–27, 1992.

[65] Y. D. I. Chen, B. B. Varasteh, and G. M. Reaven, "Plasma lactate concentration in obesity and type 2 diabetes," *Diabete et Metabolisme*, vol. 19, no. 4, pp. 348–354, 1993.

[66] N. Friedrich, K. Budde, T. Wolf et al., "Short-term changes of the urine metabolome after bariatric surgery," *OMICS*, vol. 16, no. 11, pp. 612–620, 2012.

[67] G. L. S. Pawan and S. J. G. Semple, "Effect of 3-hydroxybutyrate in obese subjects on very-low-energy diets and during therapeutic starvation," *The Lancet*, vol. 321, no. 8314-8315, pp. 15–17, 1983.

[68] R. Nosadini, A. Avogaro, and R. Trevisan, "Acetoacetate and 3-hydroxybutyrate kinetics in obese and insulin-dependent diabetic humans," *The American Journal of Physiology—Regulatory Integrative and Comparative Physiology*, vol. 248, no. 5, part 2, pp. R611–R620, 1985.

[69] J. S. Fisler, M. Egawa, and G. A. Bray, "Peripheral 3-hydroxybutyrate and food intake in a model of dietary-fat induced obesity: effect of vagotomy," *Physiology & Behavior*, vol. 58, no. 1, pp. 1–7, 1995.

[70] N. Gooda Sahib, N. Saari, A. Ismail, A. Khatib, F. Mahomoodally, and A. Abdul Hamid, "Plants' metabolites as potential antiobesity agents," *The Scientific World Journal*, vol. 2012, Article ID 436039, 8 pages, 2012.

[71] A. Perez-Cornago, L. Brennan, I. Ibero-Baraibar et al., "Metabolomics identifies changes in fatty acid and amino acid profiles in serum of overweight older adults following a weight loss intervention," *Journal of Physiology and Biochemistry*, vol. 70, no. 2, pp. 593–602, 2014.

[72] S. Wahl, C. Holzapfel, Z. Yu et al., "Metabolomics reveals determinants of weight loss during lifestyle intervention in obese children," *Metabolomics*, vol. 9, no. 6, pp. 1157–1167, 2013.

[73] P. S. Larmo, A. J. Kangas, P. Soininen et al., "Effects of sea buckthorn and bilberry on serum metabolites differ according to baseline metabolic profiles in overweight women: a randomized crossover trial," *The American Journal of Clinical Nutrition*, vol. 98, no. 4, pp. 941–951, 2013.

[74] M. J. Kim, H. J. Yang, J. H. Kim et al., "Obesity-related metabolomic analysis of human subjects in black soybean peptide intervention study by ultraperformance liquid chromatography and quadrupole-time-of-flight mass spectrometry," *Journal of Obesity*, vol. 2013, Article ID 874981, 11 pages, 2013.

[75] J. M. Miles, L. Leiter, P. Hollander et al., "Effect of orlistat in overweight and obese patients with type 2 diabetes treated with metformin," *Diabetes Care*, vol. 25, no. 7, pp. 1123–1128, 2002.

[76] J. S. Torgerson, J. Hauptman, M. N. Boldrin, and L. Sjöström, "Xenical in the prevention of diabetes in obese subjects (XENDOS) study: a randomized study of orlistat as an adjunct to lifestyle changes for the prevention of type 2 diabetes in obese patients," *Diabetes Care*, vol. 27, no. 1, pp. 155–161, 2004.

[77] H. M. Sickmann, H. S. Waagepetersen, A. Schousboe, A. J. Benie, and S. D. Bouman, "Obesity and type 2 diabetes in rats are associated with altered brain glycogen and amino-acid homeostasis," *Journal of Cerebral Blood Flow & Metabolism*, vol. 30, no. 8, pp. 1527–1537, 2010.

[78] S. Satapati, N. E. Sunny, B. Kucejova et al., "Elevated TCA cycle function in the pathology of diet-induced hepatic insulin resistance and fatty liver," *Journal of Lipid Research*, vol. 53, no. 6, pp. 1080–1092, 2012.

[79] I. H. De Boer, S. D. Sibley, B. Kestenbaum et al., "Central obesity, incident microalbuminuria, and change in creatinine clearance in the epidemiology of diabetes interventions and complications study," *Journal of the American Society of Nephrology*, vol. 18, no. 1, pp. 235–243, 2007.

[80] D. S. Hittel, Y. Hathout, E. P. Huffman, and J. A. Houmard, "Proteome analysis of skeletal muscle from obese and morbidly obese women," *Diabetes*, vol. 54, no. 5, pp. 1283–1288, 2005.

25

Diabetes Mellitus in Outpatients in Debre Berhan Referral Hospital, Ethiopia

Tesfa Dejenie Habtewold,[1] Wendwesen Dibekulu Tsega,[2] and Bayu Yihun Wale[1]

[1]*College of Health Science, Department of Nursing, Debre Berhan University, 445 Debre Berhan, Ethiopia*
[2]*College of Health Science, Department of Public Health, Debre Berhan University, 445 Debre Berhan, Ethiopia*

Correspondence should be addressed to Tesfa Dejenie Habtewold; tesfadej2003@gmail.com

Academic Editor: Marco Songini

Introduction. Diabetes mellitus is a group of metabolic diseases characterized by hyperglycemia resulting from defects in insulin secretion, insulin action, or both. Most people with diabetes live in low- and middle-income countries and these will experience the greatest increase in cases of diabetes over the next 22 years. *Objective*. To assess the prevalence and associated factors of diabetes mellitus among outpatients of Debre Berhan Referral Hospital. *Methods and Materials*. A cross-sectional study was conducted from April to June 2015 among 385 patients. Random quota sampling technique was used to get individual patients and risk factors assessment. Patients diabetes status was ascertained by World Health Organization Diabetes Mellitus Diagnostic Criteria. The collected data were entered, cleaned, and analyzed and Chi-square test was applied to test any association between dependent and independent variable. *Result*. Out of the total 385 study patients, 368 have participated in the study yielding a response rate of 95.3%. Concerning clinical presentation of diabetes mellitus, 13.3% of patients reported thirst, 14.4% of patients declared polyurea, and 14.9% of patients ascertained unexplained weight loss. The statistically significant associated factors of diabetes mellitus were hypertensive history, obesity, the number of parities, and smoking history. *Conclusion*. The prevalence of diabetes mellitus among outpatients in Debre Berhan Referral Hospital was 0.34% and several clinical and behavioral factors contribute to the occurrence of diabetes mellitus which impose initiation of preventive, promotive, and curative strategies.

1. Introduction

Diabetes mellitus is a group of metabolic diseases characterized by chronic hyperglycemia resulting from defects in insulin secretion, insulin action, or both. It is classified as type 1 diabetes, type 2 diabetes, gestational diabetes, and other types of diabetes mellitus [1]. Diabetes mellitus is the most common chronic disease among adults. The global burden of diabetes has increased twelvefold between 1985 and 2011 [2].

In 2013, 382 million people had diabetes; this number is expected to rise to 592 million by 2035. Most people with diabetes live in low- and middle-income countries and these will experience the greatest increase in cases of diabetes over the next 22 years [3, 4]. According to the international diabetes federation 2013 reports, in North America and Caribbean countries 1 in 10 adults has diabetes; in Southern and Western America 1 in 11 adults has diabetes. Similarly, in Europe 21-22 million people have diabetes [5]. Moreover, in

2013, the number of people with diabetes is estimated to be 56 million in Europe with an overall estimated prevalence of 8.5%. However, estimates of diabetes prevalence in 2013 vary widely in the 56 diverse countries in Europe from 2.4% in Moldova to 14.9% in Turkey [6].

On the contrary in 2010, 12.1 million people were to be living with diabetes mellitus in Africa and over the next 20 years the number of people with diabetes will almost double [2, 7, 8]. Based on the IDF Diabetes Atlas 2014 update the age-standardized prevalence of diabetes in the Middle East and North Africa was estimated at 10.9% and projected to increase to 11.3% by 2035 [9]. Additionally, a systematic review by Bos and Agyemang revealed that the prevalence of diabetes varied across Northern African countries ranging from 2.6% in rural Sudan to 20% in urban Egypt. Ten studies distinguished between urban and rural diabetes prevalence and all of these studies found a higher prevalence in urban areas than in rural areas [10].

According to 2011 reports of the International Diabetes Federation (IDF), the number of adults living with diabetes in Ethiopia was 3.5% [11]. Even though the national prevalence of diabetes in Ethiopia is estimated to be 2%, evidence suggests that its prevalence could be more than 5% in those older than 40 years of age in some setting [12–14]. A study by Watkins and Alemu conducted in Gondar found out most of the rural patients (77%) had type 1 diabetes whereas in urban areas only 29% had type 1 and 71% of them type 2 diabetes [15]. Generally, the global burden of diabetes mellitus has been increasing radically. The impact is high especially in developing countries in which resource is limited to identify the problem and develop need based clinical and community intervention. Therefore, the objective of this study was to assess the prevalence and associated factors of diabetes mellitus among outpatients of Debre Berhan Referral Hospital.

2. Methods and Materials

2.1. Study Setting. Debre Berhan is the capital city of North Shoa, one of the 13 zones of Amhara regional state which is located 130 KM north of Addis Ababa, Ethiopia. The foundation of the town was traced back to the regime of Atse Zereyakob. Regarding health services in the city, there are one government and one private hospital, two government health centers, five health posts, and 18 private clinics. Debre Berhan Referral Hospital is the only government hospital in the city and it is zonal referral hospital serving the population of the zone as a referral center and the place where this study was conducted [16].

2.2. Study Design and Population. A cross-sectional study was conducted from April to June 2015 among 385 patients who visited the outpatient department of Debre Berhan Referral Hospital. All outpatients who visited the hospital during the data collection period were included. Nevertheless, patients who were severely ill, not cooperative, having difficulty in hearing, and visual impairment were excluded. The hospital has many units organized to render care for clients. From these units outpatient units 1, 2, 3, and 5, dental clinic, pediatrics outpatient unit 1, and maternal health unit were selected using simple random sampling technique. To reach individual patients, random quota sampling technique was used.

2.3. Data Collection Tools and Procedures. The questionnaire has three parts: sociodemographic characteristics, WHO Diabetes Mellitus Diagnostic Criteria [17], and associated risk factors assessment. The patients' diabetes status was ascertained by considering two classic clinical symptoms and laboratory test of random blood glucose level. To classify diabetes mellitus into type 1, type 2, and gestational, classic symptoms and signs, the age of the patient, random blood sugar level, and pregnancy status were used as a criterion. The data were collected by internship nursing students and professional nurses in selected unit using pretested, structured interviewer administered questionnaire. Also, the standard "forward-backward" procedure was applied to translate the questionnaire from English into Amharic. To ensure data

quality, orientation was given for all patients, data collectors were trained, and appropriate study design and sampling technique were deliberated. Additionally, a pretest was done on 5% of respondents. The data was entered, cleaned, and analyzed. Chi-square test was applied to test any association between dependent and independent variable using significance level (α) 0.05. To calculate the exact p value, Social Science Statistics p value calculator was used [18]. Fisher's exact test was also used when the chi-square test assumption was not fulfilled. Finally, the result was presented using descriptive statement, table, and figure.

2.4. Ethical Consideration. This study was done in conformity with the ethical guidelines approved by the Institute of Medicine and Health Science of Debre Berhan University. By explaining objectives of the study and its significance, relevant permission was obtained from hospital administration office. At individual level verbal consent was obtained from all patients.

3. Result

3.1. Sociodemographic Characteristics. Out of the total 385 study participants, 368 have participated in the study yielding a response rate of 95.32%. As described in Table 1, among the patients more than half (53.26%) of them were females. The majority of respondents (30.98%) were in the age group of <30. Additionally, most of the study subjects (74.45%) were Amhara and 70.10% were married. Moreover, 27.44% of the patients were illiterate.

3.2. Diagnostic Criteria of Diabetes Mellitus. As shown in Table 2, 13.32% of patients reported polydipsia, 14.40% of patients declared polyuria, and 14.94% of patients reported unexplained weight loss. Similarly, 7.07% of the patients had random blood sugar ≥200 mg/dL. Based on these criteria the overall prevalence of diabetes mellitus in Debre Berhan Referral Hospital was 0.34%.

3.3. Factors Associated with Diabetes Mellitus. As revealed in Table 3, 6.52% of the respondents had a family history of diabetes mellitus, 2.72% were twins, and 5.43% had previously known hypertensive disease. Also, most of (82.07%) patients did not do regular physical exercise.

As shown in Figure 1, among those diabetes cases, 4 cases (15.4%) were diagnosed as type 1 diabetes mellitus, 80.77% were type 2 DM, 3.85% were gestational type of diabetes mellitus.

As portrayed in Figure 2, 15.4% of the diabetes cases were found in the age group of <30; 30.77% of the diabetes cases were found in the age group of 30–39; the other 23.07% of them were found in the age group of 40–49; and about 30.77% of the diabetes cases were found in the age group of ≥50.

Concerning nonclassical symptoms and signs, 15.4% had reported a loss of consciousness, 46.15% reported developing numbness and tingling sensation, 42.3% have blurred vision, and the other 15.4% have reported wounds that cannot heal easily. Furthermore, among the diabetes cases, 23% of them had a history of hypertension.

TABLE 1: Sociodemographic characteristics of patients in Debre Berhan Referral Hospital in June 2015.

Variables	Categories	Frequency	Percentage
Sex	Male	172	46.74
	Female	196	53.26
Age	<30	114	30.98
	30–39	112	30.43
	40–49	77	20.92
	>50	65	17.67
Ethnicity	Amhara	274	74.45
	Tigray	24	6.53
	Oromia	66	17.93
	Other	4	1.09
Religion	Orthodox	271	73.64
	Muslim	63	17.12
	Catholic	6	1.63
	Protestant	28	7.61
Marital status	Married	258	70.10
	Single	72	19.56
	Divorced	16	4.35
	Widowed	22	5.99
Educational status	Illiterate	100	27.17
	Can read and write	76	20.65
	Grade 1 to grade 8	63	17.12
	Grade 9 to grade 12	54	14.67
	Diploma and above	75	20.65
Occupational status	Government employed	76	20.65
	Self-employed	90	24.45
	Merchant	42	11.41
	Housewife	87	23.64
	Others	73	19.84
Monthly income status	≤650	189	51.36
	651–1400	75	20.38
	≥1401	104	28.26

TABLE 2: WHO diagnostic criteria to know diabetes mellitus status of patients in Debre Berhan Referral Hospital in June 2015.

Variables	Frequency	Percentage
Classic symptoms		
Thirst		
Yes	49	13.32
No	319	86.68
Polyuria		
Yes	53	14.40
No	311	84.51
Unexplained weight loss		
Yes	55	14.94
No	313	85.06
Classic sign		
RBS ≥ 200 mg/dL		
Yes	26	7.07
No	342	92.93
Others		
Fatigue		
Yes	161	43.75
No	207	56.25
Nausea and vomiting		
Yes	84	22.83
No	284	77.59
Polyphagia		
Yes	23	6.25
No	345	93.75
Headache		
Yes	148	40.22
No	220	59.78
Loss of consciousness		
Yes	15	4.08
No	353	95.92
Numbness and tingling sensation		
Yes	45	12.23
No	323	87.77
Blurring of vision		
Yes	34	9.24
No	334	90.76

3.4. *Statistical Test.* As observed from Table 4, the p value of family history of diabetes mellitus and twin delivery was greater than 0.05, consequently interpreted as there is no association of family history of diabetes mellitus and twin delivery with the occurrence of diabetes mellitus. On the other hand, hypertensive history, obesity, number of parities, and smoking history have direct association with the occurrence of diabetes mellitus. Among those associated factors hypertensive history has the highest contribution following the number of parities and obesity.

4. Discussion

To our knowledge, this study was the first in Debre Berhan. It was conducted with the aim of assessing the prevalence and associated factors of diabetes mellitus.

In this study the percentage of diabetes mellitus among children ≤ 14 years was about 3.85%. Differently in a study by the World Health Organization's multinational project for childhood initially reported in 2000 the prevalence was 19,164 cases from the population of 75.1 million people which are about 0.025% [19]. This difference might be due to variation in sample size. Also, in this study the percentage of type 1 diabetes mellitus was about 15.4%; however, a decreased prevalence of 4% of type 1 diabetes mellitus was observed in the population studied in Asia, about 3.2% in Europe and 5.3% in North America [20]. This might be due to the lifestyle difference between Ethiopia and Western countries.

Furthermore, we found out the frequency of type 1 diabetes was not high in the youngest age group (0–4 years)

TABLE 3: Associated factors among patients in Debre Berhan Referral Hospital in June 2015.

Variables	Frequency	Percentage
Family history of diabetes mellitus		
Yes	24	6.52
No	344	93.48
Twin delivery		
Identical	5	1.36
Fraternal	5	1.36
Previously hypertensive disease		
Yes	20	5.43
No	348	94.57
Activity and exercise		
Good	302	82.07
Poor	66	17.03
Obesity (BMI)		
≤24.9 kg/m^2	340	92.39
>24.9 kg/m^2	28	7.61
Number of children delivered		
<2 times	71	19.29
≥2 times	61	16.58
No	33	8.97

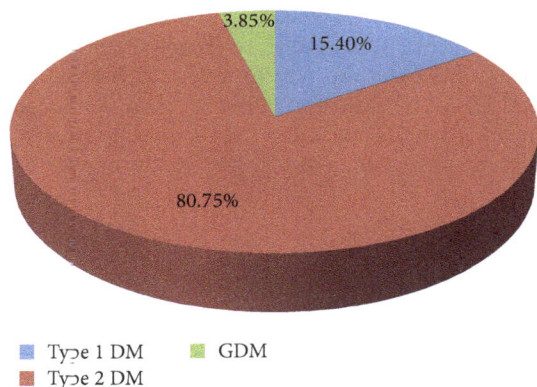

FIGURE 1: Diabetes mellitus category of patients in Debre Berhan Referral Hospital in June 2015.

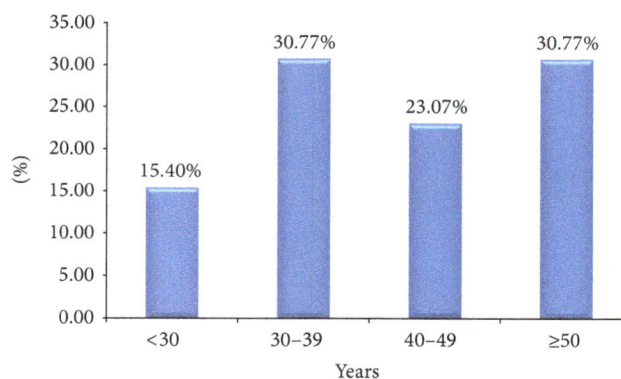

FIGURE 2: Distribution of diabetes mellitus among different age groups of patients in Debre Berhan Referral Hospital in June 2015.

and the percentage increased (15.4%) after puberty and young adulthood (15–29 years). On the contrary, a study done in Europe suggests that the prevalence rate of type 1 DM was highest in the youngest age group (0–4 years) and prevalence rates decline after puberty and appear to stabilize in young adulthood (15–29 years) [21]. This might be due to the difference in feeding habit, knowledge and health seeking behavior, and living standard.

In addition, in this study the percentage of type 2 diabetes mellitus was 80.77% but a ten-year observation at Gondar University Teaching Referral Hospital found out 49.9% were type 2 DM [22] and the prevalence study in Jimma University stated that 66.2% of the respondents were medically diagnosed as having type 2 diabetes mellitus [23].

This difference might be due to the difference in the duration of time of the study to conclude for the general population.

Concerning associated factors, numerous epidemiological studies were conducted to discriminate the different associated factors. In this study, there is no significant association between family history of diabetes mellitus and the occurrence of diabetes mellitus but a study done on the Palestinians, Iranians, and Kuwaitis documented that family history of diabetes increased the risk of the incidence by 1.6, 1.8, and 2.4 times, respectively [24–26]. In our study, however, the increased body mass index was also one of significant risk factors. This finding was consistent with WHO STEPS report [27], the study done in Israel [28] and Iran and Jordan [29]. Moreover, smoking history was a significant risk factor. This finding was in line with the study conducted in European countries [6]. Other significant risk factors of diabetes mellitus, not assessed in this study (but future researchers should consider them), are elevated triglycerides, total cholesterol, and low HDL cholesterol [30], gender and educational status [24], socioeconomic status [31], and physical inactivity [6, 27, 32, 33].

5. Strength and Limitation

The strengths of this study include a high response rate and the inclusive nature of this research as individuals could participate regardless of their demographic variation. Additionally, a reasonable sample size and culturally adapted questionnaires were used. Since it was the first study in Debre Berhan, it will provide basic information for those who have an interest. Furthermore, objective laboratory data were used to ascertain disease status of patients.

Despite these strengths, this study contains the following limitations: since the study was institutional and conducted among outpatients in only one hospital it could limit our understanding regarding the prevalence and associated factors of diabetes mellitus in the setting. Even though data collectors were blind for the study subjects, there might be selection bias. Moreover, due to cross-sectional nature of the study causal relationships between the risk factors and disease outcome could not be assumed. Furthermore, the data was

TABLE 4: Statistical test for associated factors of diabetes mellitus in Debre Berhan Referral Hospital in June 2015.

Variables	Calculated chi-square value	Degree of freedom	Odds ratio	p value
Family history of diabetes mellitus	3.6	1	2.9	0.06
Previous history of hypertension	25.25	1	9.3	**0.000**
Body mass index	9.33	1	4.36	**0.002**
Parity	11.34	1	8.95	**0.0008**
Twin delivery	0.2	1	1.46	0.65
Smoking history	5.45	1	4.33	**0.02**

analyzed manually and chi-square model which was a weak measure of association was utilized.

6. Conclusion

Diabetes mellitus and other noncommunicable diseases are becoming abundant in developing countries including Ethiopia due to lack of problem identification and intervention of these problems.

This study is targeted to know the prevalence of diabetes mellitus among outpatients in Debre Berhan Referral Hospital and associated factors that contribute to the occurrence of diabetes mellitus accompanied by initiation of preventive, promotive, and curative strategies.

Moreover, the study will help to initiate the community, health institution, and other concerned nongovernmental organizations to give emphasis to the population for controlling of diabetes mellitus. It will also give baseline information for those who aim to conduct a community-based longitudinal research in this area. Finally, mass media, zonal health office, and the Ministry of Health should work on the use of evidence-based medicine and awareness creation by developing an up-to-date guideline tailored to each specific group of the population.

Abbreviations

BMI: Body mass index
CBE: Community-based education
DBRH: Debre Berhan Referral Hospital
DBU: Debre Berhan University
DM: Diabetes mellitus
ETB: Ethiopian birr
GDM: Gestational diabetes mellitus
IDDM: Insulin dependent diabetes mellitus
IDF: International diabetes federation
OPD: Outpatient department
PI: Principal investigator
SSB: Sugar sweetened beverage
T_1 DM: Type 1 diabetes mellitus
T_2 DM: Type 2 diabetes mellitus
UKDPS: United Kingdom diabetes prospective study
WHO: World Health Organization.

Conflict of Interests

The authors declare that they have no competing interests.

Authors' Contribution

Bayu Yihun Wale conceived of the study and participated in its design. Tesfa Dejenie Habtewold participated in design and coordination of the study. Wendwesen Dibekulu Tsega helped to draft the paper. All authors read and approved the final paper.

Acknowledgments

The authors would like to thank Debre Berhan University, Department of Nursing, for creating this chance. Additionally, They would like to forward their special acknowledgment to Alelign Wondim, Bizualem Lemma, Ejinu Yizezew, and Tsgie Gebretsadik who had a crucial role during data collection and analysis of the data. The authors' recognition also goes to Debre Berhan Referral Hospital officials, Sr. Tseganesh Biyabil (Matron Nurse) and Dr. Feseha Tadesse (Medical Director), who facilitated the data collection. The authors' heartfelt gratitude and high appreciation also go to patients who were willing to take part in the study.

References

[1] A. T. Kharroubi and H. M. Darwish, "Diabetes mellitus: the epidemic of the century," *World Journal of Diabetes*, vol. 6, no. 6, pp. 850–867, 2015.

[2] J. E. Shaw, R. A. Sicree, and P. Z. Zimmet, "Global estimates of the prevalence of diabetes for 2010 and 2030," *Diabetes Research and Clinical Practice*, vol. 87, no. 1, pp. 4–14, 2010.

[3] L. Guariguata, D. R. Whiting, I. Hambleton, J. Beagley, U. Linnenkamp, and J. E. Shaw, "Global estimates of diabetes prevalence for 2013 and projections for 2035," *Diabetes Research and Clinical Practice*, vol. 103, no. 2, pp. 137–149, 2014.

[4] T. A. Harrison, L. A. Hindorff, H. Kim et al., "Family history of diabetes as a potential public health tool," *American Journal of Preventive Medicine*, vol. 24, no. 2, pp. 152–159, 2003.

[5] International Diabetes Federation, *Diabetes ATLAS*, Updated, 5th edition, 2013, http://www.idf.org/sites/default/files/Media-Information-Pack.pdf.

[6] T. Tamayo, J. Rosenbauer, S. H. Wild et al., "Diabetes in Europe: an update," *Diabetes Research and Clinical Practice*, vol. 103, no. 2, pp. 206–217, 2014.

[7] World Health Organization, *The Global Burden of Disease*, World Health Organization, Geneva, Switzerland, 2004, http://www.who.int/healthinfo/global_burden_disease/2004_report_update/en/.

[8] R. Sicree, J. Shaw, and P. Zimmet, "The global burden: diabetes and impaired glucose tolerance," April 2015, https://www.idf .org/sites/default/files/Diabetes%20and%20Impaired%20Glucose%20Tolerance_1.pdf.

[9] A. Majeed, A. A. El-Sayed, T. Khoja, R. Alshamsan, C. Millett, and S. Rawaf, "Diabetes in the Middle-East and North Africa: an update," *Diabetes Research and Clinical Practice*, vol. 103, no. 2, pp. 218–222, 2014.

[10] M. Bos and C. Agyemang, "Prevalence and complications of diabetes mellitus in Northern Africa, a systematic review," *BMC Public Health*, vol. 13, no. 1, article 387, 2013.

[11] D. R. Whiting, L. Guariguata, C. Weil, and J. Shaw, "IDF Diabetes Atlas: global estimates of the prevalence of diabetes for 2011 and 2030," *Diabetes Research and Clinical Practice*, vol. 94, no. 3, pp. 311–321, 2011.

[12] L. D. Nshisso, A. Reese, B. Gelaye, S. Lemma, Y. Berhane, and M. A. Williams, "Prevalence of hypertension and diabetes among Ethiopian adults," *Diabetes and Metabolic Syndrome*, vol. 6, no. 1, pp. 36–41, 2012.

[13] S. Alemu, A. Dessie, E. Seid et al., "Insulin-requiring diabetes in rural Ethiopia: should we reopen the case for malnutrition-related diabetes?" *Diabetologia*, vol. 52, no. 9, pp. 1842–1845, 2009.

[14] G. V. Gill, J.-C. Mbanya, K. L. Ramaiya, and S. Tesfaye, "A sub-Saharan African perspective of diabetes," *Diabetologia*, vol. 52, no. 1, pp. 8–16, 2009.

[15] P. Watkins and S. Alemu, "Delivery of diabetes care in rural Ethiopia: an experience from Gondar," *Ethiopian Medical Journal*, vol. 41, no. 1, pp. 9–17, 2003.

[16] Ministry of Urban Development and Construction, Debre Berhan City Administration, December 2015, http://www.mwud .gov.et/web/debreberehan/home.

[17] Diagnostic Criteria for Diabetes World Health Organisation (WHO) Recommendations, 2015, https://www.diabetes.org.uk/ About_us/What-we-say/Diagnosis-ongoing-management-monitoring/New_diagnostic_criteria_for_diabetes/.

[18] J. Stangroom, "Social Science Statistics: p-Value from Chi-Square Calculator," 2015, http://www.socscistatistics.com/pvalues/chidistribution.aspx.

[19] M. Karvonen, M. Viik-Kajander, E. Moltchanova, I. Libman, R. LaPorte, and J. Tuomilehto, "Incidence of childhood type 1 diabetes worldwide. Diabetes Mondiale (DiaMond) Project Group," *Diabetes Care*, vol. 23, no. 10, pp. 1516–1526, 2000.

[20] DIAMOND Project Group, "Prevalence and trends of childhood type 1 diabetes worldwide 1990–1999," *Diabetic Medicine*, vol. 23, no. 8, pp. 857–866, 2006.

[21] EURODIAB ACE Study Group, "Variation and trends in incidence of childhood diabetes in Europe," *The Lancet*, vol. 355, no. 9207, pp. 873–876, 2000.

[22] S. M. Abebe, Y. Berhane, A. Worku, and S. Alemu, "Increasing trends of diabetes mellitus and body weight: a ten year observation at Gondar university teaching referral hospital, northwest Ethiopia," *PLoS ONE*, vol. 8, no. 3, Article ID e60081, 2013.

[23] K. Ayele, B. Tesfa, L. Abebe, T. Tilahun, and E. Girma, "Self care behavior among patients with diabetes in Harari, eastern Ethiopia: the health belief model perspective," *PLoS ONE*, vol. 7, no. 4, Article ID e35515, 2012.

[24] H. Harati, F. Hadaegh, N. Saadat, and F. Azizi, "Population-based incidence of Type 2 diabetes and its associated risk factors: results from a six-year cohort study in Iran," *BMC Public Health*, vol. 9, article 186, 2009.

[25] H. S. A. Mousa, S. Yousef, F. Riccardo, W. Zeidan, and G. Sabatinelli, "Hyperglycaemia, hypertension and their risk factors among Palestine refugees served by UNRWA," *Eastern Mediterranean Health Journal*, vol. 16, no. 6, pp. 609–614, 2010.

[26] M. A. A. Moussa, M. Alsaeid, T. M. K. Refai, N. Abdella, N. Al-Sheikh, and J. E. Gomez, "Factors associated with type 1 diabetes in Kuwaiti children," *Acta Diabetologica*, vol. 42, no. 3, pp. 129–137, 2005.

[27] World Health Organization STEPS country reports, 2015, http:// www.who.int/chp/steps/reports/en/.

[28] A. Tirosh, I. Shai, A. Afek et al., "Adolescent BMI trajectory and risk of diabetes versus coronary disease," *The New England Journal of Medicine*, vol. 364, no. 14, pp. 1315–1325, 2011.

[29] M. Zindah, A. Belbeisi, H. Walke, and A. H. Mokdad, "Obesity and diabetes in Jordan: findings from the behavioral risk factor surveillance system, 2004," *Preventing Chronic Disease*, vol. 5, no. 1, article A17, 2008.

[30] K. M. V. Narayan, J. P. Boyle, T. J. Thompson, E. W. Gregg, and D. F. Williamson, "Effect of BMI on lifetime risk for diabetes in the U.S," *Diabetes Care*, vol. 30, no. 6, pp. 1562–1566, 2007.

[31] M. Maddah, "Association of diabetes with living area in Iranian women," *International Journal of Cardiology*, vol. 143, no. 1, pp. 100–102, 2010.

[32] V. R. Collins, G. K. Dowse, P. M. Toelupe et al., "Increasing prevalence of NIDDM in the Pacific Island population of Western Samoa over a 13-year period," *Diabetes Care*, vol. 17, no. 4, pp. 288–296, 1994.

[33] S. T. Win Tin, C. M. Y. Lee, and R. Colagiuri, "A profile of diabetes in Pacific island countries and territories," *Diabetes Research and Clinical Practice*, vol. 107, no. 2, pp. 233–246, 2015.

26

Conserved Metabolic Changes in Nondiabetic and Type 2 Diabetic Bariatric Surgery Patients: Global Metabolomic Pilot Study

Konrad Sarosiek,[1] Kirk L. Pappan,[2] Ankit V. Gandhi,[1]
Shivam Saxena,[1] Christopher Y. Kang,[1] Heather McMahon,[1] Galina I. Chipitsyna,[3]
David S. Tichansky,[1] and Hwyda A. Arafat[3]

[1]Department of Surgery, Thomas Jefferson University, Philadelphia, PA 19107, USA
[2]Metabolon, Inc., Research Triangle Park, Durham, NC 27713, USA
[3]Department of Biomedical Sciences, University of New England, Biddeford, ME 04005, USA

Correspondence should be addressed to Galina I. Chipitsyna; gchipitsyna@une.edu

Academic Editor: Michal Ciborowski

The goal of this study was to provide insight into the mechanism by which bariatric surgical procedures led to weight loss and improvement or resolution of diabetes. Global biochemical profiling was used to evaluate changes occurring in nondiabetic and type 2 diabetic (T2D) patients experiencing either less extreme sleeve gastrectomy or a full gastric bypass. We were able to identify changes in metabolism that were affected by standard preoperation liquid weight loss diet as well as by bariatric surgery itself. Preoperation weight-loss diet was associated with a strong lipid metabolism signature largely related to the consumption of adipose reserves for energy production. Glucose usage shift away from glycolytic pyruvate production toward pentose phosphate pathway, via glucose-6-phosphate, appeared to be shared across all patients regardless of T2D status or bariatric surgery procedure. Our results suggested that bariatric surgery might promote antioxidant defense and insulin sensitivity through both increased heme synthesis and HO activity or expression. Changes in histidine and its metabolites following surgery might be an indication of altered gut microbiome ecology or liver function. This initial study provided broad understanding of how metabolism changed globally in morbidly obese nondiabetic and T2D patients following weight-loss surgery.

1. Introduction

Diabetes is a major public health concern in the United States because of its prevalence, considerable morbidity and mortality, and economic burden with total medical costs of 245 billion dollars in 2012 alone [1, 2]. In 2010, the prevalence rate of diabetes in the US was 9.3%, affecting older population (65 years or older) even more dramatically with the rate of 25.9% [1]. Diabetes is associated with serious complications, including coronary heart disease, stroke, kidney failure, neuropathy, blindness, and amputation, and was the seventh leading cause of death in 2010 [1, 2]. Type 2 diabetes (T2D) accounts for 90–95% of all diagnosed cases [1]. Obesity is a major risk factor for T2D [2, 3], and the risk of diabetes increases directly with BMI [2, 4, 5]. According to National Center for Health Statistics (NCHS) more than one-third of US adults (34.9 percent) were obese in 2011-2012 [6]. The medical care costs of obesity in the United States are staggering, totaling about $147 billion dollars in 2008 alone [7].

Weight loss is important therapeutic goal in obese patients with T2D, because even moderate weight loss (5%) improves insulin sensitivity [2, 8]. Bariatric surgery is the most effective weight-loss therapy and has considerable beneficial effects on diabetes and other obesity-related comorbidities [2, 9–11].

Weight-loss surgery by laparoscopic sleeve gastrectomy (SG) leads to a 40–65% reduction in excess weight and, amazingly, 56% of patients achieve resolution in their type 2 diabetes and 37% see improvement in their T2D symptoms [12]. Laparoscopic gastric bypass (GB) is a more intense surgery that typically results in a 60–70% loss of excess weight and is also characterized by improvement or resolution of diabetes [9, 12, 13].

The objective of this study was to provide insight into the mechanism by which gut/stomach rerouting leads to weight loss and the improvement or resolution of diabetes. In metabolomics, an individual's metabolic state is profiled by multiplexed measurement of many low-molecular-weight metabolites [14]. Over 4,000 such metabolites have been identified in human serum [15]. Two complementary approaches, targeted and nontargeted analyses, have evolved [16]. In targeted analysis discrete groups of chemically related metabolites (e.g., amino acids) are quantified in a biological sample. In contrast, nontargeted analysis is a more qualitative approach that surveys as many different metabolites as possible [14]. Using primarily targeted approaches, multiple studies have identified higher levels of branched-chain and aromatic amino acids in insulin-resistant, obese, and T2D individuals [17]. More recent studies demonstrated that higher levels of these amino acids are predictive of progression to T2D as well as future insulin resistance and hyperglycemia [14, 18–22]. Recently, Gall and colleagues [23] used nontargeted approach to identify plasma metabolites associated with development of insulin resistance and/or glucose intolerance. Two top-ranked metabolites were an organic acid, α-hydroxybutyrate (α-HB), and a lipid, 1-linoleoyl-glycerophosphocholine (L-GPC). Ferrannini et al. proposed fasting α-HB and L-GPC levels as new biomarkers to help predict dysglycemia and T2D [14, 24]. This nontargeted global metabolomic profiling represents new tool that allows the comprehensive survey of metabolism and metabolic networks to gain insight into phenotype and identify biomarker candidates. So far this approach was used to find a way to predict the progression to T2D as well as future insulin resistance and impaired glucose tolerance by serum analysis of insulin-resistant, obese individuals who progressed to T2D [14]. We took an opposite approach utilizing bariatric surgery tool as the most promising way to affect weight loss and to rectify T2D symptoms in morbidly obese patients. The range of metabolic changes that accompany weight reduction is not fully characterized. It is not known whether metabolic response is the same for all bariatric procedures, nor is it known whether there are any differences between nondiabetic and T2D patients.

2. Research Design and Methods

2.1. Serum Samples Collection. 15 patients represented three disease-surgery groups: nondiabetic (non-T2D) receiving SG and T2D receiving either SG or GB surgery (Table 1). Blood samples were collected over the course of treatment for each patient at the following times: at baseline (BL) prior to dieting/surgery, 14 days after baseline with adherence to strict preoperation weight-loss liquid diet (preop diet), and 28 days after surgery recovery after bariatric surgery (postop). Blood samples were collected in serum separator tubes, allowed to stand at room temperature for 15–20 minutes, centrifuged at 2500 rpm for 10 minutes at 4°C, aliquoted, snap frozen in liquid nitrogen, and stored at −80°C until analysis.

2.2. Global Metabolomic Analysis. Nontargeted global metabolomic analysis was performed by Metabolon, Inc. (Durham, NC), using two independent platforms: ultrahigh performance liquid chromatography/tandem mass spectrometry (UHPLC-MS/MS) optimized for basic species or acidic species, and gas chromatography/mass spectrometry (GC/MS). General platform methods are described in details in Online Supplemental Data section (see Supplementary Methods and Materials available online at http://dx.doi.org/10.1155/2015/3467403).

Following log transformation and imputation with minimum observed values for each compound, repeated measures 2-way ANOVA with posttest contrasts was used to identify biochemicals that differed significantly between experimental groups and across study time points with statistical cut-offs for P value ($P < 0.05$). Multiple comparisons were accounted for by estimating the false discovery rate using q-values of less than 5% ($q < 0.05$) [25].

3. Results and Discussion

3.1. Metabolite Summary and Significantly Altered Biochemicals. The search continues to identify biomarkers capable of predicting the onset of T2D [14]. Genome-wide association studies have identified many T2D susceptibility genes [14, 26] but generally failed to improve risk prediction over that provided by routine clinical measures [14, 27]. Global nontargeted analysis performed in this study is the first study to provide the insight into mechanism by which bariatric surgery leads to weight loss and resolution or improvement of T2D. This approach might also be used to identify T2D biomarker candidates and find new, cost effective treatments that can replace surgery itself.

Since metabolomic profiling generates a wealth of data that must be parsed to extract information, we chose statistical cut-offs at both the level of individual metabolites—P values—and the level of multiple testing across the 476 metabolites detected in the serum samples—q-values. By narrowing in on metabolites meeting the conservative criteria of $P < 0.05$ and an estimated false discovery rate of less than 5% ($q < 0.05$), we were able to reduce the complexity of the dataset and observed a number of statistically significant changes that occurred in common in nondiabetic and T2D patients with SG or GB. Furthermore, we were able to identify concerted changes of related metabolites that pointed to areas of metabolism that were affected by standard preop diet as well as by bariatric surgery itself. A list of all 476 metabolites detected and heat map of the statistical comparisons across time and patient groups are presented in Online Supplemental Tables A1 and A2.

Comparison of serum profiles at baseline, following a preop weight reduction diet, and after weight-loss surgery revealed several key metabolic differences as highlighted below.

TABLE 1: Clinicopathological characteristics of the patients.

Average	Gastric sleeve with T2D	Gastric sleeve without T2D	Gastric bypass with T2D
M, number of patients	2	0	1
F, number of patients	3	5	4
Age, years	46 ± 12.84	45.2 ± 14.24	44.4 ± 17.57
Weight, lb	306.28 ± 46.27	250.4 ± 18.58	304.4 ± 44.11
BMI	48.74 ± 8.2	43.54 ± 4.13	47.56 ± 6.61
Fasting blood sugar, mg/dL	140.6 ± 26.03	87 ± 2.92	98.8 ± 21.71
HTN, number of patients	2	3	3

Fat mobilization and oxidation were the key signatures associated with preop diet. Prior to surgery, patients were subjected to 2-week clear liquid diet that promoted weight loss on the order of 3–5% of body weight. The preoperative liquid diet is a 14-day high protein, very low calorie diet (VLCD) designed to deplete glycogen and fat stores in the liver or "shrink the liver" which is lifted to access the stomach during surgery. This VLCD includes 800 kcal with 80 g protein and typically produces a 10–20-pound weight loss. High protein drinks with less than 200 calories and at least 20 g protein are consumed 3-4x daily; no solid food is allowed on this diet. In addition, at least 64 ounces of sugar-free decaffeinated clear liquids a day are recommended along with a multivitamin and a calcium + vitamin D supplement. Medications, such as antihyperglycemics, are adjusted during this preoperative weight-loss phase to account for decreased calorie and carbohydrate intake. The study found that patients who follow a preoperative liquid diet effectively reduced visceral fat and achieve greater weight loss [28].

Examination of preop metabolic profiles, serum samples taken immediately before surgery, showed a profound mobilization of fat as attested by statistically significant elevations of ketones, monoacylglycerols, oleate, and an acyl-carnitine (Online Supplemental Table A3, Figure 1). These are compounds associated with lipolysis and fatty acid oxidation which suggested that a major metabolic effect of the preop diet was to stimulate fat tissue triglyceride hydrolysis, transport of fatty acids to the liver, and subsequent liver fatty acid oxidation and ketogenesis to supply energy substrates for peripheral tissues. The elevation of the markers associated with lipolysis and ketone production was transient and, in most cases, returned to near baseline levels by day 28 postsurgery time point. These results suggest that 3–5% weight loss experienced by patients during preop diet is largely due to the consumption of adipose reserves for energy production.

Another interesting observation is that preop diet led to a transient elevation of alpha-hydroxybutyrate (α-HB) and its precursor alpha-ketobutyrate (Online Supplemental Table A3, Figure 1). α-HB is a sensitive biomarker of insulin resistance [23, 24] which suggests that both nondiabetic and T2D patients experienced a temporary relative increase in insulin resistance during preop diet.

Compounds that changed in a statistically significant manner after 28 days of recovery from bariatric surgery, relative to baseline, were more numerous and diverse than observed in response to the preoperation diet. 62 compounds in the postsurgery to baseline comparison represented $P < 0.05$ and showed $q < 0.05$ in at least one of the disease-surgery groups (Online Supplemental Table A4). 28 compounds showed P and q-value cut-offs across all three disease-surgery groups at the 28-day postsurgery sample collection time point relative to baseline. 13 of the compounds that changed across all three groups had fold-change increases—including 100-fold + increases for trans-urocanate, cis-urocanate, pyroglutamylvaline, and heme in most or all of the groups. The remaining fifteen compounds that changed across all three groups were reduced at the postsurgery time point compared to baseline. Levels of ascorbate and various tocopherols were substantially reduced with ascorbate showing a 12.5-fold or greater decrease in each of the groups (Online Supplemental Table A4, Figure 2). Difficulty in absorbing micronutrients, such as vitamin C, following bariatric surgery has been reported previously [29, 30] and appeared to be confirmed at a shorter follow-up time point in this study.

Glutathione and its precursors were more abundant following weight-loss surgery. Weight-loss surgery led to concerted changes in compounds related to sulfur-containing amino acid metabolism that were largely shared across the groups. Glutathione (GSH) is a tripeptide comprised of glutamate, cysteine, and glycine. These amino acids along with the recycling intermediates Cys-Gly and 5-oxoproline were increased in all groups following surgery (Online Supplemental Table A4), suggesting a greater potential availability of substrates for GSH production. Oxidized forms of glutathione and cysteine, such as the mixed heterodimer cysteine-glutathione and glutathione homodimer GSSG, were elevated following surgery (Online Supplemental Table A4, Figure 2) and could be a sign of increased oxidative stress following surgery. However, an alternate interpretation is that a greater availability of glutathione and sulfur-containing amino acids following weight-loss surgery led to the greater formation of these oxidized compounds.

Weight-loss surgery appeared to shift glucose usage away from glycolytic pyruvate production. Pyruvate—the terminal product of glucose metabolism via the glycolysis pathway—dropped sharply after bariatric surgery (Online Supplemental Table A4, Figure 3), likely indicating its more efficient mitochondrial utilization. The reduction of pyruvate was matched by increases in fumarate, in all T2D patients, and malate perhaps indicating an inadequate supply of acetyl-CoA, which is derived from pyruvate, relative to

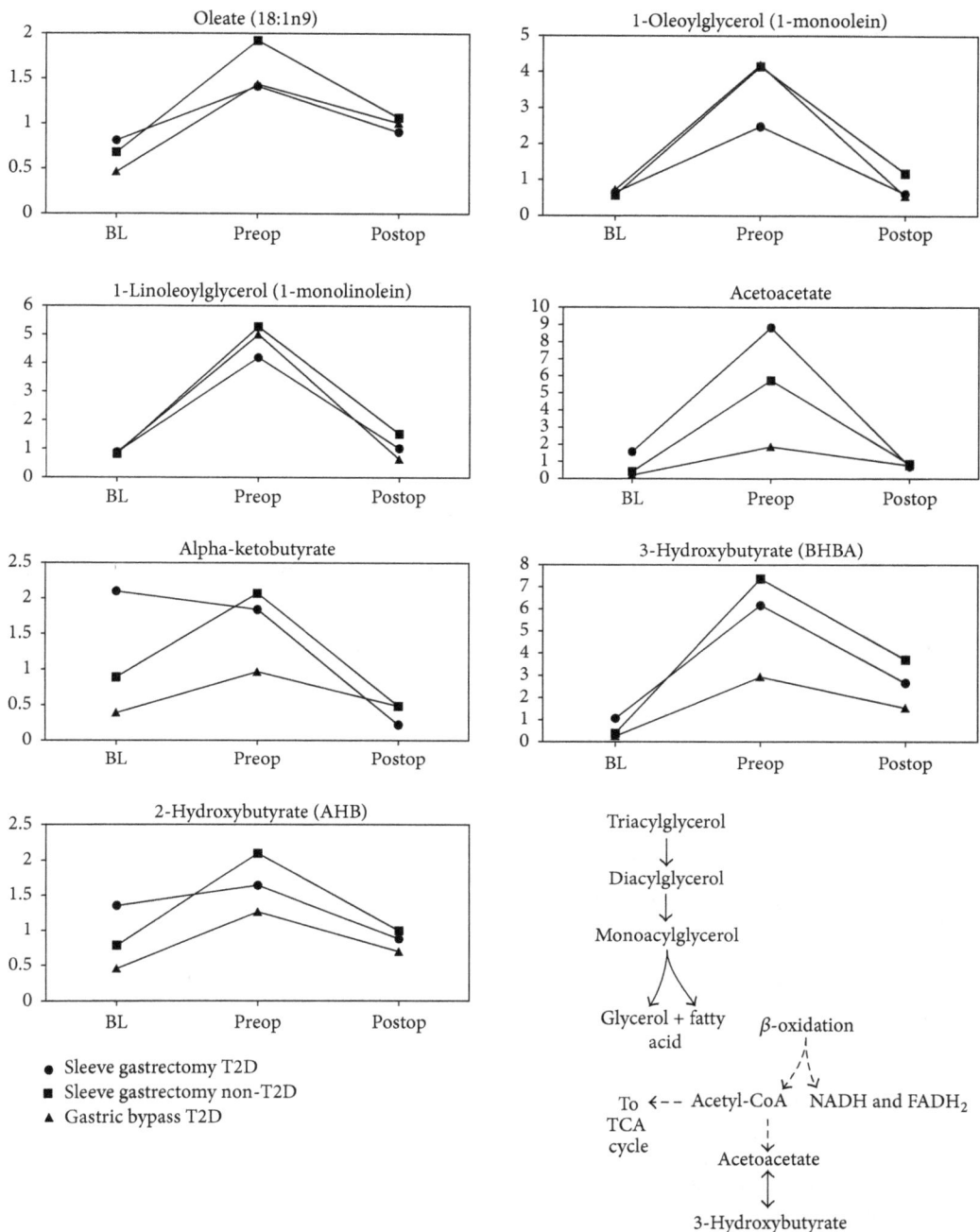

FIGURE 1: Fat mobilization and oxidation: key signatures associated with preop diet. All shown metabolites meet the conservative criteria of $P < 0.05$ and an estimated false discovery rate of less than 5% ($q < 0.05$).

the level of TCA cycle components. However, levels of the glycolytic intermediate 3-phosphoglycerate (3-PG) increased after surgery as did nonglycolytic products—glycerol and serine—potentially derived from 3-PG.

In addition to changes in pyruvate production, glucose usage via the pentose phosphate pathway (PPP) was also shifted following bariatric surgery. The PPP is a key source of pentose sugars used for nucleotide synthesis as well as NADPH which is used for reductive synthesis reactions and regeneration of reduced glutathione. PPP intermediates and

derivative pentose sugars, including ribulose-5-phosphate and xylulose-5-phosphate that are isobars that cannot be differentiated by our platform, and their nonphosphorylated products, such as xylulose, were significantly increased in all groups following surgery (Online Supplemental Table A4, Figure 3). Glucose carbons, via glucose-6-phosphate, may have been directed toward the pentose phosphate pathway in the face of the proposed decrease in glycolysis pathway activity. Glucose metabolism was likely confounded by the use of antidiabetic medications. For example, at baseline,

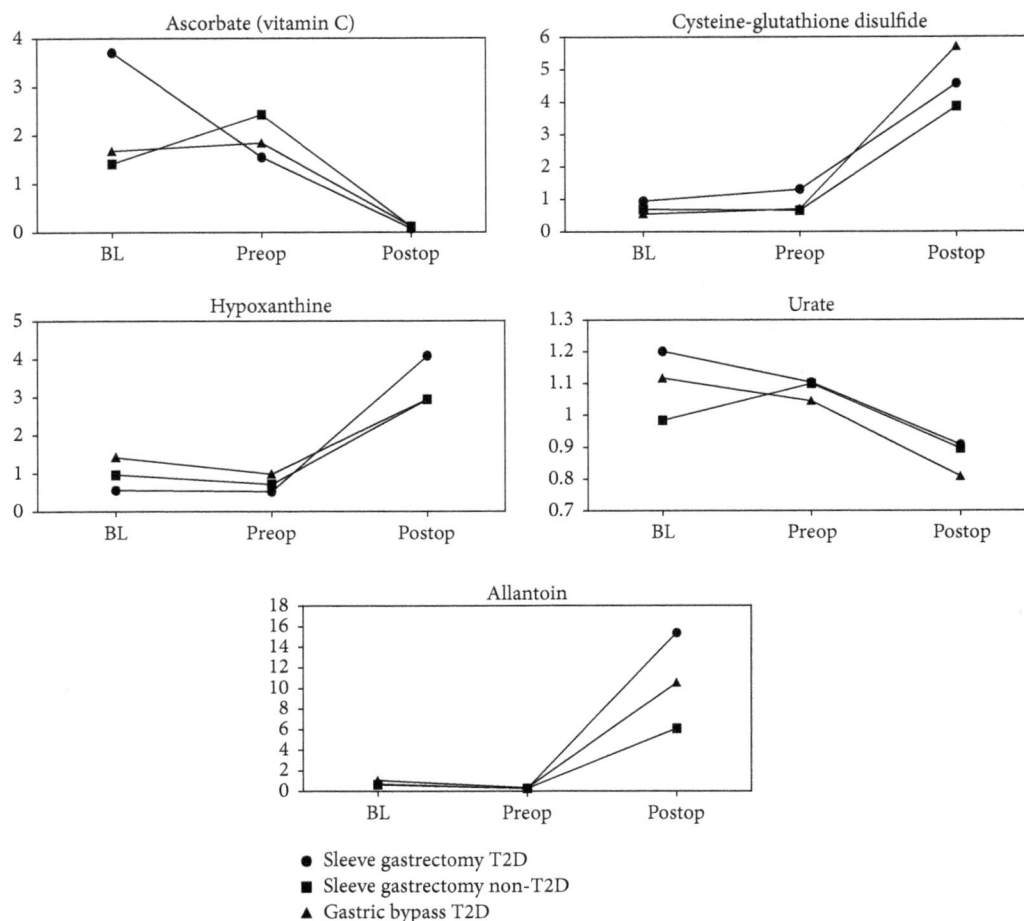

FIGURE 2: Postsurgery metabolic changes. All shown metabolites meet the conservative criteria of $P < 0.05$ and an estimated false discovery rate of less than 5% ($q < 0.05$).

metformin was detected in 100% of the T2D SG patient samples, 60% of the T2D GB samples, and none of the nondiabetic SG samples. After bariatric surgery, metformin was only detected in 20% of the T2D SG and GB serum samples. Postsurgery serum glucose levels decreased relative to baseline but this change only reached statistical significance ($P < 0.05$) in the T2D SG group (Online Supplemental Table A4, Figure 3). In total, the results suggest that bariatric surgery affected glucose metabolism through glycolytic and nonglycolytic pathways similarly for all three of the disease-surgery groups.

Increased serum heme levels were a possible indication of improved liver function following surgery. Each of the patient groups experienced an increase in serum heme levels around 100-fold compared to their respective baseline levels following surgery (Online Supplemental Table A4). A couple of interesting possibilities, such as a reduced level of heme breakdown by heme oxygenase (HO) or an increased level of synthesis by 5-aminolevulinate synthase (ALA synthase), could explain these changes. The understanding of HO-1 function has evolved beyond a simple disposal of heme to include cytoprotective, anti-inflammatory, and antioxidant functions. For instance, endogenous carbon monoxide

produced by HO-1 engages multiple signal transduction pathways to confer antiapoptotic and anti-inflammatory effects and biliverdin and bilirubin are potent antioxidants. HO activation has been shown to have insulin sensitizing and anti-inflammation effects in T2D [31]. So the increase in heme and biliverdin following surgery could represent an increase in heme oxidation by HO leading to greater antioxidant protection and insulin sensitivity. On the other hand, the greater availability of glycine, which shows a relative deficiency in T2D [23, 32], could also serve as the basis for greater heme production by ALA synthase—the rate-limiting enzyme of heme formation whose expression is repressed by glucose [33]. On the other hand, biliverdin catabolism—which can reflect red blood cell turnover and heme disposal—was less evident following surgery as indicated by reductions in bilirubin ZZ and its EE photoisomer (Online Supplemental Table A4). Together, these exciting results suggest that bariatric surgery may promote antioxidant defense and insulin sensitivity through both increased heme synthesis and HO activity or expression.

Diabetes and obesity are chronic conditions associated with elevated oxidative/inflammatory activities with a

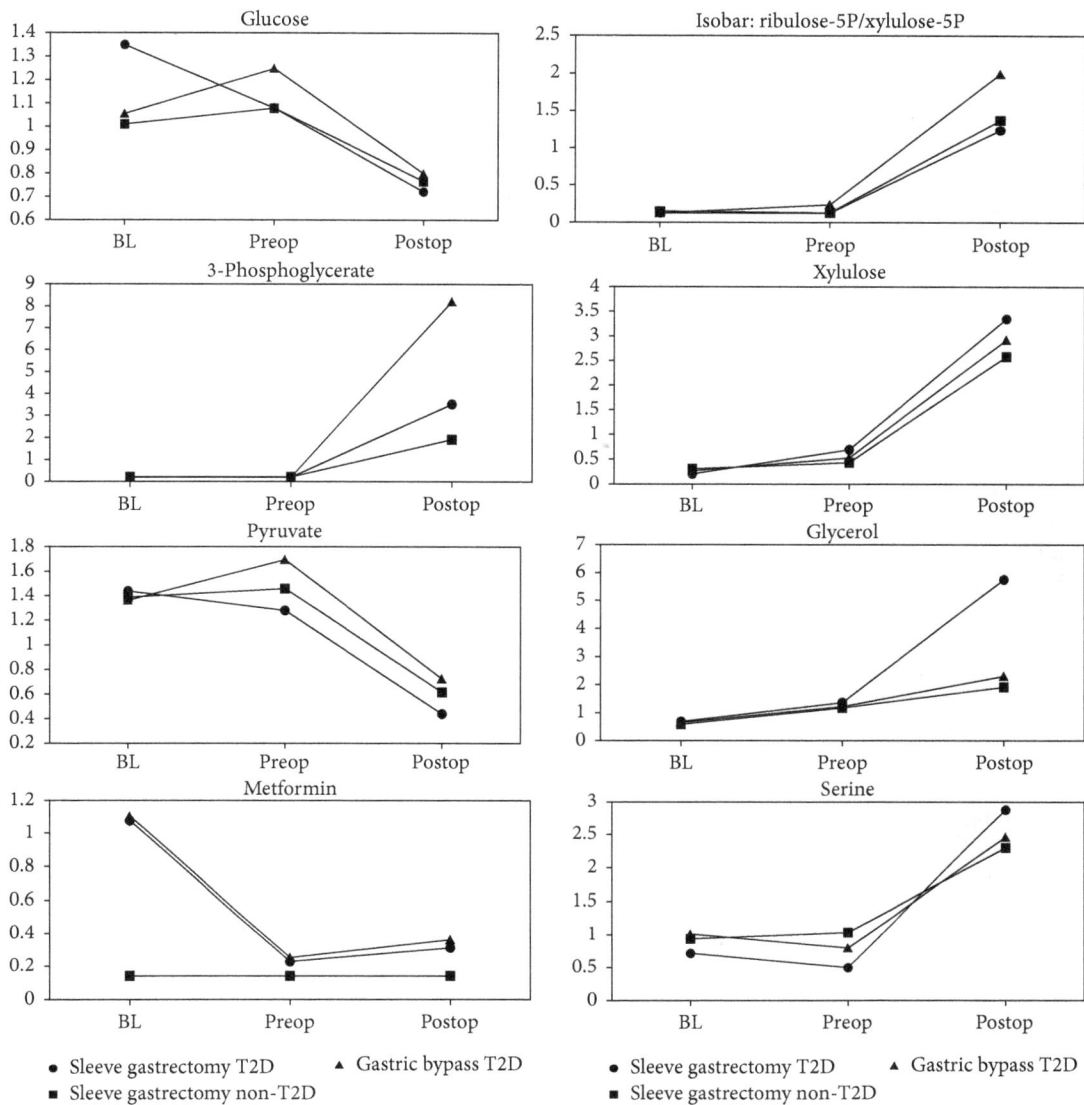

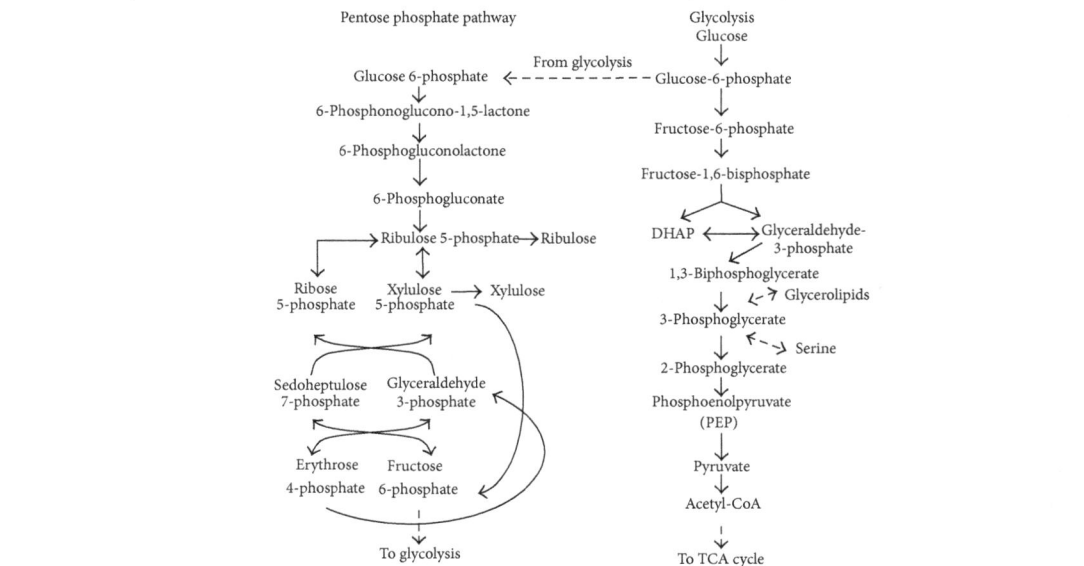

FIGURE 3: Postsurgery glucose usage shift towards pentose phosphate pathway. All shown metabolites meet the conservative criteria of $P < 0.05$ and an estimated false discovery rate of less than 5% ($q < 0.05$).

continuum of tissue insults leading to more severe cardiometabolic and renal complications including myocardial infarction and end-stage-renal damage [31]. A common denominator of these chronic conditions is the enhanced levels of cytokines like tumour necrosis factor-alpha (TNF-α), interleukin (IL-6), IL-1beta, and resistin, which in turn activates the c-Jun-N-terminal kinase (JNK) and NF-κB, pathways, creating a vicious cycle that exacerbates insulin resistance, type-2 diabetes, and related complications [31]. Emerging evidence indicates that heme oxygenase (HO) inducers are endowed with potent antidiabetic and insulin sensitizing effects besides their ability to suppress immune/inflammatory response [31]. Importantly, the HO system abates inflammation through several mechanisms including the suppression of macrophage-infiltration and abrogation of oxidative/inflammatory transcription factors like NF-κB, JNK, and activating protein-1 [31]. Thus, HO system could be explored in the search for novel remedies against T2D and its complications.

Ferrannini et al. proposed using fasting α-HB and L-GPC levels as new biomarkers to help predict dysglycemia and T2D [14, 24]. Both were detected in this study but postsurgery results do not bear out an improvement in insulin resistance based on these markers. α-HB is positively but L-GPC is negatively correlated with insulin resistance, so a postsurgery signature of improved insulin sensitivity would be expected to show a decrease of α-HB and an increase of L-GPC. Our findings showed an opposite pattern: α-HB was increased during the liquid weight-loss diet and then returned to near baseline levels after the surgery, while L-GPC levels showed significant postsurgery decrease across all three disease-surgery groups (Online Supplemental Table A4, Figure 1). There could be several reasons for this to occur, including the assumption that α-HB will drop after bariatric surgery is incorrect, or the 28-day time point is too soon to register a change. For the T2D subjects, there is the potential that metformin therapy also altered the baseline levels of α-HB and L-GPC. Future research is needed to clarify these findings.

Large increases in histidine derivatives were possibly due to altered gut microbiome composition or increased liver histidine-ammonia lyase activity. Histidine and several catabolites, such as imidazole propionate and urocanate isomers, both trans- and cis-urocanate, were significantly elevated ($P < 0.05$, $q < 0.00001$, including 100-fold + increases for trans-urocanate and cis-urocanate) in all three groups (Online Supplemental Table A4, Figure 4). Histidine is classified as an essential amino acid but gut bacteria can synthesize it, perhaps using precursors supplied by the human host. These markers may be an indication of changes in gut microbiome as the direct participation of the rat intestinal flora in the degradation of urocanate to imidazole propionate has been demonstrated previously [34].

Although the sample size was very small, these results suggested that histidine metabolites could also be important marker candidates to monitor metabolic changes associated with weight-loss surgery. Recently, Ryan and colleagues [35] found that vertical sleeve gastrectomy that led to weight loss and improvement of diabetes also resulted in changes in the gut bacteria. The researchers observed changes in several key bacterial groups that have been previously linked to the risk of T2D, and these changes were related to increase in circulating of bile acids that are known to bind to the nuclear receptor FXR. Interesting is the researches proposal that manipulating the gut bacteria might be another way to mimic the surgery [35].

On the other hand, urocanate is also formed in the liver by histidine-ammonia lyase (HAL) which converts histidine into urocanate and ammonia. Interestingly, HAL gene expression in hepatocytes can be stimulated by glucagon [36], so it is also possible that the increase of urocanate following surgery reflects a change in circulating glucagon levels. trans-Urocanate is converted to cis-urocanate by sunlight. cis-Urocanate has interesting immunosuppressive properties that are believed to help protect the skin during sun exposure and perhaps sites distal from the skin [37]. Little is known about imidazole propionate but it is a reported constituent of urine and has been proposed as a marker of intestinal dysfunction [38]. It may be useful to validate the ability of trans-urocanate, cis-urocanate, and imidazole propionate to serve as markers to monitor bariatric surgery in a larger independent cohort of patients and targeted quantitative assay. It will also be interesting to determine what, if any, utility such markers have for predicting long-term patient outcomes following surgery.

Comparing the postsurgery to the preoperation diet time point revealed 18 compounds that met the P and q-value cutoff criteria across all three disease-surgery groups (Online Supplemental Table A5). Thirteen were increased postsurgery samples relative to the samples collected at the preoperation diet time point and trans-urocanate, cis-urocanate, and pyroglutamylvaline displayed 100-fold or greater increases in nearly all of the groups.

Ascorbate and 1-linolenoylglycerol showed the greatest reductions among the 5 compounds that decreased in postsurgery samples relative to preoperation diet samples following surgery, but these reductions could also reflect altered gut absorption of these vitamins in addition to their consumption via the quenching of reactive oxygen species.

There were 29 additional compounds that represented $P < 0.05$ in all groups but did not reach $q < 0.05$ for all of the disease-surgery combinations. Histidine and several catabolites, such as imidazole propionate and urocanate isomers, were increased in T2D patients and the urocanate isomers were also likewise increased in nondiabetic patients after surgery (Online Supplemental Tables A4 and A5). Again, these results suggest that histidine metabolites could be important markers to monitor metabolic changes associated with weight-loss surgery.

4. Conclusions

Global metabolomic analysis was used to evaluate the changes occurring in nondiabetic and T2D patients experiencing either less extreme sleeve gastrectomy or a full gastric bypass. This study allowed gaining insights into the metabolic changes during both the preoperation weight-loss diet and early postsurgery recovery that accompany bariatric surgery.

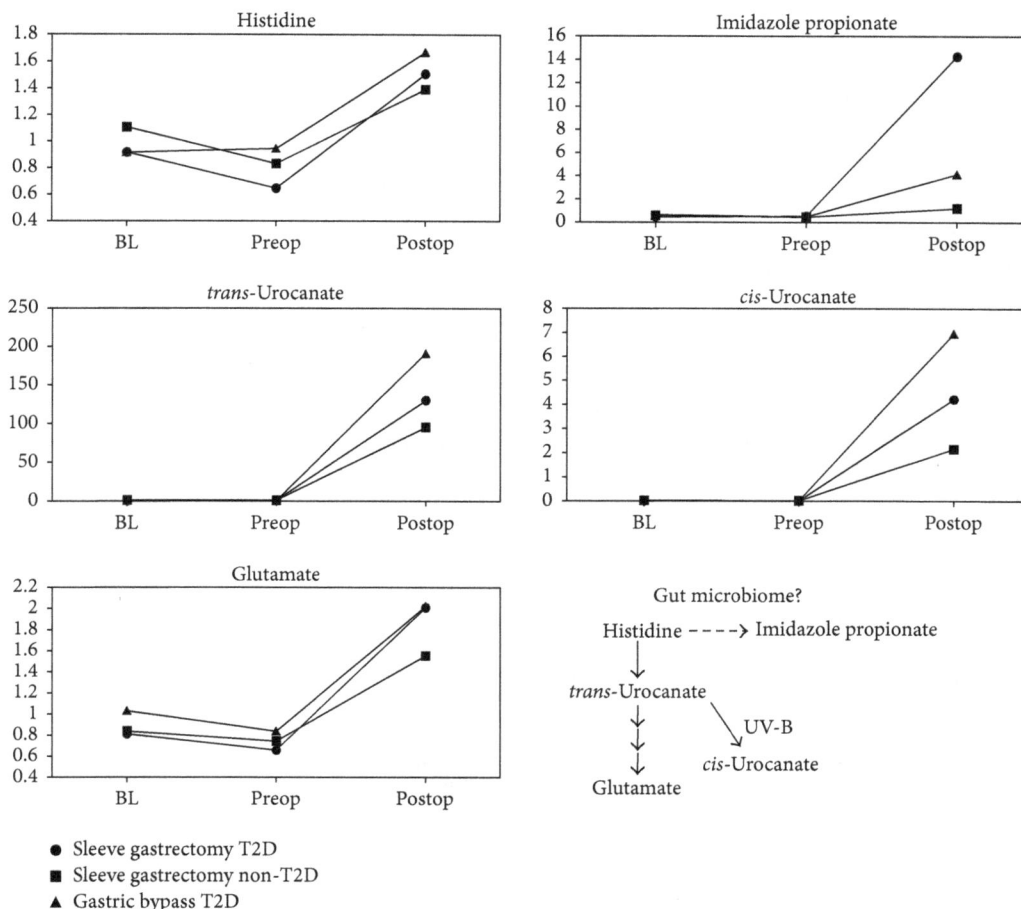

FIGURE 4: Postsurgery increase in histidine derivatives. All shown metabolites meet the conservative criteria of $P < 0.05$ and an estimated false discovery rate of less than 5% ($q < 0.05$).

To identify metabolic changes that were conserved across nondiabetic and T2D patients and different bariatric surgery procedures—sleeve gastrectomy (SG) versus gastric bypass (GB)—the metabolomic data collected for each disease-surgery combination were filtered according to statistical cut-offs for P value ($P < 0.05$) and to establish an estimated false discovery rate of less than 5% ($q < 0.05$).

It is important to point out that, despite age and sex difference, T2D status or bariatric surgery procedure, and coexistence of other associated diseases, all patients demonstrated striking similarity in major metabolome changes associated with preoperation weight-loss diet and bariatric surgery itself.

The preoperation weight-loss diet was associated with a strong lipid metabolism signature related to triglyceride hydrolysis, fatty acid oxidation, and ketone formation.

Diverse changes across a variety of metabolic areas were observed after bariatric surgery. Glucose metabolism via glycolytic and nonglycolytic pathways appeared to share a similar response across all patients regardless of baseline T2D status or the bariatric surgery procedure. Glycolysis pathway appeared to be suppressed and perhaps led to an accumulation of the TCA cycle components: malate and fumarate.

Glucose derivatives in the pentose phosphate pathway were elevated following surgery. Such increases might indicate a greater demand for pentose sugars and NADPH and the redirection of glucose-6-phosphate away from glycolysis.

Increased heme levels were a likely sign of improved antioxidant defense via the action of heme oxygenase and liver function through increased heme biosynthesis in the liver. The increased availability of glutathione precursors suggested a greater capacity to synthesize glutathione. The simultaneous postsurgery disappearance of vitamin C and surge in oxidative stress markers such as allantoin and cysteine-glutathione disulfide suggest that micronutrient status should be monitored and supported by nutritional supplementation. This initial study provided a broad understanding of how metabolism changed globally in morbidly obese subjects following weight-loss surgery. Future serum metabolomic profiling studies focusing on baseline and 28 days (or other) after surgery with a greater number of patients in each group might help to further resolve differences between diabetic and nondiabetic patients. Additionally, profiling of baseline and postsurgery fecal samples might provide a more focused manner to interrogate changes associated with gut and microbiome function. Finally, the significance of this study lays in the exploration of future treatments for obesity and T2D that can mimic bariatric surgery weight loss and improvement and resolution of T2D.

Conflict of Interests

The authors declare that they have no competing interests or other interests that might be perceived to influence the results and/or discussion reported in this paper.

Acknowledgments

The authors acknowledge research support and funding they have received from the Department of Surgery, Thomas Jefferson University Hospital, Philadelphia, PA, relevant to the work described. This work was funded by the Robert Saligman Charitable Trust.

References

[1] *National Diabetes Statistics Report: Estimates of Diabetes and Its Burden in the United States*, Department of Health and Human Services, US Centers for Disease Control and Prevention, Atlanta, Ga, USA, 2014.

[2] S. Klein, A. Ghosh, P. Y. Cremieux, S. Eapen, and T. J. McGavock, "Economic impact of the clinical benefits of bariatric surgery in diabetes patients with BMI $\geq$ 35 kg/m^2," *Obesity (Silver Spring)*, vol. 19, pp. 581–587, 2011.

[3] E. S. Ford, D. F. Williamson, and S. Liu, "Weight change and diabetes incidence: findings from a national cohort of US adults," *American Journal of Epidemiology*, vol. 146, no. 3, pp. 214–222, 1997.

[4] G. A. Colditz, W. C. Willett, A. Rotnitzky, and J. E. Manson, "Weight gain as a risk factor for clinical diabetes mellitus in women," *Annals of Internal Medicine*, vol. 122, no. 7, pp. 481–486, 1995.

[5] N. T. Nguyen, X.-M. T. Nguyen, J. Lane, and P. Wang, "Relationship between obesity and diabetes in a US adult population: findings from the national health and nutrition examination survey, 1999–2006," *Obesity Surgery*, vol. 21, no. 3, pp. 351–355, 2011.

[6] *Obesity Data*, National Health and Nutrition Examination Survey (NHANES), Centers for Disease Control and Prevention, National Center for Health Statistics (NCHS), 2014.

[7] E. A. Finkelstein, J. G. Trogdon, J. W. Cohen, and W. Dietz, "Annual medical spending attributable to obesity: payer-and service-specific estimates," *Health Affairs*, vol. 28, no. 5, pp. w822–w831, 2009.

[8] R. R. Wing, R. Koeske, L. H. Epstein, M. P. Nowalk, W. Gooding, and D. Becker, "Long-term effects of modest weight loss in type II diabetic patients," *Archives of Internal Medicine*, vol. 147, no. 10, pp. 1749–1753, 1987.

[9] W. J. Pories, M. S. Swanson, K. G. MacDonald et al., "Who would have thought it? An operation proves to be the most effective therapy for adult-onset diabetes mellitus," *Annals of Surgery*, vol. 222, no. 3, pp. 339–352, 1995.

[10] J. B. Dixon, P. E. O'Brien, J. Playfair et al., "Adjustable gastric banding and conventional therapy for type 2 diabetes," *Journal of the American Medical Association*, vol. 299, no. 3, pp. 316–323, 2008.

[11] P. R. Schauer, S. Ikramuddin, W. Gourash, R. Ramanathan, and J. Luketich, "Outcomes after laparoscopic Roux-en-Y gastric bypass for morbid obesity," *Annals of Surgery*, vol. 232, no. 4, pp. 515–529, 2000.

[12] H. Buchwald, R. Estok, K. Fahrbach et al., "Weight and type 2 diabetes after bariatric surgery: systematic review and meta-analysis," *American Journal of Medicine*, vol. 122, no. 3, pp. 248–256, 2009.

[13] J. B. Dixon, P. E. O'Brien, J. Playfair et al., "Adjustable gastric banding and conventional therapy for type 2 diabetes: a randomized controlled trial," *The Journal of the American Medical Association*, vol. 299, no. 3, pp. 316–323, 2008.

[14] W. L. Lowe Jr. and J. R. Bain, "'Prediction is very hard, especially about the future': new biomarkers for type 2 diabetes?" *Diabetes*, vol. 62, no. 5, pp. 1384–1385, 2013.

[15] N. Psychogios, D. D. Hau, J. Peng et al., "The human serum metabolome," *PLoS ONE*, vol. 6, no. 2, Article ID e16957, 2011.

[16] J. R. Bain, R. D. Stevens, B. R. Wenner, O. Ilkayeva, D. M. Muoio, and C. B. Newgard, "Metabolomics applied to diabetes research: moving from information to knowledge," *Diabetes*, vol. 58, no. 11, pp. 2429–2443, 2009.

[17] C. B. Newgard, "Interplay between lipids and branched-chain amino acids in development of insulin resistance," *Cell Metabolism*, vol. 15, no. 5, pp. 606–614, 2012.

[18] T. J. Wang, M. G. Larson, R. S. Vasan et al., "Metabolite profiles and the risk of developing diabetes," *Nature Medicine*, vol. 17, no. 4, pp. 448–453, 2011.

[19] P. Wurtz, P. Soininen, A. J. Kangas et al., "Branched-chain and aromatic amino acids are predictors of insulin resistance in young adults," *Diabetes Care*, vol. 36, no. 3, pp. 648–655, 2013.

[20] P. Würtz, M. Tiainen, V. P. Mäkinen et al., "Circulating metabolite predictors of glycemia in middle-aged men and women," *Diabetes Care*, vol. 35, pp. 1749–1756, 2012.

[21] A. Floegel, N. Stefan, Z. Yu et al., "Identification of serum metabolites associated with risk of type 2 diabetes using a targeted metabolomic approach," *Diabetes*, vol. 62, no. 2, pp. 639–648, 2013.

[22] S. E. Mccormack, O. Shaham, M. A. Mccarthy et al., "Circulating branched-chain amino acid concentrations are associated with obesity and future insulin resistance in children and adolescents," *Pediatric Obesity*, vol. 8, no. 1, pp. 52–61, 2013

[23] W. E. Gall, K. Beebe, K. A. Lawton et al., "α-hydroxybutyrate is an early biomarker of insulin resistance and glucose intolerance in a nondiabetic population," *PLoS ONE*, vol. 5, no. 5, Article ID e10883, 2010.

[24] E. Ferrannini, A. Natali, S. Camastra et al., "Early metabolic markers of the development of dysglycemia and type 2 diabetes and their physiological significance," *Diabetes*, vol. 62, no. 5, pp. 1730–1737, 2013.

[25] J. D. Storey and R. Tibshirani, "Statistical significance for genomewide studies," *Proceedings of the National Academy of Sciences of the United States of America*, vol. 100, no. 16, pp. 9440–9445, 2003.

[26] A. P. Morris, B. F. Voight, T. M. Teslovich et al., "Large-scale association analysis provides insights into the genetic architecture and pathophysiology of type 2 diabetes," *Nature Genetics*, vol. 44, no. 9, pp. 981–990, 2012.

[27] J. L. Vassy, N. H. Durant, E. K. Kabagambe et al., "A genotype risk score predicts type 2 diabetes from young adulthood: the CARDIA study," *Diabetologia*, vol. 55, no. 10, pp. 2504–2612, 2012.

[28] S. L. Faria, O. P. Faria, M. D. A. Cardeal, and M. K. Ito, "Effects of a very low calorie diet in the preoperative stage of bariatric surgery a randomized trial," *Surgery for Obesity and Related Diseases*, vol. 11, no. 1, pp. 230–237, 2015.

[29] V. R. G. da Silva, E. A. M. Moreira, D. Wilhelm-Filho et al., "Proinflammatory and oxidative stress markers in patients submitted to Roux-en-Y gastric bypass after 1 year of follow-up," *European Journal of Clinical Nutrition*, vol. 66, no. 8, pp. 891–895, 2012.

[30] S. P. Donadelli, M. V. M. Junqueira-Franco, C. A. de Mattos Donadelli et al., "Daily vitamin supplementation and hypovita-minosis after obesity surgery," *Nutrition*, vol. 28, no. 4, pp. 391–396, 2012.

[31] J. F. Ndisang, "Role of heme oxygenase in inflammation, insulin-signalling, diabetes and obesity," *Mediators of Inflammation*, vol. 2010, Article ID 359732, 18 pages, 2010.

[32] R. Wang-Sattler, Z. Yu, C. Herder et al., "Novel biomarkers for pre-diabetes identified by metabolomics," *Molecular Systems Biology*, vol. 8, article 615, 2012.

[33] C. Handschin, J. Lin, J. Rhee et al., "Nutritional regulation of hepatic heme biosynthesis and porphyria through PGC-1alpha," *Cell*, vol. 122, no. 4, pp. 505–515, 2005.

[34] A. V. Emes and H. Hassall, "The degradation of L-histidine in the rat. The formation of imidazolylpyruvate, imidazolyl-lactate and imidazolylpropionate," *Biochemical Journal*, vol. 136, no. 3, pp. 649–658, 1973.

[35] K. K. Ryan, V. Tremaroli, C. Clemmensen et al., "FXR is a molecular target for the effects of vertical sleeve gastrectomy," *Nature*, vol. 509, no. 7499, pp. 183–188, 2014.

[36] G. Alemán, V. Ortíz, E. Langley, A. R. Tovar, and N. Torres, "Regulation by glucagon of the rat histidase gene promoter in cultured rat hepatocytes and human hepatoblastoma cells," *The American Journal of Physiology—Endocrinology and Metabolism*, vol. 289, no. 1, pp. E172–E179, 2005.

[37] N. K. Gibbs and M. Norval, "Urocanic acid in the skin: a mixed blessing," *Journal of Investigative Dermatology*, vol. 131, no. 1, pp. 14–17, 2011.

[38] C. Van der Heiden, S. K. Wadman, P. K. De Bree, and E. A. K. Wauters, "Increased urinary imidazolepropionic acid, n-acetylhistamine and other imidazole compounds in patients with intestinal disorders," *Clinica Chimica Acta*, vol. 39, no. 1, pp. 201–214, 1972.

27

Tyrosine Is Associated with Insulin Resistance in Longitudinal Metabolomic Profiling of Obese Children

Christian Hellmuth,[1] Franca Fabiana Kirchberg,[1] Nina Lass,[2] Ulrike Harder,[1] Wolfgang Peissner,[1] Berthold Koletzko,[1] and Thomas Reinehr[2]

[1]Division of Metabolic and Nutritional Medicine, Dr. von Hauner Children's Hospital, Ludwig-Maximilians-University of Munich, Lindwurmstraße 4, 80337 Munich, Germany
[2]Department of Pediatric Endocrinology, Diabetes and Nutrition Medicine, Vestische Hospital for Children and Adolescents, University of Witten-Herdecke, Dr. Friedrich Steiner Strasse 5, 45711 Datteln, Germany

Correspondence should be addressed to Berthold Koletzko; office.koletzko@med.uni-muenchen.de

Academic Editor: Francisco J. Ruperez

In obese children, hyperinsulinaemia induces adverse metabolic consequences related to the risk of cardiovascular and other disorders. Branched-chain amino acids (BCAA) and acylcarnitines (Carn), involved in amino acid (AA) degradation, were linked to obesity-associated insulin resistance, but these associations yet have not been studied longitudinally in obese children. We studied 80 obese children before and after a one-year lifestyle intervention programme inducing substantial weight loss >0.5 BMI standard deviation scores in 40 children and no weight loss in another 40 children. At baseline and after the 1-year intervention, we assessed insulin resistance (HOMA index), fasting glucose, HbA1c, 2 h glucose in an oral glucose tolerance test, AA, and Carn. BMI adjusted metabolite levels were associated with clinical markers at baseline and after intervention, and changes with the intervention period were evaluated. Only tyrosine was significantly associated with HOMA ($p < 0.05$) at baseline and end and with change during the intervention ($p < 0.05$). In contrast, ratios depicting BCAA metabolism were negatively associated with HOMA at baseline ($p < 0.05$), but not in the longitudinal profiling. Stratified analysis revealed that the children with substantial weight loss drove this association. We conclude that tyrosine alterations in association with insulin resistance precede alteration in BCAA metabolism. This trial is registered with ClinicalTrials.gov Identifier NCT00435734.

1. Introduction

Obesity in childhood is strongly associated with cardiovascular risk factors (CRFs) including dyslipidemia, hyperglycaemia, and hypertension [1]. In obese children hyperinsulinaemia and other CRFs are far more commonly found than in normal weight children and adolescents [2–4]. Most metabolic consequences appear to be mediated through insulin resistance (IR) [5]; therefore improving insulin sensitivity seems even more important than weight loss [6]. "Omics" platforms, such as proteomics, transcriptomics, epigenomics, and metabolomics, provide insights into molecular changes and allow assessing biochemical alterations in the development of obesity and IR [7, 8]. While new targets or potential biomarkers are identified in humans with these approaches [9, 10], the role of known metabolites still needs to be evaluated. Particularly, the influence of amino acid (AA) metabolism on the onset of IR still needs clarification. Two recent studies have reported on the untargeted metabolomic approach to study the relation of metabolites to IR in older adults [11] and children [12]. Untargeted metabolomics involves an unbiased screening of all metabolites present in a specimen regardless of chemical class. Targeted metabolomic techniques facilitate the profiling of specific metabolites of interest in a given population, to aid in-depth analysis of metabolic processes in the context of preformed findings. Thus, clinical targeted metabolomics platforms are suitable tools to reveal associations between AA and IR. Different studies depicted associations between IR or type 2 diabetes mellitus (T2DM) and branched-chain amino acids (BCAA), aromatic amino acids (AAA), sulphur containing AA, and other AAs as well as short-chain acylcarnitines (Carn) involved in AA metabolism in adults [13–23]. BCAA were found to be positively associated with homeostasis model assessment (HOMA), an IR index, in nonobese Chinese men [15] and young Finn adults [16]. Mohorko et al. recently reported elevated serum levels of cysteine (Cys) and tyrosine (Tyr) as early biomarkers for metabolic syndrome in young adults [14] Newgard et al. showed that BCAA and short-chain Carn derived from BCAA contribute to the development of obesity-associated IR [13]. However, the majority of these studies describe relations of clinical markers to metabolites in cross-sectional settings. Furthermore, such associations are susceptible to confounders, like dietary protein intake that was shown to be higher in obese subjects than in normal weight subjects [15]. A few studies describe the prediction potential of BCAA and AAA for the onset of IR [16, 18, 24]. Although metabolomic analyses in children yield the potential to investigate the early onset of metabolic disease, studies on obese children are lacking. Recently, Newbern et al. reported an association of HOMA with a metabolic signature containing BCAA, uric acid, and long-chain Carn in adolescent boys in a cross-sectional study [25]. A combination of BCAA and AAA was associated with HOMA in obese Hispanic children [26], but only BCAA in Korean children [27]. BCAA pattern and androgen hormone pattern were associated with childhood adiposity and cardiometabolic risk, like HOMA, in another recently published cross-sectional study [12]. Longitudinal studies are necessary to explore stronger association between IR and metabolic alterations. To our knowledge, two longitudinal studies in children have been published so far, showing an association of baseline BCAA with HOMA in healthy American children [28] and in Korean children [27].

We embarked on a longitudinal study on obese children participating in a lifestyle intervention for inducing weight loss to explore the relationship between changes in AA metabolism and IR in the fasting state and after an oral glucose tolerance test (oGTT) in obese European children. Additionally, we analysed the obesity-independent associations of changes during the intervention period in makers of IR, hemoglobin A1c (HbA1c), 2 h glucose in oGTT, and changes of AA and Carn.

2. Methods

2.1. Study Written informed consent was obtained from all parents of the participants prior to inclusion in the study. The study has been performed according to the Declaration of Helsinki. The local ethics committee of the University of Witten/Herdecke in Germany approved the study (ClinicalTrials.gov Identifier NCT00435734). We studied 80 obese Caucasian children participating in the one-year lifestyle intervention "Obeldicks," which has been described in detail elsewhere [29]. Briefly, this outpatient intervention program is based on promoting regular physical activity, nutrition education, and behavior therapy including individual psychological care of the children and their families. The one-year training program was divided into three phases. In the first one, intensive phase (3 months), the children took part in the nutritional course and in the eating-behavior course

in six group-sessions, each lasting for 1.5 hours. Parents were invited to attend six evening classes. In the establishing phase (6 months), individual psychological family therapy was provided (30 minutes/month). In the last phase of the program (accompanying the families back to their everyday lives) (3 months), further individual care was possible, if and when necessary. None of the children in the current study were smokers, took any drugs, or suffered from endocrine disorders or syndromal obesity such as Prader Willi syndrome [30]. Also MC4 receptor mutation was excluded. The children studied were selected at random from the Obeldicks cohort reported previously [30] choosing 40 obese children with substantial weight loss and 40 obese children without weight loss of similar age, gender, pubertal stage, and degree of overweight. We included only children who participated in oGTT both at baseline and after one year. Substantial reduction of overweight was defined by a decrease in standard deviation score of body mass index (BMI-SDS) ≥ 0.5 based on previous studies [31], whereas no reduction of overweight was defined by a decrease in BMI-SDS < 0.15. The metabolomic profile of these children in respect to obesity status and weight loss was previously reported [32].

2.2. Measurements and Sampling. Height was measured to the nearest millimeter using a rigid stadiometer. Weight was measured unclothed to the nearest 0.1 kg using a calibrated balance scale. BMI was calculated as weight in kilograms (kg) divided by the square of height in meters (m^2). The degree of overweight was quantified using Cole's LMS method, which normalized the BMI skewed distribution and expressed BMI as a standard deviation score (BMI-SDS) [33]. Reference data for German children were used [34]. Waist circumference was measured halfway between lower rib and iliac crest.

For longitudinal analysis, blood samples were collected in the fasting state before the intervention and after 1 year. Furthermore, oGTT were performed according to current guidelines [35]. The glucose load was 1.75 g/kg with a maximum of 75 g. Blood samples were taken at 8 a.m. after overnight fasting for at least 10 hours. Following coagulation at room temperature, blood samples were centrifuged for 10 min at 8000 rpm at room temperature and aliquoted. Glucose (Boehringer, Mannheim, Germany), HbA1c (Germany Tinaquant Hemoglobin A1c Gen), and insulin (Abbott, Wiesbaden, Germany) were measured in serum by using commercially available test kits directly. Intra-assay and interassay CVs of glucose, HbA1c, and insulin were less than 5%. HOMA was used to detect the degree of IR [36]. Furthermore, serum samples were stored at –81°C and thawed at room temperature for the metabolomics assay only once.

2.3. Biochemical Measures. Metabolites were qualified and quantified with the Absolute IDQ p 150 kit (Biocrates Life Sciences AG, Innsbruck, Austria) as described previously [32]. Briefly, 10 μL of blood serum was analysed with a flow injection tandem mass spectrometer (FIA-MS/MS). An Agilent 1200 SL series high-performance liquid chromatography system (Agilent, Waldbronn, Germany) was coupled to a hybrid quadrupole mass spectrometer (QTRAP 4000, AB Sciex, Darmstadt, Germany). MS/MS analysis was run in

TABLE 1: Characteristics of participating children at start and end point of the 1-year intervention period. Characteristics are shown for all obese children ($n = 80$), children with substantial weight loss (WL, $n = 40$), and children without substantial weight loss (nWL, $n = 40$) as mean ± SD unless stated otherwise.

Parameter	All start (%)	All end (%)	WL start (%)	WL end (%)	nWL start (%)	nWL end (%)
Sex, male	36 (45%)		18 (45%)		18 (45%)	
Age (years)	11.5 ± 2.42	12.5 ± 2.42	10.6 ± 2.54	11.6 ± 2.54	12.4 ± 1.9	13.4 ± 1.9
Prepubertal	34 (42%)	26 (32%)	23 (58%)	18 (45%)	11 (28%)	8 (20%)
Early pubertal	42 (52%)	44 (55%)	17 (42%)	22 (55%)	25 (62%)	22 (55%)
Postpubertal	4 (5%)	10 (12%)	—	—	4 (10%)	10 (25%)
BMI-SDS	2.4 ± 0.45	2.1 ± 0.63*	2.4 ± 0.44	1.7 ± 0.58*	2.4 ± 0.46	2.4 ± 0.47*
Waist circumference (cm)	91.7 ± 14	89.3 ± 13.89*	87 ± 13.59	81 ± 10.99*	96.5 ± 12.88	97.3 ± 11.55
Insulin (mU/L)	19.9 ± 15.01	17 ± 12.39	18 ± 12.01	9.3 ± 3.87*	21.9 ± 17.44	25.1 ± 13.14*
Fasting glucose (mg/dL)	86.3 ± 7.38	87.1 ± 6.39	84.8 ± 7.05	85.5 ± 5.76	87.8 ± 7.47	88.8 ± 6.65
2-hour oGTT glucose (mg/dL)	132.7 ± 25.02	113.9 ± 23.94*	133.9 ± 24.26	98.9 ± 10.42*	131.4 ± 25.99	123.9 ± 24.28
HbA1C (mmol/mol Hb)	373.43 ± 32.92	372.81 ± 37.98	364.16 ± 30.12	363.77 ± 30.81	382.95 ± 33.32	382.61 ± 42.78
HOMA	4.29 ± 3.1	3.79 ± 3.2	4.01 ± 3	1.96 ± 0.81*	4.58 ± 3.21	5.57 ± 3.64*

*Significant different means between start and end point ($p < 0.05$, paired Wilcoxon rank sum test).

Multiple Reaction Monitoring mode with electrospray ionization used in both positive and negative modes. Data acquisition on the mass spectrometer was controlled by Analyst 1.5 software (AB Sciex, Darmstadt, Germany). For raw data processing, peak integration, isotope correction, calibration, and quality control, the Met IQ software package (Biocrates Life Sciences AG, Innsbruck, Austria) was used, which is an integral part of the Absolute *IDQ* kit quantifying a total of 163 metabolites. Middle- and long-chain Carn, sphingomyelins (SM), acyl-linked phosphatidylcholines, ether-linked phosphatidylcholines, and lysophosphatidylcholines were not used for the data analysis of this work, since the presented study focused on alterations in AA metabolism with respect to IR. For the presented work, we analyzed 14 short-chain Carn ($Cx:y$, hydroxyl acylcarnitines $Cx:y$-OH, oxoacylcarnitines $Cx:y$-oxo, and dicarboxylacylcarnitines $Cx:y$-DC), free carnitine (Carn C0), and 14 AA. $Cx:y$ abbreviates the lipid side chain composition, x and y denoting the number of carbons and double bonds, respectively. The sum of leucine (Leu) and isoleucine (Ile) is expressed as xLeu. Samples were integrated with the Met IQ software by automated calculation of metabolite concentrations. For the data analysis performed here, only short-chain Carn, Carn C0, and AA are used. The sum of xLeu and valine (Val) is expressed as BCAA sum. The sum of phenylalanine (Phe), tryptophan (Trp), and Tyr is expressed as AAA sum. We report all metabolite concentrations in μmol/L. In addition to the 29 metabolite concentrations and two sum parameters, eleven metabolite ratios were calculated resulting in a total of 42 metabolites and metabolite ratios.

2.4. *Statistics.* All statistical analyses were performed using the statistical software R (3.0.2) [37]. In a first step, we graphically screened for outliers and normality. An absolute metabolite concentration that lay greater than 1 standard deviation (SD) away from its nearest neighbor was considered to be an outlier and this measurement was excluded from the analysis. Principal component analysis score plots were used

as a complementary tool to ensure that no outliers remained undetected.

Differences in clinical parameters between baseline and follow-up were calculated using the paired Wilcoxon rank test. Associations between markers for insulin and glucohomeostasis were quantified using Spearman rank correlation coefficients.

The changes in the clinical markers, metabolite concentrations, and metabolite ratios over the one-year intervention are expressed as the relative difference of baseline and follow-up measurements (with the baseline values being the reference). For each time point (baseline and follow-up) as well as for the relative change, we calculated the following model to assess the association between the metabolites and the clinical parameters: (1) firstly, in order to account for the effect of obesity status on the metabolite level, we fitted age and sex adjusted robust regression models of the BMI on the metabolite using the M-estimator with Huber bisquare weighting (R package MASS); (2) subsequently, we regressed the obtained metabolite residuals on markers for IR with robust regression models using the M-estimator with Huber bisquare weighting (R package MASS). p values and estimates are taken as proxies for the strengths and directions of the associations. Results of selected clinical outcomes are represented graphically in Manhattan plots, where the $\log_{10}(p)$ values are plotted and the sign is used to indicate the direction of the relationship, as assessed by the robust regression model. Due to the small sample size and in order not to veil differences in p values, we will report the raw (unadjusted) p values. The significance level was thus set at $p < 0.05$. Bonferroni corrected p values can be obtained by multiplying the reported p values with the factor 42 (number of analytes tested). The Bonferroni corrected significance level is 0.0012.

3. Results

3.1. *Population Characteristics.* Characteristics of participating children are presented in Table 1. In all obese children,

TABLE 2: Spearman correlation coefficients of markers of insulin homeostasis in all obese children ($n = 80$) at baseline.

	Fasting glucose (mg/dL)	2-hour oGTT glucose (mg/dL)	HbA1C (mmol/mol Hb)	Insulin (mU/L)	HOMA	BMI-SDS	Waist circumference (cm)
Fasting glucose (mg/dL)	1	0.246	0.231	0.091	0.154	−0.001	0.241
2-hour oGTT glucose (mg/dL)		1	0.188	0.113	0.135	0.153	0.164
HbA1C (mmol/mol Hb)			1	0.120	0.176	0.116	0.234
Insulin (mU/L)				1	0.984	0.343	0.586
HOMA					1	0.402	0.669
BMI-SDS						1	0.445
Waist circumference (cm)							1

waist circumference and 2-hour oGTT glucose decreased significantly during the intervention period. Additionally, insulin levels and HOMA decreased in the group of 40 obese children with substantial weight loss. In contrast, insulin levels and HOMA increased in the group of obese children without substantial weight loss. Since HOMA and insulin were strongly correlated (Table 2) and HbA1C and fasting glucose showed no changes between the two time points in any of the groups, in contrast to HOMA, waist circumference, and 2 h glucose in oGTT (Table 1), we focused our data analysis on HOMA, 2-hour oGTT glucose, and waist circumference. Waist circumference showed no significant association with the metabolites. No difference between puberty and HOMA status was found at baseline ($p = 0.44$), but after the intervention period ($p = 0.036$) with pubertal children having higher HOMA values.

Associations of all clinical parameters and metabolites are reported in the Supplementary Material (available online at http://dx.doi.org/10.1155/2016/2108909).

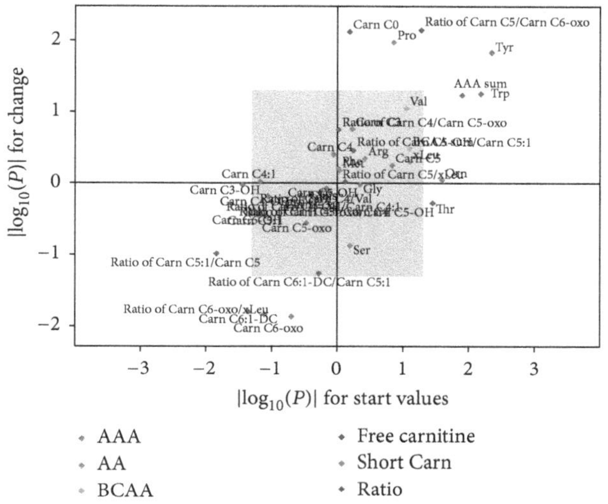

3.2. HOMA. At baseline, HOMA was positively associated with Tyr ($p = 0.004$, Figure 2), Trp ($p = 0.007$), sum of AAA ($p = 0.013$), ornithine (Orn, $p = 0.026$), and threonine (Thr, $p = 0.036$) and negatively associated with Carn C3-OH ($p = 0.036$) and the ratios of Carn C5:1/Carn C5 ($p = 0.014$) and Carn C6-oxo/xLeu ($p = 0.044$) in all obese children (Figure 1). After the end of the intervention, only Tyr was associated with HOMA in all obese children ($p = 0.044$, Figures 2 and 3). In a stratified analysis including the 40 children with substantial weight loss, HOMA was negatively associated with the ratio of Carn C6-oxo/xLeu ($p = 0.011$), Carn C6-oxo ($p = 0.023$), and Carn C4 ($p = 0.031$) and positively associated with Carn C4/Carn C5-oxo ($p = 0.041$) and Tyr ($p = 0.047$, Figure 2) at baseline. After the intervention, only Tyr was associated with HOMA ($p = 0.041$) in the children with substantial weight loss (Figures 2 and 3). Children without substantial weight loss showed different associations for HOMA. Thr ($p < 0.001$) and proline (Pro, $p = 0.0322$) were positively associated with HOMA, while the ratios of Carn C5:1/Carn C5 ($p = 0.030$) and Carn C4/Val ($p = 0.033$) were negatively associated at baseline. After the intervention, only the ratio of Carn C5-OH/Carn C5:1 was associated with HOMA ($p = 0.048$) in children without substantial weight loss (Figure 3). The significant associations

FIGURE 1: Associations of amino acids (AA) and acylcarnitines (Carn) with HOMA. Associations were calculated at baseline (x-axis) and for changes of AA and Carn to changes of HOMA during the intervention (y-axis) period in all children ($n = 80$). Displayed are the absolute log(p) values of the applied obesity-independent robust regression models for both associations. AAA, aromatic amino acids; BCAA, branched-chain amino acids.

between the relative change of HOMA during the intervention period and the relative change of AA and Carn are shown in Table 3 for all obese children (Figure 1), children with substantial weight loss, and children without substantial weight loss. The change of ratio of Carn C5/Carn C6-oxo was positively associated with change of HOMA in all three groups, while this was true for the ratio of Carn C4/Carn C5-oxo only in children with substantial weight loss. Changes of Tyr were again positively correlated with changes in HOMA in all children and children with substantial weight loss.

3.3. Two-Hour oGTT Glucose. Two-hour oGTT glucose showed different associations compared to HOMA, particularly in children with substantial weight loss. At baseline, the ratios of Carn C4:1/Carn C4 ($p = 0.011$, negative), Carn C4/Carn C5-oxo ($p = 0.023$, positive), and Carn C4/Val ($p = 0.05$, positive) as well as histidine (His, $p = 0.040$,

TABLE 3: Estimates and p values (p) of changes in metabolite concentrations which are significantly associated with changes in HOMA in at least one (sub)group (All, WL, and nWL). Change is defined as the relative change over the one-year intervention. Estimates are given with 95% confidence interval (CI). Estimates, confidence intervals, and p values were calculated with robust regression models. WL, children with substantial weight loss; nWL, children without substantial weight loss; AAA, aromatic amino acids; Carn, acylcarnitine; Pro, proline; Trp, tryptophan; Tyr, tyrosine; Val, valine, xLeu, sum of leucine and isoleucine.

Analyte	All ($n = 80$)		WL ($n = 40$)		nWL ($n = 40$)	
	Estimate [95% CI]	p	Estimate [95% CI]	p	Estimate [95% CI]	p
AAA sum	0.79 [−0.04; 1.60]	0.059	1.04 [0.29; 1.80]	0.009	0.27 [−1.40; 1.90]	0.742
Carn C0	1.10 [0.29; 1.90]	0.008	1.71 [0.88; 2.50]	<0.001	0.24 [−1.30; 1.70]	0.751
Carn C3	0.34 [−0.16; 0.83]	0.174	0.49 [0.03; 0.96]	0.036	0.24 [−0.72; 1.20]	0.615
Carn C6:1-DC	−0.33 [−0.59; −0.06]	0.015	−0.29 [−0.47; −0.10]	0.003	−0.37 [−1.10; 0.38]	0.342
Carn C6-oxo	−0.24 [−0.43; −0.05]	0.014	−0.21 [−0.35; −0.08]	0.003	−0.21 [−0.73; 0.31]	0.438
Pro	0.81 [0.19; 1.40]	0.011	0.72 [0.11; 1.30]	0.023	0.88 [−0.08; 1.80]	0.067
Ratio of Carn C4/Carn C5-oxo	0.23 [−0.09; 0.55]	0.177	0.48 [0.18; 0.77]	0.003	−0.21 [−0.86; 0.45]	0.530
Ratio of Carn C5/Carn C6-oxo	0.24 [0.07; 0.41]	0.007	0.22 [0.08; 0.35]	0.002	0.29 [0.02; 0.57]	0.041
Ratio of Carn C6:1-DC/Carn C5:1	−0.27 [−0.54; 0.01]	0.055	−0.22 [−0.41; −0.03]	0.024	−0.39 [−1.10; 0.37]	0.321
Ratio of Carn C6-oxo/xLeu	−0.19 [−0.34; −0.03]	0.016	−0.15 [−0.25; −0.04]	0.007	−0.24 [−0.84; 0.37]	0.442
Trp	0.93 [−0.02; 1.90]	0.056	1.13 [0.14; 2.10]	0.027	0.44 [−1.30; 2.20]	0.613
Tyr	0.79 [0.17; 1.40]	0.015	1.09 [0.51; 1.70]	0.001	0.28 [−0.99; 1.50]	0.651
Val	0.65 [−0.11; 1.40]	0.090	0.73 [0.07; 1.40]	0.033	0.48 [−1.10; 2.10]	0.544

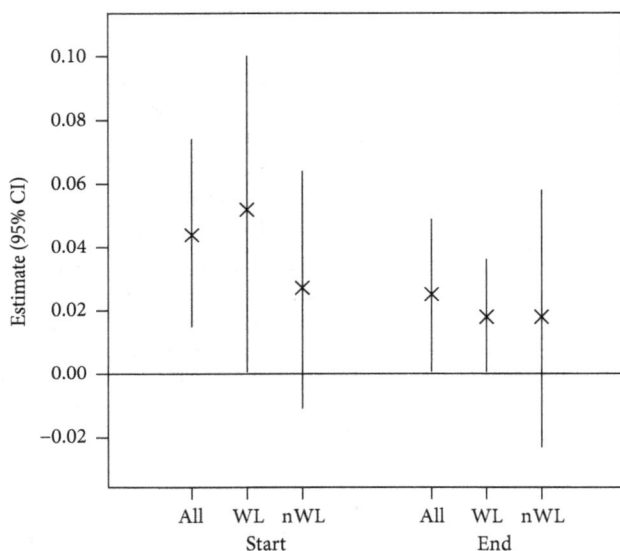

FIGURE 2: Estimates (95% CI) for associations of tyrosine with HOMA. Associations were calculated at baseline (Start) and after the intervention (End). Associations were calculated for all obese children ($n = 80$), children with substantial weight loss (WL, $n = 40$), and children without substantial weight loss (nWL, $n = 40$). 95% CI: 95% confidence interval.

negative), serine (Ser, $p = 0.043$, negative), and Carn C4 ($p = 0.049$, positive) were associated with 2-hour oGTT glucose in children with substantial weight loss, while children without substantial weight loss showed only positive associations between arginine (Arg) and 2-hour oGTT glucose at baseline. After the intervention, 2-hour oGTT glucose was associated negatively with Ser ($p = 0.048$) and Orn ($p = 0.039$) in children with substantial weight loss and with glutamine

(Gln, $p = 0.011$) and Carn C3-OH ($p = 0.012$) in children without substantial weight loss. Interestingly, changes of 2-hour oGTT glucose during the one-year intervention period were not significantly associated with changes of any of the measured metabolites, ratios, or sums in any of the groups.

4. Discussion

To our knowledge, this is the first longitudinal study analysing the relationships between metabolites and markers of glucose metabolism in obese children. Tyr is the only metabolite which was significantly associated with HOMA at baseline and after intervention. Changes of Tyr over time were also positively associated with changes of HOMA in our obesity-independent model. Thus, Tyr, rather than BCAA, seems to be associated with IR. This is in accordance with a recent study where Tyr was identified as the most important metabolite in a random forest analysis in obese children [26]. In the same study, a combination of BCAA and AAA was most strongly related to HOMA. Furthermore, Tyr was found to be a strong predictor for diabetes in South Asian men [21]. Tyr is biosynthesised endogenously by hydroxylation of Phe by phenylalanine hydroxylase in mammals [38]. Since Phe was not associated with HOMA in any of the groups at any time point, we assume that there is no confounding dietary effect on Tyr levels. Tyr stimulates insulin secretion, but other AAs are more effective in stimulating insulin release [39]. In contrast, Michaliszyn et al. showed a positive association of β-cell function and all AAs except for Tyr and citrulline in adolescents [40]. The same group reported lower AA plasma levels, except for Tyr, in diabetic adolescents [41], which is in contrast to the role of elevated AA in IR [42]. However, the effect on insulin secretion should not be driving the relation between Tyr and HOMA. An influence on Tyr metabolism appears more likely. Insulin is known to increase

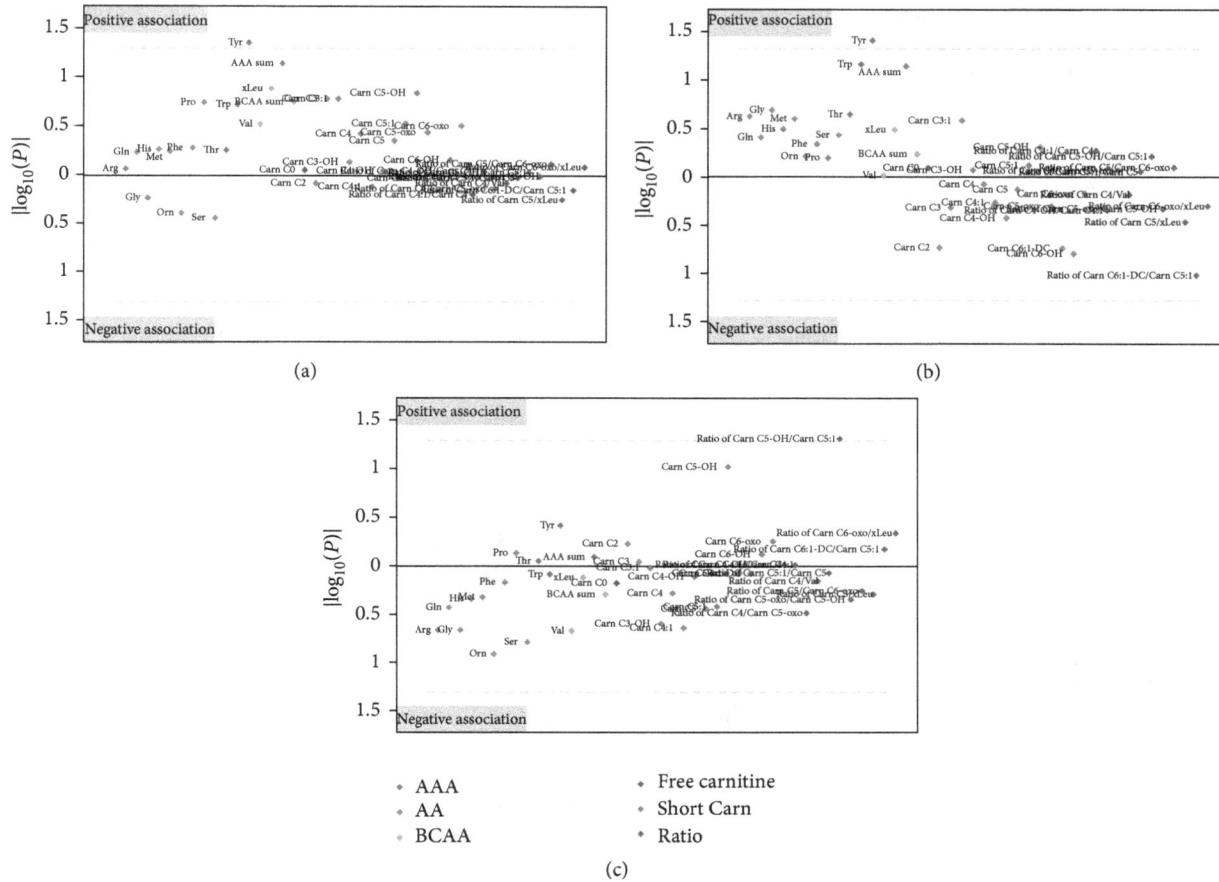

FIGURE 3: Manhattan plot for associations of amino acids (AA) and acylcarnitines (Carn) with HOMA after the one-year lifestyle intervention for all obese children (a), children with substantial weight loss (b), and children without substantial weight loss (c). Plotted are the $\log_{10}(p)$ values and the sign is used to indicate the direction of the relationship, as assessed by the robust regression model. The area below or above the dashed lines contains metabolites that are significantly related to HOMA (p values < 0.05). AAA, aromatic amino acids; BCAA, branched-chain amino acids.

tyrosine aminotransferase (TAT) activity in rat liver [43], probably by selectively slowing down the rate of degradation of TAT [44]. TAT catalyses the transamination of Tyr to p-hydroxyphenylpyruvate. This should result in lower Tyr levels. A possible inhibition of TAT may occur due to higher Cys levels. Cys is an inhibitor of TAT [19, 45]. In a recent study, only Cys and Tyr were found to be increased in nonobese adults who had one symptom of the metabolic syndrome [14]. With further progression of the metabolic syndrome, BCAA and Phe were enhanced in subjects with two or more symptoms of the metabolic syndrome. It seems that alterations in Cys and Tyr metabolism precede changes in BCAA metabolism. Thus, Tyr is a potential early marker for the onset of IR. Higher insulin levels in the IR state may still cover demands to ensure adequate glucose metabolism, but Tyr may be affected and Tyr may present an early biomarker for the onset of IR in obese children. This predictive value of Tyr was shown in previous studies in adults, along with BCAA in young adults [16, 18]. In the presented study, we could not investigate Tyr as predictor for later IR, since the "Obeldicks" study has an interventional design not a prospective one.

Contrarily, Lee et al. found BCAA, and not AAA, as predictive marker for IR in Korean children [27]. Thus, further prospective, longitudinal studies are required to unravel associations between AA and IR with respect to sex and ethnicity.

Furthermore, Tyr can affect BCAA levels, since BCAA and AA compete for the same neutral AA transporter for cellular uptake [46]. Thus, prolonged elevated Tyr levels may also result in elevated BCAA level. Many studies found altered levels of BCAA when studying obesity in adults [9], but also when looking at IR and T2DM in adults [13, 15–18, 42]. Similar results were found in a few cross-sectional studies in children [12, 25]. We found no association between HOMA and BCAA, neither at baseline nor after the intervention. A previous cross-sectional metabolomic analysis of the presented population did not find different BCAA levels between obese and normal weight children [47]. Levels of BCAA, being essential AAs, are mainly defined by the diet. Thus, higher BCAA levels later in life may result from competition for the neutral AAs transport [46], higher protein intake, and/or disturbed BCAA clearance [48]. During BCAA degradation, Val, Leu, and Ile are first degraded to the α-keto acids

C5-oxo and C6-oxo by the branched-chain amino transferase (BCAT). These keto acids are subsequently reduced by branched-chain α-keto acid dehydrogenase (BCKDH) in the rate limiting step [49]. To identify alterations of BCAA metabolism in obesity and IR, we calculated the ratios of the different steps in the BCAA degradation pathway. We found that the ratio of C6-oxo to C5 was positively associated with HOMA at baseline and in the change during the intervention period in all three groups. The ratio of C5-oxo to C4 was positively associated with HOMA only in children with substantial weight loss only. Both ratios are markers for the second, rate limiting degradation step of BCAA which is regulated by BCAA itself to keep BCAA concentrations at a constant level. Thus, this pathway may have been upregulated in our study resulting in BCAA levels not associated with HOMA. In contrast, all other ratios showed no significant association with HOMA or were negatively associated with HOMA, particularly the first step of xLeu degradation to methyl-ketopentanoate (C6-oxo) by BCAT. It was shown recently that IR subjects have a significant reduction in BCAT expression and other enzymes involved in BCAA metabolism in the adipose tissue compared to none-IR subjects [50]. Additionally, BCAT2 (mitochondrial) was significantly downregulated, whereas BCAT1 (cytosolic) was significantly upregulated in the adipose tissue of obese subjects [51]. Other mitochondrial genes of BCAA metabolism were also downregulated in adipose tissue, but not in liver or muscle tissue. Our study showed that the reduction of BCAA degradation seems to precede elevated BCAA levels in IR state or obesity in children, since no elevated BCAA were found but alterations in BCAA metabolite ratios. Thus, insulin negatively alters BCAA metabolism resulting in higher plasma BCAA in later life, when BCAA concentrations overcome their own degradation and contribute to the vicious circle of IR [52]. The analysis of metabolite profiles in children allowed us to study this early development effect of IR, but far more studies in children and early adulthood are needed to investigate the molecular changes in the early state of obesity and IR. However, BCAA and BCAA metabolism are more affected by protein-rich diet than other AAs [53], and thus diet is a known confounder, especially in obese patients with higher protein intake [15, 22]. After the intervention, in a state of homogenous lifestyle and diet, the BCAA ratios were no longer significantly associated with HOMA, except for the ratio of Carn C5-OH to Carn C5:1, which was positively associated with HOMA in children without substantial weight loss. Thus, lifestyle may have strong effect on BCAA metabolism, and the results found at baseline were hidden by the homogenous lifestyle of the studied cohort. This possible confounding effect of diet and lifestyle on BCAA metabolism has to be investigated in further studies. The nonsignificant association of HOMA and BCAA could also be result of less power of our study. Tai et al. depicted the same challenge when they found an association of IR with BCAA in a large group of Chinese men, but not in a smaller group of Indian Asian men [15]. Two-hour oGTT glucose showed different associations with AA and AA derivatives compared to HOMA. Particularly, Ser was negatively associated with 2-hour oGTT glucose. Since fewer studies exist on relations of

2-hour oGTT glucose to metabolites, we can only speculate about the underlying mechanisms. Ser and glycine (Gly) were found to be decreased in obese Hispanic children [26] and in obese Korean children [27]. The concentrations of Gly and Ser were found to be lower in diabetic than in fasted normal rats [54]. The authors concluded that the contribution of Ser to gluconeogenesis becomes proportionally higher in diabetes. Thus, an increased gluconeogenesis rate in diabetic or prediabetic patients most likely leads to decreased Ser levels. In this case, Ser seems to be the AA which is first affected by higher gluconeogenesis rate. But to unravel this relation, further studies are needed. Another explanation is the use of consumed Ser for SM synthesis, since SM are elevated in IR state [55]. Furthermore, we have to recall the relatively low reliability of 2 h glucose in oGTT [56]. Additionally, elevated 2 h glucose levels in obese children tend to normalize in follow-up even without weight loss as also demonstrated in our study [57, 58].

All the described relations between metabolites and HOMA or 2-hour oGTT glucose were driven by children with substantial weight loss. Children without substantial weight loss showed fewer and different associations. Thus, it is plausible that different metabolomic changes are associated with different types of IR. However, HOMA and 2-hour oGTT glucose did not change significantly in children without substantial weight loss during the intervention period, and thus the information in these parameters may be too little to depict associations between metabolites and clinical parameters in this group. Nevertheless, estimates for the associations between metabolites and HOMA were different at baseline, in change, and at follow-up, assuming different metabolic pattern which could be related to IR, the intervention, or weight loss. Thus, further prospective studies should focus on the relation of IR to different metabolomic patterns.

However, we were not able to differentiate the effect of diet, increased physical exercise, and weight loss on metabolites and their ratio concentrations due to our study protocol. Unfortunately, we could not perform stratified analyses to the influence of pubertal status on the associations of metabolites with IR. An explorative statistical approach showed no influence on the association of IR with Tyr, but on Carn. Further studies with larger sample number are required to determine differences in IR development with respect to puberty status. A limitation of our study is that BMI percentiles were used to classify overweight. Although BMI is a good measure for overweight, it is not a precise measure of body fat mass. Furthermore, the degree of obesity was relatively homogeneous in our obese children. Additionally, the HOMA model is only an assessment of IR [59]. Clamp studies are actually the gold standard for analysing IR. In addition to the small sample number, these facts reduced the odds to detect associations between metabolites and clinical outcomes. The relatively low sample number also reduced the statistical power of the presented data analysis, which kept us from correction for multiple testing. Among the strengths of our study are the longitudinal design and the analysed children that were naïve to drugs and other diseases and had similar lifestyle during the one-year intervention. The additional focus on ratios allowed for a closer insight into degradation pathways associated with obesity-related IR. Thus, the influence of diet and physical activity on changes of metabolite levels should be limited.

5. Conclusions

This study provides novel insights into the longitudinal interrelations of IR and obesity markers to metabolites and generates possible questions for further mechanistic studies of IR in obese children. Our cross-sectional and longitudinal analyses confirm a relationship between the Tyr and HOMA in obese children. So, Tyr and the Tyr metabolism should be focused more on in studies searching for early biomarkers and predictors in the switch from obesity to IR. In contrast, BCAA levels were negatively related to IR in cross-sectional analyses, while there was no significant association in the longitudinal analysis, which does not support a causal role of BCAA in inducing IR. Furthermore, responders to the intervention showed different associations between HOMA and AA compared to nonresponders, which appears to reflect different mechanisms for the development of obesity-induced IR. Further studies should also explore other analytes which were not determined in our study, such as p-hydroxyphenylpyruvate, fumarate, or acetoacetate that are involved in Tyr metabolism and sulfur containing AA.

Conflict of Interests

The authors declare that there is no conflict of interests regarding the publication of this paper.

Acknowledgments

The authors thank the participating children in this study. The research leading to these results has received funding from the European Union's Seventh Framework Programme (FP7/2007–2013), project EarlyNutrition under Grant Agreement no. 289346, and the European Research Council Advanced Grant ERC-2012-AdG, no. 322605 META-GROWTH. The research leading to these results has received support from the Innovative Medicines Initiative Joint Undertaking under EMIF Grant Agreement no. 115372, resources of which are composed of financial contribution from the European Union's Seventh Framework Programme (FP7/2007–2013) and EFPIA companies in kind contribution. This paper does not necessarily reflect the views of the Commission and in no way anticipates the future policy in this area. Further grant support by the German Ministry of Education and Research (Obesity Network: Grant nos. 01 01GI1120A, 01GI 1120B, and 001 GI 0825) is gratefully acknowledged.

References

[1] E. R. Pulgarón, "Childhood obesity: a review of increased risk for physical and psychological comorbidities," *Clinical Therapeutics*, vol. 35, no. 1, pp. A18–A32, 2013.

[2] G. Csábi, K. Török, D. Molnár, and S. Jeges, "Presence of metabolic cardiovascular syndrome in obese children," *European Journal of Pediatrics*, vol. 159, no. 1-2, pp. 91–94, 2000.

[3] D. S. Freedman, W. H. Dietz, S. R. Srinivasan, and G. S. Berenson, "The relation of overweight to cardiovascular risk factors among children and adolescents: the Bogalusa Heart study," *Pediatrics*, vol. 103, no. 6, part 1, pp. 1175–1182, 1999.

[4] T. Reinehr, W. Andler, C. Denzer, W. Siegried, H. Mayer, and M. Wabitsch, "Cardiovascular risk factors in overweight German children and adolescents: relation to gender, age and degree of overweight," *Nutrition, Metabolism and Cardiovascular Diseases*, vol. 15, no. 3, pp. 181–187, 2005.

[5] F. M. Biro and M. Wien, "Childhood obesity and adult morbidities," *The American Journal of Clinical Nutrition*, vol. 91, no. 5, pp. 1499S–1505S, 2010.

[6] T. Reinehr, G. de Sousa, and W. Andler, "Longitudinal analyses among overweight, insulin resistance, and cardiovascular risk factors in children," *Obesity Research*, vol. 13, no. 10, pp. 1824–1833, 2005.

[7] S. S. Coughlin, "Toward a road map for global -omics: a primer on -omic technologies," *American Journal of Epidemiology*, vol. 180, no. 12, pp. 1188–1195, 2014.

[8] N. M. R. Sales, P. B. Pelegrini, and M. C. Goersch, "Nutrigenomics: definitions and advances of this new science," *Journal of Nutrition and Metabolism*, vol. 2014, Article ID 202759, 6 pages, 2014.

[9] S. Rauschert, O. Uhl, B. Koletzko, and C. Hellmuth, "Metabolomic biomarkers for obesity in humans: a short review," *Annals of Nutrition and Metabolism*, vol. 64, no. 3-4, pp. 314–324, 2014.

[10] S. Demine, N. Reddy, P. Renard, M. Raes, and T. Arnould, "Unraveling biochemical pathways affected by mitochondrial dysfunctions using metabolomic approaches," *Metabolites*, vol. 4, no. 3, pp. 831–878, 2014.

[11] M. S. Lustgarten, L. Lyn Price, E. M. Phillips, and R. A. Fielding, "Serum glycine is associated with regional body fat and insulin resistance in functionally-limited older adults," *PLoS ONE*, vol. 8, no. 12, Article ID e84034, 2013.

[12] W. Perng, M. W. Gillman, A. F. Fleisch et al., "Metabolomic profiles and childhood obesity," *Obesity*, vol. 22, no. 12, pp. 2570–2578, 2014.

[13] C. B. Newgard, J. An, J. R. Bain et al., "A branched-chain amino acid-related metabolic signature that differentiates obese and lean humans and contributes to insulin resistance," *Cell Metabolism*, vol. 9, no. 4, pp. 311–326, 2009.

[14] N. Mohorko, A. Petelin, M. Jurdana, G. Biolo, and Z. Jenko-Pražnikar, "Elevated serum levels of cysteine and tyrosine: early biomarkers in asymptomatic adults at increased risk of developing metabolic syndrome," *BioMed Research International*, vol. 2015, Article ID 418681, 14 pages, 2015.

[15] E. S. Tai, M. L. S. Tan, R. D. Stevens et al., "Insulin resistance is associated with a metabolic profile of altered protein metabolism in Chinese and Asian-Indian men," *Diabetologia*, vol. 53, no. 4, pp. 757–767, 2010.

[16] P. Wurtz, P. Soininen, A. J. Kangas et al., "Branched-chain and aromatic amino acidsare predictors of insulinresistance in young adults," *Diabetes Care*, vol. 36, no. 3, pp. 648–655, 2013.

[17] O. Fiehn, W. T. Garvey, J. W. Newman, K. H. Lok, C. L. Hoppel, and S. H. Adams, "Plasma metabolomic profiles reflective of glucose homeostasis in non-diabetic and type 2 diabetic obese African-American women," *PLoS ONE*, vol. 5, no. 12, Article ID e15234, 2010.

[18] S. H. Shah, D. R. Crosslin, C. S. Haynes et al., "Branched-chain amino acid levels are associated with improvement in insulin resistance with weight loss," *Diabetologia*, vol. 55, no. 2, pp. 321–330, 2012.

[19] S. H. Adams, "Emerging perspectives on essential amino acid metabolism in obesity and the insulin-resistant state," *Advances in Nutrition*, vol. 2, no. 6, pp. 445–456, 2011.

[20] H.-H. Chen, Y. J. Tseng, S.-Y. Wang et al., "The metabolome profiling and pathway analysis in metabolic healthy and abnormal obesity," *International Journal of Obesity*, vol. 39, no. 8, pp. 1241–1248, 2015.

[21] T. Tillin, A. D. Hughes, Q. Wang et al., "Diabetes risk and amino acid profiles: cross-sectional and prospective analyses of ethnicity, amino acids and diabetes in a South Asian and European cohort from the SABRE (Southall And Brent REvisited) Study," *Diabetologia*, vol. 58, no. 5, pp. 968–979, 2015.

[22] P. Würtz, V.-P. Mäkinen, P. Soininen et al., "Metabolic signatures of insulin resistance in 7,098 young adults," *Diabetes*, vol. 61, no. 6, pp. 1372–1380, 2012.

[23] J. Villarreal-Pérez, J. Villarreal-Martínez, F. Lavalle-González et al., "Plasma and urine metabolic profiles are reflective of altered beta-oxidation in non-diabetic obese subjects and patients with type 2 diabetes mellitus," *Diabetology & Metabolic Syndrome*, vol. 6, article 129, 2014.

[24] T. J. Wang, M. G. Larson, R. S. Vasan et al., "Metabolite profiles and the risk of developing diabetes," *Nature Medicine*, vol. 17, no. 4, pp. 448–453, 2011.

[25] D. Newbern, P. G. Balikcioglu, M. Balikcioglu et al., "Sex differences in biomarkers associated with insulin resistance in obese adolescents: metabolomic profiling and principal components analysis," *Journal of Clinical Endocrinology and Metabolism*, vol. 99, no. 12, pp. 4730–4739, 2014.

[26] N. F. Butte, Y. Liu, I. F. Zakeri et al., "Global metabolomic profiling targeting childhood obesity in the Hispanic population," *The American Journal of Clinical Nutrition*, vol. 102, no. 2, pp. 256–267, 2015.

[27] A. Lee, H. B. Jang, M. Ra et al., "Prediction of future risk of insulin resistance and metabolic syndrome based on Korean boy's metabolite profiling," *Obesity Research & Clinical Practice*, 2014.

[28] S. E. Mccormack, O. Shaham, M. A. Mccarthy et al., "Circulating branched-chain amino acid concentrations are associated with obesity and future insulin resistance in children and adolescents," *Pediatric Obesity*, vol. 8, no. 1, pp. 52–61, 2013.

[29] T. Reinehr, G. de Sousa, A. M. Toschke, and W. Andler, "Long-term follow-up of cardiovascular disease risk factors in children after an obesity intervention," *American Journal of Clinical Nutrition*, vol. 84, no. 3, pp. 490–496, 2006.

[30] T. Reinehr, A. Hinney, G. de Sousa, F. Austrup, J. Hebebrand, and W. Andler, "Definable somatic disorders in overweight children and adolescents," *The Journal of Pediatrics*, vol. 150, no. 6, pp. 618.e5–622.e5, 2007.

[31] T. Reinehr, W. Kiess, T. Kapellen, and W. Andler, "Insulin sensitivity among obese children and adolescents, according to degree of weight loss," *Pediatrics*, vol. 114, no. 6, pp. 1569–1573, 2004.

[32] T. Reinehr, B. Wolters, C. Knop et al., "Changes in the serum metabolite profile in obese children with weight loss," *European Journal of Nutrition*, vol. 54, no. 2, pp. 173–181, 2015.

[33] T. J. Cole, "The LMS method for constructing normalized growth standards," *European Journal of Clinical Nutrition*, vol. 44, no. 1, pp. 45–60, 1990.

[34] K. Kromeyer-Hauschild, M. Wabitsch, D. Kunze et al., "Perzentile für den Body-mass-Index für das Kindes- und Jugendalter unter Heranziehung verschiedener deutscher Stichproben," *Monatsschrift Kinderheilkunde*, vol. 149, no. 8, pp. 807–818, 2001.

[35] American Diabetes Association, "Type 2 diabetes in children and adolescents," *Diabetes Care*, vol. 23, no. 3, pp. 381–389, 2000.

[36] D. R. Matthews, J. P. Hosker, A. S. Rudenski, B. A Naylor, D. F. Treacher, and R. C. Turner, "Homeostasis model assessment: insulin resistance and β-cell function from fasting plasma glucose and insulin concentrations in man," *Diabetologia*, vol. 28, no. 7, pp. 412–419, 1985.

[37] The R Project for Statistical Computing, http://www.r-project.org/.

[38] S. L. C. Woo, A. S. Lidsky, F. Guttler, T. Chandra, and K. J. Robson, "Cloned human phenylalanine hydroxylase gene allows prenatal diagnosis and carrier detection of classical phenylketonuria," *Nature*, vol. 306, no. 5939, pp. 151–155, 1983.

[39] T. Kuhara, S. Ikeda, A. Ohneda, and Y. Sasaki, "Effects of intravenous infusion of 17 amino acids on the secretion of GH, glucagon, and insulin in sheep," *American Journal of Physiology—Endocrinology and Metabolism*, vol. 260, no. 1, pp. E21–E26, 1991.

[40] S. F. Michaliszyn, L. A. Sjaarda, S. J. Mihalik et al., "Metabolomic profiling of amino acids and β-cell function relative to insulin sensitivity in youth," *The Journal of Clinical Endocrinology & Metabolism*, vol. 97, no. 11, pp. E2119–E2124, 2012.

[41] S. J. Mihalik, S. F. Michaliszyn, J. de las Heras et al., "Metabolomic profiling of fatty acid and amino acid metabolism in youth with obesity and type 2 diabetes: evidence for enhanced mitochondrial oxidation," *Diabetes Care*, vol. 35, no. 3, pp. 605–611, 2012.

[42] K. M. Huffman, S. H. Shah, R. D. Stevens et al., "Relationships between circulating metabolic intermediates and insulin action in overweight to obese, inactive men and women," *Diabetes Care*, vol. 32, no. 9, pp. 1678–1683, 2009.

[43] F. Labrie and A. Korner, "Effect of glucagon, insulin, and thyroxine on tyrosine transaminase and tryptophan pyrrolase of rat liver," *Archives of Biochemistry and Biophysics*, vol. 129, no. 1, pp. 75–78, 1969.

[44] C. J. Spencer, J. H. Heaton, T. D. Gelehrter, K. I. Richardson, and J. L. Garwin, "Insulin selectively slows the degradation rate of tyrosine aminotransferase," *Journal of Biological Chemistry*, vol. 253, no. 21, pp. 7677–7682, 1978.

[45] J. L. Hargrove, J. F. Trotter, H. C. Ashline, and P. V. Krishnamurti, "Experimental diabetes increases the formation of sulfane by transsulfuration and inactivation of tyrosine aminotransferase in cytosols from rat liver," *Metabolism*, vol. 38, no. 7, pp. 666–672, 1989.

[46] J. D. Fernstrom, "Branched-chain amino acids and brain function," *Journal of Nutrition*, vol. 135, supplement 6, pp. 1539S–1546S, 2005.

[47] S. Wahl, Z. Yu, M. Kleber et al., "Childhood obesity is associated with changes in the serum metabolite profile," *Obesity Facts*, vol. 5, no. 5, pp. 660–670, 2012.

[48] G. Marchesini, G. P. Bianchi, H. Vilstrup, M. Capelli, M. Zoli, and E. Pisi, "Elimination of infused branched-chain amino-acids from plasma of patients with non-obese type 2 diabetes mellitus," *Clinical Nutrition*, vol. 10, no. 2, pp. 105–113, 1991.

[49] J. T. Brosnan and M. E. Brosnan, "Branched-chain amino acids: enzyme and substrate regulation," *Journal of Nutrition*, vol. 136, no. 1, supplement, pp. 207S–211S, 2006.

[50] A. E. Serralde-Zúñiga, M. Guevara-Cruz, A. R. Tovar et al., "Omental adipose tissue gene expression, gene variants, branched-chain amino acids, and their relationship with metabolic syndrome and insulin resistance in humans," *Genes and Nutrition*, vol. 9, no. 6, article 431, 2014.

[51] A. Mardinoglu, C. Kampf, A. Asplund et al., "Defining the human adipose tissue proteome to reveal metabolic alterations in obesity," *Journal of Proteome Research*, vol. 13, no. 11, pp. 5106–5119, 2014.

[52] T. M. O'Connell, "The complex role of branched chain amino acids in diabetes and cancer," *Metabolites*, vol. 3, no. 4, pp. 931–945, 2013.

[53] F. F. Kirchberg, U. Harder, M. Weber et al., "Dietary protein intake affects amino acid and acylcarnitine metabolism in infants aged 6 months," *The Journal of Clinical Endocrinology & Metabolism*, vol. 100, no. 1, pp. 149–158, 2015.

[54] G. Hetenyi Jr., P. J. Anderson, M. Raman, and C. Ferrarotto, "Gluconeogenesis from glycine and serine in fasted normal and diabetic rats," *Biochemical Journal*, vol. 253, no. 1, pp. 27–32, 1988.

[55] J. M. R. Gill and N. Sattar, "Ceramides: a new player in the inflammation-insulin resistance paradigm?" *Diabetologia*, vol. 52, no. 12, pp. 2475–2477, 2009.

[56] I. M. Libman, E. Barinas-Mitchell, A. Bartucci, R. Robertson, and S. Arslanian, "Reproducibility of the oral glucose tolerance test in overweight children," *Journal of Clinical Endocrinology and Metabolism*, vol. 93, no. 11, pp. 4231–4237, 2008.

[57] M. Kleber, G. deSousa, S. Papcke, M. Wabitsch, and T. Reinehr, "Impaired glucose tolerance in obese white children and adolescents: three to five year follow-up in untreated patients," *Experimental and Clinical Endocrinology and Diabetes*, vol. 119, no. 3, pp. 172–176, 2011.

[58] M. Kleber, N. Lass, S. Papcke, M. Wabitsch, and T. Reinehr, "One-year follow-up of untreated obese white children and adolescents with impaired glucose tolerance: high conversion rate to normal glucose tolerance," *Diabetic Medicine*, vol. 27, no. 5, pp. 516–521, 2010.

[59] G. I. Uwaifo, E. M. Fallon, J. Chin, J. Elberg, S. J. Parikh, and J. A. Yanovski, "Indices of insulin action, disposal, and secretion derived from fasting samples and clamps in normal glucose-tolerant black and white children," *Diabetes Care*, vol. 25, no. 11, pp. 2081–2087, 2002.

28

Gmelina arborea Roxb. (Family: Verbenaceae) Extract Upregulates the β-Cell Regeneration in STZ Induced Diabetic Rats

Anoja Priyadarshani Attanayake,[1] Kamani Ayoma Perera Wijewardana Jayatilaka,[1] Chitra Pathirana,[1] and Lakmini Kumari Boralugoda Mudduwa[2]

[1]*Department of Biochemistry, Faculty of Medicine, University of Ruhuna, 80000 Galle, Sri Lanka*
[2]*Department of Pathology, Faculty of Medicine, University of Ruhuna, 80000 Galle, Sri Lanka*

Correspondence should be addressed to Anoja Priyadarshani Attanayake; anoja715@yahoo.com

Academic Editor: Janet H. Southerland

Gmelina arborea Roxb. (common name: Et-demata, Family: Verbenaceae) has been used traditionally in Sri Lanka as a remedy against diabetes mellitus. The objective of the present study was to evaluate antidiabetic mechanisms of the aqueous bark extract of *G. arborea* in streptozotocin induced (STZ) diabetic male Wistar rats. Aqueous bark extract of *G. arborea* (1.00 g/kg) and glibenclamide as the standard drug (0.50 mg/kg) were administered orally using a gavage to STZ diabetic rats (65 mg/kg, ip) for 30 days. The antidiabetic mechanisms of aqueous extract of *G. arborea* (1.00 g/kg) were determined at the end of the experiment. The fasting blood glucose concentration was significantly lowered and the serum insulin and C-peptide concentrations were increased by 57% and 39% in plant extract treated rats on day 30, respectively ($p < 0.05$). The histopathology and immunohistochemistry results of the plant extract treated group showed a regenerative effect on β-cells of the pancreas in diabetic rats. In addition, serum lipid parameters were improved in *G. arborea* extract treated diabetic rats. The results revealed that the aqueous stem bark extract of *G. arborea* (1.00 g/kg) showed beneficial effects against diabetes mellitus through upregulating the β-cell regeneration and biosynthesis of insulin in diabetic rats.

1. Introduction

Diabetes mellitus (DM) is one of the most common metabolic disorders worldwide [1]. The global prevalence of diabetes mellitus has shown an upward trend over the past few decades. Every ten seconds a person dies from diabetes-related causes. DM therefore has become a very serious public health problem with a heavy socioeconomic burden to most of the South Asian countries including Sri Lanka [2, 3].

DM is characterized by hyperglycemia and alteration of carbohydrate, fat, and protein metabolisms associated with absolute or relative deficiency in insulin secretion or insulin action [1]. Present pharmacological therapies aim at correcting/overcoming these defects. However, studies have consistently demonstrated that patients' adherence to present

therapeutic regimes has not been satisfactory. Regime complexity, occurrence of hypoglycemia, other side effects, lack of confidence in immediate or future benefits, and patients' education/beliefs are among the common reasons limiting compliance. Inadequacies in current treatment regimens have resulted in relying on complementary and alternative medicines for the management of diabetes [4, 5].

Gmelina arborea Roxb. (common name: Et-demata; Family: Verbenaceae) is valuable in Sri Lankan traditional medicine and a decoction of the bark of *G. arborea* is successfully employed for glycemic control and long term complications of diabetes mellitus by Ayurvedic physicians [6, 7]. Extensive research has been done for the investigations on phytochemicals, *in vivo* and *in vitro* antioxidant potentials and *in vivo* toxic effects by our research group [8, 9].

Furthermore, acute hypoglycemic and antihyperglycemic activities of the aqueous extract of *G. arborea* were studied in a graded dose range (0.25 g/kg–2.0 g/kg) in healthy (normoglycemic) and streptozotocin induced diabetic rats, respectively. Results of the acute study confirmed that the optimum effective antihyperglycemic dose of the *G. arborea* extract was 1.00 g/kg in streptozotocin induced diabetic rats [10].

In the present study, the effect of aqueous extract of *G. arborea* on selected glycemic parameters (fasting blood glucose concentration, percentage of glycated hemoglobin (HbA_{1C}) and serum concentration of fructosamine) and lipid parameters (serum concentrations of total cholesterol: TC; high density lipoprotein cholesterol: HDL-C; triglyceride: TG; low density lipoprotein cholesterol: LDL-C; very low density lipoprotein cholesterol: VLDL-C) was evaluated. In addition, the antidiabetic mechanisms of the extract were determined through the estimation of serum concentration of insulin, C-peptide, and detailed assessments of histopathology and immunohistochemistry of the pancreas. Glibenclamide was used as the standard drug in the present study and it has been widely accepted as a standard drug in diabetic animal experiments associated with mild, severe hyperglycemia [11].

The objective of the study was to determine detailed antidiabetic mechanisms of the bark extract *G. arborea* and its potency to induce β-cell regeneration in the pancreas of streptozotocin induced (STZ) diabetic rats.

2. Materials and Methods

2.1. Chemicals. D-glucose, glibenclamide, and streptozotocin were purchased from Sigma-Aldrich Company (St. Louis, MO, USA). A UV visible spectrophotometer (Gallenkamp PLC, UK) and microplate reader (Mindray, China) were used for spectrophotometric and enzyme linked immunosorbent assay (ELISA) measurements, respectively. Olympus CX 21 (Japan) microscope was used in the assessment of histopathology and immunohistochemistry of the pancreatic tissues.

2.2. Plant Material. Stem bark parts of *G. arborea* were collected during May-June 2013 from the Southern Region of Sri Lanka. Botanical identity was determined by the descriptions given by Jayaweera [6] and confirmed by comparing authentic samples at the National Herbarium, Royal Botanical Gardens, Peradeniya, Sri Lanka. A voucher specimen was preserved at the Department of Biochemistry, Faculty of Medicine, University of Ruhuna, Sri Lanka (Attanayake/2011/01).

2.3. Preparation of the Plant Extract. The bark parts of *G. arborea* were cut into small pieces and dried at 40°C until a constant weight. Powdered plant material (50.00 g) was dissolved in 400.0 mL of distilled water and refluxed for 4 h. The mixture was strained and the final volume was adjusted to 50.0 mL. The dose of 1.00 g/kg was administered orally to streptozotocin induced diabetic rats.

2.4. Animals. Healthy adult male rats of Wistar strain (200 ± 25 g, body weight) were purchased from the Medical Research Institute (MRI), Sri Lanka, and used to carry out the experiments. They were housed in standard environmental conditions at the Animal House of Faculty of Medicine, University of Ruhuna, Sri Lanka (Temp. 25 ± 2°C, relative humidity 55–65%, and 12 ± 1 h light/dark cycle). Rats were fed with standard diet (MRI rat formulae, Sri Lanka) with free access to water before and during the experiment. The rats were randomized into various groups and allowed to acclimatize for a period of seven days under standard environmental conditions before the commencement of the experiments. The animals described as fasting were deprived of food but had access for water for 12 h. All protocols used in this study were approved by the Ethics Committee of Faculty of Medicine, University of Ruhuna, Sri Lanka, guided by the Council for International Organization of Medical Sciences (CIOMS) international guiding principles of biomedical research involving animals.

2.5. Development of Diabetes Mellitus in Wistar Rats. Streptozotocin dissolved in citrate buffer (0.1 M, pH 4.4) at a dose of 65 mg/kg was administered intraperitoneally to rats fasted for 12 h. Thereafter, rats were maintained on 5% D-glucose solution for the next 24 h. Rats were allowed to stabilize for three days thereafter and on the 4th day, blood samples were drawn from tail vein to determine the blood glucose concentration to confirm the development of diabetes mellitus. Rats with fasting blood glucose concentration of 12.0 mmol/L or above were considered as hyperglycemic and from 4th day onwards they were used in the experiments [12].

2.6. Blood/Serum Glycemic Parameters in Diabetic Rats. Oral glucose tolerance test was performed in all groups on the 1st, 7th, 14th, 21st, 28th, and 30th days. The rats were given an oral dose of glucose (3.00 g/kg) 30 minutes after the administration of the plant extract. Blood samples were collected just prior to the administration of the extract/drug (0) and at 1, 2, 3, and 4 h subsequently. Blood glucose concentration was measured immediately by the glucose-oxidase method using a glucose assay kit based on the Trinder reaction [13]. The acute effect was evaluated over a 4 h period using area under the oral glucose tolerance curve [14].

The percentage of HbA_{1C} and serum concentration of fructosamine was estimated in all rats using a spectrophotometric enzyme assay kit [15, 16]. The concentrations of serum insulin and C-peptide in all rats were estimated using enzyme linked immune-sorbent assay methods [17, 18].

2.7. Serum Lipid Parameters in Diabetic Rats. The concentrations of serum TC, HDL-C, and TG were estimated in all rats using spectrophotometric enzyme assay kits [19–21]. The concentrations of serum LDL-C, VLDL-C were calculated using the Friedewald formulae [22].

2.8. Assessment of Histopathology and Immunohistochemistry of the Pancreas of Diabetic Rats. Paraffin embedded tissue blocks of the pancreas were used for the detailed assessment of histopathology and immunohistochemistry. The sections of the pancreatic tissues were stained with hematoxylin and eosin for the light microscopic examination of histopathology changes of pancreatic tissue in all rats. Histopathology score was developed for the assessment of selected histological parameters of destruction of islet cells and regeneration of islet cells [23]. The criteria for scoring the islet cell destruction were as follows: score 0 (normal): normal number of islet cells; score 1 (mild): loss of 1/3 of islet cells; score 2 (moderate): loss of 1/3 to 2/3 of islet cells; score 3 (severe): loss of more than 2/3 of islet cells. The criteria for scoring the regeneration were as follows: score 0 (none): no regeneration; score 1 (mild): regeneration of 1/3 of islet cells; score 2 (moderate): regeneration of 1/3 to 2/3 of islet cells; score 3 (prominent): regeneration of more than 2/3 of islet cells. Immunohistochemical staining was done to confirm the presence of insulin secreting cells in the islets of pancreas in all rats. Dako polyclonal guinea pig anti-insulin and Dako REAL EnVision/HRP, Rabbit/Mouse, were used for immunohistochemical staining. Islets were observed on light microscopy (high power field).

Islets were defined as being small, average, and large with an islet diameter of ≤125 μm, 126–149 μm, and ≥150 μm, respectively [24]. Four islets of each size in each rat (72 islets for each group) were chosen randomly [25]. The percentage of insulin secreting β-cells in islets and islet profile diameter were estimated [24, 25].

2.9. Statistical Analysis. Results are expressed as mean ± SEM for biochemical estimations. The quantitative data were analyzed by ANOVA followed by Dunnett's multiple comparison tests. The Kruskal-Wallis test was used for the semiquantitative analysis of histopathology score values. Results were considered to be significant at $p < 0.05$.

3. Results

3.1. Blood/Serum Glycemic Parameters. Effect of the *G. arborea* (1.00 g/kg) extract on fasting blood glucose concentration in diabetic rats is shown in Figure 1. The healthy animals were normoglycemic throughout the experimental period. The fasting blood glucose concentration of *G. arborea* treated diabetic rats was reduced significantly from the 21st day onwards for the period of 30 days ($p < 0.05$). The reduction in fasting blood glucose concentration with the administration of *G. arborea* and glibenclamide was 37% and 42% in streptozotocin induced diabetic rats at the end of the study, respectively ($p < 0.05$). The total area under the curve values of plant extract treated diabetic rats showed a statistically significant improvement of 37% on the 30th day ($p < 0.05$, Figure 2). Effect of plant extract on the percentage of HbA$_{1C}$ and concentration of fructosamine, insulin, and C-peptide in STZ diabetic rats is shown in Table 1. The diabetic rats treated with the plant extract exhibited a remarkable glycemic control as evident by a reduction in the percentage of HbA$_{1C}$. The reduction in the percentage of HbA$_{1C}$ and fructosamine was 31% and 28% in diabetic rats, respectively. However, glibenclamide treated diabetic rats

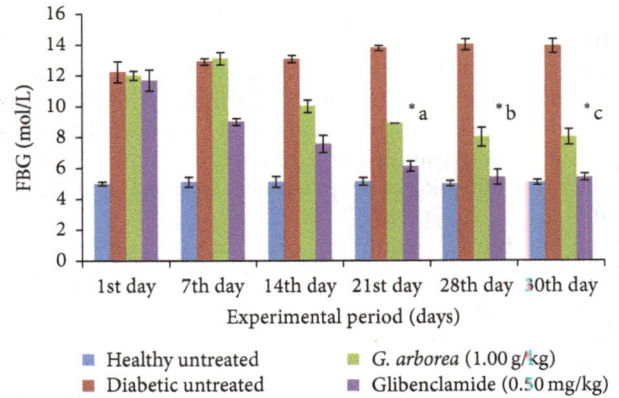

FIGURE 1: Effect of aqueous bark extract of *Gmelina arborea* (1.00 g/kg) fasting blood glucose concentration (FBG) in streptozotocin induced diabetic rats for 30 days. Data are expressed as mean ± SEM (n = 6/group). From the 21st day onwards, the fasting blood glucose concentration of *G. arborea* (1.00 g/kg) treated rats is significantly different from the fasting blood glucose concentration of diabetic untreated rats (*a, b, c).

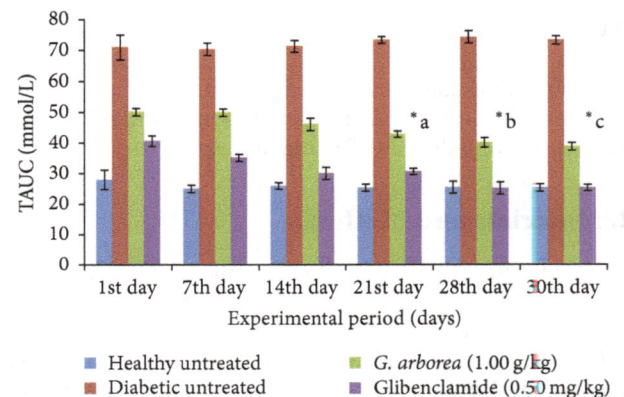

FIGURE 2: Effect of aqueous bark extract of *Gmelina arborea* (1.00 g/kg) on total area under the curve (TAUC) values in streptozotocin induced diabetic rats for 30 days. Data are expressed as mean ± SEM (n = 6/group). From the 21st day onwards, total area under the curve value of *G. arborea* (1.00 g/kg) treated rats is significantly different from the total area under the curve values of diabetic untreated rats (*a, b, c).

demonstrated a fall of 40% and 43% in the above parameters in diabetic rats. The concentrations of serum insulin and C-peptide were increased significantly by 57% and 39% in plant extract treated diabetic rats, respectively ($p < 0.05$). The concentration of serum TC, HDL-C, LDL-C, VLDL-C, and TG in streptozotocin induced diabetic rats followed by the plant treatment is shown in Table 2. The streptozotocin induced diabetic control rats had a significant elevation in the concentration of serum TC (57%), LDL-C (93%), VLDL-C (95%), and TG (94%) and a reduction in HDL-C (12%) as compared with the untreated healthy control rats. The extract of *G. arborea* treated streptozotocin induced diabetic rats showed a significant reduction in the concentration of

TABLE 1: Blood/serum glycemic parameters in diabetic rats after 30 days of treatment.

Treatment	Glycated hemoglobin (%)	Fructosamine (μmol/L)	Insulin (μIU/mL)	C-peptide (ng/mL)
Healthy untreated	4.86 ± 0.10	221.88 ± 3.10	14.23 ± 0.44	9.53 ± 0.80
Diabetic untreated	9.00 ± 0.09	405.39 ± 2.78	6.23 ± 0.09	5.75 ± 0.80
G. arborea (1.00 g/kg)	6.20 ± 0.06*	292.30 ± 2.19*	9.80 ± 0.10*	7.98 ± 0.07*
Glibenclamide (0.50 mg/kg)	5.38 ± 0.06*	230.08 ± 0.99*	11.75 ± 0.02*	8.80 ± 0.01*

The values are expressed as mean ± SEM (n = 6/group). *Statistically significant from streptozotocin induced diabetic control rats at $p < 0.05$ (ANOVA followed by Dunnett's test).

TABLE 2: Lipid profile in diabetic rats after 30 days of treatment.

Treatment	TC (mmol/L)	HDL-C (mmol/L)	LDL-C (mmol/L)	VLDL-C (mmol/L)	TG (mmol/L)
Healthy untreated	3.70 ± 0.08	1.25 ± 0.03	2.21 ± 0.02	0.22 ± 0.01	1.10 ± 0.09
Diabetic untreated	5.80 ± 0.05	1.10 ± 0.01	4.27 ± 0.18	0.43 ± 0.00	2.14 ± 0.05
G. arborea (1.00 g/kg)	4.00 ± 0.05*	1.23 ± 0.01*	2.47 ± 0.01*	0.30 ± 0.03*	1.50 ± 0.04*
Glibenclamide (0.50 mg/kg)	3.95 ± 0.06*	1.10 ± 0.09	2.63 ± 0.01*	0.22 ± 0.03*	1.12 ± 0.04*

The values are expressed as mean ± SEM (n = 6/group). *Statistically significant from streptozotocin induced diabetic control rats at $p < 0.05$ (ANOVA followed by Dunnett's test). TC: total cholesterol; HDL-C: high density lipoprotein cholesterol; LDL-C: low density lipoprotein cholesterol; VLDL-C: very low density lipoprotein cholesterol; TG: triglyceride.

serum TC (31%), LDL-C (43%), VLDL-C (25%), and TG (29%) and an elevation in HDL-C (45%) on the 30th day of study ($p < 0.05$). The concentrations of serum TC, LDL-C, VLDL-C, and TG were reduced by 32%, 38%, 49%, and 48% in glibenclamide treated diabetic rats. In contrast, there was no significant change in the concentration of serum HDL-C with the glibenclamide treatment in diabetic rats ($p > 0.05$).

3.2. Histopathology and Immunohistochemistry of the Pancreas in Diabetic Rats. As shown in Table 3 and Figure 3, the sections of the pancreas from untreated diabetic rats showed an extensive destruction of islet cells as compared with that of healthy control rats (score value of 3 versus 0). Further, there was a definite reduction in the number of islets in diabetic rats, compared with that in the healthy rats. However, hemorrhages were not observed and acinar cells were intact in the pancreatic tissues of streptozotocin induced diabetic control rats. Further, severe inflammatory cell infiltrations in islets were also observed in diabetic control rats. Immuno-histochemical staining with anti-insulin antibody confirmed a marked reduction (less than 10%) in insulin secreting cells in small, average, and large size islets in diabetic control rats (Table 4, Figure 4). The mean diameter of islets was reduced in small (15%), average (8%), and large (7%) islets in diabetic control rats as compared with the normal control rats. The sections from G. arborea extract treated diabetic rats revealed a statistically significant score value for the regeneration of islet cells with some hyperplastic islets as compared to diabetic untreated group (score value of 1 versus 0, $p < 0.05$). The number of islets was increased in plant treated diabetic rats when compared to diabetic control rats. Further the G. arborea extract produced a significant increase in the mean profile diameter in large islets (6%) as compared with the streptozotocin induced diabetic control rats.

TABLE 3: Semiquantitative analysis of pancreatic tissue on selected parameters in streptozotocin induced diabetic rats after 30 days of plant treatment.

Treatment	Destruction of islet cells	Regeneration of islet cells
Healthy untreated	0	N/A
Diabetic untreated	3	0
G. arborea (1.00 g/kg)	0*	1*
Glibenclamide (0.50 mg/kg)	1*	1*

0: none; 1: mild; 2: moderate; 3: severe/prominent.
*Statistically different from streptozotocin induced diabetic control rats at $p < 0.05$ (Kruskal-Wallis test).

4. Discussion

The present research was designed to evaluate antidiabetic effects of bark extract G. arborea (1.00 g/kg) in STZ diabetic rats. STZ diabetic rat is one of the most widely accepted models to investigate antidiabetic effects and mechanisms of action of any novel antidiabetic agents [26]. Streptozotocin (STZ) enters the pancreatic β-cells via a glucose transporter-GLUT2 and causes alkylation of DNA. The intraperitoneal injection of a single dose of STZ 65 mg/kg b. wt. exerts direct toxicity on β-cells resulting in necrosis within 48 hrs and causes permanent hyperglycemia. This causes the generation of superoxide, hydrogen peroxide, nitric oxide, and hydroxyl radicals which are responsible for β-cell damage and necrosis resulting in hyperglycemia [27–29].

Glibenclamide was used as the standard drug in the present study. It has been proposed that sulphonylureas exert antihyperglycemic effects through secretion of insulin from pancreatic β-cells and enhancement of insulin action on target tissues [30].

TABLE 4: Effect of plant extracts on percentage of insulin secreting β-cells and diameter of islets in the pancreas of streptozotocin induced diabetic rats after 30 days of treatment.

Treatment	Percentage area of insulin secreting cells in islets (%)			Diameter of islets (μm)		
	Small	Average	Large	Small	Average	Large
Healthy untreated	86.17 ± 3.54	72.00 ± 3.90	78.33 ± 7.53	86.80 ± 1.32	138.50 ± 5.57	173.16 ± 8.97
Diabetic untreated	9.17 ± 0.91	7.50 ± 1.23	6.83 ± 0.87	32.34 ± 1.55	127.43 ± 2.70	153.05 ± 0.37
G. arborea (1.00 g/kg)	$60.89 \pm 3.34^{*}$	$48.78 \pm 4.78^{*}$	$69.00 \pm 4.99^{*}$	37.12 ± 2.13	$137.00 \pm 2.07^{*}$	$164.34 \pm 2.56^{*}$
Glibenclamide (0.50 mg/kg)	$33.33 \pm 2.34^{*}$	$10.00 \pm 0.15^{*}$	$7.17 \pm 1.42^{*}$	36.10 ± 3.31	128.38 ± 1.99	154.08 ± 5.88

The values are expressed as mean $\pm$ SEM ($n = 6$/group). *Statistically significant from streptozotocin induced diabetic control rats at $p < 0.05$ (ANOVA followed by Dunnett's test).

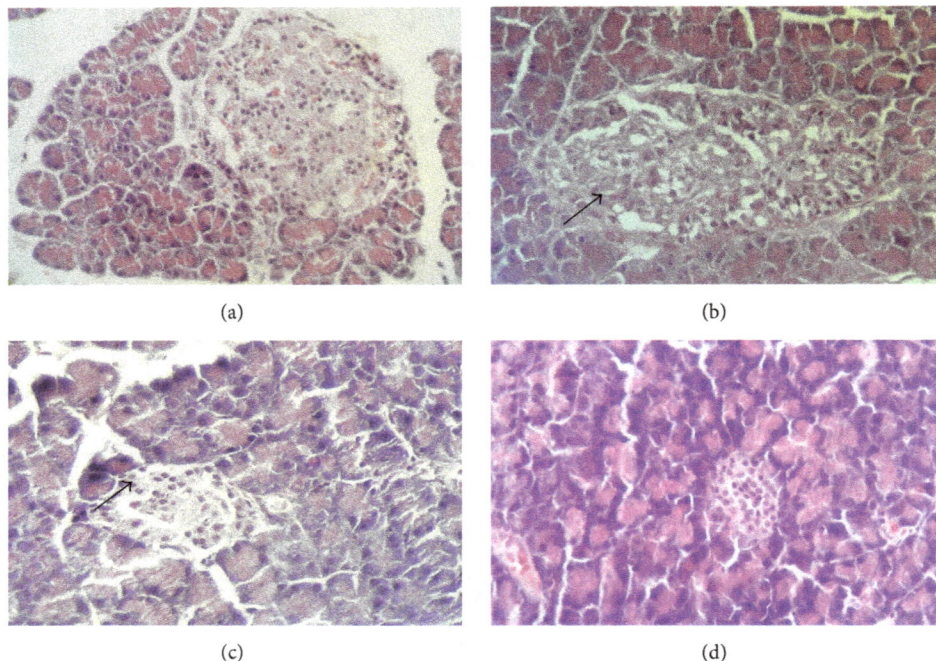

(a)

(b)

(c)

(d)

FIGURE 3: (a–d) Photomicrographs of histopathology of the pancreatic tissues, stained with hematoxylin and eosin ($\times$400). (a) Healthy control rats, islets of Langerhans with normal islet cell population. (b) Diabetic control rats, an islet with few preserved islet cells, fibrosis, and infiltration by inflammatory cells. (c) Gmelina arborea (1.00 g/kg) treated diabetic rats, restoration of pancreatic islet cells with prominent islets. (d) Glibenclamide treated (0.50 mg/kg) diabetic rats with reduced number of islet cells.

The study was performed for a period of 30 days in diabetic rats considering the life span of Wistar rats. In addition, many published studies on evaluating antidiabetic effects of medicinal plant extracts have been carried out in diabetic rats for a period of 30 days [11]. Diabetic animals showed an increase in blood glucose concentration which was reduced by the administration of G. arborea (1.00 g/kg). The antihyperglycemic activity was evident with the significant reduction of glycated hemoglobin in plant extract treated diabetic rats ($p < 0.05$). However, the reduction in the percentage of HbA$_{1C}$ in glibenclamide treated diabetic rats was superior to the reduction in G. arborea extract treated diabetic rats at the end of the study period (30th day). The possible mechanism by which the extract produced the antidiabetic action in diabetic rats may be by potentiating the insulin effect of plasma by increasing the pancreatic secretion of insulin from the existing β-cells and promoting the regeneration of β-cells [31]. The pancreatic mechanism may be predominant because in mild diabetes mellitus induced by STZ all β-cells of the pancreas are not destroyed. Therefore, the surviving β-cells retain the capacity to synthesize and secrete insulin.

A significantly deranged lipoprotein profile was observed in STZ diabetic rats. This is in agreement with previous reports [32, 33]. The serum total cholesterol concentration was increased significantly in diabetic rats. Since insulin has a potent inhibitory effect on lipolysis in adipocytes, insulin deficiency is associated with excess lipolysis and increased influx of free fatty acids to the liver [34]. The increased levels of LDL-C and VLDL-C in diabetic rats might be

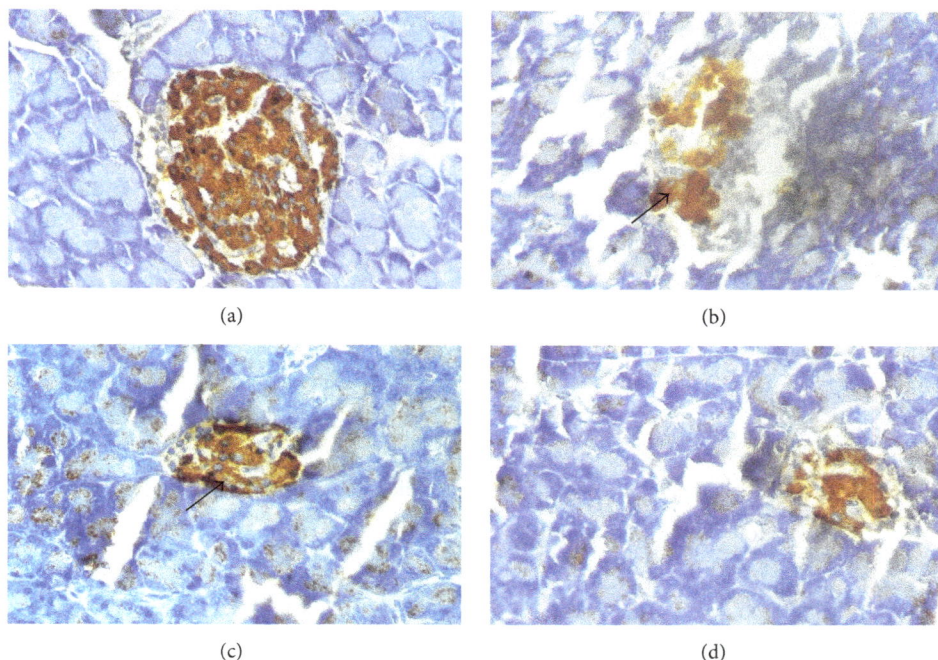

FIGURE 4: (a–d) Photomicrographs of insulin immune reactivity in pancreatic islets with anti-insulin antibody (×400). (a) Healthy control rats, a normal islet composed predominantly of insulin secreting cells. (b) Diabetic control rats, marked reduction in the number of insulin secreting β-cells due to the destruction of islet cells by streptozotocin. (c) *Gmelina arborea* (1.00 g/kg) treated (1.00 g/kg) rats, an islet with a marked increase in insulin secreting β-cells. (d) Glibenclamide treated (0.50 mg/kg) rats, mild increase in insulin secreting β-cells.

due to overproduction of LDL-C and VLDL-C by the liver due to the stimulation of hepatic triglyceride synthesis as a result of free fatty acid influx. HDL-C was also significantly reduced in diabetic rats, which indicates a positive risk factor for atherosclerosis [35]. The concentrations of serum TC, TG, LDL-C, and VLDL-C were significantly reduced in the plant extract treated diabetic rats. This could be due to the reduction in hepatic triglyceride synthesis and/or lipolysis in plant extract treated diabetic rats [36]. Furthermore, the HDL-C was significantly increased in the plant extract treated animals indicating a reversed atherogenic risk ($p < 0.05$).

The optimum pancreatic β-cell function is essential for the regulation of intracellular glucose homeostasis. Several studies have provided evidence that loss of functional β-cell mass through apoptosis and impaired proliferation consequent to hyperglycemia is central to the development of both type 1 and type 2 diabetes mellitus. Indeed, it has been considered as a hallmark of both types of diabetes mellitus. Regulation of functional β-cell mass has been considered as a critical therapeutic challenge in patients with the disease. However, islet cell regeneration has gained much interest and has been considered as a strategy to restore the loss of β-cell mass in diabetes mellitus [36–38]. Insulin and C-peptide are the products of enzymatic cleavage of proinsulin and are secreted into the circulation in equimolar concentration. After insulin is released from the pancreas it undergoes significant first-pass clearance by the liver and therefore the estimation of serum insulin concentration alone may not be sufficient to confirm the insulin secreted by the pancreas.

Therefore, estimation of both the concentrations of C-peptide and insulin has been reported to be valuable indices of insulin secretion [39]. The increment in serum insulin and C-peptide concentrations in plant extract treated rats corroborated the formation of functional islets and biosynthesis of insulin as evident through immunohistochemistry studies.

The results of the present study revealed a regeneration in the pancreatic β-cells in diabetic rats treated with the extract of *G. arborea* (1.00 g/kg). A pancreatic mechanism is possible because, in mild diabetes induced by STZ, all β-cells of the pancreas are not destroyed. The surviving β-cells retain the capacity to proliferate, synthesize, and secrete insulin [37]. The islet cell regeneration in diabetic rats with the plant treatments could be due to the replication of existing islet cells and differentiation (or neogenesis) from ductal or intraislet pancreatic precursor cells [38]. Various histopathological studies demonstrated an effective increase in the number of β-cells in the pancreas of diabetic rats treated with various plant extracts [39, 40]. The antidiabetic effects of the plant extracts are probably due to the presence of polyphenol compounds and flavonoids. Indeed, flavonoids as quercitrin and epicatechin are well documented for islet regeneration and enhancement of β-cell function *in vivo* [41].

5. Conclusions

The results confirm that the aqueous bark extract of *G. arborea* (1.00 g/kg) possesses *in vivo* antidiabetic activity through increased biosynthesis of insulin probably by β-cell regeneration in the pancreas of streptozotocin induced diabetic rats. In addition, the plant extract exerts antihyperlipidemic activities in diabetic rats. This is the first ever study to report the detailed pancreatic mechanisms of *G. arborea in vivo*. The findings of the present investigation revealed scrutinizing the therapeutic benefits of the *G. arborea* extract in the management of diabetes mellitus in traditional medicine.

Conflict of Interests

The authors declare that there is no conflict of interests regarding the publication of this paper.

Acknowledgments

The financial assistance given by University Grants Commission in Sri Lanka is greatly appreciated (UGC/ICD/CRF 2009/2/5). The authors wish to thank Dr. D. A. B. N. Gunarathne of the Department of Crop Science, Faculty of Agriculture, University of Ruhuna, Sri Lanka, for the guidance given in statistical data analysis and Mrs. B. M. S. Malkanthie, Mr. G. H. J. M. Priyashanthaand, Mr. D. G. P. Pathmabandu, and Mrs. G. G. D. D. Gunawardane, Faculty of Medicine, University of Ruhuna, Sri Lanka, for technical assistance.

References

[1] American Diabetes Association, "Standards of medical care in diabetes—2014," *Diabetes Care*, vol. 37, supplement 1, pp. S14–S80, 2014.

[2] J. E. Shaw, R. A. Sicree, and P. Z. Zimmet, "Global estimates of the prevalence of diabetes for 2010 and 2030," *Diabetes Research and Clinical Practice*, vol. 87, no. 1, pp. 4–14, 2010.

[3] O. Veiseh, B. C. Tang, K. A. Whitehead, D. G. Anderson, and R. Langer, "Managing diabetes with nanomedicine: challenges and opportunities," *Nature Reviews Drug Discovery*, vol. 14, pp. 45–57, 2015.

[4] S. Bastaki, "Diabetes mellitus and its treatment," *International Journal of Diabetes and Metabolism*, vol. 13, no. 3, pp. 111–134, 2005.

[5] R. R. Chattopadhyay, "A comparative evaluation of some blood sugar lowering agents of plant origin," *Journal of Ethnopharmacology*, vol. 67, no. 3, pp. 367–372, 1999.

[6] D. M. A. Jayaweera, *Medicinal Plants (Indigenous and Exotic) Used in Ceylon*, National Science Foundation in Sri Lanka, Colombo, Sri Lanka, 2nd edition, 1982.

[7] E. R. H. S. S. Ediriweera and W. D. Ratnasooriya, "A review on herbs used in treatment of diabetes mellitus by Sri Lankan Ayurvedic and traditional physicians," *AYU*, vol. 30, pp. 373–391, 2009.

[8] A. P. Attanayake, K. A. P. W. Jayatilaka, C. Pathirana, and L. K. B. Mudduwa, "Antioxidant activity of *Gmelina arborea* Roxb. (Verbenaceae) bark extract: *in vivo* and *in vitro* study," *Journal of Medical Nutrition and Nutraceuticals*, vol. 4, no. 1, pp. 32–38, 2015.

[9] A. P. Attanayake, K. A. P. W. Jayatilaka, C. Pathirana, and L. K. B. Mudduwa, "Sub-chronic toxicological investigation of *Gmelina*

[10] A. P. Attanayake, K. A. P. W. Jayatilaka, C. Pathirana, and L. K. Mudduwa, "Acute hypoglycemic and antihyperglycemic effects of ten Sri Lankan medicinal plant extracts in healthy and streptozotocin induced diabetic rats," *International Journal of Diabetes in Developing Countries*, vol. 35, no. 3, pp. 177–183, 2015.

[11] J. Sokolovska, S. Isajevs, O. Sugoka et al., "Comparison of the effects of glibenclamide on metabolic parameters, GLUT1 expression, and liver injury in rats with severe and mild streptozotocin-induced diabetes mellitus," *Medicina*, vol. 48, no. 10, pp. 532–543, 2012.

[12] C. F. B. Vasconcelos, H. M. L. Maranhão, T. M. Batista et al., "Hypoglycaemic activity and molecular mechanisms of *Caesalpinia ferrea* Martius bark extract on streptozotocin-induced diabetes in Wistar rats," *Journal of Ethnopharmacology*, vol. 137, no. 3, pp. 1533–1541, 2011.

[13] P. Trinder, "Determination of blood glucose using an oxidase-peroxidase system with a non-carcinogenic chromogen," *Journal of Clinical Pathology*, vol. 22, no. 2, pp. 158–161, 1969.

[14] R. D. Purves, "Optimum numerical integration methods for estimation of area-under-the-curve (AUC) and area-under-the-moment-curve (AUMC)," *Journal of Pharmacokinetics and Biopharmaceutics*, vol. 20, no. 3, pp. 211–226, 1992.

[15] E. C. Abraham, T. A. Huff, N. D. Cope et al., "Determination of the glycosylated haemoglobin (Hb$_{A1C}$) with a new micro column procedure: suitability of the technique for assessing the clinical management of diabetes mellitus," *Diabetes*, vol. 27, no. 9, pp. 931–937, 1978.

[16] R. N. Johnson, P. A. Metcalf, and J. R. Baker, "Fructosamine: a new approach to the estimation of serum glycolprotein. An index of diabetic control," *Clinica Chimica Acta*, vol. 127, no. 1, pp. 87–95, 1983.

[17] L. Andersen, B. Dinesen, P. N. Jorgensen, F. Poulsen, and M. E. Roder, "Enzyme immunoassay for intact human insulin in serum or plasma," *Clinical Chemistry*, vol. 39, no. 4, pp. 578–582, 1993.

[18] J. P. Ashby and B. M. Frier, "Circulating C-peptide: measurement and clinical application," *Annals of Clinical Biochemistry*, vol. 18, no. 3, pp. 125–130, 1981.

[19] P. Roeschlau, E. Bernt, and W. Gruber, "Enzymatic determination of total cholesterol in serum," *Zeitschrift für klinische Chemie und klinische Biochemie*, vol. 12, no. 5, article 226, 1974.

[20] G. Assmann, H. Schriewer, G. Schmitz, and E. C. Hagele, "Quantification of high-density-lipoprotein cholesterol by precipitation with phosphotungstic acid/MgCl$_2$," *Clinical Chemistry*, vol. 29, no. 12, pp. 2026–2030, 1983.

[21] A. W. Wahlefeld, "Triglycerides: determination after enzymatic hydrolysis," in *Method of Enzymatic Analysis*, H. K. Bergmeyer, Ed., pp. 1825–1831, Academic Press, New York, NY, USA, 1974.

[22] W. T. Friedewald, R. I. Levy, and D. S. Fredrickson, "Estimation of the concentration of low-density lipoprotein cholesterol in plasma, without use of the preparative ultracentrifuge," *Clinical Chemistry*, vol. 18, no. 6, pp. 499–502, 1972.

[23] Q. G. Li, R. Sun, and F. Z. Gao, "Effect of Shen Di Jiang Tang granules on diabetic rats," *China Journal of Chinese Materia Medica*, vol. 26, pp. 488–490, 2001.

[24] R. R. MacGregor, S. J. Williams, P. Y. Tong, K. Kover, W. V. Moore, and L. Stehno-Bittel, "Small rat islets are superior to large islets in in vitro function and in transplantation outcomes," *The American Journal of Physiology—Endocrinology and Metabolism*, vol. 290, no. 5, pp. E771–E779, 2006.

[25] A. A. Elayat, M. M. El-Naggar, and M. Tahir, "An immunocytochemical and morphometric study of the rat pancreatic islets," *Journal of Anatomy*, vol. 186, no. 3, pp. 629–637, 1995.

[26] A. J. F. King, "The use of animal models in diabetes research," *British Journal of Pharmacology*, vol. 166, no. 3, pp. 877–894, 2012.

[27] M. Nukatsuka, Y. Yoshimura, M. Nishida, and J. Kawada, "Importance of the concentration of ATP in rat pancreatic beta cells in the mechanism of streptozotocin-induced cytotoxicity," *Journal of Endocrinology*, vol. 127, no. 1, pp. 161–165, 1990.

[28] D. C. Almonte-Flores, N. Paniagua-Castro, G. Escalona-Cardoso, and M. Rosales-Castro, "Pharmacological and genotoxic properties of polyphenolic extracts of *Cedrela odorata* L. and *Juglans regia* L. barks in rodents," *Evidence-Based Complementary and Alternative Medicine*, vol. 2015, Article ID 187346, 8 pages, 2015.

[29] C. O. Eleazu, K. C. Eleazu, and M. A. Iroaganachi, "Effect of cocoyam (*Colocasia esculenta*), unripe plantain (*Musa paradisiaca*) or their combination on glycated hemoglobin, lipogenic enzymes, and lipid metabolism of streptozotocin-induced diabetic rats," *Pharmaceutical Biology*, pp. 1–7, 2015.

[30] J. E. Jackson and R. Bressler, "Clinical pharmacology of sulphonylurea hypoglycaemic agents: part 1," *Drugs*, vol. 22, no. 3, pp. 211–245, 1981.

[31] B. I. Patel and P. D. Sachdeva, "Anti-diabetic activity of *linaria amosissima* (wall) Janch in streptozotocin induced diabetic rats," *International Journal of Pharmacy and Pharmaceutical Sciences*, vol. 6, no. 7, pp. 166–171, 2014.

[32] S. S. Fatima, M. D. Rajasekhar, K. V. Kumar, M. T. S. Kumar, K. R. Babu, and C. A. Rao, "Antidiabetic and antihyperlipidemic activity of ethyl acetate: isopropanol (1:1) fraction of *Vernonia anthelmintica* seeds in Streptozotocin induced diabetic rats," *Food and Chemical Toxicology*, vol. 48, no. 2, pp. 495–501, 2010.

[33] R. I. Levy, "High density lipoproteins, 1978—an overview," *Lipids*, vol. 13, no. 12, pp. 911–913, 1978.

[34] R. Rajalingam, N. Srinivasan, and P. Govindarajulu, "Effects of alloxan induced diabetes on lipid profiles in renal cortex and medulla of mature albino rats," *Indian Journal of Experimental Biology*, vol. 31, no. 6, pp. 577–579, 1993.

[35] K. N. Bopanna, J. Kannan, S. Gadgil, R. Balaraman, and S. P. Rathod, "Antidiabetic and antihyperlipaemic effects of neem seed kernel powder on alloxan diabetic rabbits," *Indian Journal of Pharmacology*, vol. 29, no. 3, pp. 162–167, 1997.

[36] M. Brownlee, "Biochemistry and molecular cell biology of diabetic complications," *Nature*, vol. 414, no. 6865, pp. 813–820, 2001.

[37] T. Nishikawa, D. Edelstein, X. L. Du et al., "Normalizing mitochondrial superoxide production blocks three pathways of hyperglycaemic damage," *Nature*, vol. 404, no. 6779, pp. 787–790, 2000.

[38] M. Banerjee, M. Kanitkar, and R. R. Bhonde, "Approaches towards endogenous pancreatic regeneration," *The Review of Diabetic Studies*, vol. 2, no. 3, pp. 165–165, 2005.

[39] I. E. Juárez-Rojop, J. C. Díaz-Zagoya, J. L. Ble-Castillo et al., "Hypoglycemic effect of *Carica papaya* leaves in streptozotocin-induced diabetic rats," *BMC Complementary and Alternative Medicine*, vol. 12, article 236, 2012.

[40] A. N. Nagappa, P. A. Thakurdesai, N. Venkat-Rao, and J. Singh, "Antidiabetic activity of *Terminalia catappa* Linn fruits," *Journal of Ethnopharmacology*, vol. 88, no. 1, pp. 45–50, 2003.

[41] R. Babujanarthanam, P. Kavitha, and M. R. Pandian, "Quercitrin, a bioflavonoid improves glucose homeostasis in streptozotocininduced diabetic tissues by altering glycolytic and gluconeogenic enzymes," *Fundamental and Clinical Pharmacology*, vol. 24, no. 3, pp. 357–364, 2010.

Permissions

List of Contributors

Feng-fei Li, Wen-li Zhang, Xiao-fei Su, Jin-danWu, Jin Sun and Jian-hua Ma
Department of Endocrinology, Nanjing First Hospital, Nanjing Medical University, Nanjing 210012, China

Li-yuan Fu
Nanjing University of Chinese Medicine, Nanjing 210023, China

Lei Ye
National Heart Research Institute Singapore, National Heart Centre Singapore, Singapore 169606

Michala Prause
Immuno-Endocrinology Lab, Endocrinology Research Section, Department of Biomedical Sciences, University of Copenhagen, 2200 Copenhagen N, Denmark
Section of Cellular and Metabolic Research, Department of Biomedical Sciences, University of Copenhagen, 2200 Copenhagen N, Denmark

Christopher Michael Mayer
Hagedorn Research Institute, Novo Nordisk, 2760 Måløv, Denmark

Joachim Størling and Caroline Brorsson
Copenhagen Diabetes Research Center, Herlev University Hospital, 2730 Herlev, Denmark

Klaus Stensgaard Frederiksen
Biopharmaceuticals Research Unit, Novo Nordisk, 2760 Måløv, Denmark

Nils Billestrup
Section of Cellular and Metabolic Research, Department of Biomedical Sciences, University of Copenhagen, 2200 Copenhagen N, Denmark

ThomasMandrup-Poulsen
Immuno-Endocrinology Lab, Endocrinology Research Section, Department of Biomedical Sciences, University of Copenhagen, 2200 Copenhagen N, Denmark
Department of Molecular Medicine and Surgery, Karolinska Institutet, 17177 Stockholm, Sweden

Sebastjan Merlo
Institute of Oncology Ljubljana, Zaloška 2, Sl-1000 Ljubljana, Slovenia

Jovana NikolajeviT StarleviT, Sara Mankol, Marjeta Zorc and Daniel Petrovil
Institute of Histology and Embryology, Faculty of Medicine, University in Ljubljana, Vrazov trg 2, Sl-1000 Ljubljana, Slovenia

Marija Šantl Letonja
General Hospital Rakičan, Ulica dr. Vrbnjaka 6, Sl-9000 Murska Sobota, Slovenia

Andreja Cokan Vujkovac
General Hospital Slovenj Gradec, Gosposvetska Cesta 1, SI-2380 Slovenj Gradec, Slovenia

Nicola M. Glasson and Sarah L. Larkins
College of Medicine and Dentistry, James Cook University, 1 James Cook Drive, Townsville City, QLD 4811, Australia

Lisa J. Crossland
Discipline of General Practice, University of Queensland, Level 8 Health Sciences Building, Royal Brisbane Hospital, Herston, QLD 4029, Australia

Li-ping Han, Chun-jun Li, Bei Sun, Yun Xie, Yue Guan, Ze-jun Ma and Li-ming Chen
2011 Collaborative Innovation Center of Tianjin for Medical Epigenetics, Key Laboratory of Hormone and Development, Ministry of Health, Metabolic Disease Hospital and Tianjin Institute of Endocrinology, Tianjin Medical University, Tianjin 300070, China

S. A. Afanasiev, D. S. Kondratieva, T. Yu. Rebrova, R. E. Batalov and S. V. Popov
Federal State Budgetary Scientific Institution "Research Institute for Cardiology", 111a Kievskaya Street, Tomsk 634012, Russia

Xiaolu Xiong
Department of Endocrinology, Drum Tower Clinical Medical College of Nanjing Medical University, 53 North Zhongshan Road, Nanjing 210008, China

Anyuan Zhong
Department of Respiratory Diseases,The Second Affiliated Hospital of Soochow University, 1055 Sanxiang Road, Suzhou 215004, China

Huajun Xu
Department of Otolaryngology, Shanghai Jiao Tong University Affiliated Sixth People's Hospital,

Otolaryngology Institute of Shanghai Jiao Tong University, 600 Yishan Road, Shanghai 200233, China

ChunWang
Department of Geriatrics, Drum Tower Clinical Medical College of Nanjing Medical University, 53 North Zhongshan Road, Nanjing 210008, China

Young Gun Park and Young-Jung Roh
Department of Ophthalmology and Visual Science, Catholic University of Korea, No. 62 Yeouido-dong, Yeongdeungpo-gu, Seoul 07345, Republic of Korea

Guendalina Graffigna, Serena Barello and Julia Menichetti
Department of Psychology, Universitá Cattolica del Sacro Cuore, Largo A. Gemelli 1, 20123 Milan, Italy

Andrea Bonanomi
Department of Statistical Sciences, Universitá Cattolica del Sacro Cuore, Largo A. Gemelli 1, 20123 Milan, Italy

Kai O. Hensel, Franziska Grimmer, Markus Roskopf, Andreas C. Jenke, Stefan Wirth and Andreas Heusch
Department of Pediatrics, HELIOS Medical Center Wuppertal, Centre for Clinical & Translational Research (CCTR), Centre for Biomedical Education & Research (ZBAF), Faculty of Health, Witten/Herdecke University, Heusnerstraße 40, 42283Wuppertal, Germany

Zhan Liu, Zhi-Hong Zhao and Yu Zhang
Department of Clinical Nutrition and Gastroenterology, The First Affiliated Hospital (People's Hospital of Hunan Province), Hunan Normal University, Changsha 430070, China'

Peng Li
College of Pharmacy, Xinxiang Medical University, Xinxiang 453003, China

Zhi-MinMa
Division of Endocrinology, The Second Affiliated Hospital, Soochow University, Suzhou 215000, China

Shuang-Xi Wang
Division of Endocrinology, The Second Affiliated Hospital, Soochow University, Suzhou 215000, China
The Key Laboratory of Cardiovascular Remodeling and Function Research, Chinese Ministry of Education and Chinese Ministry of Health, Qilu Hospital, School of Medicine, Shandong University, Jinan 250012, China

Anna M. Hogendorf, Wojciech Fendler, Agnieszka Szadkowska and Wojciech Mlynarski
Department of Pediatrics, Oncology, Hematology and Diabetology, Medical University of Lodz, 91-738 Lodz, Poland

Janusz Sieroslawski
Department of Studies on Alcoholism and Other Dependencies, Institute of Psychiatry and Neurology, 02-957Warsaw, Poland

Katarzyna Bobeff, KrzysztofWegrewicz, Kamila I. Malewska and Maciej W. Przudzik
Students' Scientific Circle at the Department of Pediatrics, Oncology, Hematology and Diabetology, Medical University of Lodz, 91-738 Lodz, Poland

Malgorzata Szmigiero-Kawko, Beata Sztangierska and MalgorzataMysliwiec
Department of Pediatrics, Diabetology and Endocrinology, Medical University of Gdańsk, 80-211 Gdańsk, Poland

Alberto Mimenza Alvarado and Sara Aguilar Navarro
Geriatrics Department, National Institute of Medical Sciences and Nutrition Salvador Zubirán, Vasco de Quiroga No. 15, Colonia Section XVI, Delegación Tlalpan, 14000 Mexico, DF, Mexico

Xue Cai
Department of Ophthalmology, Dean McGee Eye Institute, Oklahoma University Health Sciences Center, Oklahoma City, OK 73104, USA

James F. Mc Ginnis
Department of Ophthalmology, Dean McGee Eye Institute, Oklahoma University Health Sciences Center, Oklahoma City, OK 73104, USA
Department of Cell Biology, Oklahoma University Health Sciences Center, Oklahoma City, OK 73104, USA
Oklahoma Center for Neuroscience, Oklahoma University Health Sciences Center, Oklahoma City, OK 73104, USA

Shenghui Wu
Department of Epidemiology & Biostatistics, University of Texas Health Science Center at San Antonio, Laredo Campus, Laredo, TX 78045, USA

Susan P. Fisher-Hoch, Belinda Reninger, Kristina Vatcheva and Joseph B.Mc Cormick
Division of Epidemiology, School of Public Health, University of Texas Health Science Center at Houston, Brownsville Campus, Brownsville, TX 78520, USA

Carlos K. H. Wong, Fang-Fang Jiao, Esther Y. T. Yu, Yvonne Y. C. Lo, Colman S. C. Fung and Cindy L. K. Lam
Department of Family Medicine and Primary Care, The University of Hong Kong, Ap Lei Chau, Hong Kong

Shing-Chung Siu and Ka-Wai Wong
Department of Medicine and Rehabilitation, Tung Wah Eastern Hospital, Causeway Bay, Hong Kong

Daniel Y. T. Fong
School of Nursing, The University of Hong Kong, Pokfulam, Hong Kong

Akira Mima
Department of Nephrology, Nara Hospital, Kindai University Faculty of Medicine, Nara 630-0293, Japan

Jia Sun, Hua Zhang, Yuting Ruan and Hong Chen
Department of Endocrinology, Zhujiang Hospital, Southern Medical University, Guangzhou, China

Jinhua Luo
Department of Geratology,The Affiliated Hospital of Guangdong Medical College, Guangdong Medical College, Zhanjiang, Guangdong, China

Liangchang Xiu
Department of Epidemiology and Medical Statistics, School of Public Health, Guangdong Medical College, Dongguan, Guangdong, China

Bimei Fang
Second Clinical School of Medicine, Southern Medical University, Guangzhou, China

Ming Wang
Nephrology Center of Integrated Traditional Chinese and Western Medicine, Zhujiang Hospital, Southern Medical University, Guangzhou, China

Koffi Alouki and Hélène Delisle
TRANSNUT,WHO Collaborating Centre on Nutrition Changes and Development, Department of Nutrition, Faculty of Medicine, University of Montreal, 2405 Chemin de la Côte Sainte-Catherine, Montreal, QC, Canada H3T 1A8

Clara Bermúdez-Tamayo
Institut de Recherche en Santé Publique de l'Université de Montréal (IRSPUM), University of Montreal, 7101 Avenue du Parc, 3é Etage, Montréal, QC, Canada H3N 1X9

Mira Johri
Centre de Recherche du Centre Hospitalier de l'Université de Montréal (CRCHUM), Tour Saint-Antoine, 850 Rue Saint-Denis, Montréal, QC, Canada H2X 0A9
Department of Health Administration, School of Public Health (ESPUM), Faculty of Medicine, University of Montreal, 7101 Avenue du Parc, 3é Etage, Montréal, QC, Canada H3N1X9

Kristine Kloster-Jensen, Afaf Sahraoui, Aksel Foss and Hanne Scholz
Department of Transplant Medicine, Oslo University Hospital, P.O. Box 4950, 0424 Oslo, Norway
Institute for Surgical Research, Oslo University Hospital, P.O. Box 4950, 0424 Oslo, Norway
Institute of Clinical Medicine, University of Oslo, P.O. Box 1171, Blindern, 0318 Oslo, Norway

Nils Tore Vethe
Department of Pharmacology, Oslo University Hospital, P.O. Box 4950, 0424 Oslo, Norway

Olle Korsgren
Science for Life Laboratory, Department of Immunology, Genetics and Pathology, Uppsala University, Box 815, 75108 Uppsala, Sweden
Department of Clinical Immunology, Genetics and Pathology, Rudbeck Laboratory, Uppsala University Hospital, 75185 Uppsala, Sweden

Stein Bergan
Department of Pharmacology, Oslo University Hospital, P.O. Box 4950, 0424 Oslo, Norway
School of Pharmacy, University of Oslo, P.O. Box 1171, Blindern, 0318 Oslo, Norway

Michelle T. Barati, Susan Isaacs, Daniel W. Wilkey and Michael L. Merchant
Kidney Disease Program, Department of Medicine, University of Louisville, Louisville, KY 40202, USA

James C. Gould
Kidney Disease Program, Department of Medicine, University of Louisville, Louisville, KY 40202, USA
Harvard Medical School, Boston, MA 02115,USA

Sarah A. Salyer
Tuskegee University School of Veterinary Medicine, Tuskegee, AL 36088, USA

Tim Johansson and Sophie Keller
Institute of General Practice, Family Medicine, and Preventive Medicine, Paracelsus Medical University, 5020 Salzburg, Austria

Henrike Winkler
Paris Lodron University, 5020 Salzburg, Austria

Thomas Ostermann
Centre for Integrative Medicine, University of Witten/Herdecke, 58448 Witten, Germany

RaimundWeitgasser
Department of Internal Medicine, Wehrle-Diakonissen Hospital, 5026 Salzburg, Austria
Paracelsus Medical University, 5020 Salzburg, Austria

Andreas C. Sönnichsen
Institute of General Practice and Family Medicine, University of Witten/Herdecke, 58448Witten, Germany

Ranjita Misra
Department of Social & Behavioral Sciences, Robert C Byrd Health Science Center, School of Public Health, West Virginia University, 3313A, Morgantown, WV 26506-9190, USA

Cindy Fitch
Programs and Research, Extension Service, West Virginia University, P.O. Box 6031, 812 Knapp Hall, Morgantown, WV 26506-6031, USA

David Roberts
WVU Extension Service, Lincoln and Boone Counties Extension Agent, Hamlin, WV, USA

Dana Wright
WVU Extension Services, 815 Alderson Street, Williamson, WV 25661, USA

Najla Gooda Sahib Jambocus and Nazamid Saari
Faculty of Food Science and Technology, Universiti Putra Malaysia, 43400 Serdang, Selangor, Malaysia

Amin Ismail
Faculty of Medicine and Health Sciences, Universiti Putra Malaysia, 43400 Serdang, Selangor, Malaysia

Alfi Khatib
Department of Pharmaceutical Chemistry, Kulliyyah of Pharmacy, International Islamic University Malaysia, 25200 Kuantan, Pahang, Malaysia

Mohamad Fawzi Mahomoodally
Department of Health Sciences, Faculty of Science, University of Mauritius, 230 Réduit, Mauritius

Azizah Abdul Hamid
Halal Products Research Institute, Universiti Putra Malaysia, 43400 Serdang, Selangor, Malaysia

Tesfa Dejenie Habtewold and Bayu Yihun Wale
College of Health Science, Department of Nursing, Debre Berhan University, 445 Debre Berhan, Ethiopia

Wendwesen Dibekulu Tsega
College of Health Science, Department of Public Health, Debre Berhan University, 445 Debre Berhan, Ethiopia

Konrad Sarosiek, Shivam Saxena, Christopher Y. Kang, Heather McMahon, David S. Tichansky and Ankit V. Gandhi
Department of Surgery, Thomas Jefferson University, Philadelphia, PA 19107, USA

Kirk L. Pappan
Metabolon, Inc., Research Triangle Park, Durham, NC 27713, USA

Galina I. Chipitsyna and Hwyda A. Arafat
Department of Biomedical Sciences, University of New England, Biddeford, ME 04005, USA

Christian Hellmuth, Franca Fabiana Kirchberg, Ulrike Harder, Wolfgang Peissner and Berthold Koletzko
Division of Metabolic and Nutritional Medicine, Dr. von Hauner Children's Hospital, Ludwig-Maximilians-University of Munich, Lindwurmstraße 4, 80337 Munich, Germany

Nina Lass and Thomas Reinehr
Department of Pediatric Endocrinology, Diabetes and Nutrition Medicine, Vestische Hospital for Children and Adolescents, University of Witten-Herdecke, Dr. Friedrich Steiner Strasse 5, 45711 Datteln, Germany

Anoja Priyadarshani Attanayake, Kamani Ayoma Perera Wijewardana Jayatilaka and Chitra Pathirana
Department of Biochemistry, Faculty of Medicine, University of Ruhuna, 80000 Galle, Sri Lanka

Lakmini Kumari BoralugodaMudduwa
Department of Pathology, Faculty of Medicine, University of Ruhuna, 80000 Galle, Sri Lanka